AF856523

Handbuch der experimentellen Pharmakologie

Handbook of Experimental Pharmacology

Heffter-Heubner New Series

Herausgegeben von/Editorial Board

G.V.R.Born Cambridge · O.Eichler Heidelberg · A.Farah Rensselaer, NY · H.Herken Berlin · A.D.Welch Memphis, TN

Beirat/Advisory Board

E. J. Ariëns · Z. M. Bacq · P. Calabresi · S. Ebashi · E. G. Erdös
V. Erspamer · U. S. von Euler · W. S. Feldberg · G. B. Koelle
O. Krayer · T. A. Loomis · H. Rasková · M. Rocha e Silva · F. Sakai
J. R. Vane · P. G. Waser · W. Wilbrandt

Vol. XVI/3

Springer-Verlag New York · Berlin · Heidelberg 1975

Experimental Production of Diseases

Part 3

Heart and Circulation

With Contributions by

E. Betz · R. J. Bing · H. G. Borst · Y. K. Byon · R. Carlson
H.-J. Döring · A. Fleckenstein · A. Grollman · S. Heyden · S. Ikeda
M. S. Islam · J. Janke · H.-G. Lasch · K. Loßnitzer · H. Meisner
G. Müller-Berghaus · J. Gy. Papp · H. D. Schmidt · L. Szekeres
H. Tillmanns · W. T. Ulmer · M. Weil · M. M. Winbury

Edited by

J. Schmier · O. Eichler

With 154 Figures

Springer-Verlag New York · Berlin · Heidelberg 1975

Professor Dr. JOHANNES SCHMIER, Direktor der Abteilung für experimentelle Chirurgie, Chirurgische Universitäts-Klinik, 6900 Heidelberg 1

Professor Dr. OSKAR EICHLER, 6900 Heidelberg-Schlierbach, Gutleuthofweg 18

ISBN-13: 978-3-642-45469-1 e-ISBN-13: 978-3-642-45467-7
DOI: 10.1007/978-3-642-45467-7

Library of Congress Cataloging in Publication Data. Main entry under title: Experimental production of diseases. (Handbook of experimental pharmacology: New series; v. 16/3). Bibliography: p. Includes index. CONTENTS: —pt. 3. Heart and circulation. 1. Pathology, Experimental. I. Betz, Eberhard, 1926— II. Schmier, Johannes, 1922— III. Eichler, Oskar, 1898— IV. Series: Handbuch der experimentellen Pharmakologie: New series; v. 16/3 [DNLM: 1. Cardiovascular diseases. 2. Pharmacology. QV34 H236 v. 16 pt. 3] QP905.H3 vol. 16, pt. 3[RB125] 615'.1'08s [616.07'07'2] 75-28458

This work is subject to copyright. All rights are reserved, whether the whole or part of the material is concerned, specifically those of translation, reprinting, re-use of illustrations, broadcasting, reproduction by photocopying machine or similar means, and storage in data banks.

Under § 54 of the German Copyright Law where copies are made for other than private use, a fee is payable to the publisher, the amount of the fee to be determined by agreement with the publisher.

© by Springer-Verlag Berlin · Heidelberg 1975.
Softcover reprint of the hardcover 1st edition 1975

The use of general descriptive names, trade marks, etc. in this publication, even if the former are not especially identified, is not be taken as a sign that such names as understood by the Trade Marks and Merchandise Marks Act. may accordingly be used freely by anyone.

Table of Contents

Experimental Coronary Disease — Models and Methods of Drug Evaluation.
M. M. Winbury. With 10 Figures

Genetic Induction of a Cardiomyopathy. K. LOSSNITZER. With 11 Figures

Basic Actions of Ions and Drugs on Myocardial High-Energy Phosphate Metabolism and Contractility. A. FLECKENSTEIN, H. J. DÖRING, J. JANKE, and Y. K. BYON. With 49 Figures

Experimental Models of Hemorrhagic Shock. R. CARLSON and M. H. WEIL

List of Contributors

E. Betz, Professor Dr., Physiologisches Institut der Univ., D-7400 Tübingen

R. J. Bing, M. D., Professor of Medicine, University of Southern California, Huntington Memorial Hospital, Pasadena, CA 91105/USA

H. G. Borst, Professor Dr., Chirurgische Klinik, Medizinische Hochschule, D-3000 Hannover

Y. K. Byon, Dr., Senior Research Fellow, Physiologisches Institut der Universität, D-7800 Freiburg

R. Carlson, M. D., Ph. D., Center for Critically Ill, University of Southern California, School of Medicine, Los Angeles, CA 90027/USA

H.-J. Döring, Dr., Associate Professor of Physiology, Physiologisches Institut der Universität, D-7800 Freiburg

A. Fleckenstein, Professor Dr., Physiologisches Institut der Universität, D-7800 Freiburg

A. Grollman, M. D., Ph. D., Professor of Experimental Medicine, The University of Texas, Southwestern Medical School, Department of Experimental Medicine, Dallas, TX 75235/USA

S. Heyden, Professor Dr., Department Community Health Sciences, Duke University Medical Center, Durham, NC 27710/USA

S. Ikeda, Dr., University of Southern California, Huntington Memorial Hospital, Pasadena, CA 91105/USA

M. S. Islam, Dr., Silikose-Forschungsinstitut der Bergbau-Berufsgenossenschaft, Medizinische Abteilung, D-4630 Bochum

J. Janke, Dr., Associate Professor of Physiology, Physiologisches Institut der Universität, D-7800 Freiburg

H.-G. Lasch, Professor Dr., Zentrum für Innere Medizin am Klinikum der Justus Liebig-Universität, D-6300 Gießen

K. Lossnitzer, Privatdozent Dr., Universität Ulm, Zentrum für Innere Medizin und Kinderheilkunde, D-7900 Ulm

H. Meisner, Privatdozent Dr., Deutsches Herzzentrum München, Klinik für Herz- und Gefäßchirurgie, D-8000 München

G. Müller-Berghaus, Professor Dr., Zentrum für Innere Medizin am Klinikum der Justus Liebig-Universität, D-6300 Gießen

J. Gy. Papp, Dr., University Medical School of Szeged, Institute of Pharmacology, 6701 Szeged/Hungary

H. D. Schmidt, Professor Dr., Physiologisches Institut der Freien Universität, D-1000 Berlin

L. Szekeres, Professor Dr., University Medical School of Szeged, Institute of Pharmacology, 6701 Szeged/Hungary

H. Tillmanns, Dr., University of Southern California, Huntington Memorial Hospital, Pasadena, CA 91105/USA

W. T. Ulmer, Professor Dr., Medizinische Abteilung des Silikose-Forschungsinstitutes der Bergbau-Berufsgenossenschaft, D-4630 Bochum

M. Weil, Professor Dr., Presbyterian Hospital, Los Angeles, CA 90046/USA

M. M. Winbury, Professor, Warner-Lambert Research Institute, Division of Biological Research, Morris Plains, NJ 07950/USA

Experimental Coronary Disease - Models and Methods of Drug Evaluation

M. M. WINBURY

With 10 Figures

A. Introduction

Animal models of coronary disease have many deficiencies. They do not duplicate the disease seen in man, which is slow in onset and may take several decades to develop. It is for that reason we find many different models of angina pectoris or myocardial infarction, and many methods for evaluation of coronary drugs.

The term coronary disease is a generic one and indefinite, for it can refer to a functional state, an anatomical disorder, or both. The basic problem is an inadequate blood supply relative to tissue requirements and, as will be seen later, we are specifically concerned with the supply of oxygen and substrate required for maintenance of tissue function and integrity. Angina pectoris is coronary insufficiency, usually associated with excess requirements. On the other hand, myocardial infarction results when the blood supply to a region is reduced below the minimum compatable with tissue viability. In both cases the central theme is myocardial ischemia, in one case transitory, in the other prolonged. The clinical spectrum may range from angina of effort to myocardial infarction. Both are frequently associated with progressive narrowing of the major branches of the coronary artery by atherosclerosis. This encroaches on the lumen of the vessel and on the compensatory mechanisms. When vessel stenosis and tissue hypoxia become critical, collateral development may limit or prevent damage when the normal pathway of blood supply is severely compromised.

I. Definitions

1. **Angina pectoris** is the most common form of coronary heart disease or myocardial ischemia. There is usually a specific syndrome consisting of radiating chest pain brought on by exertion, emotional episodes, or other activities that increase sympathetic discharge and increase the oxygen requirement of the heart. Specific electrocardiographic changes in the ST segment and/or T wave accompany the stress-induced pain. The attack is transitory and will disappear on cessation of the stress and/or treatment with nitroglycerin. In fact, the relief of the symptoms by nitroglycerin is frequently considered a diagnostic criterion.

Regional myocardial ischemia is the underlying mechanism of angina pectoris. There is an imbalance between oxygen supply and demand most likely due to an increased demand. This leads to temporary left ventricular failure, a decrease in left ventricular compliance and a rise in left ventricular end-diastolic pressure. These changes are observed during diagnostic stress tests such as the Masters "two-step", bicycle ergometer or treadmill exercise, or atrial pacing. Pretreatment with nitroglycerin or other nitrates will prevent the coronary insufficiency or permit a greater amount of work before signs of angina appear. Beta adrenergic blockers are effective against exercise-induced angina but not against pacing-induced angina, because the decrease in heart rate is an important facet of the oxygen sparing action.

Severe coronary atherosclerosis is not always found in patients with angina pectoris and this has lead to a renewed interest in spasm of the coronary artery (HELLSTROM, 1973), particularly in the variant forms of angina (PRINZMETAL'S variant) where the pain occurs during rest. Recently, ELIOT and BRATT (1969) described a group of young women having evidence of coronary insufficiency (angina pectoris) with normal coronary arteriograms. However, there was an abnormal oxyhemoglobin dissociation with delayed-release characteristics leading to focal hypoxia.

The transmural distribution of blood flow in the left ventricular wall is an important factor in tissue oxygenation. Studies in dogs have demonstrated the extreme vulnerability of the subendocardium to any reduction of coronary perfusion (WINBURY et al., 1971a). Although coronary perfusion rates through the left ventricle are homogeneous, the deeper subendocardial region is in critical balance and relatively hypoxic. With any decrease in coronary perfusion subendocardial oxygen tension will show a corresponding decrease, as illustrated in Fig. 1. Likewise, with any impairment of the ability of the coronary system to autoregulate, an increase in oxygen requirement will have a more profound effect in the subendocardium.

2. Coronary artery disease is an anatomic definition frequently based on coronary arteriograms. There are various methods of quantitating coronary artery disease based on the degree of stenosis of each of the three major vessels—left anterior descending, left circumflex, and right coronary. The severity of angina pectoris may not be related to the severity of the disease and the number of vessels involved. Likewise, angina pectoris or myocardial infarction may occur in the absence of any major obstructive lesion.

Nonetheless, coronary atherosclerosis can produce changes in the coronary arteries which prevent the response to normal physiological stimuli and in this way can produce limitations of coronary blood flow. Under these circumstances reserve compensatory mechanisms are exhausted and perfusion becomes more pressure-dependent (HOOD, 1971).

The disease is usually confined to the larger vessels that can be visualized under cineangiography (GENSINI et al., 1971). Small-vessel disease has been described but is rare compared with large-vessel disease. The large-vessel disease can lead to infarction of a region and/or angina pectoris, or produce no damage if an adequate collateral circulation has developed between a normal and the ischemic region. We must remember that the large-artery stenosis develops over many years as a result of coronary atherosclerosis. If the timing and degree of ischemia is appropriate, collateral circulation can develop sufficiently to limit or prevent damage in the ischemic region when flow is reduced to a critical point (SCHAPER, 1971).

3. Myocardial infarction occurs when the severity and duration of ischemia reaches a critical level that produces irreversible changes in the ischemic region. There has been controversy concerning the duration of deprivation of blood flow (total anoxia) a region can tolerate before irreversible changes occur and lead to cell death. In experimental infarction in the dog there is stratification of tissue perfusion, with the central zone having <5% of normal while the border zone may have a perfusion rate 75% of normal (WINBURY et al., 1971 b).

Coronary artery disease with partial or total occlusion is frequently the cause of infarction. However, there are many cases of infarction or sudden death without any occlusion or thrombosis. In fact, it has been suggested that thrombosis occurs secondary to the infarct and reflex vasospasm of a major vessel may be the precipitating factor (HELLSTROM, 1973; BAROLDI, 1973).

The hemodynamic consequence of myocardial infarction can be devastating if large areas of the left ventricle are involved. Left ventricular failure is frequently present even in the absence of clinical signs and with a normal blood pressure. When large areas of the left ventricle are infarcted, cardiogenic shock can develop as a result of the decreased contractility and left ventricular failure accompanied by tachycardia and intense peripheral vasoconstriction. Therapy for cardiogenic shock is poor and has not reduced mortality in spite of improved monitoring and coronary care units. The major problem is the large area of left ventricle that has been damaged and is therefore nonfunctional.

In recent times there has been revived interest in reducing the size of experimental infarcts in the dog by drug interventions. These studies will be considered in detail later. However, the major problem is translation of the results from dog to man.

II. Common Role of Subendocardial Ischemia

Common to myocardial infarction and angina pectoris is subendocardial ischemia (GUY and ELIOT, 1970, 1973; HOOD, 1971). In a high percentage of cases, focal infarction starts in the endocardial layer; many are not associated with a recent coronary occlusion. The blood supply to the subendocardium is dependent upon vessels that are subjected to the periodic throttling during systole which makes the region extremely susceptible to ischemic insult. Most of the problems are associated with an inappropriate or maldistribution of blood flow between the subepicardium and subendocardium, as illustrated in Fig. 1.

There are compensatory mechanisms in the subendocardium, such as greater capillary density and greater arteriolar conductance, yet the "nutrient" circulation is just capable of keeping pace with demand. When there is a major imbalance in the supply:demand ratio, "nutrient" circulation becomes inadequate. Details in Section C below.

III. Objective of the Presentation

According to the Coronary Heart Disease Task Group Panel Report of 1973 (Vol. 4, Part 1) there is no adequate animal model that duplicates human coronary heart disease, and they recommended that effort be directed toward the development of an animal model for myocardial infarction, sudden death, and arrhythmias due to coronary artery disease. Although not mentioned in their recommendations, we can add to this a model of angina pectoris.

Relevance of model, methods, and species to disease in man. Throughout the years many models have been studied and used in an attempt to better understand the consequences of coronary occlusion and to evaluate drugs. These have included abrupt or gradual occlusion by ligation, balloons around or in the artery,

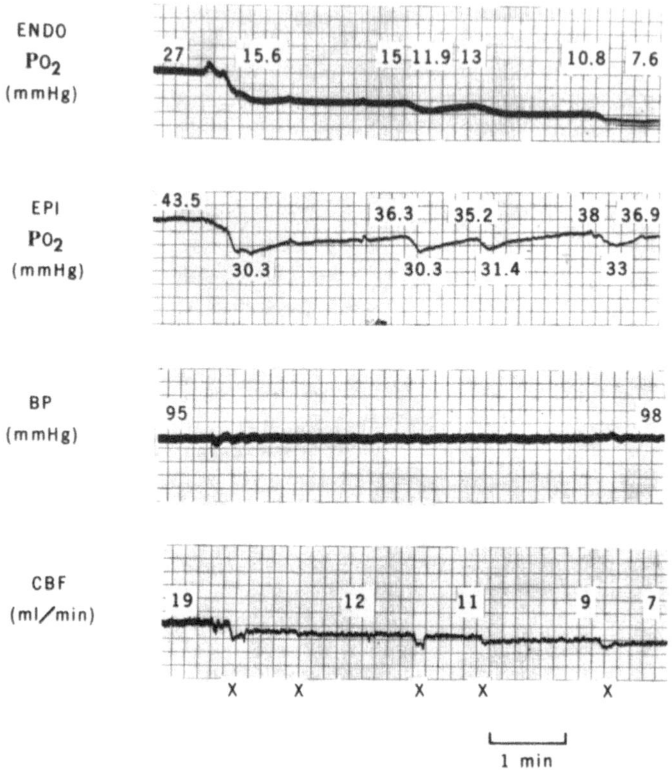

Fig. 1. Effect of decrease in coronary blood flow (CBF) on subendocardial (ENDO) and subepicardial (EPI) oxygen tension (pO_2). Polarographic electrodes were inserted to a depth of 9 and 3 mm, respectively, into the free wall of the left ventricle. At X a small clamp around the anterior descending branch was tightened. BP equals blood pressure. Note the stepwise decline in ENDO pO_2 with each decline in CBF. The EPI pO_2 tends to recover after each decrease in flow indicating autoregulation or interarterial anastomoses. From WINBURY et al. (1971a) with permission

injection of mercury, steel balls, small or large particles and procedures for thrombosing specific vessels. Some of the procedures such as injection of small particles (lycopodium spores, microspheres, or starch) produce "global" myocardial ischemia which may be accompanied by pump failure and a "shock-like" syndrome. Others produce regional ischemia, which may or may not be accompanied by "cardiogenic shock".

There are questions about the relevance of the different models to myocardial infarction in man. Each method has proponents and logical arguments for its validity but the fact that there are so many models indicates that no one procedure is universally acceptable. Certainly, the disease in man develops over a long period and the myocardial infarction is the culmination of this slowly progressing process of atherosclerosis. Therefore, there are the questions of slow or rapid occlusion, and the site (major or branch vessel).

Many of the original studies were in open-chest dogs. This, of course, markedly alters the hemodynamics and now more investigators use intact, closed-chest animals.

The species used is of great importance. Most of the investigations have been in dogs, yet that species has certain features that differ from man. There is a difference in the major regions of the left ventricle supplied by the right coronary and the branches of the left coronary (SCHAPER, 1971). The distribution in the pig is more like that in man. Of greater importance is the difference in the effect of abrupt occlusion in the two species. A high percentage of the pigs, but not dogs, fibrillate at an early stage after occlusion. At 24 and 48 h most dogs have a multifocal ventricular tachycardia, but few pigs have such a rhythm (WINBURY et al., 1962). Some showed nodal rhythm or heart block. At 4 to 5 days after occlusion both the pig and dog are sensitive to the arrhythmogenic properties of epinephrine, whereas prior to occlusion the major effect observed was sinus bradycardia. There is a major difference in the normal anastomotic and collateral circulation between the two species which may explain the difference in the sensitivity to ventricular fibrillation following abrupt coronary occlusion. The dog has a well-developed subepicardial interarterial anastomotic circulation and the potential for rapid recruitment of preformed collateral vessels. These do not seem to be well developed in the pig, and the collaterals are subendocardial in the pig and man (SCHAPER, 1971).

Models of angina pectoris can be produced in rabbits made atherosclerotic by cholesterol feeding. Stress produced by ergonovine, hypoxia, or atrial pacing causes a significant ST-segment change, suggestive of coronary insufficiency (RINZLER et al., 1956; WINBURY et al., 1961). The pacing-induced changes can be prevented by nitrates (LEE and BAKY, 1973). These methods are discussed in Section I.

Finally, we consider other approaches to evaluation of drugs, primarily antianginal agents, based on various theoretic aspects of the effect of nitrates in coronary insufficiency. It is generally accepted that coronary arteriolar dilatation is not an effective approach to the treatment of angina pectoris (WINBURY, 1964; CHARLIER, 1971; PARRATT, 1974). Rather, the distribution of the myocardial blood flow and the relation to tissue oxygen requirement is of greater importance. This is discussed in Sections B and C that follow.

Methods for the study of nutritional circulation have been reviewed by this author (WINBURY, 1971a) and will not be considered except for specific purposes.

Recently, SZEKERES' group (CSIK et al., 1973; SZEKERES, 1974) and ours (unpubl.) have been attempting with some success to duplicate pacing-induced ECG changes in dogs having a compromised coronary circulation. The long-range value of this model is yet to be established.

B. Pathophysiology of Myocardial Ischemia

The myocardium is flow-dependent and extracts a high and relatively fixed percentage of the oxygen from the arterial blood. It has highest extraction of any organ except that of skeletal muscle during heavy work. The arterioles and precapillary sphincters provide a fine regulatory mechanism to maintain an adequate oxygen supply for tissue function. These autoregulatory mechanisms function adequately in the normal heart; however, in the presence of coronary disease regional autoregulatory mechanisms may fail because they have reached the limits of their reserve. Thus, a critical balance is maintained, which can be easily upset by increased demand or decreased blood flow to the potentially ischemic region.

The systems analysis in Fig. 2 provides some index of the many factors involved. We consider only the major ones below. The central theme is the tissue oxygen tension which depends upon the O_2 demand/O_2 supply ratio. Myocardial hypoxia occurs when the balance is upset and demand exceeds the capacity of the diseased vessels to deliver oxygen (angina pectoris) or the degree of coronary artery disease becomes so severe that delivery is inadequate for maintenance of regional tissue viability (myocardial infarction).

I. Regulation of Tissue Oxygen Tension (pO_2)

The supply of oxygen to the tissue (right side, Fig. 2) is dependent on: (1) proper arterial saturation at the lungs; (2) adequate coronary inflow (coronary blood flow); (3) proper distribution between epicardium and endocardium; (4) capillary circulation; (5) transport from blood to tissue; and (6) transport to mitochondria (Moss, 1971). Much of this scheme is based on the original concept of KROGH (1936), who provided a mathematical treatment for the radial gradient from the capillary blood to the tissue in which metabolism acts as an infinite sink for the oxygen. A more recent modification by KETY (1957) takes into account the longitudinal gradient from the arterial to venous end of the capillary.

The O_2 demand (left side, Fig. 2) is dependent on: (1) cardiac fiber length; (2) diastolic wall tension (ventricular volume and end-diastolic pressure—preload); (3) systolic pressure and wall tension (intraventricular pressure—afterload); (4) contractile state; and (5) heart rate and ejection time (Ross, 1971; HOOD, 1971).

The presence of a transmural gradient of oxygen tension in the dog has been well established by many groups (Moss, 1968; KIRK and HONIG, 1964; HONIG et al., 1967; WINBURY, 1971 b; WINBURY et al., 1971 a). The lower oxygen tension of the subendocardium can be explained within the framework of the factors in the previous paragraph. There is no absolute perfusion deficit per se since perfusion appears to be homogeneous. However, there is a greater metabolic requirement in the subendocardium resulting in a relatively hypoxic state. Thus, the distribution between the epicardium and endocardium assumes a central role in the maintenance of subendocardial function.

II. Autoregulation

Autoregulation results from feedback circuits to maintain an adequate tissue oxygen tension by adjustment of blood flow rate and the capillary surface area available for diffusion from blood to the tissue.

1. **Arteriolar autoregulation** is the major mechanism by which the rate of blood flow and oxygen delivery keeps pace with the myocardial metabolic requirements. An increase in myocardial oxygen consumption will usually be accompanied by an increased coronary blood flow due to arteriolar vasodilatation. Under normal circumstances there is a large autoregulatory reserve and flow can be increased three- to fourfold. The strongest stimulus to arteriolar autoregulatory vasodilatation is tissue hypoxia. When there is impairment of coronary flow due to atherosclerosis of large vessels, arteriolar autoregulation will diminish arteriolar resistance and reserve will be reduced.

Proper arteriolar tone is important for the appropriate distribution of blood flow. Potent coronary arteriolar dilators like carbochromen or dipyridamole have the ability to produce maximal arteriolar dilatation and impair arteriolar autoregulation. The excessive dilatation in the normal regions will divert blood flow

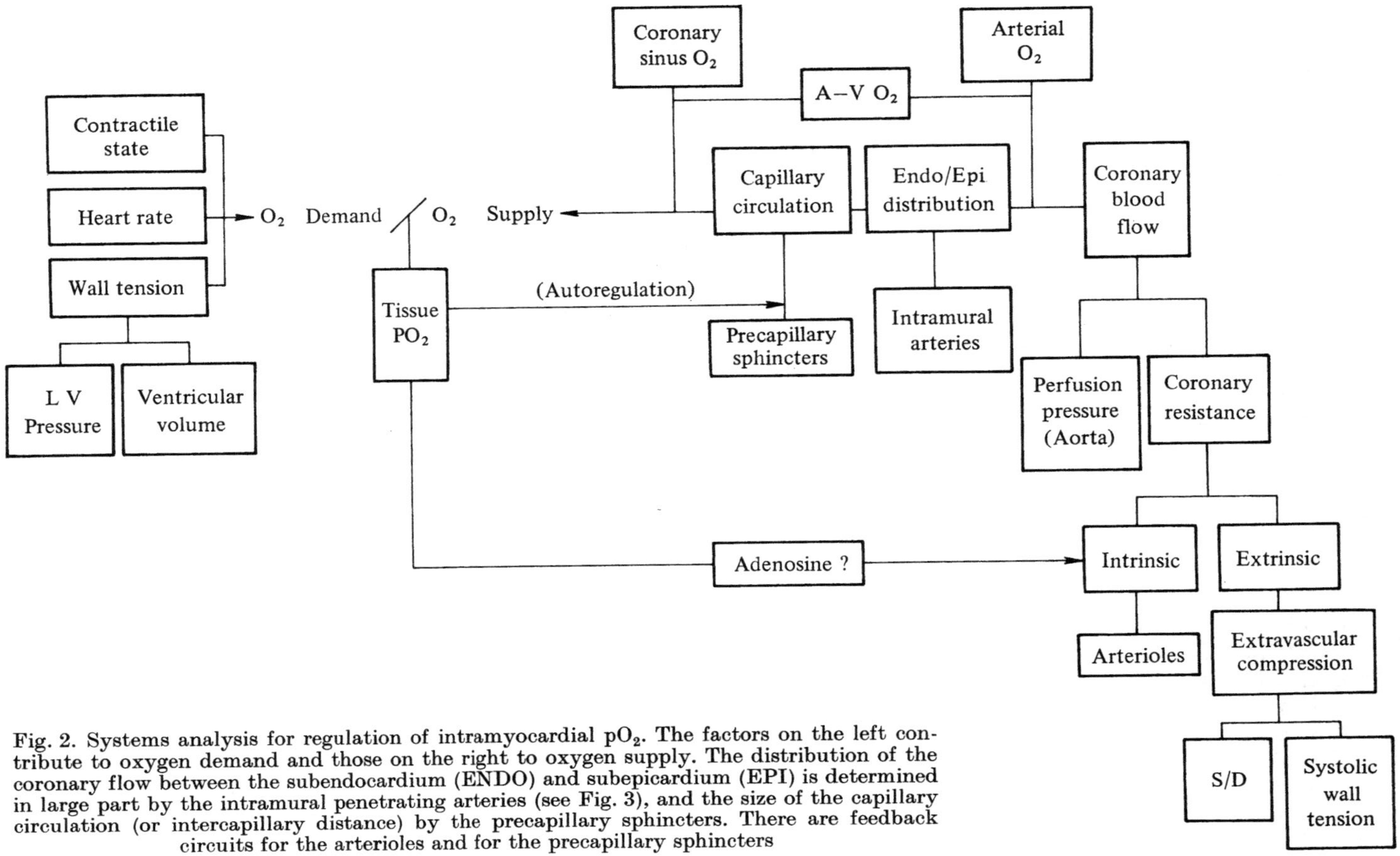

Fig. 2. Systems analysis for regulation of intramyocardial pO_2. The factors on the left contribute to oxygen demand and those on the right to oxygen supply. The distribution of the coronary flow between the subendocardium (ENDO) and subepicardium (EPI) is determined in large part by the intramural penetrating arteries (see Fig. 3), and the size of the capillary circulation (or intercapillary distance) by the precapillary sphincters. There are feedback circuits for the arterioles and for the precapillary sphincters

from the ischemic regions and produce "coronary steal" and "paradoxical angina" (Winbury et al., 1969; Rowe, 1970; Wilcken et al., 1971).

It is believed that adenosine released from ATP breakdown is the mediator of arteriolar autoregulation (Berne, 1964). However, this is not universally accepted and some believe that the arteriolar smooth muscle can respond to pO_2 (Gellai et al., 1973).

2. Precapillary sphincters regulate the size of the capillary bed and surface area available for diffusion. This has been called the "nutritional" circulation because it is at the capillary interface that the exchange process with the tissue is initiated. The precapillary sphincters are sensitive to interstitial pO_2 and are continually opening and closing. The percentage open at any one time will govern tissue oxygenation and nutrition.

Under normal circumstances the percentage of myocardial capillaries open ranges from 60 to 85% and as tissues become hypoxic capillary recruitment will occur (Howe and Winbury, 1973). The lower values for capillarity (60–75% open) are based on small-vessel blood content (Howe and Winbury, 1973; Weiss and Winbury, 1974) and the higher values (75–85%) on ^{86}Rb transport in the dog (Winbury, 1967, 1971a). With recruitment, not only is the surface area for diffusion increased but the diffusional distance between the capillary and tissue cells is decreased. Furthermore, the velocity of blood flow in each capillary is diminished and offers a greater chance for equilibrium to be established between the capillary blood and tissues, particularly for permeability-limited substances.

Studies of regional capillarity based on small-vessel blood content show that the subendocardium has a higher percentage of capillaries open than the subepicardium. No doubt this is a compensatory response to the lower subendocardial oxygen tension. Although recruitment of capillaries seems a logical method for improvement of tissue nutrition, the question arises as to what percentage of the myocardial capillaries are not functioning (closed) at any one time.

III. Effect of Antianginal Drugs

Both the nitrates and beta adrenergic blocking agents diminish myocardial oxygen requirement and, as shown in Sections C, D, E and F, elevate subendocardial oxygen tension by redistribution of blood flow in the left ventricular wall to maintain subendocardial perfusion at the expense of the subepicardium.

1. Nitrates decrease demand (Fig. 2) by peripheral venous pooling (preload) and a decrease of aortic pressure (afterload). The result is decreased wall tension during systole (aortic and intraventricular systolic pressure) and diastole (end-diastolic size and pressure); ventricular compliance is increased. There may be reflex tachycardia and increased contractile state (Ross, 1971; Hood, 1971).

Coronary blood flow is usually unchanged or decreased slightly, but regional perfusion of ischemic regions may be markedly improved. It has been generally accepted that the transient arteriolar dilator effect is of little significance. Recently it has been proposed that the prolonged dilatation of the intramural penetrating arteries may be of great importance in the favorable transmural redistribution of blood flow in the left ventricular wall (Winbury et al., 1969). This would not necessitate any change in coronary blood inflow. However, the superb studies of Ganz and Marcus (1972) in man challenge the role of a coronary effect. Intracoronary injection of nitroglycerin did not relieve pacing-induced angina in spite of an increase in coronary sinus flow, yet intravenous injection relieved the pacing-induced angina in face of a decrease in coronary sinus flow. They concluded that the peripheral effect of nitroglycerin and the decrease in oxygen requirement were the critical factors.

2. Beta adrenergic blockers increase end-distolic pressure and volume as well as wall tension. However, heart rate, contractility, and intraventricular systolic pressure are reduced. Coronary blood flow is usually diminished or unchanged. Coronary arteriolar resistance and intramural artery resistance are increased. Regional perfusion is maintained in the subendocardium even though oxygen requirement is diminished.

C. Subendocardium and Effect of Drugs

Although it has been well known that the subendocardium of the left ventricle is extremely susceptible to ischemia and infarction, only in recent years has attention been focused on that region. An editorial by GUY and ELIOT (1970) calls the left ventricular subendocardium "A Physiologic Enigma" because it is "the weakest link in the chain of survival". About 60% of myocardial infarctions are subendocardial (endo) with the vast majority not associated with recent coronary arterial occlusion. Transmural gradients exist in oxygen tension (endo lower), oxygen consumption (endo higher), systolic and diastolic wall tension (endo higher) and capillary density (endo higher) (MOIR, 1972; ARMOUR and RANDALL, 1971; KIRK and HONIG, 1964; MOSS, 1968; WINBURY et al., 1971a). All of these facts suggest that the subendocardium is in a critical balance and extremely susceptible to stress-induced ischemia, especially when there is some impairment of the normal circulation. Under those circumstances the compensatory mechanisms such as arteriolar and precapillary autoregulatory reserve may be extremely limited and any increase in oxygen requirement or decrease in perfusion pressure will lead to regional hypoxia.

I. Anatomy of Circulation through Left Ventricular Wall

A schematic diagram of the blood supply through the left ventricular wall is presented in Fig. 3. This is based on the descriptions of FULTON (1965) and ESTES et al. (1966). The epicardial (surface) arteries are extramural and give off perpendicular branches, the intramural penetrating vessels. These are about 100 μm in diameter and do not change size in going from epicardium to endocardium. Branches are given off to the epicardium (A), the endocardium (B), and a subendocardial plexus that serves as a collateral pathway when a major vessel is blocked (e.g. surface epicardial artery between regions I and II). Arteriolar conductance (1/R) and open capillary density is greater in the subendocardium than the subepicardium as a result of arteriolar and precapillary sphincter autoregulation, in response to the lower oxygen tension. The penetrating intramural arteries do not participate in autoregulation but do respond to drugs (Section D.II.).

Transmural distribution of blood flow. The distribution of blood flow between the subepicardium (A) and subendocardium (B) is a result of regional arteriolar resistances and intramural penetrating artery resistance (WINBURY et al., 1969). The parallel superficial and deep regions compete for the available blood flow. Since oxygen tension in the deeper region is approximately one half that in the

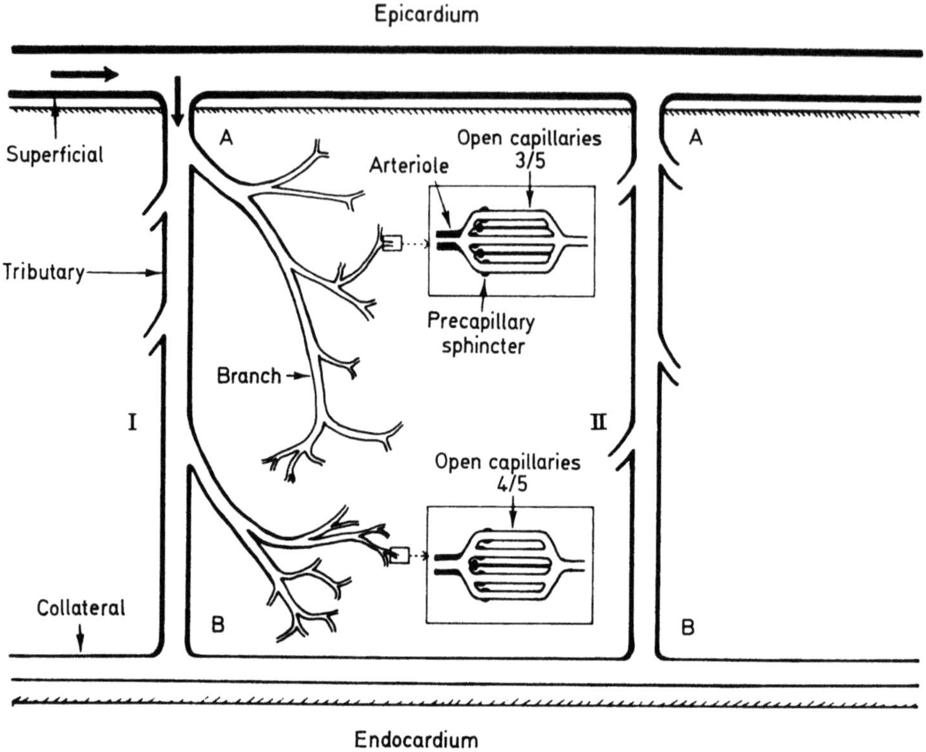

Fig. 3. Arterial blood supply through wall of the left ventricle. The superficial and intramural penetrating (tributary) arteries are large arteries and respond differently than the arterioles. A represents subepicardium and B subendocardium. The microcirculation for each region is illustrated in the insert. Arteriolar resistance is lower and more capillaries are open in the subendocardium. From WINBURY et al. (1969) with permission

superficial region, arteriolar resistance is low and the intramural penetrating vessels are limiting to subendocardial perfusion.

Perfusion of the deeper region occurs during diastole because, during systole, intramyocardial wall tension in the deeper region exceeds the perfusion pressure and flow ceases. The subendocardial perfusion therefore is dependent on diastolic duration and the diastolic perfusion gradient (BECKER and PITT, 1971a; BUCKBERG et al., 1972; PARRATT, 1974). An increase in end-diastolic pressure and diastolic wall tension will reduce the diastolic perfusion gradient. Likewise, shortening of the period of diastole (tachycardia) will have a similar effect. During stress induced by exercise there is a rise in end-diastolic pressure, tachycardia, and decreased left ventricular compliance. All of these changes will tend to diminish the subendocardial diastolic perfusion gradient and result in subendocardial hypoxia, even when arteries are not obstructed.

II. Basal State of Left Ventricular Subepicardium and Subendocardium

1. Transmural gradients. The transmural gradients are depicted schematically in Fig. 4. There is general agreement that the subendocardial *oxygen tension* is considerably below that of the subepicardium whether measured by small (or

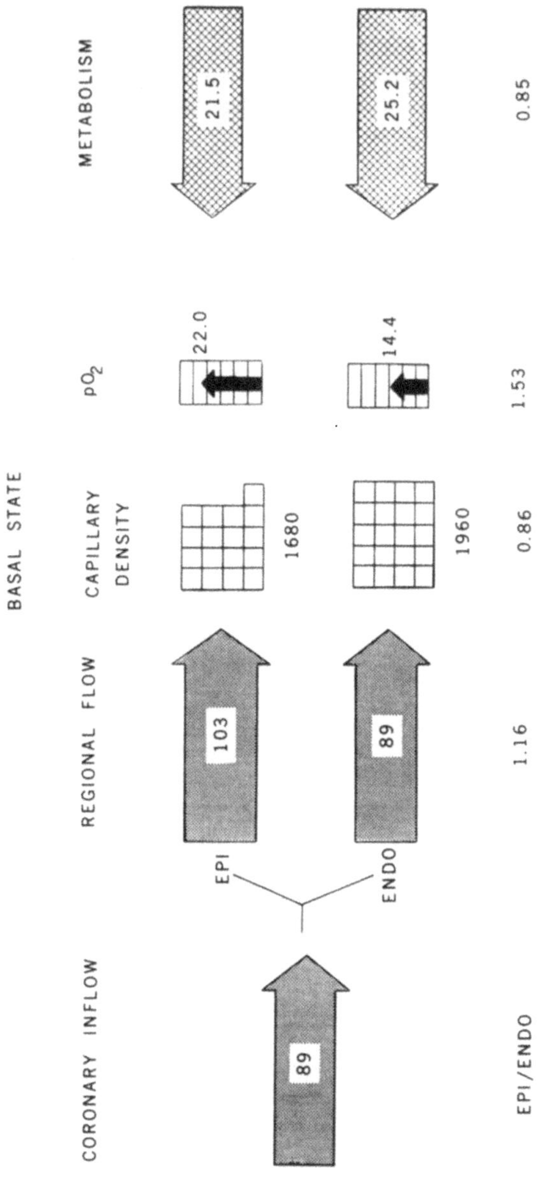

Fig. 4. Basal state of coronary hemodynamics and metabolism in left ventricular wall. Coronary inflow and regional flow are expressed in ml/min/100 g. The EPI/ENDO ratio does not differ from 1.0. Capillary density is based on small-vessel blood content and pO_2 on the mean values from many animals. The metabolism is a relative value and considerably higher than the "true" metabolism. It is calculated on the basis of the KETY (1957) modification of the KROGH (1936) equation. The higher ENDO oxygen consumption would be expected in view of the lower pO_2, greater capillary density, and normal perfusion

micro) oxygen electrodes or by mass spectrometer. The magnitude of the gradient and absolute levels of pO_2 may differ somewhat depending upon the depth of the electrodes or mass spectrometer cannula and the percentage of oxygen in the respired gas. However, the epi/endo ratio is greater than one in every animal and may be as great as two (KIRK and HONIG, 1964; MOSS, 1968; WINBURY et al., 1971a; LOISANCE and OWENS, 1973; WHALEN et al., 1973). In addition, there is a reverse gradient for pCO_2 with an epi/endo ratio of 0.97 (LOISANCE and OWENS, 1973).

There has not been universal agreement regarding regional *perfusion.* The difference between the two regions in Fig. 4 is not significant and later studies by our group based on hydrogen clearance measured with hydrogen electrodes in each region show homogeneous perfusion (GROSS and WINBURY, 1973).

When washouts of depot injections (extravascular) were used, the subepicardium was frequently 25% higher than the subendocardium, but when intravascular methods were used (^{86}Rb, microspheres) perfusion was homogeneous or the subendocardium was higher (see references in WINBURY, 1971b; MOIR, 1972).

The open *capillary density* is based on terminal small-vessel blood content, which can be used as an index of open capillary density using appropriate correction factors. There is an overall gradient from the superficial to deep regions of the left ventricle. The ratio of epi/endo was 0.86, which indicates a greater open capillary density in the subendocardium under basal conditions (HOWE and WINBURY, 1973; MYERS and HONIG, 1964). Assuming a capillary density of 2500/mm^2 (RENKIN, 1967; HORT, 1968) we can estimate that about 66% of capillaries are open in the subepicardium and 77% in the subendocardium.

The relative *metabolism* (oxygen consumption) was estimated on the basis of the KETY (1957) modification of the KROGH (1936) equation. Although the values of oxygen consumption are a gross overestimation, the greater requirement in the subendocardium is probably correct. Such factors as greater fiber length and greater wall tension would contribute to the differential.

We can conclude that under normal conditions perfusion through the left ventricular wall is homogeneous but that, because of a greater oxygen requirement, subendocardial pO_2 is lower than subepicardial pO_2. The greater open-capillary density is not adequate to compensate for the greater oxygen requirement and the subendocardium is relatively hypoxic.

2. Decreased perfusion has profound effects on subendocardial oxygen tension. The experiment shown in Fig. 1 illustrates this point very clearly. The autoregulatory reserve in both regions was determined by stepwise reduction in flow in the left anterior descending artery by gradual occlusion (WINBURY et al., 1971a). With each decrease in coronary blood flow, subendocardial pO_2 decreased stepwise. Subepicardial pO_2 decreased transiently but returned toward the control value in a short time, as would be expected with autoregulation. The subepicardial pO_2 was well maintained until flow decreased more than 50%. At that point subendocardial pO_2 had reached an almost minimal level. This demonstrates the vulnerability of the subendocardium and how infarction can occur even in the presence of some coronary flow. BECKER et al. (1973) studied the transmural gradient in acutely ischemic regions by microspheres. In the middle of the ischemic region flow was markedly reduced in both layers, but to a greater extent in the subendocardium. At the border of the ischemic zone subepicardial flow was nearly normal but subendocardial flow was still quite low.

Acute occlusion of a coronary artery is followed by an abrupt drop of subendocardial pO_2 to a plateau of about 1–4 Torr within 30 sec, while the subepicardial pO_2 decreases much more gradually over many minutes (WINBURY et al., 1971a).

3. Nitrates and beta adrenergic blockers have similar effects on average coronary blood flow (electromagnetic flowmeter), regional oxygen tension, and regional metabolism, as illustrated in Fig. 5 (WINBURY and HOWE, 1973). There is a significant decrease in coronary blood flow and subepicardial perfusion; subendocardial perfusion is unchanged. On the other hand, pO_2 is selectively increased in the subendocardium with no significant change in the subepicardium. Capillary density is not altered significantly by nitroglycerin, but is decreased in both

COMPARISON OF CHANGES AFTER NITRATES OR BETA BLOCKERS

	CORONARY INFLOW		REGIONAL FLOW	CAPILLARY DENSITY	pO_2	METABOLISM
NITROGLYCERIN	−4.4*	EPI	−16*	+90	+0.6	−2.9*
		ENDO	−1	0	+5.0*	−3.4*
BETA BLOCKER	−16*	EPI	−14*	−240*	−3.9	−2.0*
		ENDO	+3	−210*	+4.1*	−3.2*

Fig. 5. Changes in coronary hemodynamics and metabolism produced by nitrates and beta adrenergic blockers. Both types of drug decrease EPI perfusion and metabolism, but preserve ENDO perfusion and elevate ENDO pO_2. In addition, beta adrenergic blockade decreased capillary density. The * indicates significance at $p < 0.05$

regions by beta adrenergic blockade (Howe and Winbury, 1973). Finally, calculated regional oxygen consumption is diminished by both drugs but to a greater extent in the subendocardium (Winbury and Howe, 1973; Winbury et al., 1972).

The preservation of subendocardial perfusion at the expense of subepicardial perfusion is an example of favorable redistribution of blood flow, particularly in face of the diminution of oxygen consumption (Becker et al., 1971; Winbury et al., 1972; Gross and Winbury, 1973). This would explain the elevation of the oxygen tension effected by these agents in the relatively hypoxic subendocardium.

The hemodynamic effects of nitrates and beta adrenergic drugs have already been considered in Sections B.III.1 and B.III.2. Both types of drug diminish the tension time index as well as increase the diastolic pressure time interval (DPTI). The nitrates increase DPTI by diminution of left ventricular end-diastolic pressure and the beta adrenergic blockers by prolongation of diastole. Autoregulation is a requisite for blood-flow redistribution by beta adrenergic blockers but not by nitrates. Carbochromen, at a dose which produces maximal coronary arteriolar dilatation, prevents the decrease in epi/endo perfusion ratio by beta adrenergic blockers but not by nitrates (Gross and Winbury, 1973; Winbury et al., 1972).

There are several theories about the mechanism of the transmural redistribution of blood flow within the left ventricular wall. Among those suggested for the nitrates are preferential dilatation of the large intramural penetrating arteries, a decrease in systolic extravascular compression, and a decrease in diastolic wall tension and end-diastolic pressure, thereby increasing the diastolic perfusion gradient (Winbury et al., 1969, 1971a, c; Becker et al., 1971; Parratt, 1974). The beta adrenergic blockers are more difficult to understand. However, the fact that autoregulation is a requisite for redistribution by beta adrenergic blockers and that coronary arteriolar resistance is increased suggests that the ratio of epicardial to endocardial arteriolar resistance is involved. Since the subepicardium is well oxygenated, the decrease in myocardial metabolism would be expected to lead to increased arteriolar tone in that region by autoregulation. The relatively hypoxic subendocardium would not be expected to change. The ratio of the arteriolar resistances in the two regions would now favor perfusion of the subendocardium.

D. Regional Resistance — Large and Small Coronary Arteries

I. Quantitative Angiography

Coronary arteriograms in patients and animals show that nitrates increase the diameter of the visualized vessels (100 μm or >) but do not increase the rate of dye clearance, while dipyridamole does not alter vessel diameter but accelerates dye clearance.

This suggests that the primary action of dipyridamole is on the small resistive (arteriolar) vessels while the nitrates act on the large vessels (see Fig. 3).

GENSINI and co-workers (1971) described a technique for measurement of coronary vasomotion in intact animal and man. Motion pictures were taken at the rate of 80 frames/sec using a 6-in. Philips intensifier and an Arriflex-Philips camera with Kodak double X 35 mm film. To prevent possible blurring, each frame was exposed for 4 msec. After development the film was viewed and measured with a Vanguard Motion Analyzer by positioning the cross-hairs on the image and activating a switch to record the frame number and X-Y coordinates on a punch card. At least three cardiac cycles (approximately 120 frames) were measured for each visualization. The cards were run through an 1130 IBM computer, which plotted the results as either metric values or percentage variation.

For studies in dogs, anesthesia was induced with thiopental sodium and after intubation respiration was maintained with a Harvard respirator. Nitrous oxide in oxygen was used for anesthesia for the remainder of the experiment. The left coronary artery was catheterized with a $7^1/_2$ F Sones coronary catheter (USCI Corp.) via the right carotid artery. Two to four control angiograms were made using a Cordis injector to deliver 4 ml of contrast medium (Renografin 76, Squibb) at 100 psi. Groups of animals received a nitrate or an equal volume of saline intravenously or directly into the coronary artery. An oral group was given the nitrate through a gastromy. Arteriograms were repeated at frequent intervals over 240 min.

Isosorbide dinitrate (ISDN), intracoronary 1 mg and intravenous 2 mg, produced a similar degree of vasodilatation (about 7% increase in arterial diameter). When 40 mg was given directly into the stomach as four crushed 10-mg tablets, significant vasodilatation was noted within 2 to 3 min, reached a peak at 30 min and was still present at 180 min.

Similar studies were carried out in sedated patients; half of the group had normal coronary arteries. The right and left coronary arteries were selectively catheterized and visualized with 6 ml Renografin for each injection. The patient received drug after the diagnostic procedure and arteriograms were taken and analyzed as described above. ISDN, 5 mg sublingual, produced marked vasodilatation (15%) 7 to 12 min postdrug. A similar change (17%) was observed with a 5-mg tablet chewed and swallowed. There was a greater increase in vessel diameter in the normal subjects than in those with CAD. A dose of 10 mg chewed and swallowed produced a greater effect (22% increase) than 5 mg.

The margin of error in the procedure was determined *in vitro* and *in vivo* with steel ball bearings and catheters of known diameter. The margin of error was less than ± 80 μm. Since the vessels studied were 3 to 4 mm in diameter, the error was less than 2 to 3%.

II. Large and Small Arteries *in vivo*

Fig. 3 illustrates the anatomy of the coronary macro- and microcirculation through the left ventricular wall. The larger intramural penetrating arteries (and surface epicardial arteries) serve a different purpose than the resistive arteriolar vessels. The larger vessels have more of a conduit and distribution function while the arterioles have a flow regulatory function for the region they subserve. For these reasons it is not surprising that these portions of the coronary arterial circulation may respond differently to various neurohumoral agents and drugs.

Furthermore, one of the possible mechanisms for redistribution of blood flow is a change in the large intramural artery resistance. Certainly, a decrease in resistance would favor distribution of blood flow toward the subendocardium, which is most vulnerable to infarction. Also, the coronary angiograms suggested large-vessel dilatation by nitrates but not by dipyridamole. It had been previously established that nitroglycerin does not increase coronary flow in the angina patient when the attack is relieved. Furthermore, dipyridamole does not have a beneficial effect in angina (see WINBURY et al., 1969, for references). Therefore, we decided to investigate the effects of large and small coronary arteries *in vivo*.

1. Principle. The resistances of the large surface coronary arteries, the intramural penetrating arteries and their branches, and the arterioles can be considered as resistances in series. It is not possible to isolate the various segments but rather one can arbitrarily determine the large-surface-artery resistance and the "total" coronary resistance. The large-surface-artery resistance (RL) is assumed to reflect the properties of the intramural penetrating vessels, and "total" resistance (RT) primarily the resistance of the arterioles. One can calculate small-vessel resistance (RS = RT − RL) but since RL is normally about 5% of RT it does not seem necessary under most conditions. RL and RT can be determined in a preparation where aortic pressure and coronary blood flow are permitted to vary (WINBURY et al., 1969) or where coronary flow is held constant (COHEN and KIRK, 1973).

2. Method. Large dogs were anesthetized, the trachea intubated and positive pressure respiration was started. Aortic pressure was determined with an arterial transducer connected to a large-bore polyethylene catheter advanced into the arch from the left carotid artery. The chest was opened in the 5th left interspace and the pericardium opened. A small branch of the left anterior descending branch (about 0.5 mm) close to the apex was isolated and cannulated centrally after ligation with a Bard Intracath gauge-17 catheter connected to a second arterial pressure transducer. Under normal circumstances the pressure gradient between the aorta and peripheral coronary catheter was about 5 mm Hg. Coronary blood flow in the main artery was determined with a close-fitting electromagnetic flowmeter probe (1.5 or 2 mm diameter). The transducers for measuring aortic pressure (Pa), central peripheral coronary pressure (Pc) and coronary blood flow (Q) were fed into an on-line computer, which provided a direct continuous record of Pa; Pc; pressure gradient, Pg (Pa-Pc); Q; RL (Pg/Q); RT (Pa/Q); and the ratio RL/RT, as illustrated in Figs. 6 and 7. Intravenous injections of drugs were administered over a period of one minute.

Other authors have used a constant-flow technique (COHEN and KIRK, 1973) in which the left main coronary artery was cannulated with a modified GREGG cannula and perfused by a pump with blood from a femoral artery. The perfusion system between the pump and coronary artery contained an extracorporeal electromagnetic flow probe, a site for intracoronary injections and a side arm for measurement of proximal coronary pressure. A small branch of the left anterior descending or left circumflex coronary artery was cannulated centrally and the

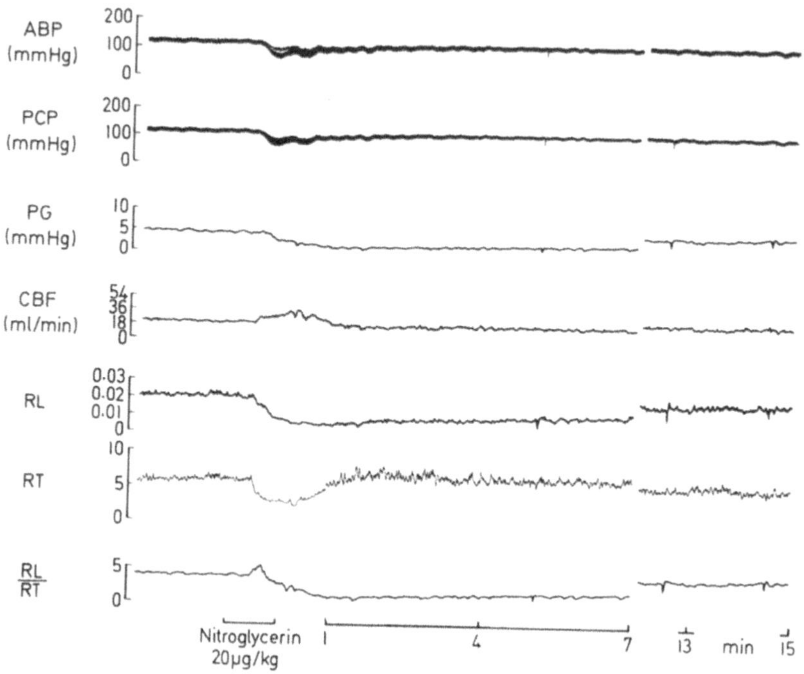

Fig. 6. Effect of nitroglycerin on large (RL) and total (RT) coronary arterial resistance. ABP = aortic blood pressure; PCP = proximal peripheral coronary pressure; PG = pressure gradient (ABP-PCP); CBF = coronary blood flow; RL/RT = ratio of resistance × 100. Normally, RL is about 5% of RT. Nitroglycerin caused a prolonged decrease in RL, but a transient decrease in RT followed by a secondary rise. RL/RT was decreased after an initial rise

distal portion ligated. Proximal and distal coronary pressure as well as the proximal–distal pressure gradient were recorded continuously. At constant coronary flow, distal pressure and the proximal–distal gradient are proportional to small artery (RS) and large artery (RL) resistances, respectively.

3. Nitrates versus potent coronary dilators. *Nitroglycerin*, 10 to 20 µg/kg intravenously, in the preparation with variable flow and pressure produced a prolonged decrease in RL but only a transient decrease in RT followed by a more prolonged increase. RL/RT was decreased for as long as 15 min due to the prolonged effect on RL (Fig. 6). Coronary blood flow rose during the infusion but gave way to a decline as aortic pressure was reduced.

Similar prolonged effects on RL and RL/RT were observed after intracoronary injection of 8 µg. Likewise, when coronary flow was constant, intracoronary injection of 18 µg produced a prolonged decrease in RL and a transient effect on RS (COHEN and KIRK, 1973).

The decrease in RL produced by nitroglycerin was observed even when autoregulation of the small resistive vessels was exhausted by previous administration of a potent coronary arteriolar dilator like carbochromen, or by hypoxia.

Potent coronary dilators like *carbochromen*, *nifedipine* or *dipyridamole* can produce maximal arteriolar dilatation (RT) and a marked increase in coronary blood flow (Fig. 7). At the maximal effective dose arteriolar resistance is minimal

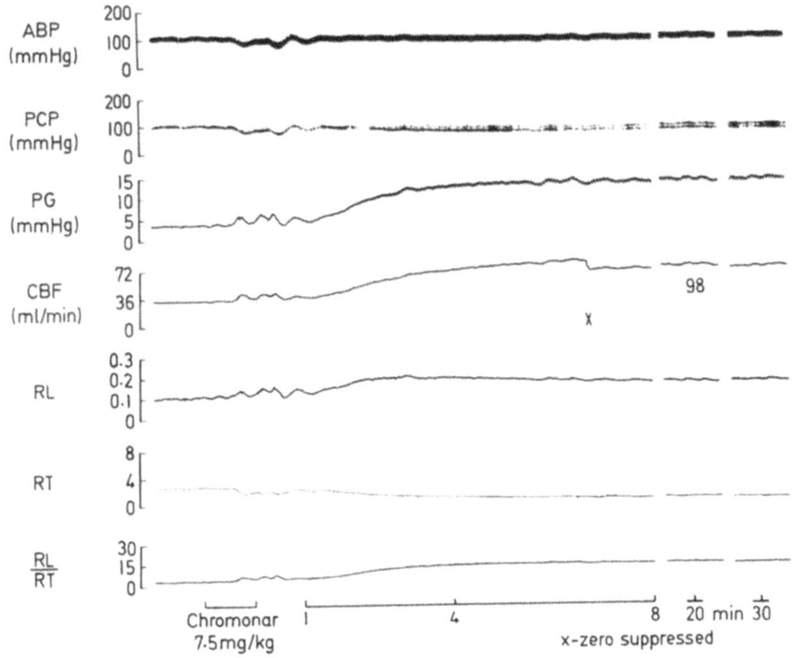

Fig. 7. Effect of carbochromen (Chromonar) on large (RL) and total (RT) coronary arterial resistance. This drug produced prolonged coronary arteriolar dilatation, decreased RT and elevated CBF. X on CBF record indicates change in scale factor

and equal to that during the peak of reactive hyperemia following temporary coronary occlusion. Thus, autoregulation was impaired. RL was elevated by each of the agents.

4. Beta adrenergic blockers. *Propranolol*, 0.5 mg/kg, produced a slight decline in aortic pressure, coronary blood flow, and heart rate. RL and RT increased slightly; the increase was relatively greater in RT.

5. Physiological studies. The arterioles demonstrate excellent *autoregulation* but the large vessels do not. After a short occlusion RS (or RT) declined to a minimum value at the peak of reactive hyperemia. During that time RL could account for more than 20% of RT and be limiting for flow to an ischemic or hypoxic region. Carbochromen produced arteriolar dilatation equal to that following occlusion, but the nitrates had no such effect.

When coronary perfusion pressure was changed over a broad range, RS increased as pressure increased—*autoregulation*—but RL decreased as pressure rose—*passive distensibility* (WINBURY et al., 1969).

6. Role in action of antianginal agents. The small resistive arteries (arterioles) are involved in the fine local autoregulatory adjustment of myocardial oxygen supply to the requirement. In ischemic regions, autoregulatory reserve may be exhausted because of nearly maximal dilatation of arterioles. The intramural penetrating arteries (large) are not involved in metabolic autoregulation but determine blood flow distribution, particularly to the subendocardium. Like the other vessels within the left ventricular wall, the penetrating vessels are subjected to systolic extravascular compression and may be influenced by diastolic wall tension in the deeper portions of the myocardium. Nitrates have a selective prolonged vasodilator effect on the intramural penetrating arteries and would favor or preserve blood flow to the relatively hypoxic subendocardium. Potent coronary dilators would have the opposite effect and produce coronary "steal" by producing arteriolar dilatation in well-oxygenated subepicardium.

Beta adrenergic blockade increases arteriolar resistance, probably to a greater extent in the subepicardium, as an autoregulatory response to the diminution of metabolism. In this way, perfusion of the hypoxic subendocardium will be preserved.

III. Large and Small Arteries *in vitro*

SCHNAAR and SPARKS (1972) demonstrated that helical strips of coronary arteries of different diameters respond differently to drugs. Large arteries (2 mm OD) had a greater sensitivity to nitroglycerin and sodium nitrite than small arteries (0.5 mm OD). Adenosine caused greater relaxation of small vessels than of large vessels.

Large (2 mm OD) and small (550 µm OD) arteries were dissected from the myocardium and helical strips prepared. Those from large arteries were 1 cm long and 1.5 to 2 mm wide, those from small arteries 2 mm long and 0.3 to 0.5 mm wide. The strips were mounted in the same bath of physiological salt solution with the potassium concentration elevated to 35 mM to produce resting tone. The strips were attached to a fixed point and a force transducer with a tension of 1.6 g on the large artery and 0.12 g on the small artery. Bath temperature was 37° C; a 95% O_2-5% CO_2 gas mixture was used for aeration. The strips were treated with various concentrations of a drug for 3 min, then washed three times with the high potassium solution. After the last dose the passive tension was determined by bathing the strips in calcium-free solution containing 4 mM EGTA.

The response was calculated as a percentage of the relaxation in calcium-free solution. The difference between the resting tension before each injection and that in the absence of calcium was considered the maximal relaxation, or 100%. In this way it was possible to compare the responses of the different size strips.

Results show that over the concentration range 4.4×10^{-8} M to 1.38×10^{-4} M nitroglycerin produced greater relaxation of the large vessels than of the small vessels. In general, sodium nitrate showed a similar effect. Adenosine produced a greater effect on small arteries over the concentration range of 3.74×10^{-8} M to 1.17×10^{-4} M.

These studies tend to support the *in vivo* finding that nitroglycerin has a preferential dilator effect on large coronary arteries. However, the vessels used in the *in vitro* studies were much greater in size than those used *in vivo*. In the intact animal the large vessel cannulated is 0.5 mm and the small resistive vessels would be arterioles. Nonetheless, there may well be a gradient of activity and duration in response to drugs with changing vessel size.

E. Regional Tissue Oxygen Tension

In a review prepared more than ten years ago this author concluded that intramyocardial oxygen tension really measured a function of blood flow. It was suggested that intracellular recordings might be of great value (WINBURY,

1964). There has been much progress since that time and now methods are available to measure intracellular pO_2 as well as interstitial pO_2. What is important is that there is a gradient of pO_2 in the left ventricular wall and drugs can have different effects on pO_2 at various depths.

I. Principle and Determinants of Oxygen Tension

Intramyocardial oxygen tension is related to the balance between supply and demand at the tissue level. The determinants are: arterial oxygenation, tissue blood flow, intercapillary distance and tissue oxygen consumption (KROGH, 1936; KETY, 1957).

Oxygen tension can be increased by a decrease in intercapillary distance (recruitment), a decrease in metabolism, or an increase in tissue blood flow. On a theoretical basis the intercapillary distance and tissue oxygen consumption have a greater influence than tissue blood flow but from a practical standpoint we find tissue blood flow (*via* redistribution to ischemic or hypoxic regions) and metabolism are the primary factors.

II. Approaches

The polarographic method for determination of pO_2 is used by many groups. Some employ microelectrodes with either a recessed or coated tip, others use larger electrodes that may have a coated or bare tip. It is beyond the scope of this review to consider the arguments in favor of various sizes and types of tips, intracellular versus extracellular, etc. Suffice it to say that valuable information has been acquired by each approach.

Recently the mass spectrometer has been adapted for measurement of blood and tissue gas tensions of O_2, CO_2, and foreign gases. Small probes have been designed for use in various tissues and applied to the myocardium (LOISANCE and OWENS, 1973, 1974; FURUSE et al., 1973).

III. Polarographic Method

Bare-tipped platinum electrodes insulated with Teflon were used by KIRK and HONIG (1964), MOSS (1968) and WINBURY et al. (1971a) to determine pO_2 in the superficial and deep regions of the left ventricle. KADATZ (1969) and DIEDEREN and KADATZ (1973) used semimicro (15 to 25 µm tip diameter) glass-insulated electrodes at a superficial depth.

The eletrodes used by our group were made from 20 mm lengths of Teflon coated platinum–iridium wire with a diameter of 177 µm. To assure proper insulation and bonding, the wire was quadruple-coated with Teflon insulation; this increased the outer diameter to 254 µm. Insulation was removed from 0.2 to 0.3 mm of the tip of each electrode and lead wires were soldered to the distal end. Each electrode was calibrated in saline equilibrated with various concentrations of oxygen to yield pO_2 values equivalent to those expected in the tissue. Electrodes were selected for similarity of response curves and cemented together at the distal end with one tip 6 mm above the other. The twin electrode was plunged into an area supplied by the anterior descending branch, avoiding regions with obvious blood vessels. The tips were usually 3 and 9 mm below the epicardial surface but the actual depth was verified at the end of each experiment. Electrolysis was discontinued every 20 to 30 min to allow recovery of the electrode. However, in some studies we used continuous electrolysis and found normal responses.

The platinum electrodes were polarized at −0.6 V relative to a reference silver–silver chloride electrode placed under the skin at the operative site. Current flow was measured by an amplifier consisting of a high gain amplifier and a feedback resistor. The output went through a filter and inverting amplifier and was recorded on a direct-writing instrument. It was possible to measure changes of < 1 Torr.

In addition to the pO_2, coronary blood flow was recorded by an eletromagnetic flowmeter and aortic pressure with a transducer.

Nitrates, carbochromen and beta adrenergic blockers. As mentioned in Section C.II.1, there was a significant transmural gradient of pO_2 in the left ventricular wall with the epicardium (epi) almost twice that of the endocardium (endo). WEISS et al. (1973) reported the epi pO_2 was 24 and endo pO_2 14 Torr before any drug intervention. Other reports from our group show similar values. The effect of *nitroglycerin* is given in Table 1 (modified from WEISS et al., 1973). Oxygen tension initially declined in both regions as blood pressure fell. This was followed by a selective rise in endo pO_2 to about 5 Torr above control at 4 to 7 min and a gradual return of epi pO_2 to normal. The rise in endo pO_2 lasted for as long as 15 min. A similar selective rise in endo pO_2 can be produced by nitroglycerin, even if perfusion pressure and coronary blood flow are reduced to exhaust autoregulatory reserve in the subendocardium as in Fig. 1 (WINBURY et al., 1971a) or after maximal coronary arteriolar dilatation produced by dipyridamole or carbochromen (WEISS et al., 1973). Furthermore, intracoronary injection of nitroglycerin elevated endo pO_2 even in the absence of any change in coronary blood flow (WEISS and WINBURY, 1972).

Carbochromen produced a marked increase in coronary blood flow, which was slow in onset but of long duration (> 1 h). The changes in blood pressure, coronary

Table 1. Effect of nitroglycerin, 20 μg/kg i.v., on intramyocardial oxygen tension

	Blood pressure mm Hg	CBF ml/min	Oxygen tension (Torr)		
			Epi	Endo	Epi/Endo
Control	115/91	36.7	25.6	13.3	2.17
NG 1–2 min	95/67	36.3	23.7	11.4	2.63
Δ	−20[a]/−24[a]	−0.4	−1.9	−2.1[a]	+0.46
NG 4–7 min	110/87	34.7	25.2	18.2	1.55
Δ	−5/−4	−3.4[a]	−0.4	+4.9[a]	−0.62[a]

[a] Significantly different from zero: $p < 0.05$.

Table 2. Effect of carbochromen, 5–10 mg/kg i.v., on intramyocardial oxygen tension

	Blood pressure mm Hg	CBF ml/min	Oxygen tension (Torr)		
			Epi	Endo	Epi/Endo
Control	119/95	32.4	22.9	15.4	1.57
Ch 15–30 min	115/86	90.3	30.3	15.2	2.10
Δ	−4/−9	+58.5[a]	+7.4[a]	0.0	+0.52[a]

[a] Significantly different from zero: $p < 0.05$.

Table 3. Effect of bunolol, 0.2 mg/kg i.v., on intramyocardial oxygen tension

	Blood pressure mm Hg	HR b/min	CBF ml/min	Oxygen tension (Torr)		
				Epi	Endo	Epi/Endo
Control	123/103	119	21.4	22.7	15.3	1.44
B 10 min	121/101	101	19.3	20.2	19.1	1.07
Δ	−2/−2	−18[a]	−2.1	−2.5	+3.8[a]	−0.37[a]

[a] Significantly different from zero: $p < 0.05$.

blood flow, and intramyocardial oxygen tension are given in Table 2 (modified from Weiss et al., 1973). Epi pO_2 increased consistently but endo pO_2 decreased in half the animals and increased in the others.

Carbochromen produced maximal arteriolar dilatation and abolished autoregulation. *Dipyridamole* (250 µg/kg i.v.) was also capable of abolishing arteriolar autoregulation and markedly increased coronary blood flow, but there was no significant change in epi or endo pO_2. The comparison of nitrates with highly effective coronary arteriolar dilators indicates that the selective elevation of subendocardial oxygen tension by the nitrates is not a result of arteriolar dilatation.

Kadatz (1969) and Diederen and Kadatz (1973) compared dipyridamole, papaverine and nitroglycerin in normal and chronically occluded (ameroids) regions with bare-tip electrodes 15 to 25 µm in diameter. They reported that dipyridamole and papaverine consistently increased pO_2 in both regions but nitroglycerin had a variable effect. We can offer no explanation for the difference in the results except that they measure only epi pO_2.

Beta adrenergic blockade with propanolol, 1 mg/kg i.v., produced a selective increase in endo pO_2 in about two thirds of the animals; epi pO_2 did not change or decreased. *Bunolol*, 0.2 mg/kg i.v., produced the selective endo increase in a higher percentage of the animals. The results are given in Table 3. The mean increase in endo pO_2 produced by bunolol was 3.8 Torr and by propanolol 1.9. Other changes included a decrease in heart rate, contractile force, coronary blood flow, and blood pressure. The epi/endo pO_2 ratio decreased. Thus, beta adrenergic blocking agents and nitrates had a similar effect on regional intramyocardial pO_2.

IV. Mass Spectrographic Method

A medical mass spectrometer (Medspect MS-8 or RMS 2, Scientific Research Instruments, Baltimore, Md.) has been developed which permits alternate reading of different gases from two different sites at 5-sec intervals (Loisance and Owens, 1973, 1974; Furuse et al., 1973). Two sampling cannulas were connected to a single instrument by stainless tubing. The spectrometer was usually programmed to read pO_2 and pCO_2 in two myocardial regions or in blood. The sampling cannulas used by Furuse et al. (1973) were made of 22-gauge stainless steel tubing encased in a thin Teflon membrane. Other cannulas were designed with a series of 5 holes in the metal tubing (about 350 µm OD) which has also covered by Silastic (Roberts et al., 1972). The cannula from the heart was connected to the Medspect with tubing made of Saran. This is gas-impermeable and flexible. The gases are ionized in the spectrometer and identified by their respective masses. The spectrometer and cannulas were calibrated in a saline bath equilibrated with various concentrations of the gas.

The size of the sampling cannula and choice of membrane is of particular importance. The smaller the diameter of the sampling cannula, the less the tissue damage; for that reason OWENS' group developed a cannula equivalent to a 30-gauge needle (about 300 μm OD). Holes were placed in the cannula to increase the "sampling window". When this cannula is used with mass spectrometer MS 8, the rate of gas withdrawal is 1.1×10^{-6} ml/sec. This is slow enough to allow small Silastic-covered cannulas to be used in tissues, but larger ones cannot be used because at the higher sampling rate oxygen would be withdrawn more rapidly than it could be supplied by the blood, and tissue pO_2 would fall. Large cannulas can be coated with Teflon, which is less permeable, but small Teflon-coated cannulas had very long response times and were not practical (ROBERTS et al., 1972).

1. Multiple gas measurement and perfusion. LOISANCE and OWENS (1973, 1974) also determined myocardial washout of argon, as an index of local perfusion. The dog was placed on a mixture of 5% argon and 95% room air until pAr in the myocardium reached a plateau. The animal was then returned to room air and the slope of decay determined.

In the studies of LOISANCE and OWENS (1973, 1974) cannulas were placed in the epicardium (2 mm) and endocardium (10 mm) in the region of the left anterior descending coronary artery. Partial pressures of O_2 and CO_2 in epi and endo were recorded alternately. In addition, argon clearance was measured by determining the desaturation curve of both regions simultaneously.

Perfusion appeared to be homogeneous with an epi/endo ratio of 0.97. However, the epi/endo ratio for pO_2 was 1.24, in general agreement with the polarographic data. The absolute values are higher by spectrometer than by oxygen electrode. Epi and endo pO_2 were 37 and 27 by spectrometer and 24 and 14 by oxygen electrode, respectively. Epicardial pCO_2 (61) was lower than endocardial (64).

2. Nitrates. Nitroglycerin, 20 μg/kg i.v. over one minute, produced an increase in endo pO_2 and a slight decrease in epi pO_2. Both epi and endo pCO_2 were reduced. Perfusion rate was decreased slightly in both regions but the epi/endo ratio did not change.

The effect of degree of occlusion was studied by FURUSE et al. (1973). A cannula made of 22-gauge tubing was inserted into the region supplied by the left anterior descending coronary artery and another into the circumflex region. Reduction of the circumflex lumen by 50 to 60% did not alter circumflex blood flow, pO_2, or pCO_2. Severe obstruction of 70 to 90% diminished blood flow by 35% and pO_2 by 50%, and elevated pCO_2 by 100%.

LOISANCE and OWENS (1973) determined the effect of complete ligation of the anterior descending branch on the epicardium and endocardium and the subsequent action of nitroglycerin on the normal and ischemic region (LOISANCE and OWENS, 1974). Perfusion of both epi and endo was reduced; the decrease was greater in endo. Oxygen tension was decreased at both depths but more rapidly and severely in the endo, similar to the findings of WINBURY et al. (1971a). PCO_2 increased to a considerably greater extent in endo. Infusion of nitroglycerin produced a large and selective increase in endo pO_2 but no change in epi pO_2. Endo pCO_2 diminished, but not epi pCO_2. There were no changes in epi or endo perfusion.

3. Advantages and disadvantages. Certainly the mass spectrographic method has proven useful for measurement of intramyocardial, intra-arterial and intravenous gas tensions in absolute terms. Several gases and sites can be determined at rapid intervals (2 sec) by appropriate switching. Tissue perfusion rates can be determined by conventional washout procedures. This is not possible with oxygen electrodes or hydrogen electrodes. Even though the same electrode can be used, it must be polarized at a different voltage for each gas.

The cannulas for mass spectrometry have been reduced in size so that they produce no greater damage than the small oxygen electrodes. The choice of membrane (Teflon or Silastic) must take into account the amount of gas removed relative to the partial pressure in the tissue. The long stainless steel tube from the tissue to the spectrometer could cause tissue damage in moving tissue but this has been solved in part by use of Saran tubing.

The response time of the mass spectrometer is slow compared to that of the oxygen electrode. There is a delay from the time of change in the tissue or blood to the first change in reading (ROBERTS et al., 1972). This delay differs for different gases because of the permeability characteristics of the Silastic membrane. With the small cannula system, the response time delay for O_2 is 12.1 sec, for CO_2 13.9 sec, and for argon 12.5 sec. However, time required to reach equilibrium is 108 sec for O_2, 127 sec for argon, and 140 sec for CO_2. If the small cannula is covered with Teflon the response is too long to be practical. However, since the changes are usually gradual, transit and equilibrium time is not a serious problem with the Silastic membrane.

On an overall basis we must conclude that the mass spectrometer has much to offer in biological application, providing the equipment is reliable and can be easily serviced. The ability to measure several gases at rapid intervals outweighs the delay in reaching equilibrium.

V. Conclusions — Regional Oxygen Tension

Changes in regional oxygen tension are important in the evaluation of drugs for treatment of coronary disease. There is a transmural gradient in the left ventricular wall and the subendocardium is relatively hypoxic. Likewise, there are gradients in oxygen tension from normal to ischemic zones. Drugs can influence these gradients in different ways. Nitroglycerin causes a selective increase in subendocardial oxygen tension in normal and ischemic regions. In contrast, carbochromen causes an increase in subepicardial oxygen tension and a marked rise in coronary sinus oxygen tension. Thus, venous pO_2 does not reflect intramyocardial pO_2.

F. Regional Blood Flow and Perfusion

Mean coronary blood flow can be measured by various transducers, such as the recording rotameter or electromagnetic flowmeter, or by coronary sinus outflow measured directly, by indicator dilution, or other techniques (see KADATZ, 1971; CHARLIER, 1971). These procedures provide an index of average left ventricular blood flow but provide no index of regional differences. The normal region or area with a high rate of blood flow will predominate, but it may be that the drugs do not affect flow in those regions. Redistribution of flow may not affect average or mean flow.

There is considerable controversy about the responsiveness of normal and anginal patients to nitrates and to potent coronary dilators. It is beyond the scope of this article to discuss this point in detail other than to emphasize the fact that the majority of investigators find that sublingual nitroglycerin does not increase average coronary blood flow in the anginal patient even during relief of an attack. The recent studies of GANZ and MARCUS (1972) demonstrated that intracoronary nitroglycerin in anginal patients increased coronary sinus outflow but did not relieve pacing-induced angina pectoris. However, intravenous nitroglycerin produced relief of angina in spite of a decrease in coronary blood flow.

This highlights the problem of peripheral versus coronary effects but does not consider the possibility of changes in regional perfusion. Another possible factor —nutritional versus non-nutritional circulation—is related to regional perfusion. It has been covered extensively in a previous review (WINBURY, 1971a) and will be touched on only superficially where necessary.

I. Epicardium and Endocardium

There is a lack of agreement about the homogeneity of perfusion of the left ventricular wall. Washout of intramyocardial depots of radioactive diffusible tracers suggests 25% lower perfusion of the subendocardium. Procedures involving uptake of diffusible tracers from the blood (^{86}Rb) or use of microspheres indicate homogeneous perfusion or slightly higher for the subendocardium. Our procedure with hydrogen electrodes has recently indicated homogeneous perfusion. The same was true when regional perfusion was measured by mass spectrometry.

In all cases there is agreement that coronary occlusion (either partial or total) has a more profound effect on subendocardial perfusion and oxygenation. Nitroglycerin usually improves the epi/endo perfusion ratio.

Regional perfusion can be measured by the SAPIRSTEIN principle using a tracer (^{86}Rb) taken up by the tissue (reviewed by WINBURY, 1971a) or trapped in the arterioles (microspheres). The washout of a foreign gas such as hydrogen can be determined polarographically with electrodes in the epicardium and endocardium, or argon by mass spectrometer with cannulas in those regions. Microspheres can be used in unanesthetized animals; as many as four to five procedures can be done, depending on the capability of the detection equipment to separate the nuclides. Clearance of hydrogen by polarography or of argon by mass spectrography requires anesthetized, open-chest dogs.

II. Microsphere Method

The principle of the microsphere method is that the fractional distribution of an indicator well mixed at the root of the aorta is in proportion to the fraction of the cardiac output received by the organs or regions. Inherent in this hypothesis is that the tracer does not escape from the region (DOMENECH et al., 1969). If the cardiac output or flow to any organ (reference flow) is known, flow to other regions can be estimated. RUDOLPH and HEYMANN (1967) did some of the original work to establish the use of labeled microspheres by studies on the fetus of sheep or goat.

The microspheres are manufactured by the Nuclear Products Division of the Minnesota Mining and Manufacturing Company. The nuclide label is incorporated within the sphere and not lost in the surrounding fluid. The original studies were on 50 μm spheres but others have used considerably smaller sizes. The nuclides used were ^{125}I, ^{51}Cr, ^{85}Sr and ^{46}Sc. The measurement of radioactivity and preparation of nuclides is well described in the several reports discussed below and they should be consulted for details. The method was validated in a physical model having four branching tubes with differing flow rates. Further, there do not appear to be any shunt pathways since the spheres remain in the section of the circulation (arterial or venous) into which they are injected.

DOMENECH and coworkers (1969) provided the definitive data for the method and an index of the limitations. Different-sized spheres were used as follows: large ^{125}I, 56.0 μm; ^{141}Ce, 60.0; ^{51}Cr, 60.9; ^{85}Sr, 55.8; ^{91}Nb, 50.9; ^{46}Sc, 55.0: medium ^{125}I, 22.4; ^{85}Sr, 20.5 and small ^{85}Sr, 14.1. The total number given varied from 7,000 to 160,000, with radioactivity of 1 to 2 μCi. The spheres were suspended in a 20% solution of dextran with a small amount of Tween 80 to prevent clumping. Before injection into the left atrium the spheres in dextran were stirred in a small mixing chamber and flushed through the catheter with about 15 to 20 ml saline.

Reference flow was collected from an artery, starting a few seconds before injection, and for some time after injection, depending on the size of the spheres. After completion of the experiment the animal was sacrificed and the heart excised and washed to remove surface blood. It was split open and sections taken from the free ventricular wall and septum and divided into inner (endocardial) and outer (epicardial) layers. Radioactivity of each sample was counted in a well scintillation detector connected to a 400-channel pulse-height analyzer.

Successive injections of large or small microspheres produced no consistent hemodynamic effects (DOMENECH et al., 1969; FORTUIN et al., 1971). Over 99% of the large microspheres were recovered in the reference sample within one minute. With small microspheres only 85 to 92% appeared in the reference sample within one minute; the remainder was found over the next 4 min. Comparison of total coronary flow calculated from large microspheres with directly measured coronary venous return to the right heart in a right heart bypass showed a reasonably good correlation with a slope of 1.02.

DOMENECH et al. (1969) and FORTUIN et al. (1971) demonstrated no difference in the distribution of large and small microspheres to large regions of the heart such as atria, right or left ventricular free walls or septum. However, there were differences in the distribution of large and small microspheres to small regions like epicardium or endocardium. There was usually a gradient across the ventricular walls with the inner layers having a higher concentration per gram than the outer layers. The inner/outer ratio for the left ventricular free wall was greater with large microspheres (50 μm) than with medium or small microspheres (20 or 15 μm).

Several groups established that there is no shunting of spheres through the heart. DOMENECH et al. (1969) found less than 0.5% of the total radioactivity in the coronary venous blood even during marked vasodilatation and with small microspheres. FORTUIN et al. (1971) reported less than 1%, BECKER et al. (1973) less than 0.03% in the coronary sinus, and SUGISHITA et al. (1971) reported no coronary arteriovenous shunting.

The microsphere method has been established as a reliable method for determination of regional blood flow. However, DOMENECH and co-workers (1969) do not feel that large spheres (50 to 60 μm) are as reliable for small regions of the myocardium as small spheres (15 μm). The difference between the inner and outer ratio may be explained by axial streaming and a shorter transit time for large spheres. However, most workers have used microspheres no greater than 15 μm in diameter and in many cases found the inner/outer ratio close to one. Since the microspheres are trapped in the arterioles, the flow determined by this method should agree with metered flow but may not always agree with flow determined by clearance of a diffusible indicator.

Ischemia and drugs on distribution of myocardial blood flow. Fortuin et al. (1971) and Sugishita et al. (1971), as well as the previous work of Domenech et al. (1969), used the microsphere method to study the distribution of myocardial blood flow and the effect thereon of drugs in anesthetized, open-chest dogs. The microspheres were injected through a catheter in the left atrium. In some cases coronary blood flow and aortic flow were recorded by electromagnetic flowmeters.

The animals were killed with a large dose of pentobarbital or potassium chloride. The heart was removed, washed free of blood, blotted dry, and cut into various sections of left and right ventricular free wall, septum, atria, etc. The free ventricular walls were divided into epicardial and endocardial halves. Each sample was weighed and counted for the isotopes present by gamma spectrometry. Sugishita et al. (1971) determined regional myocardial blood flow in ml/min/100 g on the basis of amount of radioactivity injected, aortic blood flow, regional radioactivity and regional sample weight. Fortuin et al. (1971) merely used the ratio of activity, which can be misleading, particularly after drug intervention.

All three groups found flow in the left ventricle higher than in the right ventricle and equal to the interventricular septum. Left ventricular endocardium was higher than epicardium (range 1.17 to 1.28) for 15 μm spheres. Becker et al. (1971, 1973) and Gross and Winbury (1973) found ratios close to one.

The left ventricle endo/epi ratio was decreased by isoproterenol, increased by propranolol, not changed 30 sec after nitroglycerin but increased at 5 min (Becker et al., 1971; Fortuin et al., 1971). The change in the ratio after propranolol was due to a decrease in epi from 82 to 73 ml/min/100 g with no change in endo, 77 to 78 ml/min/100 g (Gross and Winbury, 1973). The effect of antianginal drugs on normal and ischemic regions was evaluated by Becker et al. (1971). Five seconds after occlusion of the circumflex artery microspheres were injected into the left atrium and the occlusion was maintained for a total of 35 secs. Perfusion of the ischemic area was 20% that of the normal region and the endo/epi ratio decreased from 1.17 to 0.76. Thus, endocardial flow in the ischemic region was markedly diminished. Although nitroglycerin (5 min before occlusion) or propranolol did not increase the relative perfusion of the ischemic region (still 20% of normal), the endo/epi ratio was increased significantly in the ischemic as well as in the normal region.

Becker et al. (1973) used 15 μm microspheres to map the pattern of blood flow at various intervals after coronary occlusion. Spheres were injected into the left atrium after mechanical mixing for at least 3 min. A timed blood sample was collected from the brachial or femoral artery for 1 to 3 min after the injection. At 30 and 60 min after occlusion there was stratification of flow in the ischemic zone with maximal flow reduction in the center. Just outside the ischemic zone was a border of hyperemic tissue. Transmural distribution of flow in the ischemic area showed a disproportionate reduction in the endocardium. When flow was 60% of normal the endo/epi ratio was about one, but dropped linearly with the decrease in flow. This is similar to the changes in oxygen tension shown in Fig. 1. Surface electrograms show a correlation between ST segment changes and flow reduction. This question is considered in Section O.

Collateral flow measured by microspheres (Becker and Pitt, 1971b) 4 to 8 weeks after placing an ameroid constrictor (p. 45) on the left circumflex coronary artery showed no significant difference between the normal and "ischemic" areas. The ratio of microsphere concentration of the region supplied by the left anterior descending to the left circumflex was about 1.0 both in the control group and in animals with ameroids, whether or not infarction was present.

III. Hydrogen Clearance with Electrodes

We are indebted to the work of AUKLAND et al. (1964) for the demonstration of the use of hydrogen electrodes for measurement of regional blood flow based on blood-tissue exchange of an inert diffusible tracer (gas). The theory and principles of the use of diffusible tracers is discussed *in extenso* in a previous review by this author (WINBURY, 1971a) and will not be considered here except where necessary.

Hydrogen polarography resembles oxygen polarography (Section E.III); the current generated by the conversion of molecular hydrogen (H_2) to hydrogen ions is proportional to the partial pressure of hydrogen in the medium. The measuring system must be of low resistance for the current to be linearly related to the hydrogen concentration. The oxidation occurs at +0.24 V, a point at which there is minimal interference with oxygen or pH.

Tissue electrodes and intravascular electrodes have been described by various groups (AUKLAND et al., 1964, 1967; NEELY et al., 1965; KOYAMA and MARUTANI, 1971; GROSS and WINBURY, 1973). The tissue electrode of AUKLAND and co-workers (1964, 1967) was constructed of 0.8 mm platinum wire, tapered at the tip and coated with several layers of insulating lacquer and a layer of silicone rubber. The insulation was removed from the tip leaving a bare area 1 to 3 mm in length. NEELEY's group (1965) used electrodes of similar size and construction. Our electrodes (GROSS and WINBURY, 1973) were the same as those used for oxygen polarography and were constructed of 177 µm platinum wire quadruple-coated with Teflon insulation and freed of insulation at the tip for 0.2 to 0.3 mm. The OD with insulation was about 250 µm. *In vitro* calibration by WEISS (unpubl.) and by GROSS and WINBURY (1973) demonstrated a linear response to hydrogen concentration as did the other groups mentioned earlier in this paragraph. Likewise, at 0.2 to 0.3 V, oxygen, pH, and ascorbic acid had minimal effects relative to what would be expected in the tissue.

We used a pair of electrodes, as for oxygen, with one inserted to a depth of 3 mm and the other 9 mm. The electrodes remained fixed in position because the free end separated in a "wishbone" fashion when inserted into the tissue. A silver-chloride reference electrode implanted sub-cutaneously was polarized at +0.25 V. Current was measured by an electrometer which consisted of a high-gain amplifier with a feedback resistor. The amplifier output went through a filter and inverting amplifier and was recorded on a direct-writing instrument.

For determination of hydrogen clearance the dogs were respired with a gas mixture containing 2% H_2 in room air until each electrode reached a plateau (tissue 100% saturated). Then the hydrogen was discontinued and the epicardial and endocardial desaturation curves followed until a low plateau was recorded (tissue 0% saturated). A semilogarithmic plot of relative H_2 concentration (percentage) *vs.* time yielded a $T^1/_2$ which was used to calculate tissue perfusion (KETY, 1960; AUKLAND et al., 1964, 1967; NEELY et al., 1965; WINBURY, 1971a; WINBURY et al., 1972; GROSS and WINBURY, 1973). The curve was a single mono-exponential and flow was determined from the equation:

$$\text{Clearance (ml/min/100 g)} = 0.693/T^1/_2\,\text{(min)} \times 100.$$

The tissue/blood partition coefficient and specific gravity of the myocardium were assumed to be 1.00 (AUKLAND et al., 1964). Curves that were not mono-exponential after the initial 30 to 40 sec of desaturation were discarded.

The validity of the method was established by coronary venous outflow (AUKLAND et al., 1964; NEELY et al., 1965), by pump perfusion of the left coronary artery at various rates (WINBURY et al., 1972), by electromagnetic flowmeter and by microspheres (GROSS and WINBURY, 1973).

Antianginal agents, coronary dilators and hypoxia on transmural distribution. Transmural perfusion of the left ventricle is almost homogeneous based on hydrogen clearance in epicardium and endocardium (Winbury and Howe, 1973). Although the epi/endo perfusion ratio (note that this is the reverse of the microsphere ratio data) averaged 1.10 in the first study and 1.05 in the second, there were values less than 1.0. Therefore, the slightly greater epi perfusion may lack biological significance. It is of interest that in both studies as metered coronary flow (average) increased, epi perfusion was favored, and the epi/endo ratio increased.

Of interest are the effects of *nitrates* (nitroglycerin and pentaerythritoltrinitrate) and *beta adrenergic blockers* (propranolol, bunolol, and practolol). Both classes of drug decreased epi perfusion but left intact endo perfusion. Average coronary blood flow decreased. This is illustrated in Fig. 5, which is based on the data in Winbury et al. (1972) and Gross and Winbury (1973). It is important to note that the nitrate observations were made at 4 to 7 min after completion of the infusion, which time there is a steady state and endo pO_2 is elevated.

Chromonar produced a greater increase in epi than endo perfusion; 93 to 246 ml/min/100 g epi, 93 to 191 endo, respectively. The epi/endo ratio increased from 1.03 to 1.32. Coronary blood flow (flowmeter) increased out of proportion to perfusion, 97 to 311 ml/min/100 g (Gross and Winbury, 1973). It has been suggested that this could be due to a type of physiological shunting or a decrease in the efficiency of the nutritional circulation (Winbury et al., 1972; Marshall and Parratt, 1973b). We did find that when coronary blood flow was increased by a physiological stimulus, such as hypoxia induced by breathing 10% oxygen, coronary blood flow and epi clearance increased to the same extent (57 ml/min/100 g) and endo clearance increased more than flow (70 ml/min/100 g), bringing the epi/endo ratio down from 1.40 to 1.20. These studies show that perfusion can increase markedly and in proportion to coronary blood flow. We found the same to be true when we increased flow by pump perfusion. Apparently, potent coronary dilators increase the velocity of blood flow through certain capillary beds—possibly short beds—so that equilibrium cannot be attained; this is a form of shunting. Certainly, the failure of tissue oxygen tension to increase markedly in spite of the rise in coronary sinus oxygen tension would suggest this to be the case (Winbury et al., 1972).

The important information obtained by regional H_2 clearance is the decline in epi perfusion with maintenance of endo perfusion by nitrates and *beta* adrenergic blockers, and the failure of tissue perfusion to parallel average inflow after potent coronary dilators and the greater rise in epi perfusion, i.e. "coronary steal".

IV. Mass Spectrometer

The principles and use of the mass spectrometer were considered in Section E.IV. Tissue pO_2, pCO_2, and argon clearance can be determined simultaneously in epicardium and endocardium. The results are described in E.IV.2 and will not be repeated here.

V. Conclusions — Regional Flow

It has been demonstrated that compounds can alter the transmural distribution of coronary flow by different means. In some cases the change is favorable, in others unfavorable. The nitrates and *beta* adrenergic blockers cause a favorable redistribution and preserve perfusion in the relatively hypoxic subendocardium which, coupled with a decreased oxygen requirement, leads to a better balance between oxygen supply and demand, as evidenced by a rise in tissue pO_2. The subepicardial perfusion is decreased, no doubt as an autoregulatory response to the diminished oxygen requirement.

Potent coronary dilators like dipyridamole or carbochromen produce a maldistribution by arteriolar dilatation in normal regions which thereby deprives hypoxic regions of an adequate blood supply.

It should be kept in mind that microspheres may measure a different function than diffusible tracers. The former could measure total flow, the latter nutrient flow.

G. Other Methods for Measurement of Coronary Blood Flow

KADATZ (1971) and CHARLIER (1971) have discussed various other methods for determination of coronary blood flow in anesthetized and conscious animals. Only a few will be considered here. If information on other methods is desired, the above references should be consulted. Methods using electromagnetic flowmeters, Doppler ultrasonic flowmeters, rotameters and methods for direct collection of coronary sinus outflow have been reviewed extensively. We introduce here some of the newer approaches.

I. Thermodilution

The basic rationale of local thermodilution is considered in the reports of FRONEK (1973) and GANZ et al. (1971). Injection of a fluid miscible with blood at a lower temperature serves as an indicator. The resulting change in temperature measured downstream is related to the volume of dilution or rate of blood flow. The heat lost by the blood is equal to the heat gained by the indicator. Local thermodilution in a single vessel, with the injection and sensing sites close to each other, has several advantages. Flow can be measured in a single vessel at fast repetition rates without the problem of recirculation since the entire blood stream and body acts as a "sink" for the indicator. Mixing of the indicator must be complete within the few millimeters between the injection site and the sensing device. Special catheters have been designed which can be placed in specific vessels, such as the coronary sinus, and remain in place for a considerable period of time. The location of the injection site and sensing thermistor is dictated by whether one is measuring upstream or downstream flow.

Another application is implantation of several catheters in side branches, for example of the aorta, and placing the thermistor distally. This permits measurement of different flows because, as with any dilution technique, the area under the dilution curve is related inversely to the blood flow at the site of injection. A bolus or continuous injection can be used. Continuous injection has the advantage of a temperature steady state; therefore dynamic changes in flow can be easily detected because the temperature change is the only variable.

GANZ and co-workers (1971) have developed special catheters for determination of coronary sinus blood flow in man by continuous thermodilution. The technique was applied to the study of nitroglycerin in man by GANZ and MARCUS (1972). The equation derived for coronary sinus blood flow (CSBF) is

$$\mathrm{CSBF} = V_I \times \left(\frac{T_B - T_I}{T_B - T_M} - 1\right) \times 1.08$$

where V_I = volume of injectate in ml/min; T_B, T_I, T_M = temperature of blood, injectate, and mixture of blood and injectate in °C, respectively. The derivation of the equation can be found in GANZ et al. (1971) and will not be considered further. During measurement, 5% dextrose in water at room temperature is injected at a constant rate of about 40 ml/min. The resulting fall in temperature is inversely related to the rate of CSBF. It was established that the volume of blood flow was not affected by the injection.

Two types of catheter were used (Wilton Webster Mfg. Co., Altadena, Calif.) in the initial studies. The design for a single flow rate was an outer catheter 100 cm long with a 2.3 mm OD and 1 mm ID. An inner nylon tubing of 0.75 mm ID and separated from the inner wall by an insulating air space was used for injection of the indicator. The nylon tube was tapered at the tip to an injection orifice of 0.4 to 0.5 mm. An opening in the outer catheter 20 mm proximal to the closed tip was joined to the orifice of the inner catheter. An external thermistor on the shaft of the outer catheter, 10 to 15 mm proximal to the injection orifice and on the same side, measured T_B before and T_M during indicator infusion. T_I was measured by a thermistor inside the nylon tubing close to the orifice. A lead band proximal to the external thermistor served for location under fluoroscopy. The distal 45 to 50 mm of the catheter was bent to an angle of 45 to 60° to facilitate insertion and stabilization of the catheter in the coronary sinus.

The thermistors were incorporated into one arm of a Wheatstone bridge and the temperature change during injection was amplified by a dc amplifier and recorded directly.

In vitro studies showed that injectate flow rates of 35 and 55 ml/min were required at blood flow rates up to 300 and 500 ml/min, respectively. The accuracy was determined *in vitro* (model studies) and *in vivo* (open-chest dog). The slope of the regression equation was 0.99 ($r = 0.99$) in model experiments and *in vivo* in the jugular vein and the coronary sinus of the dog.

Coronary sinus blood flow was determined in 14 normal subjects and in 35 with the clinical diagnosis of coronary artery disease confirmed by arteriography. In normal subjects the values varied between 83 and 158 ml/min with a mean of 122. Patients with coronary disease ranged from 92 to 167 ml/min with a mean of 128. There is no difference between normal and coronary artery disease patients.

A special catheter was devised for simultaneous measurement of blood flow in the coronary sinus and great cardiac vein. The catheter had the injection orifice at the tip and two external thermistors, 10 mm (great cardiac vein) and 30 mm (coronary sinus) from the tip. Experiments in animals demonstrated adequate mixing at the level of both thermistors. Great cardiac vein flow averaged about 68 ml/min which is about 65% of total coronary sinus flow.

GANZ and MARCUS (1972) studied the effect of intracoronary and intravenous nitroglycerin on pacing-induced angina and coronary sinus blood flow. A single external thermistor catheter was inserted into the coronary sinus under fluoroscopic control from the left antecubital vein. A 5% solution of dextrose in water was injected into the coronary sinus at a rate of about 40 ml/min. Arterial pressure, ECG (V_5) and femoral artery and coronary sinus lactate were determined under control conditions and pacing to produce angina. Nitroglycerin, 75 µg, was injected intracoronary during pacing-induced angina through a Judkins catheter in the left coronary artery or into the right coronary artery through a modified Bourassa catheter during the pacing-induced angina. In 6 patients nitroglycerin was given intravenously in a dose of 0.2 mg while pacing was continued.

Left coronary injection of nitroglycerin in 5 subjects with normal coronary arteriograms elevated CSBF by an average of 83% for a period of less than 1 min.

Twenty five patients with typical angina pectoris had coronary artery disease. Pacing-induced angina was associated with myocardial lactate production or low extraction and significant ST segment depression in 17 patients. Nitroglycerin did not relieve the angina in any of the patients, whether injected into the left or right coronary artery; in 14 patients CSBF was increased to a higher level. Pacing alone caused a marked increase in CSBF and intracoronary injection of nitroglycerin at rest also did so, but did not elevate flow above the pacing level.

Intravenous injection of nitroglycerin relieved the angina which was unaffected by preceding intracoronary administration in all 6 patients. CSBF and arterial pressure fell before the relief was noted. These data suggest that the direct action of nitroglycerin on the coronary arteries is of little importance in the relief of angina pectoris. Possibly the peripheral actions which cause a reduction in myocardial oxygen requirement (venous pooling and reduction in left ventricular end-diastolic pressure) are the significant factors.

II. Heat Dissipation and Heat Production

Myocardial thermal conductivity and metabolic heat production has been used extensively for measurement of regional myocardial blood flow and metabolism by Grayson (1952), Grayson and Haigh (1954), Grayson and Parratt (1966), Grayson et al. (1971), Uchida and Ueda (1971) and Grayson et al. (1973). In principle a small recorder, which consists of an electrically heated filament and a thermocouple to measure the temperature, is inserted into the left ventricular wall; the heat loss from the heated element is a measure of local blood flow. The use of the method in various species is described by Grayson and Parratt (1966).

The relative measure of myocardial (tissue) blood flow is thermal conductivity. The ability to dissipate heat from a local source is a function of the blood flow in the region of the heated elements. The unit consists of a heater and a constantan wire–copper recording thermo-couple in close proximity to the heater. This is placed in the myocardium through a needle track. The difference between the thermal conductivity of living and dead (no blood flow) myocardial tissue is a linear function of blood flow. Details of the procedure can be obtained from the afore-mentioned papers and a brief summary will suffice for this review.

A coil of copper wire heats a thermocouple of copper–constantan. The reference junction is a thermocouple without the heating coil encased in plastic tubing and placed in the aortic arch. The temperatures recorded are the differentials between the myocardium and aortic blood. Cyclic current is applied to the heater coils and measurement made of the temperature changes produced.

Heat clearance, which is a function of local myocardial blood flow, is based on the thermal conductivity difference between perfused and non-perfused tissue.

Heat production in the tissue is based on the myocardial "corrected" temperature. This is myocardial temperature corrected for blood flow change, with heat losses and blood temperature controlled. In a recent paper Grayson et al. (1973) questioned the validity of heat clearance, but not xenon clearance, as a function of nutritional blood flow. The removal of a diffusible foreign tracer is a function of capillary circulation whereas thermal conductivity is a physical process and dependent on total fluid movement in the vicinity of the probe. They suggest that heat production is probably more like xenon clearance. However, this proposal is difficult to accept since increased metabolic heat production does not insure greater capillary circulation. It is obvious that the heat clearance and metabolic heat production data must be interpreted with caution. Heat clearance is dependent upon total regional flow, which would include arteriovenous anastomoses, physiological shunts, and other high-velocity flow regions which can act as a "heat sink", but where the blood flow may not be available for exchange with the tissues. Skin is an excellent example of such a region.

H. Blood Flow and Metabolism of Ischemic Region

There are various approaches to estimation of blood flow in ischemic regions. Any region deprived of blood flow via the normal pathway is dependent on collateral circulation for survival (see Fig. 3). Measurement of collateral flow has been the subject of many investigations but there is no unanimity of opinion as to the best procedure for evaluation of collateral function and development of collateral circulation.

The anatomic demonstration of the development of collateral vessels has been discussed extensively by SCHAPER (1971) in his monograph on the collateral circulation. Postmortem injection of the coronary bed with an X-ray-opaque medium and "unrolling" of the heart is a popular and useful technique. Others have injected the coronary tree with a plastic material which will fill vessels to 40 μm in diameter. The tissue is then dissolved away with potassium hydroxide leaving a cast of the coronary tree. By using plastics of different colors, one can see collateral or anastomotic interconnectors. However, anatomic demonstration of collateral vessels provides no information about their function under intact living conditions. Thus we must resort to collateral flow, or retrograde flow, or pressure.

One of the earliest and most frequently used procedures is measurement of back flow and/or back pressure from the distal end of a severed coronary artery. Others have used the distribution of a diffusible tracer or the clearance of a tracer from the ischemic region. More recently, collateral flow has been measured in unanesthetized dogs by clearance techniques or back-flow methods.

I. Retrograde Blood Flow (Back Flow)

The definitive report on measurement of collateral circulation by retrograde blood flow is that of KATTUS and GREGG (1959). The factors that affect retrograde flow were determined in order to design a method that would provide a reliable index of collateral function.

After anesthesia of the dogs with pentobarbital, a left thoracotomy was performed under positive-pressure artificial respiration. A metal cannula was passed into the left main coronary artery via the left subclavian artery and aorta. At a distance of 1 to 1.5 cm from the bifurcation of the left coronary artery the anterior descending branch or circumflex branch was ligated and the distal portion cannulated. This distal vessel could be perfused in an antegrade fashion or used to measure retrograde flow.

The cannula in the main left coronary was perfused from a perfusion reservoir of donor arterial blood at a constant pressure or directly from the recipient's carotid artery; flow was measured with a recording rotameter. Normally, the outflow from the rotameter supplied the entire left coronary bed (left main coronary and proximal portion of sectioned branch via the brass cannula plus the distal branch via a separate cannula). When retrograde flow was measured, the inflow tube to the distal severed branch was clamped and retrograde flow from the distal branch was measured in a graduate from a side arm. Perfusion of the remainder of the left ventricle was antegrade through the cannula in the main left coronary artery. Cannulas were placed in one or both femoral arteries and connected to a common reservoir for stabilization of blood pressure. Heparin was used to prevent coagulation (10 mg/kg initial dose, followed by 5 mg/kg every 30 to 40 min).

In the majority of dogs retrograde flow varied between 1 and 3 ml/min at physiological perfusion pressure. Perfusion pressure was varied by altering the height of the perfusion reservoir, or in the case of self-perfusion, by aortic clamping or hemorrhage. Retrograde flow varied with perfusion pressure, indicating that interventions aimed at altering retrograde flow must be performed at constant perfusion pressure.

Perfusion of the left coronary bed with desaturated blood from the coronary sinus produced a marked increase in antegrade coronary flow but retrograde flow was reduced slightly. Reactive hyperemia was produced by occlusion of the total left coronary inflow for 15 to 30 sec. Release of the clamp was followed by a marked increase in inflow, but not in retrograde flow, indicating that the collateral circulation did not participate in autoregulation as evidenced by reactive hyperemia.

Nitroglycerin was infused into the left coronary inflow at the rate of 60 μg/min. At constant pressure (reservoir) retrograde flow was unchanged or slightly decreased and coronary flow showed a transient increase at the start of the infusion. In self-perfusion experiments retrograde flow followed perfusion pressure.

Histamine as a single dose of 50 μg or an infusion of 50 μg/min in self-perfusion animals caused an increase in coronary flow in face of a fall in blood pressure, but retrograde flow declined slightly or was unchanged. Intracoronary *norepinephrine*, 10 to 20 μg/min at constant perfusion pressure, did not alter retrograde flow or antegrade flow. However, intravenous infusion at the same rate to self-perfused dogs increased blood pressure, coronary flow, and retrograde flow.

Physiological studies showed that heart rate did not alter retrograde flow. However, distention of the heart by aortic constriction was not accompanied by the increase in retrograde flow expected on the basis of the rise in perfusion pressure. This suggests that myocardial stretch and increased wall tension inhibited retrograde flow.

The flow measured by the retrograde technique no doubt over-estimates collateral flow since it is collected at atmospheric pressure. Furthermore, the retrograde blood is equal to arterial blood in oxygen content, indicating that it has not traversed a capillary bed. Some consider this a "potential flow" which does increase on chronic occlusion (SCHAPER, 1971). However, the functional significance of retrograde flow is still to be clarified.

II. Collateral Flow and Metabolism of Ischemic Region

PARRATT's group recently described a procedure in open-chest dogs that permits simultaneous study of blood flow, oxygen extraction, and oxygen consumption in acutely infarcted regions and normal regions of the left ventricle (LEDINGHAM et al., 1973; MARSHALL and PARRATT, 1973a, b; PARRATT et al., 1973). Blood flow in the normal region was monitored by an electromagnetic flowmeter on the appropriate artery and venous samples were taken from the coronary sinus. In the infarcted region blood flow was determined either by ^{133}Xe clearance or retrograde flow or pressure, and venous samples were taken directly from the vein draining the infarcted region.

Greyhound dogs were initially anesthetized with thiopental sodium (20 mg/kg i.v.) and the trachea intubated. Positive pressure respiration was maintained with an air mixture containing 0.5 to 1.0% trichlorethylene to maintain a steady state of anesthesia. The volume of respiration was adjusted to maintain arterial pO_2 at about 100 Torr and pCO_2 between 30 and 40 Torr.

Catheters were placed into the descending aorta, right atrium and coronary sinus under fluoroscopic guidance for blood sampling and/or pressure measurement. In some studies a catheter tip transducer was inserted into the left ventricle via the left carotid for left ventricular pressure and dP/dt. Cardiac output was determined by dye dilution with indocyanine green injected into the right atrium and blood was withdrawn from the aorta through a densitometer.

After left thoracotomy, the anterior descending branch (LAD) and circumflex branch (LC) of the left coronary artery were isolated as well as a major branch of the vein that parallels the LAD. Blood flow in the LC (normal region) was determined by a flowmeter placed around the vessel. The coronary vein draining the infarct was catheterized with a Longdwel Teflon catheter inserted about halfway between the tip of the atrium and apex of the heart. The LAD was ligated in the same location after administration of lidocaine. The distal portion of the artery was catheterized with a Portex nylon catheter (OD 1.34 mm). This could be used to measure peripheral coronary pressure, peripheral coronary flow (retrograde flow), or ^{133}Xe clearance. For the latter, ^{133}Xe (about 90 μ Ci in 1.2 ml) was injected into the infarct and clearance measured from the ischemic region using a collimator with a narrow acceptance angle.

The most pronounced hemodynamic change observed 2 to 3 h *after acute ligation of the LAD* was a decrease in cardiac output and calculated cardiac work. LVEDP and peripheral resistance were significantly elevated even though various pressures, dP/dt, coronary flow in the normal region, and myocardial oxygen consumption were unchanged (MARSHALL and PARRATT, 1973a). Although there were immediate changes in coronary vein pO_2, pCO_2, pH and oxygen content after ligation, at 2 to 3 h pO_2, pCO_2, pH and oxygen content were similar in the venous blood (infarct) and coronary sinus (normal region). Blood flow in the infarcted region was about 20% of normal.

Highly effective coronary dilators such as *carbochromen or dipyridamole* have a different effect in the normal and ischemic regions. Coronary flow in the normal region was increased markedly. This was accompanied by a decrease in coronary resistance, oxygen extraction and consumption, and an increase in coronary sinus oxygen content.

Infarct blood flow (^{133}Xe clearance), peripheral coronary flow and peripheral coronary pressure were unchanged after carbochromen or dipyridamole in spite of the marked rise in the oxygen content of the venous blood draining the ischemic area. These results were interpreted to indicate that the potent coronary arteriolar dilators do not improve perfusion of the ischemic region. This may be due to a decrease in the diastolic perfusion gradient or failure to prevent the rise in LVEDP. The increase in venous pO_2 from the infarct suggests the opening of vessels that do not provide for tissue nutrition (MARSHALL and PARRATT, 1973b; PARRATT et al., 1973).

Other studies showed that *norepinephrine and oxyfedrine* increased blood flow in the ischemic region as well as the normal region. Peripheral coronary pressure and flow were also elevated. These drugs increased the transventricular diastolic perfusion gradient, which is an important determinant of subendocardial perfusion (LEDINGHAM et al., 1973; MARSHALL and PARRATT, 1973a).

These procedures have the advantage of comparison of normal and ischemic regional blood flows and metabolism simultaneously. All too frequently coronary sinus blood has been used for study of ischemic regions. Without isolation of that portion of the coronary venous blood draining the ischemic region the results would be misleading, since the greater portion of the sinus blood represents normal areas.

III. Collateral Flow in Unanesthetized Dogs

With the development of small flow and pressure transducers and synthetic materials compatible with animal tissues, methods have been developed for the study of the coronary circulation under normal and abnormal conditions. A long series of important contributions on experimental coronary insufficiency and collateral flow in unanesthetized dogs have come from GREGG'S group (KHOURI et al., 1971; ELLIOT et al., 1968; PASYK et al., 1971; KHOURI, 1973; GREGG, 1972; ELLIOT, 1973).

In a recent volume on chronic cardiovascular instrumentation KHOURI (1973) and BOND et al. (1973) discussed in detail the techniques and problems involved in implanting flow transducers on the coronary artery and aorta, occluders on coronary arteries, and catheters in the coronary sinus. KHOURI (1973) points out that stabilization of a flow transducer on the main left coronary artery is no problem, but that particular vessel is very short and suitable for transducer placement in only one out of three or four dogs. Therefore, the left anterior descending or left circumflex branch has been used most frequently. The coronary artery branch is dissected free for 1 cm near the origin. A snug-fitting transducer is then placed on the proximal end of the freed vessel. This is followed by a 2 to 3 mm wide strip of Ivalon sponge and a zero-occluding cuff. The transducer and occlusion cuffs are oriented and stabilized by attachment of the cables and tube to the pericardium. BOND and coworkers (1973) prefer placement of the flow probe on the descending branch since the vessel is oriented in the long axis of the heart and permits easier stabilization of the probe. They find a snare occluder more efficient than a balloon. A special snare designed to permit tension on a nylon line placed under the vessel is passed through a Silastic tube in the chest wall. The external tube is capped to prevent pneumothorax but permits occlusion of the vessel when required.

ELLIOT (1973) has recently evaluated four different approaches to the study of the collateral circulation following gradual occlusion of the circumflex branch of the left coronary artery. In the first group of experiments gradual occlusion was produced by an ameroid constrictor (ELLIOT et al., 1968). The dogs were anesthetized with pentobarbital sodium, 30 mg/kg, placed under artificial respiration and the left thorax was opened in the 5th interspace. The pericardium was opened parallel to the phrenic nerve. A vinyl tube was implanted in the aortic arch for blood pressure. A length of the circumflex artery was freed from the surrounding tissue and the flow transducer was placed close to the origin, followed by the pneumatic cuff for zero flow and the ameroid constrictor. Distal to the constrictor a vinyl tube was implanted with the tip facing downstream. The cables and tubes (except for the coronary tube) were brought out through the incision and run in a subcutaneous tunnel to the back. The coronary tube was ultimately brought out through the incision and skin at the middle of the left chest and protected by a canvas jacket after closing the chest cavity and reducing the pneumothorax. The coronary tube was filled with heparin each day to prevent clotting. Aortic pressure, circumflex blood flow and peripheral coronary pressure were recorded before and during cuff occlusion. The first few days after surgery the ameroid had not closed; therefore peripheral circumflex pressure equalled aortic pressure and the blood flow pattern was normal. Temporary cuff occlusion was accompanied by a fall in peripheral coronary pressure to 2 mm Hg. Release of the occlusion was followed by reactive hyperemia, indicating good arteriolar reserve. By 21 days there was an aortic-coronary pressure gradient, a reduced and less phasic coronary flow, and peripheral coronary pressure during cuff occlusion was now up to 28 mm Hg. Reactive hyperemia was somewhat reduced (ELLIOT et al., 1968). The difficulty of this procedure was inability to predict closure of the ameroid constrictors.

A KHOURI Hg constrictor (see L.IV) was used in the second series, rather than an ameroid constrictor, to control the rate of occlusion. Stepwise, gradual occlusion over 5 days produced an early rise in peripheral coronary pressure and a further marked increase when circumflex flow was severely compromised. Reactive hyperemia was abolished at this later stage. Blood flow in the anterior descending branch increased progressively as circumflex flow decreased (GREGG, 1972). When flow in the circumflex branch decreased to zero, mean coronary pressure and peripheral coronary pressure were equal and almost 80% of the control coronary pressure, indicating collateral development (PASYK et al., 1971; ELLIOT, 1973).

The effect of circumflex occlusion on ^{133}Xe clearance was determined by injecting the isotope as a bolus into the intracoronary tube and recording the washout curve with a scintillation counter. Control values obtained with the hydraulic occluder open averaged about 40 ml/min/100 g. Collateral flow prior to chronic occlusion was determined either by acute obstruction of the vessel and injection of ^{133}Xe 15 to 20 sec later, or by first injecting the ^{133}Xe and producing the acute temporary obstruction 45 sec later. In the latter procedures, the first curve is the normal flow and the second, slower curve the collateral flow. Both techniques gave a control collateral flow of 15 to 18 ml/min/100 g. By the second or third day of chronic occlusion the collateral flow had risen to the control value of about 40 ml/min/100 g, and peripheral coronary pressure had increased to 40 mm Hg. These studies on ^{133}Xe clearance and peripheral coronary pressure provide only indirect indices of collateral flow. Therefore, a method was developed to measure retrograde flow in the unanesthetized state.

Retrograde flow was determined in conscious animals by a technique that attempted to duplicate the backflow method described in Section H.I. The left common carotid artery was cut high up in the neck, brought down into the thoracic cavity, and anastomosed to the circumflex branch. Measurement of retrograde flow was made through a Silastic tube connected to the cranial thyroid artery as far as possible from its origin from the carotid artery. A special valve located in the caudo-scapular region was used to fill the retrograde tube with heparin and for measurement of retrograde pressure and retrograde flow. A flowmeter, pneumatic cuff, and mercury constrictor were applied to the carotid inflow shunt proximal to the retrograde flow tube. Inflation of the pneumatic cuff gave a measure of peripheral coronary pressure and retrograde flow. As the central inflow to the circumflex was reduced by the mercury constrictor, there was a parallel rise in peripheral coronary pressure and flow. Several questions raised about the backflow technique have been considered in Section H.I.

An alternative procedure was developed which provided a direct measure of collateral flow in a peripheral branch of the circumflex artery (ELLIOT, 1973). Close to the origin of the circumflex artery from the left common coronary artery were placed, first, a mercury constrictor, then a *central* pneumatic cuff, followed by an intracoronary Silastic tube. Beyond this point, either between branches or on marginal branches were placed a flowmeter probe followed by a *distal* pneumatic

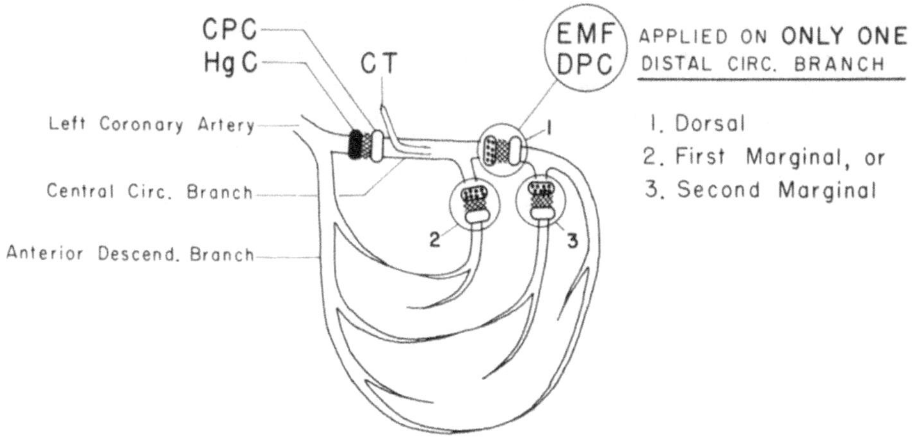

Fig. 8. Technique for determination of collateral flow in a branch of the circumflex coronary artery. HgC = Khouri Hg constrictor; CPC = central pneumatic cuff; CT = intracoronary tube; EMF = flowmeter; DPC = distal pneumatic cuff. From ELLIOT (1973) with permission

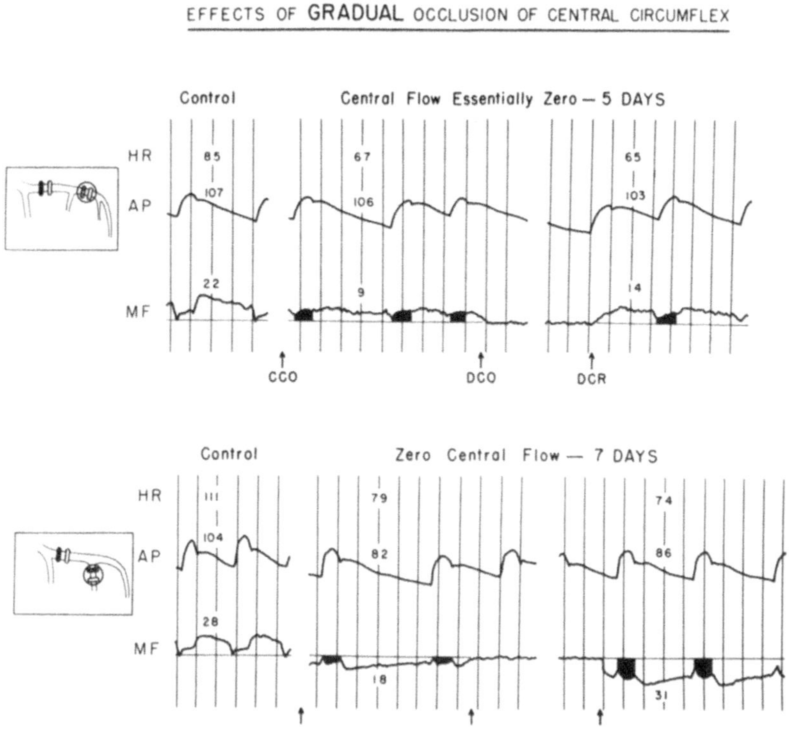

Fig. 9. Comparison of response to occlusion of main branch or marginal branch. The inset on left indicates site of flowmeter and pneumatic cuff. HR = heart rate; AP = aortic pressure; MF = blood flow; CCO = central cuff occlusion at arrow; DCO = distal cuff occlusion at arrow; and DCR = distal cuff released at arrow. Note reversed flow pattern (lower) on CCO and enhancement by DCR, indicating development of retrograde flow. From ELLIOT (1973) with permission

cuff, as illustrated in Fig. 8. Chronic circumflex occlusion was produced by the mercury constrictor with the central pneumatic cuff. Collateral flow was determined by inflating the central pneumatic cuff and then the distal cuff, and estimating blood flow in the metered branch. Gradual occlusion of the main branch of the circumflex over 4 to 7 days was studied as well as rapid occlusion over 6 to 12 h. Gradual occlusion resulted in good collateral development evidenced by retrograde blood flow, which was in the reverse direction in the marginal branch (Fig. 9). This procedure offers many possibilities but requires excellent surgical and animal-care facilities. Also, one must remember that flow is measured in only one branch and represents epicardial flow which has not traversed the capillary bed.

GREGG (1972) described the effect of nitroglycerin in normal and coronary insufficient circulation monitored by electromagnetic flowmeters on the arteries serving both regions in unanesthetized dogs. Intracoronary bolus injection (1 to 60 μg) or infusion (6 to 120 μg/min) increased coronary flow without major change in hemodynamics. Intravenous infusion (600 μg/min) or bolus injection (300 μg) as well as sublingual treatment produced an increase in coronary flow before systemic hemodynamic effects were observed.

Coronary insufficiency of the circumflex region was produced by the hydraulic occluder and collateral function was determined by changes in peripheral coronary pressure of the ischemic region. If intravenous nitroglycerin increases this pressure, dilatation of the collaterals is assumed, but if peripheral coronary pressure decreases, dilatation of the distal circumflex bed is assumed.

During the first day of abrupt occlusion of the circumflex branch nitroglycerin had no effect on peripheral coronary pressure. Several days later nitroglycerin decreased the peripheral coronary pressure. Again there was dilatation of the ischemic bed but not of the collateral vessels.

I. Atherosclerosis Model

Many investigators have been interested in developing a model of coronary heart disease by production of coronary atherosclerosis. The rabbit has been used successfully by several groups. When rabbits are fed high cholesterol diets, aortic and coronary atherosclerosis develops and the animals show characteristic ST segment changes under stress conditions (see WINBURY, 1964, for review of literature). After investigation of various methods—*ergonovine* or *hypoxia*—for production of coronary insufficiency in these animals and of the failure of nitrates to prevent the ST-segment depression, it was concluded that the animals were in generalized circulatory insufficiency and did not offer a suitable test model for antianginal drugs.

Atrial Pacing

Recently LEE and BAKY (1973) refined the method and were able to produce ST-segment changes by *atrial pacing* in atherosclerotic rabbits. Nitroglycerin, but not dipyridamole, attenuated the electrocardiographic changes.

Three-month-old male New Zealand White rabbits were fed a diet of Purina rabbit chow containing 2% cholesterol. Under local anesthesia a polyvinyl (14-gauge) catheter was inserted into the right precava for a distance of 6 to 7 cm, filled with heparin, and plugged. On the subsequent experimental days the animal was put into a "pseudohypnotic" state and restrained. Surface electrocardiographic leads were taken from the chest and sternum. The heart was paced with a bipolar electrode advanced through the precava catheter. The pacing rate was at least 100 beats/min above the normal rate to a maximum of about 410 beats/min. Animals could be paced repeatedly over a period of several weeks.

Animals maintained on the cholesterol diet for 4.5 months or longer displayed good ST-segment depression on pacing, but nitroglycerin, 20 mg/kg i.v., did not attenuate the response. In agreement with previous work, these animals had severe generalized atherosclerotic involvement (see WINBURY, 1964).

Animals tested after 6 weeks to 4 months of cholesterol feeding exhibited reproducible ST-segment depression with pacing. These animals showed a lesser degree of atherosclerotic involvement than the previous group. Nitroglycerin, about 200 μg/kg administered bucally, or 10 to 100 μg/kg i.v., prevented or attenuated the ST segment depression due to pacing. Dipyridamole, 250 μg/kg i.v., did not prevent or attenuate the ST-segment depression. In fact, the ST-segment depression due to pacing was greater after dipyridamole in a few animals.

These studies demonstrate that at early stage of atherosclerosis the coronary insufficiency induced by pacing can be altered by nitroglycerin. However, at later stages the insufficiency becomes so generalized that nitroglycerin has no effect. This type of coronary insufficiency is more diffuse than that usually seen in man. Yet the electrocardiographic changes produced by stress resemble those typical of angina pectoris. The difficulty in using this model for study of new therapeutic agents lies in predicting the degree of atherosclerotic involvement.

J. Diffuse Coronary Occlusion — Small Vessels

Injection of small particulate matter into the coronary tree will cause an occlusive process, primarily at the arteriolar level, which resembles diffuse atherosclerotic disease (WEBER et al., 1972). This type of involvement leads to chronic or acute failure of the myocardium or cardiogenic shock. In either case "pump" failure results from chronic generalized coronary insufficiency. Various forms of particulate materials have been used to produce such a condition. These include lycopodium spores, starch suspensions or large plastic spheres injected in large quantity into the base of the aorta or directly into a specific coronary artery.

I. Ischemic Heart Failure and Cardiogenic Shock by Starch Suspensions, Lycopodium Spores or Small Microspheres

1. Starch embolization was produced by repeated injection of 1 to 4 ml of 3.3% suspension of potato starch in physiological saline (ROOS and SMITH, 1948). The starch particles ranged from 12 to 72 μm and were largely ovoid in shape. The 3.3% suspension contained approximately 10^6 granules per ml.

Dogs were anesthetized with pentobarbital and placed under artificial respiration. The chest was opened by splitting the sternum and after hemostasis heparin was injected intravenously. Arterial blood pressure was determined from the right carotid artery and right atrial pressure by a water manometer connected to the atrial appendage. The starch suspension was shaken vigorously before the injection of 1 to 4 ml into the left ventricle. The aorta was occluded during the injection so that the embolizing particles entered the coronary bed. Injections were repeated at 1- to 7-min intervals until the desired effect was achieved.

After the injections, white mottled areas were seen on the epicardial surface of both ventricles but there were no significant hemodynamic changes until more than three injections had been given. Subsequent injections led to definite myocardial insufficiency with a rise in right atrial pressure, progressive cardiac dilatation and hypotension. Ultimately, pulmonary edema developed. The experiments usually terminated in death due to "pump" failure.

2. **Selective injection of lycopodium spores** into individual coronary arteries was used by GUZMAN et al. (1962) to produce a type of cardiogenic shock. The previously described procedure using starch suspensions (ROOS and SMITH, 1948) did not selectively embolize one coronary artery and there was "spill over" of particles into the systemic circulation. Furthermore, the present procedure does not necessitate opening the thorax, which of itself has a significant hemodynamic effect, nor are the coronary arteries or the perivascular nerves disturbed.

Dogs were anesthetized with morphine and a combination of Dialurethane and pentobarbital sodium. A no. 7, 8, or 9 double-lumen catheter was passed into the right heart and pulmonary artery via a jugular vein and another into the left heart via a femoral artery for left ventricular and left atrial pressures. Cardiac output was determined by dye dilution; Evans blue was injected into the pulmonary artery, and the concentration in aortic blood was determined in an aliquot continuously passed through a recording densitometer. The ECG (V_3) and pressures (pulmonary arterial, left atrial, left ventricular and aortic) were recorded continuously. The left anterior descending coronary artery was catheterized under fluoroscopy. For embolization 0.2 ml of a 1% suspension of lycopodium spores or glass microspheres were injected into the artery and immediately flushed in with 2 ml of blood. The spores or spheres ranged from 30 to 40 μm in size.

In normal dogs initial embolization produced a sharp decrease in cardiac output and blood pressure to shock levels and elevation of left atrial pressure, left ventricular end-diastolic pressure, pulmonary artery pressure, and peripheral resistance. Some of the animals died within a few minutes; others showed incomplete recovery. Subsequent injections of spores or microspheres resulted in progressive and persistent changes, and death usually occurred after the second or third embolization. Bilateral vagotomy did not alter the effects of embolization; however, in animals with intact vagi, atropine pretreatment attenuated the changes in cardiac output and blood pressure. Electrocardiographic changes following embolization consisted of initial ST-segment depression followed by elevation.

Histological studies showed spores present in arterioles, either singly or as aggregates of 3 to 10 spores. The blocked arterioles ranged from 40 to 500 μm. The size of vessels blocked overlaps the range in the studies of AGRESS et al. (1952), but they used much larger spores. The method and results of AGRESS et al. (1952) and JACOBEY et al. (1962) are considered below (Section J.II).

3. Diffuse myocardial lesions were produced in unanesthetized calves by injection of **plastic microspheres** 6 to 14 μm in diameter into the left main coronary artery by WEBER et al. (1972). Hemodynamic abnormalities produced by injection of 4 and 5 mg/kg of microspheres included elevation of left ventricular end-diastolic pressure, decreased stroke volume, cardiac output, dP/dt, mean ejection rate, and left ventricular ejection time, and prolongation of pre-ejection period.

Three-month-old calves were anesthetized with sodium thiamylal and maintained with halothane after endotracheal intubation. The surgery was performed 3 to 7 days before microsphere embolization. The left side of the thorax was opened in the fifth intercostal space. The mammary artery was cannulated with Teflon tubing and the tip was advanced distally to the junction with the brachiocephalic artery. After incision of the pericardium, a flow probe was placed around the base of the aorta and flow recorded with a Biotronex 610 flowmeter. The coronary sinus was cannulated with fluorinated silicone (Dow Corning) tubing by way of the hemiazygous vein.

An implantable pressure transducer (WITTAKER model 1017) inserted through a stab incision in the left ventricle monitored intraventricular pressure. Surface electrograms were obtained with electrodes attached directly to the epicardial surface.

A Teflon coronary arterial catheter with a flared tip was inserted into the left main coronary artery and secured in place by a purse-string suture. Microsphere injections were made through this catheter.

The incision was closed in layers and lead wires and catheters exteriorized for monitoring, taking blood samples, or microsphere injections. The coronary sinus and coronary artery catheters were kept patent by a slow drip of heparinized saline.

The microspheres were made of styrene divinyl benzene copolymer (Dow Chemical) and were 6 to 14 μm in diameter (average 7.5). They were suspended in a solution of 17% glucose in a volume of 200 ml. Two dosages of microspheres were given, 4 or 5 mg/kg into the left coronary artery over a period of 4 to 6 h. These studies were conducted in the unanesthetized state. Lactate levels were determined in coronary sinus and arterial blood as well as venous levels of creatine phosphokinase.

There were no significant hemodynamic changes during the slow microsphere injection, but by the end of the first day end-diastolic pressure was elevated after both dose levels and persisted throughout the observation period (up to 28 days). The group receiving the higher dose of microspheres showed other hemodynamic abnormalities, both at rest and during stress induced by angiotensin. The changes at rest were those associated with failure of the myocardium, e.g. decrease in peak systolic pressure, stroke volume, cardiac output, dP/dt, and mean ejection rate. Long-term survivors showed myocardial hypertrophy and increased wall thickness. Infarction was observed in many regions of the left ventricle.

Most of the spheres were found lodged in terminal arterioles; this resembles small-vessel disease with generalized failure. It is not clear whether a well-developed collateral circulation is of value in preventing the myocardial damage observed in small-vessel disease.

II. Large Spheres — Intra-Aortic

AGRESS et al. (1952) described a procedure for the controlled embolization of the coronary circulation in the closed-chest dog by injection of selective sized spheres. The most effective size to produce protracted shock was approximately 325 μm in diameter. JACOBEY et al. (1962) used the same basic procedure to produce a standardized coronary occlusion that could be used to study the therapy of coronary occlusion.

In the original study of AGRESS et al. (1952) four sizes of spheres (Dow Chemical) were used: 190, 325 and 450 μm obtained by screening through standard mesh sieves, and a fourth group ranging from 190 to 247 μm. The spheres were suspended in a 15% solution of acacia and injected rapidly with a screw-driven syringe.

A special catheter was introduced into the left carotid artery and advanced to the level of the coronary ostia. The catheter was constructed of stainless steel tubing and had a double lumen and sliding inner tube. An inflatable balloon was attached near the tip of the inner tube and the tip of the outer tube. The balloon could be stretched for passage through small vessels by sliding the inner tube or it could be inflated with saline through the outer tube. While advancing the catheter into the aorta to the level of the coronary ostia the balloon was stretched, but released once the catheter was in place. For sphere injection the balloon was inflated with saline until the peripheral pulse disappeared and the spheres were injected via the inner tube. A unit dose of 26 spheres/kg was injected until shock or death. Prior to injection the sphere suspension was shaken vigorously and the screw-driven syringe was attached to the inner tube of the catheter. The balloon was inflated prior to injection and for 15 sec after completion.

After anesthesia with morphine and pentobarbital the femoral artery was cannulated for recording blood pressure by a Statham transducer. Right atrial pressure was determined with a catheter passed down the left external jugular vein. The left internal carotid artery was used to pass the steel catheter into the aorta.

Various suspension media were studied; with 15% acacia 95% of the injected spheres entered the coronary circulation. Radioautographs of spheres labeled with ^{131}I show even distribution to the various chambers, with the greatest concentration in the epicardial region. However, the smaller the spheres, the greater the concentration in the endocardial region.

Agress et al. (1952) concluded that blood pressure alone is not an adequate criterion for cardiogenic shock. They adopted the following criteria: (1) blood pressure decrease of about 30%; (2) maintenance of fall for at least 30 min; (3) ECG evidence of severe ischemia; (4) absence of arrhythmias that could account for the fall in blood pressure.

Chronic studies with mixed-size spheres injected in a single dose of 3 to 4 mg/kg showed only one acute death among 8 animals treated; the others survived for 2 to 60 days, despite evidence of ischemia and infarction.

Acute studies with different sized spheres were carried out to evaluate the effect of the different sizes. Mixed-size spheres (190 to 247 μm) at doses ranging from 4 to 11 mg/kg in divided doses produced death, in all cases as a result of ventricular fibrillation. The 190 μm size produced death by ventricular fibrillation, cardiac arrest, or heart block. Spheres of 325 μm produced no immediate fibrillation and an average fall in blood pressure of 30%. Later deaths were by ventricular fibrillation. The large spheres of 450 μm in diameter caused immediate ventricular fibrillation in a few animals and only a 9% fall in blood pressure; none were considered to be in severe shock.

This procedure can produce cardiogenic shock. It did so most consistently with the 325 μm spheres. The authors concluded that the specific effect is correlated with occlusion of vessels of a specific size, but not with the number of spheres per gram of heart muscle.

Jacobey et al. (1962) used the same basic procedure with spheres ranging from 297 to 350 μm (average 324) in diameter. A dose of 4 to 10 mg/kg of spheres was given in three equal parts at 10-min intervals. They determined mortality rate, arterial pressure for 1 h or longer, ECG continuously for several hours and at intervals for one month (animals killed at that time), and serum lactic dehydrogenase. If animals survived for more than 4 h, postmortem coronary arteriograms were made with barium sulfate and gelatin.

There was a sigmoid dose–response curve for mortality; all animals survived the low dose of spheres and all died at the larger doses. The duration of survival was also related to the magnitude of the dose. Early deaths were due to ventricular fibrillation with about 60% preceded by primary shock. Serum lactic dehydrogenase showed a significant rise at $3^1/_2$ h, reached a peak 1 day after coronary occlusion, and returned to normal values in 3 days.

At autopsy, spheres were found in the secondary and tertiary coronary arterial branches. Animals surviving for longer than 12 h had infarcts in the left ventricular wall, interventricular septum, and right ventricle.

The authors concluded that therapeutic interventions to prevent death of the compromised myocardium must be made in the early stages of infarction. This could be accomplished by increasing blood flow to the ischemic region through utilization of collateral circulation and/or reducing the myocardial oxygen requirement. This assumes that there is a preexisting collateral network, not fully utilized prior to the occlusion. Such may be the case in the dog but it is questionable in man. Nonetheless, there is revived interest in reducing the size and severity of the infarct by use of nitrates and alpha adrenergics (see Section O). The latter studies are not based on diffuse myocardial occlusion of smaller vessels but rather on occlusion of a branch.

K. Acute Ligation

I. Two-Stage Ligation in the Anesthetized Dog

In 1950 Harris described the "two-stage" coronary ligation procedure in dogs, which has been used extensively for antiarrhythmic studies. The animals develop delayed ventricular ectopic rhythms, which can be suppressed by quinidine, procaine amide, etc. This "two-stage" ligation method was developed to avoid the early ventricular fibrillation frequently observed after an abrupt occlusion of a major coronary artery of the left ventricle. The incidence of ventricular fibrillation varies among laboratories and can range from as low as 0% to as high as 100% (see Schaper, 1971, for references). Much depends on the method of anesthesia, ventilation, location of occlusion, and other factors that are difficult to define.

The dogs were anesthetized with morphine (2 mg/kg) and barbital sodium necessary for surgery (180 mg/kg i.v.). In later studies pentothal and pentobarbital sodium were used, but there was no difference between the barbiturates on development of the ectopic rhythms. The chest was opened by midline incision and the anterior descending coronary artery was freed a few mm below the edge of the left atrial appendage. Preliminary experiments with acute ligation resulted in ventricular fibrillation within a few minutes.

Thus, the "two-stage" procedure was developed. A double ligature was passed beneath the freed coronary artery and the first ligature was tied around the artery and a 20-gauge needle along the side. The needle was immediately withdrawn allowing some flow in the anterior descending artery. Thirty minutes later the other ligature was tied so as to permanently occlude the artery without development of ventricular fibrillation. The procedure was modified so that the chest was opened in the fourth interspace, and the wound closed in layers after the ligations. The animals survived and developed multifocal ventricular ectopic rhythms by about 18 h, which usually persisted for 48 h.

The heart rate did not change for the first 4 h but then gradually increased with an increase in the frequency of ectopic beats until all were ectopic and ventricular in origin. The maximum frequency occurred during the first day and was as high as 250/min. At 48 h the rate had diminished to 160, but almost 100% of the beats were ectopic. This activity gradually subsided over the next several days. On autopsy the majority of animals demonstrated infarction in the area of occlusion.

II. Two-Stage Ligation in the Anesthetized Pig

There is a difference in the location of the collateral circulation of the dog and pig, and whether or not it can be functional under normal circumstances (SCHAPER, 1971). In the canine there are epicardial interconnections between arterial branches which can enlarge considerably; in the swine there is a subendocardial plexus which does not afford protection against abrupt cessation of blood flow in a major coronary branch. It was for these reasons that WINBURY et al. (1962) determined the effect of partial ligation on a subsequent total ligation in the pig.

Male "minipigs" from the Hormel Institute were anesthetized with pentothal sodium and administered a mixture of ether in oxygen under positive-pressure respiration through an endotracheal tube. After a left thoracotomy in the third or fourth interspace, the left anterior descending branch was dissected free at the origin and ligatures were placed under the artery. Partial ligation (18- to 20-gauge needle) or total ligation (in one stage or two stages) were performed after a stabilization period. In most "two-stage" procedures 30 min elapsed between the partial and total occlusion. In a few cases there was a 2-week interval between the partial occlusion and total occlusion.

The response of the pig was considerably different from that of the dog. In the first place, about one third fibrillated after partial occlusion and more than one half after a one-stage total occlusion. Almost all of these animals could be defibrillated electrically but about half later succumbed to heart failure. None of the survivors had an ectopic ventricular tachycardia similar to that seen in the dog. There was a high incidence of heart block following total occlusion, either one-stage or two-stage. In the majority of these animals sinus rhythm returned within 3 to 14 days. All of the animals with total occlusion had infarction with scar formation in the region normally served by the anterior descending branch.

III. Monkey, Unanesthetized

A method for induction of myocardial infarction in the unanesthetized monkey, *Macaca mulatta*, was described by HILL et al. (1972). General anesthesia was induced with 0.5 to 1.25% halothane vaporized with 40% nitrous oxide and 60% oxygen. A polyvinyl catheter was advanced to the aorta from the femoral artery for blood pressure. The thorax was opened in the midline under artificial respiration with the anesthetic mixture; a flow probe (Biotronex) was placed around the aorta, and a catheter placed in the left atrial appendage and secured with a purse string suture. A nylon ligature snare was placed around the left anterior descending coronary artery about 2 to 3 mm below the origin. A polyvinyl tube with a flared tip was passed through a stab incision in the sixth intercostal space and the ends of the snare brought out through the tube. The flared end was sutured to the pericardium and the tube filled with petroleum jelly to form an air seal. The aortic probe wires and atrial catheter were brought out through the chest and the thorax was closed. The animal was placed in a special suit to protect the leads and allowed to recover from surgery for several days.

During the experiment the monkey was placed in a restraining chair and ECG electrodes were sutured to the four limbs and to V_1, V_3 and V_5 positions. After recording the steady state, the snare was gradually tightened over a period of 1 to 2 min with continuous recording of ECG and blood pressure. The endpoint was the presence of an injury current in any of the precordial leads. At various intervals after occlusion the following were recorded: (1) 9-lead ECG, (2) aortic blood flow, (3) left atrial pressure, (4) aortic pressure, and (5) heart rate. Serious arrhythmias were treated by dc countershock.

Of the 26 "successful" monkeys, 11 died within $6^1/_2$ h from a syndrome resembling cardiogenic shock. The other 15 survived for more than 12 h and in many cases were killed 24 to 98 h after infarction.

The ECG showed immediate evidence of myocardial ischemia, especially in the precordial leads. At 30 min the Q waves appeared and a QS pattern, corresponding to infarction of the anterior and part of the lateral wall of the left ventricle, developed. Right bundle branch block was noted in a number of animals. PVC complexes were common after occlusion. Likewise, reversible ventricular fibrillation occurred in 18 animals.

This procedure is similar to that used in other species and causes similar hemodynamic and electrocardiographic changes. It would have some similarity to "sudden death" in man, which most frequently is caused by ventricular fibrillation.

L. Gradual or Controlled Occlusion

A number of procedures have been developed in recent years to produce a more gradual occlusion in order to compromise coronary flow more slowly. This is presumed to resemble the slow atherosclerotic process that occurs in man, finally leading to a critical decrease in flow and myocardial ischemia. Ameroids, developed by LITVAK et al. (1957) and VINEBERG et al. (1960), have been used extensively (see SCHAPER, 1971, for references) in the chronic preparation but the exact time of complete vessel closure is not known unless there is a flowmeter around the coronary artery, as described by ELLIOT et al. (1968). Furthermore, the process is irreversible.

Hydraulic or mercury occluders around the coronary artery can provide some degree of control and can be reversed. These also require flowmeters on the vessel to judge the degree of vessel occlusion (BOND et al., 1973; KHOURI et al., 1967; HOOD et al., 1970).

An intracoronary balloon technique was used by CORDAY et al. (1974) and MEERBAUM et al. (1974). The intracoronary balloon method is basically a variation of the hydraulic or mercury occluder placed around the vessel.

I. Ameroids

Ameroid is a product made of compressed casein, cured in formalin for hardening. It is hygroscopic and gradually swells as water is taken up. LITVAK et al. (1957) and VINEBERG et al. (1960) described the use of ameroid constrictors to produce gradual occlusion of a coronary artery.

The constrictors were made from round bars of ameroid 6 mm in diameter and about 5 mm in length. A 3 mm lumen was drilled through the center of the rod and a 0.5 mm wide longitudinal slot was cut to permit placement over the artery. In order to direct the swelling inward to reduce the inner lumen, a steel casing was slipped over the outside of the ameroid. *In vitro* studies showed that a dry ameroid constrictor placed in saline reduced the central lumen from 3 mm to 1.65 mm in 16 days, and to 1.57 mm in 26 days. Coating the ameroid constrictors with petroleum jelly reduced the rate of water absorption and swelling so that the central lumen was reduced to 1.98 mm in 32 days.

The ameroids were sterilized immediately prior to use by soaking in 1:1000 benzalkonium chloride for several hours. VINEBERG et al. (1960) and LITVAK et al. (1957) used similar procedures for placement of constrictors on the coronary arteries of dogs. After anesthesia and intubation the thorax was opened in the sixth intercostal space while the animal was maintained under artificial respiration. The pericardium was incised and the region where the constrictor was to be placed was infiltrated with a 1% solution of procaine hydrochloride. The anterior descending and/or circumflex branch was dissected free from the underlying tissue for a length of about 2 cm and all small branches were doubly ligated and cut. The vessel was raised by ligatures under each end and the ameroid with the steel jacket slipped on the vessel. The slotted opening was turned to face the operator so that traction would keep the vessel in place. In the original studies both branches of the left coronary artery were used. Other workers have used single or multiple branches in the dog or pig (see SCHAPER, 1971, for reference).

The major objection to this procedure is the inability to control the rate of occlusion. Unless a flowmeter is placed on the artery, as done by ELLIOT and co-workers (1968), the reduction in flow cannot be estimated. Nonetheless, the procedure is useful for the study of chronic occlusion and myocardial infarction.

II. Dicetyl Phosphate

Dicetyl phosphate placed on a gelatin sponge around an artery will cause development of granulation tissue and gradual closure of the lumen. ASADA et al. (1962) used such a procedure to produce gradual occlusion of the left anterior descending coronary artery of the dog.

Surgery was done under intravenous thiopental. Under artificial respiration the left chest wall was opened, the pericardium incised, and the proximal portion of the descending branch isolated. A gelatin sponge containing dicetyl phosphate was fixed in place on this portion of the vessel and the chest closed. Granulation tissue progressively developed around the sponge and encroached on the lumen. The lumen closed completely within 4 to 6 weeks and was maintained. The narrowing and closure of the vessel was confirmed by injecting a barium-agar mixture and cutting the heart open to lay the ventricles flat for X-rays.

Animals were subjected to progressive anoxia tests. The oxygen concentration of the inspired gas was progressively lowered until some electrocardiographic change appeared. At that point an arterial blood sample was taken for oxygen saturation. Normal dogs averaged 49% saturation and occlusion dogs 71%. This hypoxia test is similar to the LEVY test used clinically.

Animals treated with dipyridamole 1.2 to 1.5 mg/kg daily for 30 to 280 days could be reduced to 58% saturation, which is between the control and occlusion values.

III. Inflatable Balloon

GREGG'S group has used inflatable balloons around the coronary arteries for producing zero flow in order to calibrate the flow probe in unanesthetized animals (GREGG, 1972; PASYK et al., 1971; ELLIOT, 1973; ELLIOT et al., 1968; KHOURI et al., 1967 and KHOURI, 1973).

The zero cuff (balloon) is separated from the flow transducer by a strip of Ivalon sponge. On the other hand, BOND et al. (1973) have had problems with the balloon occluders and favor a snare for use in unanesthetized dogs.

KHOURI and GREGG (1967) described the procedure for construction of an occlusive cuff for determination of zero flow. Basically, the occluder is an inflatable elastic bag covered with a nonstretchable material on the outside. A circular stainless steel form with a 2.2 mm gap is used as the mold. There is a detachable stem to facilitate preparing the cuff. The form is first dipped in a coagulator solution of 25% calcium nitrate in ethanol, then immersed in latex solution for the appropriate time (about 15 sec) to give the desired thickness. The excess is shaken off and the latex cured under a heat lamp. The outer portion of the occluder is reinforced with a piece of fine nylon fabric cemented to the outside. The balloon occluder is dipped in latex a few more times to strengthen the walls.

After removal of the stem, the cuff is stripped from the form and cured by boiling for 1 h in a 5% solution of formaldehyde. A length of polyvinyl chloride tubing is cemented into the stem opening. This is used for inflation of the occluder. The cuff is tied around the outside of the vessel, a few mm distal to the flow probe. The end of the inflating tube is attached at skin level to a special stainless steel coupler through which the air is injected.

IV. Hydraulic Occluders

KHOURI et al. (1968) modified the zero occlusive cuff described in Section L.III above for gradual, controlled occlusion of a coronary artery. Likewise, HOOD et al. (1970) employed a hydraulic occluder to produce a gradual myocardial ischemia leading to infarction.

The technique of HOOD et al. (1970) involved gradual inflation of a Brunswick-Barger balloon cuff (Brunswick Mfg. Co., Quincy, Mass.) by a microinfusion pump. Surgery on the dogs was carried out under pentobarbital sodium anesthesia using a Harvard respiratory pump for artificial respiration. The left anterior descending coronary artery was dissected free and the occlusive balloon was fixed around the vessel about 1 cm from the origin. The Silastic tubing from the balloon was exteriorized posteriorly. The chest was closed and the animal permitted to recover for several weeks.

Gradual occlusion was produced by attaching the tubing from the balloon to a Sage model 172 microflow infusion pump. This produced a very slow inflation of the balloon cuff with fluid. The time to produce occlusion averaged about 1 h (range: 15 min to 2 h).

The onset of occlusion and ischemia was determined from continuous electrocardiographic monitoring. In several animals aortic, right atrial, pulmonary arterial, or left ventricular pressures were recorded from indwelling chronic catheters or catheters inserted under local anesthesia. The first signs of occlusion were T-wave and ST-segment changes as well as tachycardia. After a latent period of at least $3^1/_2$ h typical multifocal ventricular tachycardia appeared and persisted for about 2 days.

The hydraulic occluder of KHOURI et al. (1968) is made from the standard zero occlusive cuff but with a heavier latex wall. The outer wall of the cuff is enclosed in a tight-fitting silver capsule so that the expansion of the cuff is directed toward the blood vessel contained therein. The entire system is filled with mercury and the cuff is expanded by a micrometer piston. Temporary occlusion for determination of reactive hyperemia was produced with the zero occluder. For more prolonged gradual or stepwise partial occlusion the mercury occluder was used.

Normally, the flow transducer was placed around the artery close to the origin. This was followed by the pneumatic occlusive cuff and finally the adjustable hydraulic occluder was placed a few mm distal as described in Section H.III.

As the coronary artery was gradually constricted, reactive hyperemia after a 10 sec occlusion decreased. As the degree of constriction was increased to reduce resting coronary flow, reactive hyperemia disappeared, suggesting exhaustion of vasodilator reserve. Flow in the other major branch of the left coronary artery increased. The flow response to isoproterenol, nitroglycerin and dipyridamole was diminished in the vessel with partial occlusion (KHOURI et al., 1968).

V. Intracoronary Balloon

A closed-chest technique for reversible coronary occlusion by means of an intracoronary balloon was described by CORDAY et al. (1974) and the effect produced by such an occlusion by MEERBAUM et al. (1974). A double-lumen balloon catheter was selectively placed in a coronary artery and the vessel occluded by inflation of the balloon. The distal end of the catheter permitted blood sampling or administration of substances into the ischemic region.

Dogs were maintained under light anesthesia with morphine followed by pentobarbital sodium. Artificial respiration was instituted to provide adequate arterial oxygenation. The animal was heparinized for the duration of the study. A modified Fogarty or Swan-Ganz no. 4F catheter (Edwards Labs., Santa Ana, Calif.) was used for occlusion of a coronary artery and blood sampling and pressure determination distal to the occlusion. The catheter was placed in the left coronary artery under fluoroscopy through an angiographic cannula. The balloon was inflated with Hypaque to permit observation of the exact location and degree of distension. After complete occlusion there was a sharp drop in distal coronary pressure. The distal lumen was also used for estimation of retrograde blood flow, or the intracoronary electrogram was recorded by a platinum wire protruding beyond the lumen of the catheter.

A GANZ et al. (1971) coronary sinus catheter was used to measure sinus outflow by thermodilution (see Section G.I). Another double-lumen balloon catheter was advanced through the coronary sinus deep into the great cardiac vein close to the site of occlusion of the anterior descending artery. This was used to collect blood from the great cardiac vein; contamination with coronary sinus blood was prevented by inflation of the balloon in the sinus before collection was started.

Heart rate and rhythm were obtained from precordial leads. A transducer-tip catheter was advanced into the left ventricle for pressures and dP/dt. Cardiac output was determined by a thermodilution catheter. Total coronary sinus flow was determined with the cardiac vein balloon deflated but regional sinus flow (normally perfused) with the great cardiac vein balloon inflated.

Selective coronary occlusion was accomplished in 102 animals, of which 29 fibrillated within 30 min to 3 h. After occlusion there was a significant reduction in lactate extraction of the ischemic zone; often there was lactate production.

The distal coronary pressure on occlusion was about 43 mm Hg, a decrease of about 70% of the unoccluded value. Retrograde arterial blood has a high arterial saturation, as demonstrated by others (see Section H). The intracoronary electrocardiogram showed marked ST-segment elevation after occlusion.

The authors suggest that this method has many advantages over previously described procedures, because of the possibility of selective occlusion that can be reversed, and also permits local infusion of drugs. Actually the intracoronary balloon technique has limitations like those of other groups. In fact, the method developed by GREGG's group has many advantages in the long run.

Hemodynamic and metabolic data obtained with the intracoronary balloon method of occlusion were reported by MEERBAUM et al. (1974). On the basis of average values during 3 h of occlusion, there was a rise in left ventricular end-diastolic pressure and systemic vascular resistance and a decrease in left ventricular dP/dt, cardiac output, stroke work and coronary sinus blood flow. Metabolism differed in the ischemic and normal region. Lactate balance nearly became lactate production and a substantial loss of potassium occurred in the ischemic zone. The A-V O_2 difference increased slightly in both the normal and ischemic regions. The significance of the same increase in both regions is not clear.

M. Gradual or Acute Thrombosis

Of the various procedures for production of experimental myocardial infarction, the one that does tend to simulate the pathophysiology in man is a gradual narrowing of the coronary vessel as a result of thrombosis. Obviously, in man this is superimposed on a background of atherosclerosis and possibly platelet defects with the initial development of a "white" thrombus.

Different procedures have been used and we shall consider thrombosis produced by (1) a spiral in the coronary artery, (2) application of an electrical current to the endothelial lining of the artery, and (3) placement of a small magnet around the artery and injection of iron particles.

I. Spiral Coils

One of the first descriptions of a procedure for producing a thrombus in the coronary artery by a spiral wire coil in anesthetized dogs is that of Blair et al. (1964). The animals were anesthetized with pentobarbital sodium, intubated and put under positive-pressure respiration. The heart was approached through the fourth intercostal space and the pericardium opened over the proposed site of implantation in the left anterior descending artery. The region of the artery was cleared of perivascular fat, and the adventitia of the artery infiltrated with 1% procaine. A spiral made of 3 to 6 turns of aluminum-magnesium alloy (Aluminum Co. of America) and sharpened at the end was inserted into the artery by gradually turning the spiral to avoid damage to the vessel. The insertion was made in a retrograde fashion. Caution was taken to avoid the septal artery since blockade of this branch resulted in 100% mortality.

The thorax was closed and blood samples for SGOT, and 12-lead electrocardiograms were taken prior to surgery and daily thereafter until significant changes developed. A group of animals with a straight wire in the coronary artery was compared with the group having the coil.

All of the animals with the spiral wire implant developed a thrombus and infarct with 85% survival. Infarction occurred within 8 to 10 days. With a straight wire all developed a thrombus, but 20% did not infarct and only 65% survived. This group showed wide variation in the time of infarction: 2 to 12 days.

Electrocardiographic changes were typical of anterior infarction with ST-segment elevation in several leads. However, the electrocardiographic changes were not as reliable as the SGOT elevation for the onset and development of infarction.

The thrombosis resulting from the straight wire differed from that of the spiral. The straight-wire thrombus was loose and did not completely block the vessel lumen. The spiral thrombus adhered to the intima of the vessel and completely blocked the lumen.

The technique was modified by Kordenat et al. (1972) to permit placement of the thrombogenic coil into the coronary artery by a catheter without the necessity of opening the thorax. The coil was made of copper or magnesium alloy and the onset of infarction could be adjusted from 1 h to several days.

The coil was placed in the artery by means of a double-catheter system. An outer radiopaque (Formcath) catheter 30 cm in length had a preformed tip which enabled positioning at right angles to the plane of the coronary ostia. A vinyl inner catheter of approximately 50 cm could be advanced into the main left coronary artery and selectively directed into the descending, circumflex, or septal branch. The double-catheter assembly was passed down the left carotid artery into the aortic root and the selective catheterization performed with the inner catheter.

The copper or magnesium alloy wire (0.02 in. diameter) was formed into a coil of 2 to 6 turns around a 16-gauge needle. The two standard lengths of wire used varied from 4 to 6 mm and 8 to 12 mm.

The dogs were lightly sedated and the skin over the left carotid artery infiltrated with lidocaine to permit a cutdown. Prior to placement of the catheter assembly in the artery, the inner catheter was extended beyond the tip of the outer catheter and the wire coil placed approximately 2 to 3 mm from the end of the inner catheter.

After placement into the carotid artery, the catheter assembly was advanced into the aorta and the tip positioned at the left coronary ostium. The assembly was directed into the desired branch and the position verified by injection of a small amount of contrast media through the inner catheter. The tip of the outer catheter was held in position and the inner catheter gently pulled back, releasing the coil to float down the lumen of the selected vessel. The location of the coil was determined by the length and diameter. The position was considered "proximal" if the coil was 1 to 2 cm beyond the origin of the main branch and "distal" when the coil was at midpoint or beyond in the major vessel. Coils 4 to 6 mm in length lodged in the "distal" portion of the major left coronary arteries while coils of 8 to 12 mm remained in the "proximal" position.

Copper wire was more thrombogenic than magnesium. One to two loops of copper formed an obstructing thrombus 2 to 5 h after placement; with more loops there was complete thrombus in 1 h. Thrombus formation could be delayed by anticoagulants. Magnesium coils usually required 24 to 48 h before signs of infarction were noted. Thrombosis in the proximal portion of the vessel caused infarction in about 25% of the left ventricle while thrombosis in the distal sites caused infarction in about 10% of the ventricle.

II. Electric Induction of Thrombosis

SALAZAR (1961) reported a procedure for induction of coronary thrombosis in the intact dog by passage of an electric current through the coronary artery wall by means of an intraluminal electrode.

Dogs were lightly anesthetized and a coronary catheter was passed into either the anterior descending or circumflex coronary artery via the carotid artery. A Teflon-coated stainless steel electrode exposed for about 3 mm at the tip was advanced through the catheter under fluoroscopic guidance into the desired region of the artery. The intraluminal electrode was connected to the positive side of a circuit that was completed by a negative electrode on the chest. A direct current from a 3-V dry cell was the current source. The intensity was set from 100 to 900 μA by a 100,000-Ohm Helipot potentiometer. Current was maintained until there was electrocardiographic evidence of myocardial ischemia. The presence of an occlusion was confirmed by an arteriogram. Then the electrode and catheter were removed and the wounds closed. All hearts were studied at the time of spontaneous death or when animals were sacrificed at intervals between 8 h and 16 days after infarction.

Occlusion of a major coronary branch was induced after 18 to 93 min of current flow. Examination of the occluded vessel showed that the thrombus extended a short distance proximal to the electrode contact and a longer distance downstream, and often extended into side branches. There was intimal and subintimal injury at the point of electrode contact and the thrombus was firmly attached to the vessel wall. The tissue showed changes characteristic of myocardial infarction.

Unipolar electrograms with the intraluminal electrode as an epicardial lead showed marked ST-T changes long before changes were seen in the limb leads. This procedure was used by WEISSE et al. (1971, 1972) for comparison of anti-arrhythmic agents (1971) and study of the effect of nitrate infusions (1972). In these studies the method was modified to permit estimation of coronary blood flow by ^{85}Kr clearance. In addition, a comparison was made between infarction produced by thrombus formation and a wedged catheter.

Dogs were anesthetized with morphine and pentobarbital or pentobarbital alone, intubated, and placed in the right lateral decubitus position. A Harvard respirator was used for ventilation. Coronary occlusion was induced by thrombus formation in either branch of the left coronary artery. The catheter was advanced into the descending (1 cm) or circumflex (2 cm) branch via the carotid artery. The electrode wire was advanced 2 to 4 mm beyond the catheter tip and was attached to the positive terminal of a 6-V dry cell; the negative terminal went to the chest wall. A current of 300 to 800 μA produced thrombosis in 30 to 60 min in the descending artery and 45 to 90 min in the circumflex. Occlusion was demonstrated angiographically to be complete in two thirds of the dogs, and over 75% occluded in the remainder.

Abnormal rhythms occurred in most of the animals. Ventricular ectopic beats were observed within 5 to 10 min following ST-segment elevation. Ventricular tachycardia and fibrillation were seen within 4 h in untreated animals.

Procainamide (10 mg/kg per dose), lidocaine (3 mg/kg per dose) or diphenylhydantoin (5 mg/kg per dose) were evaluated after the appearance of ectopic beats (treatment) or after ST-segment elevation before ectopic beats (prophylaxis and treatment). The drug dosage was repeated in both groups until cessation of the arrhythmia or death of the animal.

Prophylactic administration showed no advantage over treatment only. Procainamide was superior to both lidocaine and diphenylhydantoin. However, there was a marked hypotensive effect. The 4-h survival rates for treatment only were: procainamide—80%, lidocaine—45% and diphenylhydantoin—56%.

Two methods were used for production of occlusion by WEISSE et al. (1972). Main branch obstruction of the left anterior descending artery was accomplished by thrombus formation with a somewhat modified catheter and a procedure that permitted injection beyond the site of thrombus formation. The electrode was proximal to the catheter tip. A slow saline infusion kept the opening patent for isotope injection to determine collateral flow. This procedure was compared with occlusion produced by wedging a catheter in a small coronary side branch. This is discussed in Section N. Suffice it to say that the wedging procedure produced a smaller area of infarction. The thrombus produced a more severe effect because of the larger area of the left ventricle involved, but in general there were similar hemodynamic effects after either form of occlusion. Therefore, the effects of these procedures will be discussed together below.

All dogs showed evidence of ischemia and infarction (ST-segment elevation and Q waves). In the few animals that developed ventricular arrhythmias procainamide was effective in restoring normal rhythm. Hemodynamic changes in both groups consisted of decreases in cardiac index, left ventricular work, dP/dt, and ejection fraction. Thrombus obstruction in addition produced decreases in heart rate and aortic pressure and increases in left ventricular end-diastolic pressure.

Infusion of isosorbide dinitrate to both groups with infarction decreased aortic pressure and left ventricular end-diastolic pressure. Coronary collateral flow was approximately 30 to 40% of the control value. After 30 min of isosorbide dinitrate infusion, the dogs with catheter wedging showed a slight but significant increase in collateral flow and a narrowing of the aorta—coronary sinus oxygen difference. The animals with thrombus occlusion did not respond with an increased collateral flow, although the oxygen difference did narrow.

These studies add to the confusion about the effect of nitrates on collateral flow and their role in myocardial infarction. No doubt there was a decreased oxygen requirement in both groups as a result of a decreased preload and afterload. However, coronary collateral flow increased only in the wedged-catheter group. Nonetheless, there may have been a more favorable redistribution of flow within the ischemic region.

III. Magnet and Iron Particles

A unique procedure for producing coronary thrombosis in the dog was to place a small magnet around the left anterior descending artery and to inject iron particles several days later. The iron particles picked up by the region with the magnet produced occlusion and subsequent myocardial infarction (ELZINGA et al., 1969).

The magnets placed around the vessel were machined from Alinco V cylindrical bars. The finished magnet was half a cylinder with an inner radius of 3.5 mm and a length of 7.11 mm. The bars were magnetized after machining and were sterilized in Germicide. The iron powder (General Aniline and Film Corp., Linden, N.J.) had a mean particle diameter of about 4 µm. The particles were autoclaved and suspended in saline at 1 g/10 ml. To place the magnet, animals were anesthetized, the chest was opened under artificial respiration and the artery isolated for 7 mm at the bifurcation. The magnet was placed over the artery and tied in place with sutures under the artery and over the magnet.

The magnet control animals or particle control animals showed no evidence of thrombosis or myocardial infarction. In dose-response studies it was found that 0.2 gm/kg of iron produced thrombosis and myocardial infarction in all dogs with magnets. Blood enzyme levels were elevated and all animals had severe arrhythmias with ST-segment elevation. Small doses of iron produced electrocardiographic changes but serum enzyme levels were normal.

N. Other Means of Occlusion

Various other procedures have been used to block the coronary arteries. These range from injecting large steel balls, mercury, steel or plastic cylinders, or rolls of lead foil into the coronary artery. Each procedure has a proponent, but it is obvious that no one method is a panacea since so many have been developed and used by only a few groups.

I. Mercury Injection into Coronary

Mercury has been injected directly into a major branch of the left coronary to produce embolization and a model of cardiogenic shock and/or "pump" failure (LLUCH et al., 1969; LUMICAO et al., 1971; CHANDRARATNA et al., 1973). The procedures were similar, yet there is no agreement among these three groups as to whether or not mercury embolization is an adequate model of cardiogenic shock. All groups do agree about progressive failure of the left ventricle as a pump and the inability to maintain an adequate cardiac output.

The dogs were lightly anesthetized during all or part of the procedure of placement of catheters and embolization. In one study some of the animals were kept under light anesthesia during the first 24 to 36 h of the study (CHANDRARATNA et al., 1973). The circumflex branch of the left coronary artery was embolized by all groups; in one study the anterior descending branch was also embolized in a few dogs.

The left main coronary artery was catheterized in the usual fashion under fluoroscopic guidance and then the catheter was advanced into the circumflex branch. Small amounts of contrast medium were injected to identify the branch and verify the position of the catheter. Mercury in a volume of 0.2 ml was flushed into the artery with a volume of 2 to 2.5 ml of normal saline and the catheter was withdrawn into the aorta for recording aortic pressure. In addition, cardiac output, pulmonary artery, right ventricular and left ventricular pressures were determined. Indocyanine green was injected into the right atrium or pulmonary artery for cardiac output; blood was drawn from the aorta through a recording densitometer and returned to the animal.

Within a few minutes after embolization there was evidence of myocardial ischemia (ST-segment elevation), ventricular arrhythmias and ventricular fibrillation. Hemodynamic alterations consisted of a rapid decrease in aortic pressure and cardiac output with a concomitant increase in heart rate and left ventricular end-diastolic pressure.

LUMICAO et al. (1971) determined ventricular function by constructing Starling curves before and after embolization. Heart rate was held constant by electrical pacing; left ventricular end-diastolic pressure was increased by infusions of dextran. The rise in stroke volume and stroke work with the rise in end-diastolic pressure was markedly depressed after mercury embolization. The depression of the ventricular function curves could be a result of a decreased functional myocardial mass, or decreased contractility, or both.

II. Steel Balls into Coronary

Occlusion of the circumflex branch of the left coronary was produced by injection of steel balls of 1.1 mm diameter through selective catheterization (RIBEI-LIMA, 1964). Dogs were anesthetized with pentobarbital and prepared for recording of atrial, ventricular, pulmonary, arterial, and aortic pressures as well as for determination of cardiac output by dye dilution. The coronary sinus was intubated for determination of coronary blood flow and levels of various metabolites. The left circumflex artery was catheterized with a No. 7 radiopaque catheter under fluoroscopic control and a control arteriogram obtained. The ball bearings were then injected into the intubated artery. Two doses were used, 2 to 3 balls/kg or 4 to 5/kg, and were washed in with 3 ml of saline. A second coronary arteriogram was obtained within 5 min of embolization and the catheter withdrawn into the aorta.

The hemodynamic changes produced by the occlusion were a fall in cardiac output, aortic pressure, and coronary blood flow. When the animals were sacrificed 3 to 5 days later, large infarcts were observed. However, these animals were not in heart failure since left ventricular end-diastolic pressure was not consistently elevated.

III. Lead Foil into Coronary

This is another variation of a "partial occlusive device" (POD) which can be placed into any of the three major coronary arteries by means of selective catheterization. The procedure produces a stenosis of the vessel rather than an occlusion and the ischemia is more gradual in onset and permits a higher survival rate than acute occlusion. This method has been used successfully in pigs with a mortality as low as 33% (JOHNSRUDE and GOODRICH, 1969).

The catheter assembly consisted of three components. An outer 190 polyethylene catheter (ID 1.2 mm and OD 1.7 mm) was preformed in hot water in accordance with the shape required to enter the selected coronary artery from the aorta. A French No. 3 radiopaque Teflon tube of 0.9 to 1.0 mm was threaded through the polyethylene catheter. Finally, a slightly longer thin steel wire of 0.4 mm OD was inserted into the Teflon tubing to temporarily remove the curve and permit insertion through the carotid artery. The POD was made from a small strip of lead foil 0.125 mm thick which was rolled into a tube having an ID of 0.9 to 1.0 mm. This was encased in heat-shrinkable plastic tubing and then threaded over the inner Teflon core at the distal end and held in place by gently heat-flaring the end of the Teflon tubing.

The catheter assembly was inserted into either carotid artery and advanced into the ascending aorta under fluoroscopic guidance. The inner steel wire was then removed and the catheter assembly with the POD attached resumed its original shape and was advanced into the target vessel. The position was verified by injection of contrast medium through the inner Teflon tube. The inner tube was then gradually withdrawn while the outer tube was held in place. This dislodged the POD. A second injection of contrast medium verified the location and patency of the POD. If the POD was made smaller in OD by omitting the plastic coating, it would go further down the artery and affect a smaller region.

IV. Steel Cylinder in Coronary

NAKHJAVAN et al. (1968) produced myocardial infarction in dogs by directing a stainless steel cylinder into the anterior descending or circumflex artery by a closed-chest technique. The procedure is somewhat similar to that described in the previous section, using a cylinder of lead foil.

The stainless steel cylinders were 4 mm in length, 3.25 mm OD diameter and 2 mm ID, and were smoothly tapered for ease of insertion. They were siliconized to inhibit fibrin and clot formation. Dogs were anesthetized with morphine i.m. followed by pentobarbital sodium i.v. The animals were heparinized and a No. $7^1/_2$ F radiopaque J-shaped polyethylene catheter was inserted into a coronary artery via the left carotid, and selective left coronary cineangiograms were obtained. A Teflon-coated guide wire was passed down the catheter and inserted into the circumflex or anterior descending branch of the left coronary. This served to place the steel cylinder in the selected branch. The catheter was removed after placement of the guide wire and the cylinder inserted over the guide wire. The outer catheter was then reinserted and used to push the cylinder to the desired position in the coronary branch. The catheter was then withdrawn and followed by removal of the guide wire. The heparin dosage of 1.5 mg/kg i.v. every 4 h was continued for 3 days after insertion of the cylinder. At night, concentrated heparin was given subcutaneously. Coronary cineangiograms were repeated periodically and electrocardiograms were recorded at frequent intervals.

This procedure does not produce an acute occlusion, and infarction follows a fairly uniform pattern. Electrocardiographic abnormalities appeared after 6 to 8 h and were controlled by procainamide. After this some of the animals developed signs of heart failure. The overall mortality rate was 50% but only a few died during the first 24 h; there were no immediate deaths due to arrhythmias. All of the animals showed evidence of myocardial infarction.

V. Catheter Tip in Coronary

HAMMER and PIŠA (1962) produced gradual occlusion of a main coronary artery in closed chest dogs with a Kifa catheter tip. The basic system was a catheter with a tip that could be separated and would remain behind in the coronary artery after selective catheterization. The tip of a Kifa catheter was narrowed, tapered and then severed from the main body of the catheter 5 to 8 mm from the end. A thinner catheter was threaded through the main catheter and tip and advanced into the descending or circumflex artery. The tip was separated by pulling the inner catheter back. Thus the coronary artery was closed off slowly by thrombotic closure of the lumen in the tip and in the vessel itself.

A modification of this procedure was described by COHEN and ELDH (1973) to permit immediate or delayed occlusion of a coronary artery in the dog. Anesthesia was induced by pentobarbital sodium (30 mg/kg) and after a control angiogram one of the two occlusion systems was introduced through the femoral artery.

For delayed occlusion, a 3 to 5 mm length of tapered Kifa tubing was passed into the selected artery by a coaxial catheter system. This had an outer preformed red Kifa catheter (United States Catheter and Instrument Corp., Glens Falls, N.Y.) of No. 6.6 F size, like that used for angiography, and an inner Teflon catheter (Becton Dickinson and Co., Rutherford, N.J.) with an OD of 0.039 in. The inner catheter extended beyond the tip of the Kifa catheter and carried the occluding tubing. After the dual catheter system had been manuevered into the desired coronary artery under fluoroscopy an infusion of intravenous lidocaine (1 mg/min) was started. To release the occluding plug, the inner tube was gradually withdrawn while keeping the outer catheter in position.

To produce immediate occlusion, a guide wire of 0.021 in. diameter was used instead of the inner catheter and the occluding plug was heat-sealed and impaled on the wire. Release of the plug was effected in the same way once the outer catheter was located in the proper artery. Again lidocaine infusion was started just prior to release of the occluder, and bolus doses of 50 mg were injected when runs of ventricular ectopic beats appeared.

Only a few of the animals died and all but one had well-developed collaterals based on repeat coronary angiograms. All of the animals with immediate occlusion (solid plug) had transmural infarction, but with the hollow plug 7 out of 8 had either no, or minimal infarction. Serial coronary angiography indicated that the hollow plug became occluded by thrombosis at about 4 h but there was no electrocardiographic change. Presumably the progressive occlusion promoted opening of already present collateral pathways, which prevented severe infarction.

VI. Wedging Catheter in Coronary

WEISSE et al. (1972) compared the effect of infusions of isosorbide dinitrate on infarction produced by thrombus formation (Section M.II) with infarction produced by catheter wedging in a small coronary side branch. The wedging method is described below.

The dogs were anesthetized in the usual manner with pentobarbital sodium. A Sones catheter with a single end hole was passed into the left anterior descending or circumflex branch under fluoroscopic control. The catheter was advanced into a small branch, producing ischemia in a relatively limited small region. After wedging, peripheral coronary pressure was recorded and collateral flow evaluated by washout curves of ^{85}Kr injected into the ischemic region via the wedged catheter.

The major difference in the response to isosorbide dinitrate of animals with myocardial infarction due to wedged-catheter occlusion compared with thrombus occlusion of the main branch is in collateral flow and resistance. The wedged group showed a significant increase in coronary collateral flow and a decrease in resistance after 30 min of nitrate infusion, whereas the thrombus group showed no significant change in collateral flow or resistance.

O. Surface Electrograms after Occlusion

In recent years there has been a revival of recording epicardial electrograms from normal and ischemic regions after various physiological and pharmacological interventions. The primary objective of the majority of the recent studies was to determine the area and severity of infarction by summation of ST-segment and T-wave changes following temporary or semi-chronic occlusion of a branch of the left coronary artery. The changes in the electrogram are assumed to reflect changes in regional perfusion and oxygenation; if the ischemia is maintained for too long a period, cell damage and loss of protein enzymes can occur.

In the past many investigators used surface electrograms to determine the limits and size of the ischemic zone, and whether or not collateral development had been sufficient to prevent subsequent signs of ischemia. In some of our unpublished studies in pigs we outlined the ischemic region after partial occlusion of the left anterior descending coronary artery. After 2 weeks recovery, the thorax was reopened but there was no evidence of myocardial ischemia. However, when the vessel was occluded completely, marked ST-segment elevation was again observed and the region of ischemia was as great as previously observed, indicating that the partial occlusion did not induce sufficient collateral growth to protect against subsequent total occlusion.

I. Electrograms in Open-Chest Dogs

MAROKO et al. (1971) described a procedure for determination of multiple surface electrograms on the anterior surface of the dog heart before and during temporary or semi-chronic occlusion of a branch of the left anterior descending coronary artery. BLEIFELD et al. (1973a, b, 1974) and WENDT et al. (1974) have done essentially the same with a somewhat different procedure for obtaining the electrogram from the epicardial surface. Moreover, WENDT et al. (1974) made transmural recordings at various depths in the free wall of the left ventricle.

In the studies of MAROKO et al. (1971) the heart was suspended in a pericardial cradle and a branch of the left anterior descending coronary artery periodically occluded. Arterial pressure, limb leads, and 10 to 14 surface epicardial leads were recorded. The electrograms were recorded at specific sites with particular landmarks by a hollow electrode 4 mm in diameter. In some cases a cotton wick soaked in saline was placed in the hollow portion of the electrode to reduce the contact pressure. The sites selected for recording were near bifurcations of arteries or veins so that the electrode could be easily repositioned at the same spot. Electrograms were recorded before occlusion and at 5, 10, 15 and 20 min after occlusion. In most cases blood flow was restored after this period and another test not performed until conditions had returned to normal. This usually required about 45 min.

The electrograms from the ischemic region showed ST-segment elevation. The degree of elevation is assumed to reflect the degree of ischemia, and the number of sites with ST-segment elevation reflects the area of ischemia. An elevation of 2 mV (2 mm) was considered a significant effect. The sum (Σ) of the ST-segment elevation serves as an index of the global myocardial ischemia. The average ST-segment elevation ($\overline{ST}$) was used for comparison of the effect of drugs and interventions. The correlation between ST-segment elevation at 15 min and CPK activity, histological changes, and glycogen content demonstrated early structural signs of necrosis, glycogen depletion, and decreased CPK activity 24 h later (MAROKO et al., 1971, 1972).

The mean ST-segment elevations were reproducible, indicating that $\overline{ST}$ could be used for comparative purposes. Isoproterenol infusion (0.25 to 0.50 μg/kg/min) increased the number of sites with ST-segment elevation, $\overline{ST}$, and ΣST when started before occlusion, or after it had been established. Tachycardia alone and hypotension alone had similar effects but to a lesser degree. Ouabain and glucagon increased the severity of ST-segment elevation. Propranolol and practolol (LIBBY et al., 1973) decreased the extent and severity of ischemia. Elevation of arterial pressure with methoxamine decreased $\overline{ST}$, ΣST, and the number of sites involved.

In a series of reports BLEIFELD and associates (1973a, b; 1974) described a method for recording epicardial electrograms with fixed electrodes and the effect of drugs on the response to occlusion. This type of procedure has the advantage of obtaining a continuous record at the same site. Nine gold electrodes 2 mm in diameter were placed 5 mm apart in openings on a thick (1 mm) rubber band 50×11 mm. This was sewn to the left ventricular surface in a region that included a branch of the left circumflex artery.

The electrogram from each electrode was unipolar with a central Wilson terminal, or bipolar according to Wahl. Occlusion for 20 min produced ST-segment elevation in the ischemic region. When occlusion was maintained for 3 h and isoproterenol was infused at the rate of 0.4 μg/kg/min, the degree of ST-segment elevation was increased. Dipyridamole, 0.12 mg/kg/min, had no influence on the ST-segment elevation of the ischemic region, even though coronary blood flow was markedly elevated in the normal region (BLEIFELD and IRNICH, 1973a). In a subsequent, more comprehensive study on dipyridamole BLEIFELD et al. (1974) confirmed the previous work. There was no significant change in the severity and extent of myocardial ischemia estimated by ΣST during infusion of 0.2 mg/kg/min dipyridamole.

Nitroglycerin was found to be without a protective effect against occlusion-induced ST-segment elevation, even when blood pressure was stabilized and heart rate controlled (BLEIFELD et al., 1973b). This is contrary to the results reported by SMITH et al. (1973) in closed-chest dogs. The experimental design of this study of BLEIFELD et al. (1973b) was similar to that previously described with epicardial electrograms recorded from 6 sites by gold electrodes set in a thick rubber band. One branch of the left anterior descending coronary artery was occluded for 20 min before and after nitroglycerin, with and without stabilization of blood pressure by a clamp on the aorta, and constant heart rate by pacing. Nitroglycerin (0.5 mg/kg) infused over 20 min did not significantly alter average ST-segment elevation, whether blood pressure decreased, or heart rate increased, or both values were controlled.

Transmural electrograms were investigated by WENDT et al. (1974). Surface electrograms were recorded from small beaded platinum electrodes in a 5 by 5 mm plastic plate sutured to the surface of the left ventricle in a region perfused by a small branch of the left anterior descending coronary artery; this was occluded periodically for 5-min periods. Transmural electrograms were recorded with stainless steel wires covered with Teflon, except for 1 to 2 mm at the end, inserted to an average depth of 10.2 mm. In a special study on ST-segment changes with ischemia at various depths in the left ventricular free wall, 6 Teflon-coated steel electrodes of various lengths were arranged concentrically around a surface electrode in a Plexiglass plate.

Considerable variability was observed in the epicardial ST-segment elevation during the first 5-min period of occlusion. A 30- to 45-min period was permitted between subsequent occlusions. The ΣST segment during the subsequent 5-min occlusion periods (usually 4) was less than the initial stage, but occlusions 2, 3, 4 and 5 were quite consistent and could be used for drug studies. The control ΣST-segment elevation in the subendocardium was higher than in the epicardial tracings. As with the epicardium, subendocardial ΣST elevation during the first occlusion was greater than during the 2, 3, 4 and 5th occlusions. In every animal the ΣST segment shifts were higher in the intramural than epicardial recordings.

Infusion of isoproterenol (0.25 and 1 μg/kg/min), started 5 min before occlusion and continued during the occlusion, markedly increased both epicardial and subendocardial occlusion responses. Furthermore, the increase in heart rate and decrease in blood pressure due to isoproterenol during the control period was accompanied by a significantly greater increase in the level of the intramyocardial injury current, suggesting subendocardial hypoxia in the absence of occlusion.

Norepinephrine was infused for 10 min at doses of 0.1 and 1.0 μg/kg/min. The lower dose tended to reduce the occlusion-induced ST-segment elevation, but the higher dose elevated the control ΣST-segment elevation (before occlusion) to a greater degree in the subendocardium and produced a greater occlusion response in both regions.

An increase in heart rate by pacing raised the occlusion-induced epicardial and subendocardial ST-segment elevation above the non-paced occlusion values. Beta adrenergic blockade by propranolol, 1 mg/kg i.v., significantly lowered the ST-segment elevations during occlusion, with a somewhat greater reduction in the epicardial recordings. When heart rate was returned to the pre-propranolol level by pacing, the occlusion ST-segment response returned to almost the same as the pre-propranolol level in the epicardial and intramural recordings.

Multiple-depth electrograms suggested variability in the degree of ST-segment displacement during occlusion. The author interprets these findings to indicate heterogeneity of intramyocardial ischemia during coronary artery occlusion. This may be related to regional differences in blood supply or the presence of functioning interarterial anastomosis.

In general, these studies have demonstrated the similarity of the epicardial and subendocardial response to occlusion and the changes produced in the occlusion response by the various interventions. Thus, the epicardial recording primarily reflects the subendocardial ischemia and can be used to evaluate the effect of various interventions on the response to ischemia.

II. Closed-Chest Conscious Dogs

Redwood et al. (1972) described a method for recording the degree and extent of ischemic injury in unanesthetized closed-chest dogs. The essential features of this procedure are similar to those described in the previous section, but it has the advantage of being a chronic, unanesthetized preparation.

The dogs were prepared for surgery by anesthesia with thiamylal sodium and maintained with halothane and oxygen. After the left thorax had been opened to expose the heart, the anterior descending artery was isolated between 2 and 3 cm from the origin. An inflatable silicone rubber balloon was tied around the artery and the inflation tube brought out onto the chest wall. The electrogram was recorded at multiple sites (12) with Teflon-insulated wires implanted at depths of 3 to 5 mm below the epicardial surface in the region of distribution of the left anterior descending coronary artery. The portion of wire implanted was free of insulation and kept in the myocardium by "hooking" the bare wire through the epicardium and holding the bare end in place by attachment of a small round lead "BB". (Lead shot approximately 2.5 mm in diameter.) The Teflon-coated lead wires were attached to a multi-outlet plug sutured to the chest wall. Pacing wires were attached to the left and right atrium; the pericardium was closed loosely and the thorax sutured after reduction of the pneumothorax.

The dogs were studied 5 to 7 days postoperatively under sedation with morphine and diazepam. The myocardial electrograms were recorded as unipolar leads with the limb leads as the indifferent electrodes. The sensitivity was set at 5 mV/cm. The results were the summated (Σ) ST-segment elevation, as done by others. Arterial pressure was recorded by an indwelling femoral artery catheter.

Rapid occlusion by the balloon was followed by the start of ST-segment elevation within 1 min; on release of the balloon the ST segment returned to control within 2 min following occlusion for 5 min. ST-segment elevation was greatest in the central ischemic zone and minimal on the periphery. There was good reproducibility of ΣST-segment elevation for 5 min or 15 min occlusion, even if there were several interventions between consecutive occlusions.

ΣST elevation after 5 min occlusion was correlated with heart rate. Thus, tachycardia enhanced the ST elevation if increased by pacing or by atropine. When heart rate was lowered by vagal stimulation, the same relationship obtained between change in heart rate and change in ST segment elevation.

Blood pressure was inversely related to the occlusion ΣST-segment elevation. At constant heart rate, occlusion during hypotension produced significantly greater increases in ST-segment elevation than at normotension.

In a subsequent study by the same group (Smith et al., 1973), the effects of nitroglycerin, hemorrhage, alpha adrenergic blocking agents, and alpha agonists on blood pressure, heart rate, and electrograms were determined in a similar preparation.

Nitroglycerin infusion, 200 to 400 μg/min, *reduced* the ΣST elevation due to 15 min occlusion, despite the hypotension and tachycardia. Production of the same degree of hypotension by phlebotomy caused an *increase* in ΣST elevation, not a decrease. Likewise, increasing heart rate by pacing *raised* the occlusion ΣST elevation.

When arterial pressure was increased by phenylephrine, the occlusion ΣST-segment elevation was less than that at normal blood pressure. Administration of nitroglycerin with methoxamine or phenylephrine resulted in a greater reduction in occlusion-induced ΣST than did nitroglycerin alone. The alpha agonists prevented the hypotension due to nitroglycerin and the reflex tachycardia. The improved pressure would lead to better perfusion of some portions of the ischemic zone and the reduction in heart rate would tend to reduce oxygen requirement. However, nitroglycerin has some other beneficial component—possibly decreased preload and diastolic wall stress, or redistribution of blood flow toward the subendocardium, particularly in the ischemic region.

P. Contractility of Ischemic Zone

Collateral function after catheter-tip occlusion was investigated by COHEN et al. (1973). Gradual occlusion of the anterior descending coronary artery was produced by the open Kifa catheter tip technique (Section N.V) several weeks before study of the effect of nitroglycerin on collateral function and contractile force of the ischemic region. Coronary angiograms taken a few days prior to the functional study demonstrated complete occlusion of the anterior descending artery at the level of the plug, but there was retrograde filling from other patent arteries.

The principle of the procedure was to lower perfusion pressure in the normal arteries until contractile force was significantly depressed in the ischemic zone but well maintained in the normal region. Intracoronary injection of nitroglycerin improved the contractile force of the ischemic region and decreased the pressure gradient between the normal artery and peripheral portion of the occluded artery, even though coronary perfusion pressure was constant. When both regions were ischemic due to a greater reduction in perfusion pressure and coronary flow, nitroglycerin had minimal effects on contractile force and the pressure gradient across the occlusion. This suggests that nitroglycerin improves collateral circulation and flow when there is a gradient between the region of the occluded vessels and the region with normal vessels.

For the study of collateral function the animals were anesthetized $2^1/_2$ to 4 weeks after occlusion. They were heparinized, ventilated with oxygen, and the left thorax opened. The main left coronary artery was cannulated with a double-lumen cannula. Blood from the aorta entered one shaft of the cannula through side holes and, after passing through an external loop, was returned to the left coronary artery through the other lumen. The external circuit contained an external flow probe, a pressure transducer for perfusion pressure from a side arm, a pump for perfusion, and a Starling resistance distal to the pump, which was connected to the femoral artery. The pump flow rate was maintained at a level such that flow was maintained through the extracorporeal circuit and back to the coronary artery, as well as through the Starling resistance. Perfusion pressure was varied by adjustment of the Starling resistance. The anterior descending coronary artery distal to occlusion was cannulated with a 20-gauge needle for measurement of retrograde pressure. Strain gauges for measurement of contractile force were attached to the normal and ischemic regions.

By lowering the coronary perfusion pressure gradually, it was possible to decrease the pressure gradient across the occlusion, and the contractile force of the ischemic region while maintaining the contractile force in the normal region. Intracoronary injection of 18 μg of nitroglycerin via the extracorporeal circuit increased coronary blood flow, retrograde pressure, and contractile force in the ischemic region to practically the control level, and decreased the pressure gradient across the occlusion. Contractile force in the normal region was not affected.

Likewise, nitroglycerin had no effect on contractility of either region when flow was not compromised.

If perfusion pressure was markedly lowered so that contractile force was compromised in both regions due to ischemia, nitroglycerin had no effect on contractile force in either region or on retrograde pressure of the occluded region. This represents "global" myocardial ischemia, where all collateral and resistance vessels are maximally dilated and nitroglycerin can produce no further effect.

This method has advantages over several others in that nitroglycerin was demonstrated to have a selective effect in the ischemic region, as would be expected in a region dependent on an auxiliary blood supply (collateral circulation). The ability to dilate the resistance vessels (arterioles) is of minor importance and with nitroglycerin is transient. However, the ability to dilate the collaterals and/or conducting or penetrating vessels is of importance in improving perfusion of an ischemic region.

Q. Partial Occlusion and Pacing in Dog

One of the more recently developed methods for diagnosis of anginal threshold in man and evaluation of various forms of therapy is the atrial pacing technique. This procedure permits the manipulation of one of the factors involved in coronary insufficiency and does not require whole-body exercise, with the multitude of factors which can influence the results. The heart rate is increased in steps until the patient develops pain and/or electrocardiographic signs of coronary insufficiency. Such a technique is suitable for use in animals and should be particularly valuable for evaluation of new therapeutic agents if the end-point is as sharp as in man. Atherosclerotic rabbits were paced by LEE and BAKY (1973) as described in Section I.I. The animals developed ST-segment changes when heart rate was accelerated. This change in the electrocardiogram could be prevented by nitroglycerin but not by dipyridamole. However, one of the problems with that procedure was that, if animals had been on the cholesterol diet for too long, nitrates did not prevent the ST-segment changes. In recent years it occurred to SZEKERES' group and our group that atrial pacing in dogs with a portion of the coronary bed critically compromised would be a useful and reproducible procedure for the evaluation of antianginal drugs. Obviously, the mechanism of the beneficial effect of these drugs would not involve a decrease in heart rate, as is the case with the beta adrenergic blockers. In this procedure the objective is to prevent coronary insufficiency brought on by an increase in myocardial oxygen requirement; it is not to determine the effects on myocardial ischemia and infarction due to cessation of blood flow to a region as in Section O.

The method of CSIK et al. (1973) and SZEKERES et al. (1975) is the same and involves a bypass of blood flow between the subclavian artery and the anterior descending artery. Flow to the coronary artery was gradually diminished just short of producing ST-segment elevation in epicardial leads from the area perfused. In our procedure (WINBURY and WILKES, unpubl.) a small clamp was placed around the distal portion of the anterior descending branch and the clamp was gradually tightened to the point where any further occlusion would cause epicardial electrogram changes.

Dogs were anesthetized with pentobarbital sodium and artificially respired through an endotracheal tube. The left thorax was opened in the 4th or 5th intercostal space and the left anterior descending coronary artery isolated in the central portion of the left ventricle. SZEKERES et al. (1975) and CZIK et al. (1973) ligated

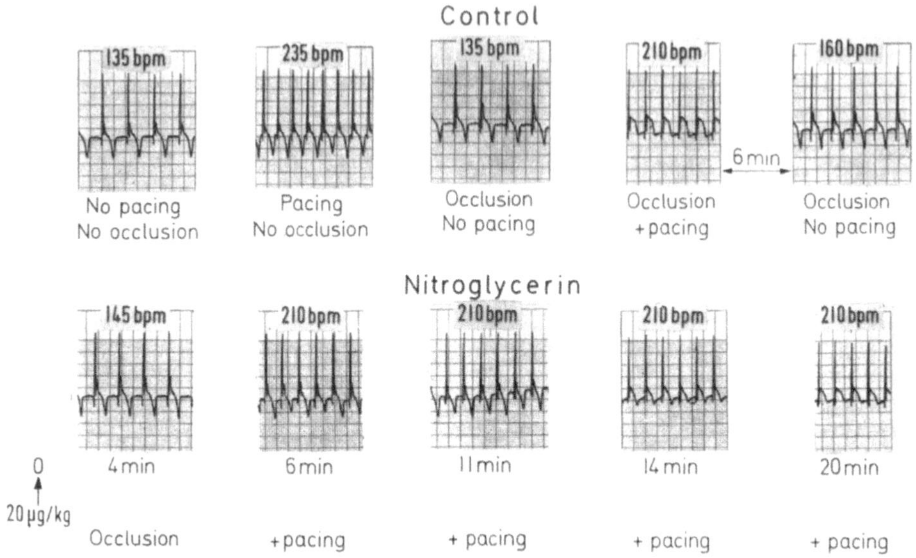

Fig. 10. Effect of nitroglycerin on pacing-induced ST-segment elevation in ischemic region. The left anterior descending coronary artery was partly occluded (upper row, occlusion; no pacing), but ST segment was not altered; pacing at 75 beats/min above control (occlusion + pacing) produced significant ST-segment elevation. Nitroglycerin prevented the pacing-induced ST-segment elevation for at least 11 min (lower row)

the vessel and cannulated the distal portion, which was then perfused from the right subclavian artery. Coronary blood flow was determined by a flow probe on the distal portion of the cannulated coronary artery. Our group used a similar procedure for a few experiments using the carotid artery for the blood supply.

Szekeres et al. (1975) used 3 silver electrodes in a rubber band, similar to the method of Bleifeld and Irnich (1973), sutured to the epicardial surface. We had two small electrodes embedded in a small piece of plastic sutured to the epicardium in the central portion of the region supplied by the compromised vessels.

After a stabilization period coronary blood flow was reduced by gradual constriction until there was minimal change in the ST segment. The degree of occlusion was such that an increase of 50 to 100 beats/min would produce marked ST-segment elevation during a 5-min pacing period. We found that pacing could be repeated at 15- to 30-min intervals with reproducible results. However, after nitroglycerin the intervals between consecutive pacing periods were shorter and pacing was continued for only 2 min, since earlier studies showed that the ST segment usually reached its peak by that time.

An example of a study is given in Fig. 10. Occlusion or pacing alone produced no ST-segment change. After occlusion, increasing heart rate from 135 to 210 beats/min (upper section, panels 3 and 4) produced the ST-segment elevation typical of coronary insufficiency in the dog. Nitroglycerin, 20 µg/kg, was administered over a 1-min period. This produced a slight decline in blood pressure and increase in heart rate. Pacing at the same rate that had previously produced the marked ST-segment change caused no change at 6 and 11 min after nitroglycerin. By 14 min, pacing-induced ST-segment elevation again started and was back to the predrug value by 20 min. The duration of protection varied from 20 to 60 min in our hands.

SZEKERES et al. (1975) administered nitroglycerin at the rate of 2 μg/kg/min over 10 min. Under these circumstances they found protection against the electrocardiographic changes for as long as 90 min. Nitroglycerin also protected against T-wave elevation. Dipyridamole at 6 μg/kg/min for 10 min did not provide any protection against the ST-segment or T-wave changes during pacing.

One of the problems that may be encountered with this procedure in dogs is the presence of an extensive interarterial anastomatic circulation. This could prevent the production of coronary insufficiency, even when the branch of the anterior descending is completely occluded. When we encountered this, it was necessary to use another region of the left ventricle in order to produce pacing-induced ST-segment elevation. It would be of interest to carry out such studies in pigs because the collateral circulation is normally sparse in that species.

SZEKERES et al. (1975) also determined changes in hemodynamic and metabolic parameters during pacing and drug interventions. During pacing, increases were noted in left ventricular end diastolic pressure, dP/dt, PRI (HR × MAP). However, the values were still within the normal range. Stroke volume and left ventricular work were diminished. The coronary hemodynamics and metabolism in the region perfused by the constricted artery were not markedly affected during pacing.

Both nitroglycerin and dipyridamole reduced basal left ventricular work in the non-paced heart. During pacing, animals treated with nitroglycerin showed an increase in left ventricular end-diastolic pressure and work, whereas dipyridamole treatment caused reductions in those parameters as well as dP/dt during pacing.

The drugs had different effects on the coronary circulation and myocardial metabolism. Nitroglycerin increased coronary flow in the compromised region and elevated oxygen consumption at normal heart rate and during pacing. Dipyridamole had no significant effect on coronary flow or oxygen consumption during the basal or paced heart rate. One of the most significant effects of nitroglycerin on the region perfused by the constricted vessels was on lactate uptake. Nitroglycerin increased lactate uptake in the normal heart and reduced the pacing-induced diminution of myocardial lactate uptake. Dipyridamole exerted no such protective effect.

The combination of myocardial metabolism and ST-segment changes has many advantages and can be of great value in explaining the mechanism of action. Even without the coronary hemodynamic and metabolic studies, this procedure has much to offer as a model of coronary insufficiency or angina pectoris, and for the screening of new therapeutic agents.

R. Summary and Conclusions

A number of procedures for the production of experimental coronary disease in animals have been described, but few if any of these are adequate models of coronary heart disease in man. Some of the procedures depend upon slow occlusion of a major coronary branch whereas others depend on rapid occlusion. These methods usually produce ischemia and/or infarction of a specific region of the heart and may cause failure of the myocardium as a pump, cardiogenic shock, ventricular fibrillation, ventricular tachycardia, or no marked decrease in myocardial function.

A number of procedures produce diffuse blockade of small vessels with particulate matter, such as starch suspensions, lycopodium spores, or microspheres. The diffuse ischemia is not typical of coronary disease in man, nor is the functional impairment that results in the animal.

Some of the more recent methods that may hold promise as "models" are those that determine the function of the ischemic zone after adequate time for collateral development. Myocardial function of the ischemic zone is based on contractile force, which was improved by nitroglycerin. Another useful model depends on local ST-segment changes produced by atrial pacing; the region that showed the ST change was partially ischemic. Nitroglycerin prevented or attenuated the local electrocardiographic change.

Methods for evaluation of antianginal drugs are also considered in relation to the action of organic nitrates and beta adrenergic blockers. Both agents are postulated to act by similar mechanisms namely, reduction in the oxygen requirement of the heart and favorable redistribution of blood flow to maintain perfusion of the subendocardium and provide a better balance between oxygen supply and demand in that region.

The subendocardium is relatively hypoxic compared with the subepicardium, even though perfusion throughout the left ventricular wall is homogeneous and open capillary density is greater in the subendocardium. Nitroglycerin and beta adrenergic blocking drugs alter the left ventricular transmural gradients by a selective increase in subendocardial oxygen tension with no change in local perfusion, but a decrease in subepicardial perfusion with no change in oxygen tension. Oxygen requirement is presumed to decrease to a greater extent in the subendocardium.

Intramyocardial oxygen tension was measured polarographically with small electrodes in the specific regions or by mass spectrometry with small cannulas in the subepicardium and subendocardium. Similar changes were observed with either method. Local tissue perfusion was determined by similar procedures using washout of a foreign gas (hydrogen or argon).

References

AGRESS, C. M., ROSENBERG, M. J., JACOBS, H. I., BINDER, M. J., SCHNEIDERMAN, A., CLARK, W. J.: Protracted shock in the closed-chest dog following coronary embolization with graded microspheres. Amer. J. Physiol. **170**, 536–549 (1952).

ARMOUR, J. A., RANDALL, W. C.: Canine left ventricular intramyocardial pressures. Amer. J. Physiol. **220**, 1833–1839 (1971).

ASADA, S., CHIBA, T., OSAWA, K., NAKAMURA, K., MURAKAWA, S.: Experimental studies of the effect of long-term oral administration of persantin. Jap. Circ. J. **26**, 849–855 (1962).

AUKLAND, K., BOWER, B. F., BERLINER, R. W.: Measurement of local blood flow with hydrogen gas. Circ. Res. **14**, 164–187 (1964).

AUKLAND, K., KIIL, F., KJEKSHUS, J., SEMB, G.: Local myocardial blood flow measured by hydrogen polarography; distribution and effect of hypoxia. Acta physiol. scand. **70**, 99–111 (1967).

BAROLDI, G.: Viewpoint of a human pathologist on the current coronary problem. In: Current Topics in Coronary Research (eds. C. M. BLOOR, R. A. OLSSON), p. 141–149. Advances exp. Med. Biol. Vol. 39. New York: Plenum Press 1973.

BECKER, L. C., FERREIRA, R., THOMAS, M.: Mapping of left ventricular blood flow with radioactive microspheres in experimental coronary artery occlusion. Cardiovasc. Res. **7**, 391–400 (1973).

BECKER, L. C., FORTUIN, N. J., PITT, B.: Effect of ischemia and antianginal drugs on the distribution of radioactive microspheres in the canine left ventricle. Circ. Res. **28**, 263–269 (1971).

BECKER, L., PITT, B.: Regional myocardial blood flow, ischemia and antianginal drugs. Ann. clin. Res. **3**, 353–361 (1971a).

BECKER, L. C., PITT, B.: Collateral blood flow in conscious dogs with chronic coronary artery occlusion. Amer. J. Physiol. **221**, 1507–1510 (1971b).

BERNE, R. M.: Regulation of coronary blood flow. Physiol. Rev. **44**, 1–29 (1964).

BLAIR, E., NYGREN, E., COWLEY, R. A.: A spiral wire technique for producing gradually occlusive coronary thrombosis. J. thorac. cardiovasc. Surg. **48**, 476–485 (1964).

BLEIFELD, W., IRNICH, W.: Methode zur epikardialen EKG-Registrierung. Z. Kardiol. **5**, 424–432 (1973).

BLEIFELD, W., WENDE, W., BUSSMANN, W. D., MEYER, J.: Influence of nitroglycerin on the size of experimental myocardial infarction. Naunyn-Schmiedeberg's Arch. Pharmacol. **277**, 387–400 (1973).

BLEIFELD, W., WENDE, W., MEYER, J., BUSSMANN, W. D.: Einfluß einer Vasodilatation durch Dipyridamol auf die Größe des akuten experimentellen Herzinfarktes. Z. Kardiol. **63**, 115–128 (1974).

BOND, R. F., MANNING, E. S., GONZALEZ, R. R., JR.: Methods for chronically implanting coronary artery blood flow probes, arterial occluders and coronary sinus catheters. In: Chronically Implanted Cardiovascular Instrumentation (ed. E. P. MCCUTCHEON), p. 281–288. New York: Academic Press 1973.

BUCKBERG, G. D., FIXLER, D. E., ARCHIE, J. P., HOFFMAN, J. I. E.: Experimental subendocardial ischemia in dogs with normal coronary arteries. Circulat. Res. **30**, 67–81 (1972).

CORDAY, E., LANG, T.-W., MEERBAUM, S., GOLD, H., HIROSE, S., RUBINS, S., DALMASTRO, M.: Closed chest model of intracoronary occlusion for study of regional cardiac function. Amer. J. Cardiol. **33**, 49–59 (1974).

DOMENECH, R. J., HOFFMAN, J. I. E., NOBLE, M. I. M., SAUNDERS, K. B., HENSON, J. R., SUBIJANTO, S.: Total and regional coronary blood flow measured by radioactive microspheres in conscious and anesthetized dogs. Circulat. Res. **25**, 581–596 (1969).

ELIOT, R. S., BRATT, G.: The paradox of myocardial ischemia and necrosis in young women with normal coronary arteriograms. Relation to abnormal hemoglobin–oxygen dissociation. Amer. J. Cardiol. **23**, 633–638 (1969).

ELLIOT, E. C.: Hemodynamic evidence of the development of coronary collateral circulation in conscious dogs. In: Current Topics in Coronary Research (eds. C. M. BLOOR, R. A. OLSSON), p. 173–190. Adv. Exp. Med. Biol. Vol. 39. New York: Plenum Press 1973.

ELLIOT, E. C., JONES, E. L., BLOOR, C. M., LEON, A. S., GREGG, D. E.: Day-to-day changes in coronary hemodynamics secondary to constriction of circumflex branch of left coronary artery in conscious dogs. Circulat. Res. **22**, 237–250 (1968).

ELZINGA, W., KAUFMAN, W., UPRIGHT, D., POWELL, D.: A new animal model myocardial infarction. In: Artificial Heart Program Conference Proceedings (ed. R. HEGYELI), p. 689–699. U.S. Dept. Health, Education and Welfare. Bethesda, Md.: Natl. Heart and Lung Inst. 1969.

ESTES, E. H., ENTMAN, M. L., DIXON, H. B., II, HACKEL, D. B.: The vascular supply of the left ventricular wall. Amer. Heart J. **71**, 58–67 (1966).

FORTUIN, N. J., KAIHARA, S., BECKER, L. C., PITT, B.: Regional myocardial blood flow in the dog studied with radioactive microspheres. Cardiovasc. Res. **5**, 331–336 (1971).

FRONEK, A.: Thermodilution in chronic experimentation. In: Chronically Implanted Cardiovascular Instrumentation (ed. E. P. MCCUTCHEON), p. 77–86. New York: Academic Press 1973.

FULTON, W. F. M.: The Coronary Arteries. Springfield, Illinois: Charles C. Thomas 1965.

FURUSE, A., BRAWLEY, R. K., GOTT, V. L.: Effects of isoproterenol, L-norepinephrine, and glucagon on myocardial gas tensions in animals with coronary stenosis. J. thorac. cardiovasc. Surg. **65**, 815–824 (1973).

GANZ, W., MARCUS, H. S.: Failure of intracoronary nitroglycerin to alleviate pacing-induced angina. Circulation **46**, 880–889 (1972).

GANZ, W., TAMURA, K., MARCUS, H. S., DONOSO, R., YOSHIDA, S., SWAN, H. J. C.: Measurement of coronary sinus blood flow by continuous thermodilution in man. Circulation **44**, 181–195 (1971).

GELLAI, M., NORTON, J. M., DETAR, R.: Evidence for direct control of coronary vascular tone by oxygen. Circulat. Res. **32**, 279–289 (1973).

GENSINI, G. G., KELLY, A. E., DA COSTA, B. C. B., HUNTINGTON, P. P.: Quantitative angiography: The measurement of coronary vasomobility in the intact animal and man. Chest **60**, 522–530 (1971).

GRAYSON, J.: Internal calorimetry in the determination of thermal conductivity and blood flow. J. Physiol. **118**, 54–72 (1952).

GRAYSON, J., HAIGH, A. L.: Internal Calorimetry — An Automatic Recorder. J. Physiol. **124**, 49P–51P (1954).

GRAYSON, J., IRVINE, M., PARRATT, J. R.: Effect of carbochromen and dipyridamole on blood flow and heat production in the normal and ischaemic canine myocardium. Cardiovasc. Res. **5**, 41–47 (1971).

GRAYSON, J., PARRATT, J. R.: A species comparison of the effects of changing perfusion pressure on blood flow and metabolic heat production in the myocardium. J. Physiol. **187**, 465–488 (1966).

GRAYSON, J., ROBERTSON, M., SCOTT, C.: Heat clearance and heat production studies in acute experimental coronary occlusion. Cardiovasc. Res. **7**, 220–225 (1973).

GREGG, D. E.: Coronary vasodilator effects of nitroglycerin during coronary insuffiency. In: The Study of the Systemic, Coronary and Myocardial Effects of Nitrates (ed. G. G. GENSINI), p. 292–296. Springfield, Ill.: Charles C. Thomas 1972.

GROSS, G. J., WINBURY, M. M.: Beta adrenergic blockade on intramyocardial distribution of coronary blood flow. J. Pharmacol. exp. Ther. **187**, 451–464 (1973).

GUY, C., ELIOT, R. S.: The subendocardium of the left ventricle: A physiologic enigma. Chest **58**, 555–556 (1970).

GUY, C. R., ELIOT, R. S.: The pathophysiologic vulnerability of the subendocardium of the left ventricle. In: Myocardial Infarction: A New Look at an Old Subject (ed. J. H. K. VOGEL), p. 42–52. Advances in Cardiol. Vol. 9. Basel: S. Karger 1973.

GUZMAN, S. V., SWENSON, E., MITCHELL, R.: Mechanism of cardiogenic shock. Circ. Res. **10**, 746–752 (1962).

HAMMER, J., PISA, Z.: A method of isolated, gradual occlusion of a main branch of a coronary artery in closed-chest dogs. Amer. Heart J. **64**, 67–70 (1962).

HARRIS, A. S.: Delayed development of ventricular ectopic rhythms following experimental coronary occlusion. Circulation **1**, 1318–1328 (1950).

HELLSTROM, H. R.: Vasospasm in ischemic heart disease — A hypothesis. Perspect. Biol. Med. **16**, 427–440 (1973).

HILL, J. D., MALINOW, M. R., MCNULTY, W. P., OCHSNER, A. J., III: Experimental myocardial infarction in unanesthetized monkeys. Amer. Heart J. **84**, 82–94 (1972).

HONIG, C. R., KIRK, E. S., MYERS, W. W.: Transmural distributions of blood flow, oxygen tension and metabolism in myocardium. Mechanisms and adaptation. In: Coronary Circulation and Energetics of the Myocardium (ed. G. MARCHETTI, B. TACCARDI), p. 31–46. Basel: S. Karger 1967.

HOOD, W. B., JR.: Pathophysiology of ischemic heart disease. Progr. cardiovasc. Dis. **14**, 297–320 (1971).

HOOD, W. B., JOISON, J., KUMAR, R., KATAYAMA, I., NEIMAN, R. S., NORMAN, J. C.: Experimental myocardial infarction. I. Production of left ventricular failure by gradual coronary occlusion in intact conscious dogs. Cardiovasc. Res. **4**, 73–83 (1970).

HORT, W.: Capillarization of the myocardium under normal and pathological conditions. In: Oxygen Transport in Blood and Tissues (eds. D. W. LÜBBERS, U. C. LUFT, G. THEWS, E. WITZLEB), p. 150–158. Stuttgart: Thieme 1968.

HOWE, B. B., WINBURY, M. M.: Effect of pentrinitrol, nitroglycerin and propranolol on small vessel blood content of the canine myocardium. J. Pharmacol. exp. Ther. **187**, 465–474 (1973).

JACOBEY, J. A., TAYLOR, W. J., SMITH, G. T., GORLIN, R., HARKEN, D. E.: A new therapeutic approach to acute coronary occlusion. I. Production of standardized coronary occlusion with microspheres. Amer. J. Cardiol. **9**, 60–73 (1962).

JOHNSRUDE, I. S., GOODRICH, J. K.: An experimental partial occlusive device for vessels delivered by arterial catheter. Amer. Heart J. **77**, 805–808 (1969).

KADATZ, R.: Sauerstoffdruck und Durchblutung im gesunden und koronarinsuffizienten Myokard des Hundes und ihre Beeinflussung durch koronarerweiternde Pharmaka. Arch. Kreisl. Forsch. **58**, 263–293 (1969).

KADATZ, R.: Agents acting on coronary blood vessels. In: Screening Methods in Pharmacology (ed. R. A. TURNER, P. HEBBORN). Vol. 2, p. 41–60. New York: Academic Press 1971.

KATTUŞ, A. A., GREGG, D. E.: Some determinants of coronary collateral blood flow in the open-chest dog. Circulat. Res. **7**, 628–642 (1959).

KETY, S. S.: Determinants of tissue oxygen tension. Fed. Proc. **16**, 666–670 (1957).

KETY, S. S.: Theory of blood-tissue exchange and its application to measurement of blood flow. In: Methods in Medical Research (ed. H. D. BRUNNER). Vol. 8, p. 223–227. Chicago, Ill.: Year Book Publishers 1960.

KHOURI, E. M.: Implantation of flow transducers on the left coronary artery and central aorta. In: Chronically Implanted Cardiovascular Instrumentation (ed. E. P. MCCUTCHEON), p. 257–262. New York: Academic Press 1973.

KHOURI, E. M., GREGG, D. E.: An inflatable cuff for zero determination in blood flow studies. J. appl. Physiol. **23**, 395–397 (1967).

KHOURI, E. M., GREGG, D. E., LOWENSOHN, H. S.: Experimental coronary insufficiency. In: Coronary Circulation and Energetics of the Myocardium (ed. G. MARCHETTI, B. TACCARDI), p. 250–258. Basel: S. Karger 1967.

KHOURI, E. M., GREGG, D. E., LOWENSHON, H. S.: Flow in the major branches of the left coronary artery during experimental coronary insufficiency in the unanesthetized dog. Circulat. Res. **23**, 99–109 (1968).

KHOURI, E. M., GREGG, D. E., McGRANAHAN, G. M., JR.: Regression and reappearance of coronary collaterals. Amer. J. Physiol. **220**, 655–661 (1971).
KIRK, E. S., HONIG, C. R.: Nonuniform distribution of blood flow and gradients of oxygen tension within the heart. Amer. J. Physiol. **207**, 661–668 (1964).
KORDENAT, R. K., KEZDI, P., STANLEY, E. L.: A new catheter technique for producing experimental coronary thrombosis and selective coronary visualization. Amer. Heart J. **83**, 360–364 (1972).
KOYAMA, T., MARUTANI, Y.: A hydrogen catheter electrode for the determination of blood flow through organ tissue and coronary blood flow under continuous hypoxia. Jap. J. Physiol. **21**, 209–228 (1971).
KROGH, A.: Anatomy and Physiology of Capillaries. New Haven: Yale University Press **1936**.
LEDINGHAM, I. McA., MARSHALL, R. J., PARRATT, J. R.: Drug-induced changes in blood flow in normal and ischaemic regions of the canine myocardium. Brit. J. Pharmacol. **47**, 626–627 P (1973).
LEE, R. J., BAKY, S. H.: The influence of nitroglycerin and dipyridamole on pacing-induced ST segment depression in unanesthetized, atherosclerotic rabbits. J. Pharmacol. exp. Ther. **184**, 205–212 (1973).
LIBBY, P., MAROKO, P. R., COVELL, J. W., MALLOCH, C. I., ROSS, J., BRAUNWALD, E.: Effect of practolol on the extent of myocardial ischemic injury after experimental coronary occlusion and its effect on ventricular function in the normal and ischemic heart. Cardiovasc. Res. **7**, 167–173 (1973).
LITVAK, J., LAMBROS, E. S., VINEBERG, A. M.: The experimental production of coronary artery insufficiency and occlusion. Amer. Heart J. **53**, 505–518 (1957).
LLUCH, S., MOGUILEVSKY, H. C., PIETRA, G., SHAFFER, A. B., HIRSCH, L. J., FISHMAN, A. P.: A reproducible model of cardiogenic shock in the dog. Circulation **39**, 205–218 (1969).
LOISANCE, D. Y., OWENS, G.: A new device for recording pO_2, pCO_2, and blood flow in focal areas of the myocardium. Amer. J. Surg. **125**, 496–500 (1973).
LOISANCE, D., OWENS, G.: Etude pharmacologique par spectrométrie de masse de la perfusion myocardiaque. 1. Effets de la nitroglycérine. Coeur Méd. inter. **13**, 125–131 (1974).
LUMICAO, B. G., RUSSELL, R. O., RACKLEY, C. E.: Left ventricular performance in dogs with selective coronary embolization with mercury. Amer. J. med. Sci. **261**, 27–39 (1971).
MAROKO, P. R., KJEKSHUS, J. K., SOBEL, B. E., WATANABE, T., COVELL, J. W., ROSS, J., JR., BRAUNWALD, E.: Factors influencing infarct size following experimental coronary artery occlusions. Circulation **43**, 67–82 (1971).
MAROKO, P. R., LIBBY, P., BLOOR, C. M., SOBEL, B. E., BRAUNWALD, E.: Reduction by hyaluronidase of myocardial necrosis following coronary artery occlusion. Circulation **46**, 430–437 (1972).
MARSHALL, R. J., PARRATT, J. R.: The effect of noradrenaline on blood flow and oxygen consumption in normal and ischemic areas of myocardium. Amer. Heart J. **86**, 653–662 (1973a).
MARSHALL, R. J., PARRATT, J. R.: The effects of dipyridamole on blood flow and oxygen handling in the acutely ischemic and normal canine myocardium. Brit. J. Pharmacol. **49**, 391–399 (1973b).
MEERBAUM, S., LANG, T.-W., CORDAY, E., RUBINS, S., HIROSE, S., COSTANTINI, C., GOLD, H., DALMASTRO, M.: Progressive alterations of cardiac hemodynamic and regional metabolic function after acute coronary occlusion. Amer. J. Cardiol. **33**, 60–68 (1974).
MOIR, T. W.: Subendocardial distribution of coronary blood flow and the effect of antianginal drugs. Circulat. Res. **30**, 621–627 (1972).
MOSS, A. J.: Intramyocardial oxygen tension. Cardiovasc. Res. **3**, 314–318 (1968).
MOSS, A. J.: Oxygenation of the heart. Hosp. Pract. **6**, 104–111 (1971).
MYERS, W. W., HONIG, C. R.: Number and distribution of capillaries as determinants of myocardial oxygen tension. Amer. J. Physiol. **207**, 653–660 (1964).
NAKHJAVAN, F. K., SHEDROVILZKY, H., GOLDBERG, H.: Experimental myocardial infarction in dogs. Description of a closed-chest technique. Circulation **38**, 777–782 (1968).
National Heart, Blood Vessel, Lung and Blood Program, Vol. IV; Panel Reports: Part 1, Report of the Heart and Blood Vessel Diseases Panel, U.S. Dept. of Health, Education and Welfare. Public Health Service. National Heart and Lung Institute, April 6, 1973.
NEELY, W. A., TURNER, M. D., HARDY, J. D., GODFREY, V. D.: The use of the hydrogen electrode to measure tissue blood flow. J. surg. Res. **5**, 363–369 (1965).
PARRATT, J. R.: Pharmacological approaches to the therapy of angina. Adv. Drug Res. **9**, 103–134 (1974).
PARRATT, J. R., LEDINGHAM, I. McA., McARDLE, C. S.: Effect of a coronary vasodilator drug (carbochromen) on blood flow and oxygen extraction in acute myocardial infarction. Cardiovasc. Res. **7**, 401–407 (1973).

Pasyk, S., Bloor, C. M., Khouri, E. M., Gregg, D. E.: Systemic and coronary effects of coronary artery occlusion in the unanesthetized dog. Amer. J. Physiol. **220**, 646–654 (1971).
Redwood, D. R., Smith, E. R., Epstein, S. E.: Coronary artery occlusion in the conscious dog. Effects of alterations in heart rate and arterial pressure on the degree of myocardial ischemia. Circulation **46**, 323–332 (1972).
Renkin, E. M.: Blood flow and transcapillary exchange in skeletal and cardiac muscle. In: Coronary Circulation and Energetics of the Myocardium (ed. G. Marchetti, B. Taccardi), p. 18–30. Basel: S. Karger 1967.
Ribeilima, J.: Selective embolization of the coronary arteries. A hemodynamic, metabolic and radiologic study. Proc. Soc. exp. Biol. Med. **117**, 367–369 (1964).
Rinzler, S. H., Travell, J., Karp, D., Charleson, D.: Detection of coronary atherosclerosis in the living rabbit by the ergonovine stress test. Amer. J. Physiol. **184**, 605–612 (1956).
Roberts, M., Thomas, D. D., Owens, G., Vilinskas, J., O'Rourke, J.: A new small-diameter mass spectrometer cannula for medical use. Medical Res. Eng. **11**, 27–28 (1972).
Roos, A., Smith, J. R.: Production of experimental heart failure in dogs with intact circulation. Amer. J. Physiol. **153**, 558–566 (1948).
Ross, R. S.: Pathophysiology of coronary circulation. Brit. Heart J. **33**, 173–184 (1971).
Rowe, G. G.: Inequalities of myocardial perfusion in coronary artery disease ("coronary steal"). Circulation **42**, 193–194 (1970).
Rudolph, A. M., Heymann, M. A.: The circulation of the fetus in utero: Methods for studying distribution of blood flow, cardiac output and organ blood flow. Circulat. Res. **21**, 163–184 (1967).
Salazar, A. E.: Experimental myocardial infarction. Induction of coronary thrombosis in the intact closed-chest dog. Circulat. Res. **9**, 1351–1356 (1961).
Schaper, W.: The Collateral Circulation of the Heart. Amsterdam: North-Holland 1971.
Schnaar, R. L., Sparks, H. V.: Response of large and small coronary arteries to nitroglycerin, $NaNO_2$ and adenosine. Amer. J. Physiol. **223**, 223–228 (1972).
Smith, E. R., Redwood, D. R., McCarron, W. E., Epstein, S. E.: Coronary artery occlusion in the conscious dog. Effects of alterations in arterial pressure produced by nitroglycerin, hemorrhage and alpha-adrenergic agonists on the degree of myocardial ischemia. Circulation **47**, 51–57 (1973).
Somani, P., Bachand, R. T., Hardman, H. F., Laddu, A. R.: Nutritional circulation in the heart (II). A reappraisal of the effect of nitroglycerin on myocardial hemodynamics, oxygen consumption and nutritional blood flow in the isolated supported heart preparation. Europ. J. Pharmacol. **8**, 1–13 (1969).
Sugishita, Y., Kaihara, S., Yasuda, H., Iio, M., Murao, S., Ueda, H.: Myocardial distribution of blood flow in the dog: Studies by the labeled microsphere. Part I. Method. Jap. Heart J. **12**, 50–59 (1971).
Szekeres, L., Csik, V., Udvary, E.: Nitroglycerin and dipyridamole on cardiac metabolism and dynamics in a new experimental model of angina pectoris. J. Pharmacol. exp. Ther. In press (1975).
Uchida, Y., Ueda, H.: Evaluation of the use of heated cross-thermocouples for assessments of regional myocardial blood flow. Jap. Heart J. **12**, 562–574 (1971).
Vineberg, A., Mahanti, B., Litvak, J.: Experimental gradual coronary artery constriction by ameroid constrictors. Surgery **47**, 765–771 (1960).
Weber, Karl T., Malinin, T. I., Dennison, B. H., Fuqua, J. M., Speaker, D. M., Hastings, F. W.: Experimental myocardial ischemia and infarction. Production of diffuse lesions in unanesthetized calves. Amer. J. Cardiol. **29**, 793–802 (1972).
Weiss, H. R., Howe, B. B., Winbury, M. M.: Differential effects of chromonar and nitroglycerin on intramyocardial oxygen tension. Europ. J. Pharmacol. **22**, 249–255 (1973).
Weiss, H. R., Winbury, M.: Intracoronary nitroglycerin, pentaerythritol trinitrate and dipyridamole on intramyocardial oxygen tension. Microvasc. Res. **4**, 273–284 (1972).
Weiss, H. R., Winbury, M. M.: Nitroglycerin and chromonar on small-vessel blood content of the ventricular walls. Amer. J. Physiol. **226**, 838–843 (1974).
Weisse, A. B., Moschos, C. B., Passannante, A. J., Khan, M. I., Regan, T. J.: Relative effectiveness of three anti-arrhythmic agents in the treatment of ventricular arrhythmias in experimental acute myocardial ischemia. Amer. Heart J. **81**, 503–510 (1971).
Weisse, A. B., Senft, A., Khan, M. I., Regan, T. J.: Effect of nitrate infusions on the systemic and coronary circulations following acute experimental myocardial infarction in the intact dog. Amer. J. Cardiol. **30**, 362–370 (1972).
Wendt, R. L., Canavan, R. C., Michalak, R. J.: Effects of various agents on regional ischemic myocardial injury: Electrocardiographic analysis. Amer. Heart J. **87**, 468–482 (1974).
Whalen, W. J., Nair, P., Buerk, D.: Oxygen tension in the beating cat heart in situ. In: Oxygen Supply; Theoretical and Practical Aspects of Oxygen Supply and Microcirculation

of Tissue (ed. M. KESSLER, D. F. BRULEY, L. C. CLARK, JR., D. W. LUBBERS, I. A. SILVER, J. STRAUSS), p. 199–201. Munich: Urban & Schwarzenberg 1973.

WILCKEN, D. E. L., PAOLONI, H. J., EIKENS, E.: Evidence for i.v. dipyridamol (Persantin) producing a "coronary steal" effect in the ischemic myocardium. Austr. N.Z. J. Med. **1**, 8–14 (1971).

WINBURY, M. M.: Experimental approaches to the development of antianginal drugs. In: Advances in Pharmacology (ed. S. GARATTINI, P. A. SHORE), p. 1–82. New York: Academic Press 1964.

WINBURY, M. M.: Role of myocardial nutritional circulation in evaluation of antianginal agents. In: Problems in Laboratory Evaluation of Antianginal Agents (ed. M. M. WINBURY), p. 26–40. Amsterdam: North-Holland 1967.

WINBURY, M. M.: Use of radioisotopic tracers in the study of nutritional circulation. In: Radionuclides in Pharmacology, vol. 1 (ed. Y. COHEN), p. 399–488. International Encyclopedia of Pharmacology and Therapeutics, Section 78. Oxford: Pergamon Press 1971a.

WINBURY, M. M.: Redistribution of left ventricular blood flow produced by nitroglycerin. An example of integration of the macro- and microcirculation. Circulat. Res. **28** and **29** (Suppl. I), 140–147 (1971b).

WINBURY, M. M., HAUSLER, L. M., PRIOLI, N. A., ZITOWITZ, L.: Effects of epinephrine on cardiac rhythm in the miniature pig before and after coronary occlusion. J. Pharmacol. exp. Ther. **138**, 287–291 (1962).

WINBURY, M. M., HOWE, B. B.: Protection of the left ventricular subendocardium by nitrates and beta-adrenergic blockers. In: Symposium on Pharmacodynamics of Circulation (abstract), Bratislava, Smolenice, Nov. 11–13, 1973.

WINBURY, M. M., HOWE, B. B., HEFNER, M. A.: Effects of nitrates and other coronary dilators on large and small coronary vessels: An hypothesis for the mechanism of action of nitrates. J. Pharmacol. exp. Ther. **168**, 70–95 (1969).

WINBURY, M. M., HOWE, B. B., WEISS, H. R.: Effect of nitroglycerin and dipyridamole on epicardial and endocardial oxygen tension — Further evidence for redistribution of myocardial blood flow. J. Pharmacol. exp. Ther. **176**, 184–199 (1971a).

WINBURY, M. M., LOSADA, M., KISSIL, D., HOWE, B. B., PENSINGER, R. R.: Pentaerythritoltetranitrate and dipyridamole on cardiac nitritive flow and blood content. Amer. J. Physiol. **220**, 1558–1563 (1971b).

WINBURY, M. M., WEISS, H. R., HOWE, B. B.: Effects of beta adrenoreceptor blockade and nitroglycerin on myocardial oxygenation. Europ. J. Pharmacol. **16**, 271–277 (1971c).

WINBURY, M. M., WEISS, H. R., HOWE, B. B.: Inhomogeneity of oxygen tension, tissue perfusion and small-vessel blood content in the left ventricle — Effect of nitrate and nonnitrate coronary dilators. In: Myocardial Blood Flow in Man — Methods and Significance in Coronary Disease (ed. A. MASERI), p. 37–52. Torino: Minerva Medica 1972.

WINBURY, M. M., WOLF, J. K., CRONIN, M. T. I.: Effect of 10% oxygen on the electrocardiogram of the atherosclerotic rabbit. Amer. J. Physiol. **200**, 642–646 (1961).

Experimental Induction of Hypertension

A. Grollman

With 3 Figures

A. Introduction

The present chapter describes the experimental procedures used to induce an elevation of the systemic arterial blood pressure. Such elevations in blood pressure are designated as "hypertension", a term used also to designate several clinical disorders referred to more specifically as hypertensive cardiovascular disease. An elevated blood pressure may complicate many disorders such as poliomyelitis, intracranial disturbances, disorders of the adrenal, arteriovenous fistulae, hyperthyroidism, *etc.* and may occur as a physiological response especially to physical and mental stimuli. The most common cause of an elevation in arterial blood pressure in man is atherosclerosis which, by reducing the elasticity of the vascular system, necessitates a rise in pulse pressure in order to maintain an adequate blood flow through the tissues. An elevation in blood pressure accordingly reflects only a change in one parameter of the circulation in response to a variety of pathologic disorders as well as to physiologic alterations of the organism (Grollman, 1969).

Failure to appreciate the diversity of pathogenetic and physiologic factors responsible for an observed elevation in blood pressure has led to much confusion not only clinically but in experimental studies as well. It is apparent that the induction of an elevation in blood pressure need not imply that one has produced an analogue of a clinical disorder occurring in the human being. Despite this obvious fact, the literature is replete with instances in which an elevation in blood pressure produced by a given procedure is presented to support an assumed cause of hypertensive disease as it occurs in the human being. For example, the rise in pressure induced by audiogenic stimuli (Yeakel et al., 1948) or by restraint of rats and monkeys (Lamprecht et al., 1973), has been cited as evidence that essential hypertension is of neurogenic origin instead of the inevitable consequence of psychic stress, a well-established cause of an elevation in blood pressure; the rise in blood pressure produced by the injection of fluids (Braun-Menéndez and Covian, 1948) has been cited as evidence that renoprival hypertension (Grollman et al., 1949) is due to expansion of the extracellular fluid volume.

Contrariwise, different procedures may induce elevations in blood pressure which are pathogenetically and clinically identical. There is, for example, good evidence to indicate that essential hypertension in the human being may be the result of some basic renal defect induced by such diverse procedures as bilateral nephrectomy and chronic nephritis (Grollman, 1959). Only when the pathological manifestations (arteriolosclerosis and cardiac hypertrophy), hemodynamic changes (diastolic hypertension and increased peripheral resistance) and the clinical course of the experimental procedure are shown to be the same as those of the disorder occurring in the human being can the former be considered as the analogue of the human disease.

The important clinical disorders which are characterized by an elevation in blood pressure have been reproduced in the experimental animal, and our present concepts of their pathogenesis have been derived largely from a study of these animal models. The view has often been expressed that observations on the experimentally induced disorder are not applicable to the human being, but there is, in fact, a remarkable identity in the disorder as observed in the experimental animal and in man (GROLLMAN, 1953). A consideration, therefore, of the various experimental procedures used to induce hypertensive states in experimental animals is of considerable importance in understanding the etiologic and pathogenetic factors concerned in hypertensive disease of man.

Numerous procedures are available for inducing an elevation in blood pressure in experimental animals. In some of these, the elevation in blood pressure is acute in onset and transient; in others, it develops more slowly and is chronic. In the case of some of the commonly used procedures, the pathogenesis and mechanism maintaining the hypertension change with time. Hence the results obtained using different experimental models and at different times following its induction will differ (GROLLMAN and KRISHNAMURTY, 1971).

The dog (GOLDBLATT et al., 1934; GROLLMAN, 1946) and rat (SELYE, 1943; OKAMOTO, 1972) are the laboratory animals most commonly used for the study of hypertension. The mouse (SOKABE, 1968), rabbit (DRURY, 1938; GROLLMAN, 1944b), sheep (FUNDER et al., 1970), goat (GOLDBLATT et al., 1943), monkey (GOLDBLATT, 1937) and hamster (STROIA et al., 1954) have been used to a lesser extent. The chicken has been used, since, like the human being, it is subject to severe atherosclerosis (GROLLMAN et al., 1963); the frog, for the production of renoprival hypertension (GROLLMAN and GROLLMAN, 1960); the guinea pig, to study the effect of spontaneous nephrosclerosis (TAKEDA and GROLLMAN, 1970); and the opossum, a marsupial, to demonstrate the effects of certain procedures during the extra-uterine stages of embryonic life (GROLLMAN, 1970a). The choice of animals used for a given experiment will depend on the nature of the problem under investigation. For obvious reasons the laboratory rat has been the animal of choice for most experimental studies.

The induction of hypertension in experimental animals serves two principal purposes. It provides models for the study of the uncomplicated hemodynamic and other characteristics of the disorder, which is not always possible in man, and suggests probable mechanisms for the pathogenesis of the various forms of hypertensive disease. For either purpose the condition induced must be a true analogue of the disorder as it occurs in the human being and not simply an elevation in the arterial blood pressure unrelated to the clinical condition under investigation. Before accepting a given preparation as an analogue of the human disease, the same criteria should be applied in experimental studies that one requires to identify the clinical disorder in the human being.

Rather than simply describing seriatim the various procedures used for inducing hypertension experimentally, an attempt will be made to classify the available methods according to the clinical disorder which they mimic. This, however, is not always possible and hence can only be partially followed in the present chapter. The methods used for inducing well-established models of the hypertensive diseases encountered in the human being will be described first, followed by other procedures which induce an elevation in blood pressure which may or may not be related to the spontaneously occurring disorders in the human.

B. Experimental Induction of Essential Hypertension

That form of hypertensive cardiovascular disease, euphemistically designated as "essential", constitutes by far the most prevalent form of chronic diastolic hypertension in the human being. It is congenital in origin and is characterized clinically by a gradual increase in systolic and diastolic arterial blood pressure; the absence of any appreciable interference with the excretory function of the kidney; characteristic pathological changes (arteriolosclerosis and cardiac hypertrophy); and hemodynamically by an increase in peripheral resistance with a normal cardiac output. It is an inheritable disease (PLATT, 1960) with a high incidence in certain races (e.g. the Negro) and absent only in rare isolated aboriginal groups (for review, *cf.*, GROLLMAN, 1973b). Its presence is already evident in early childhood, the blood pressure gradually increasing with age. An analogous condition having the above characteristics may be produced experimentally and occurs spontaneously in several laboratory animals.

I. Spontaneous Genetically Determined Hypertension

Although spontaneously occurring diastolic hypertension has only recently received widespread attention, it is of greatest interest since, like essential hypertension, its counterpart in the human being, it is genetically determined and has the same characteristic features as does the human disorder. Hence such animals may serve as experimental models for the study of the human disease (OKAMOTO, 1972).

SMIRK and HALL (1958) and ALEXANDER et al. (1959) first produced genetically determined colonies of hypertensive rats and rabbits, respectively, by selective inbreeding, but their studies did not elicit wide attention. The production and study of readily reproducible genetically determined colonies of spontaneous hypertensive rats by OKAMOTO and AOKI (1963) attracted wide interest and led to the production of readily reproducible colonies of hypertensive animals which are now available commercially and widely utilized. For experimental use, animals purchased or obtained from established colonies can be bred in the laboratory or may be developed from other strains (BEN-ISHAY et al., 1972).

The usually encountered colony of laboratory rats manifests a wider variation in blood pressure than one would anticipate to occur as a result simply of normal physiologic variations. Arbitrarily, only those animals with systolic pressures of 150 mm Hg or more are usually considered as hypertensive, but it is more probable that animals with systolic blood pressures over about 100 ± 10 are actually mildly hypertensive. This conclusion is confirmed by the fact that by selective inbreeding of animals with the highest and lowest blood pressures one can obtain hypertensive and normotensive colonies, respectively, which subsequently breed true. It is probable also that other animal species manifesting wide variations in their basal blood pressure carry the genetic defect responsible for the development of hypertensive disease and if inbred will produce spontaneous hypertensive colonies.

OKAMOTO and AOKI (1963) developed their spontaneous hypertensive rats by mating a male Wistar rat with a blood pressure of 145 to 175 mm Hg and a female of the same strain with a blood pressure of 130 to 140 mm Hg. The most severe hypertensive animals of subsequent litters were then mated, resulting in hypertension and its characteristic cardiovascular lesions in the third generation and thereafter. After 20 generations of sibling inbreeding an inbred strain was established in which hypertension occurred in all animals at maturity. It was thus established that genetic factors to a degree of 80 to 90% were responsible for the development of the hypertension, environmental factors (such as salt feeding) playing only a minor role in its pathogenesis. Hemodynamic and other studies support the conclusion that the spontaneous hypertensive rat is a model for human essential hypertension (OKAMOTO, 1972).

II. Teratogenic Induction of Hypertension

Another form of hypertension which resembles essential hypertension of the human being and the spontaneous inherited hypertension just described may be induced by treatment of pregnant rats during certain critical periods of embryonic development. Although the term "teratogenic" has generally been confined to its literal meaning of morphologic "monstrosities", it may justifiably be broadened to include disorders such as hypertensive disease. GROLLMAN and GROLLMAN (1962) demonstrated that subjecting pregnant rats to dietary and hormonal measures known to induce hypertension in the adult results in the birth of offspring which are normotensive in early life but gradually develop hypertension with age (Table 1).

Although not occurring spontaneously, this procedure for inducing hypertension resembles essential hypertension of man in being congenital in origin and having the other basic characteristics of the latter disorder of which it may be considered an experimental model.

Table 1. Effect of drugs and diets administered to pregnant rats on the blood pressure of their offspring at one year of age. (After GROLLMAN and GROLLMAN, 1962)

Experimental procedure	Systolic blood pressure		p value of difference between experimental and control groups
	Range mm Hg	Mean ± S.D. mm Hg	
Controls	98–128	114 ± 7.4	
Aldosterone (0.05 mg/day SC)	125–160	140 ± 9.5	< 0.001
Cortisone (1.0 mg/day i.m.)	140–150	144 ± 4.8	< 0.001
Desoxycorticosterone (1.0 mg/day i.m.)	120–155	142 ± 8.1	< 0.001
Progesterone (1 mg/day i.m.)	130–155	142 ± 6.5	< 0.001
Chlorothiazide (166 mg/day p.o.)	130–155	145 ± 9.3	< 0.001
Low K intake	130–140	136 ± 4.8	< 0.001
High Na intake	135–160	148 ± 6.7	< 0.001
Choline-free diet plus 5% ethanol	135–155	150 ± 8.7	< 0.001
NaCl (1%) as drinking water	110–130	116 ± 7.9	> 0.3 < 0.4

C. Surgical Induction of Chronic Sustained Diastolic Hypertension

A number of surgical procedures are available which produce experimental models of essential hypertension. Unlike the previously described procedures, these involve manipulation of the kidney or its blood supply and are not congenital in origin. They, therefore, are not strictly speaking analogues of essential hypertension. Moreover, during their early post-operative period they may give rise to the surgically remediable type of hypertension to be described later or progress rapidly to the malignant type rather than to the chronic stage of diastolic hypertension characteristic of essential hypertension. Despite these differences, these procedures usually terminate as chronic elevations in blood pressure with the hemodynamic and pathological characteristics of essential hypertension and have been widely used as experimental models of this disease.

The first procedures introduced for the induction of chronic hypertension in experimental animals consisted in partial removal of the kidneys or in interfering with the blood supply to these organs (for a review of the earlier literature see GROLLMAN, 1973c). The most consistently effective of these procedures was that of CHANUTIN and FERRIS (1932) who ablated the poles of both kidney after clamping the renal pedicle for a few minutes to prevent excessive bleeding. The high mortality and short survival time of the animals has rendered this procedure obsolete.

I. The Goldblatt Procedure

The classic study of GOLDBLATT et al. (1934) attracted wide attention and stimulated the modern experimental investigation of hypertension. For the first time it was possible to induce an elevation of blood pressure in dogs without damaging the kidney grossly or interfering with its excretory function. The procedure of GOLDBLATT et al. consisted of constricting one renal artery by an adjustable clamp and after a period of a week or more extirpating the opposite kidney. One could also apply clamps to both kidneys, thereby producing what subsequent workers have designated as the "two-kidney" as opposed to the "one-kidney" Goldblatt dog, in which only one renal artery was constricted.

The method of GOLDBLATT et al. (1934) consists of applying a silver clamp similar to the commonly used Hoffmann clamp over the renal artery exposed through an incision in the flank along the costal margin. The clamp is then partially closed in order to occlude the renal artery to about two-thirds of its normal diameter. Occasionally the constriction of only one kidney suffices to induce hypertension. In most instances, however, it is necessary to remove the contralateral kidney or apply a clamp to its artery in order to induce hypertension. When the clamp is applied too tightly, vascular necrosis suggestive of human malignant hypertension occurs together with the death of the animal in uremia.

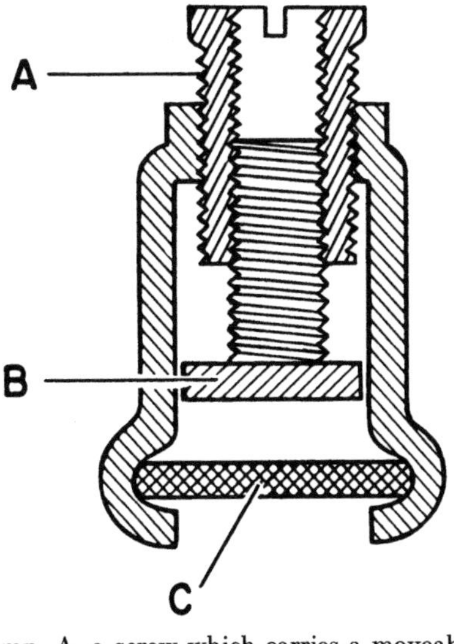

Fig. 1. The Goldblatt Clamp. A, a screw which carries a moveable plate, B; C, a removeable plate. The clamp is inserted around the renalartery. The latter, in place between B and C, is compressed by means of a special screw-driver. (After GOLDBLATT et al., 1934)

If applied too loosely, the blood pressure will fail to rise even after removal of the opposite kidney.

An early rise in blood pressure following the application of a Goldblatt clamp is due to the liberation from the kidney of a circulating pressor agent which is presumably responsible for the observed rise in blood pressure. Removal of the kidney at this time results in a resumption of the normotensive state. Should the animal survive this early stage of renovascular or surgically remediable hypertension, a chronic stage of hypertension ensues which is not accompanied by the presence of a circulating pressor agent, and nephrectomy no longer abolishes the elevation in blood pressure (EBIHARA and GROLLMAN, 1968).

Goldblatt's procedure has been applied with success to the dog, cat, monkey, sheep, goat, rabbit and, by the use of a miniature clamp, to the rat, but has been largely replaced by the simpler methods to be described next.

II. Other Procedures for Constricting the Renal Artery

Instead of using a miniature adjustable clamp of the type used by GOLDBLATT in the dog, it is simpler and more convenient to use the method of DRURY (1938) for smaller animals such as the rat or rabbit. In this procedure a wire, approximately one third the diameter of the normal renal artery, is placed along the artery and a loop of silk thread tied tightly around the artery and wire, proximal to its junction with the adrenal artery. The left kidney, being more accessible, is used preferably, but if the right one is used, the loop is placed proximally to the point at which the vessel runs dorsally to the inferior vena cava. After tying the loop, the wire is withdrawn.

As in the case of the Goldblatt clamp, it is difficult to judge the extent of the constriction, and the mortality is high or there is failure to develop hypertension even when contralateral nephrectomy is performed. For this reason the use of the figure-of-eight procedure or the application of a clip as described next is preferred for the induction of chronic hypertension. Drury's procedure, however, is the method of choice for inducing acute surgically remediable renovascular hypertension to be described later.

A convenient and widely used procedure for constricting the renal artery consists of applying a U-shaped strip of silver ribbon over the artery. For rats weighing about 150 g, a clip with an inside diameter of 0.22 mm is prepared by

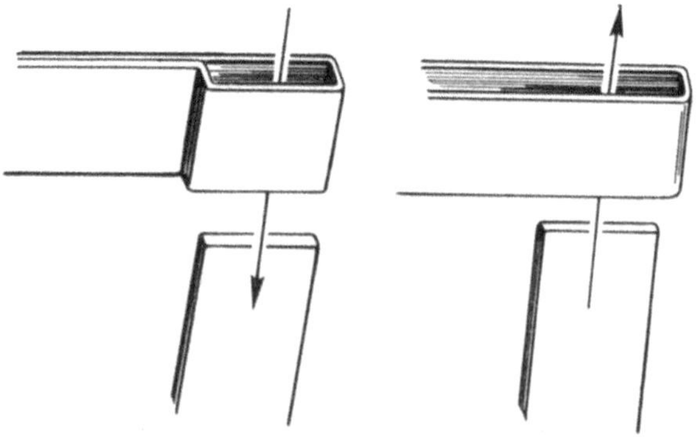

Fig. 2. Procedure used for molding a silver ribbon (1.5 × 0.1 mm) shown on the left, over a metal form to produce the clip, shown on the right, which is slipped over the renal artery. (After SOKABE, 1968)

bending a thin silver ribbon about 0.5 mm thick and 1 mm wide over a metal plate 0.22 mm in width (LEDINGHAM, 1956; FLOYER, 1955; BROOKS et al., 1972). A similar procedure is used in the rabbit or other animals by using a clip with an internal diameter approximately two-thirds that of the renal artery. As in the case of the Goldblatt procedure, it is necessary to remove the contralateral kidney either at the time of the application of the clip or subsequently to induce hypertension except in a small percentage of the animals in which hypertension (presumably because of the pre-existence of some degree of hypertension) follows without removing the untouched kidney. The development of hypertension can also be expedited by substituting 0.9% NaCl solution (preferably with 2% glucose) for the drinking water.

Hypertension may also be produced by partial occlusion of the abdominal aorta above the origin of both main renal arteries (GOLDBLATT et al., 1939) presumably by interfering with the blood supply to the kidneys. When the ligature is placed between the sites of exit of the two renal arteries, hypertension may also result with the formation of SELYE's "endocrine" kidney.

III. Application of a "Figure-of-Eight" Ligature

A simple procedure for inducing chronic hypertension in the mammal, which has been used in the mouse, rat, dog, cat, rabbit and hamster, is the application of a ligature to deform the parenchyma of the kidney (GROLLMAN, 1944a). In this method a cotton thread (in the smaller rodent) or umbilical tape (in larger animals) is passed over the poles and body of the kidney and drawn taut to distort the kidney. The kidney need not be removed from its normal position and an attempt is made not to remove or rupture the capsule. This is readily accomplished in the larger mammals, but in the rat it may be necessary to remove the capsule by gentle traction.

After anesthetizing the animal the kidney is exposed through a lumbar incision. In the dog, the tape is passed through the capsular connective tissue of the under surface of the kidney in order to fix it firmly in position. In the rat or mouse,

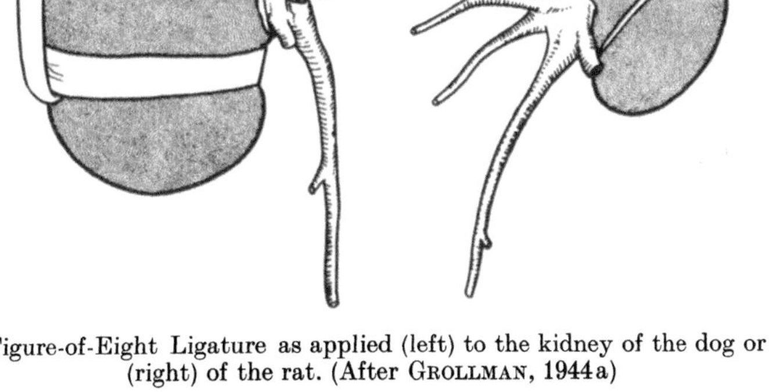

Fig. 3. The Figure-of-Eight Ligature as applied (left) to the kidney of the dog or rabbit and (right) of the rat. (After GROLLMAN, 1944a)

cotton thread (No. 8 gauge) is used; for the dog and rabbit or larger mammal, sterile umbilical tape is used. The ligature is tightened sufficiently to deform the normal bean-shape of the kidney without cutting into the renal parenchyma, and care is taken to avoid the ureter and blood vessels which emerge from the hilus.

Rats 130 to 180 g in weight or dogs are anesthetized by the injection intraperitoneally of 60 mg of sodium pentobarbital per kg of body weight supplemented when necessary by the use of ether during the operative procedure. The kidneys are approached through an incision made parallel to the costal margin beginning in the costovertebral angle. After separating the lumbar muscles, the kidney is delivered through the incision by gentle external pressure. After performing the necessary surgical procedure, the kidney is replaced in its usual position and the incision closed with cotton or silk. In the case of the rat, the skin may be brought in apposition by the use of skin clips.

In about 10 to 20% of the animals, hypertension develops gradually during the next 3 to 6 months without further manipulations. If the second kidney is also compressed, about half of the animals will develop hypertension. By removing the contralateral kidney, hypertension of a more severe degree develops rapidly. By following the course of the blood pressure and applying a ligature or removing the contralateral kidney as indicated, it is possible to induce stable chronic hypertension and avoid an acute, rapidly developing malignant hypertension.

IV. Infarction of the Kidney

Focal infarction of the kidney results in an elevation of blood pressure in the rat and affords an effective method for producing a colony of experimental hypertensive animals (LOOMIS, 1946). The development of hypertension is accelerated by removing the contralateral kidney and replacing the animal's drinking water with 1% sodium chloride. Alternatively, one can infarct both kidneys. The blood pressure reaches hypertensive levels within about 4 to 8 weeks (SOKABE and GROLLMAN, 1963b).

Infarction of the kidney is produced by ligating one of the small arterial branches of the renal artery at the hilus of the kidney. The artery is freed from its surrounding fibrous tissue by gentle dissection, and a silk ligature is passed under it and tied. Blanching of the triangular area supplied by the artery reflects the extent of the infarction which need be only a millimeter in width. Ultimately only a hair-line scar is noted at the site of the infarction.

Infarction of the kidney does not induce hypertension in the dog as it does in the rat, suggesting that some mechanism specific for the rat is concerned in its pathogenesis. This difference in response concerns the immune mechanism which is much more readily activated in the rat than in the dog. That this is the case has been demonstrated by WHITE and GROLLMAN (1964a) who showed that results similar to those noted after infarction were obtainable by injecting homologous renal tissue; this finding had been noted by others but was attributed to the effects of renin (MASSON et al., 1962).

As indicated later, the hypertension induced by infarction of the kidney is the experimental model of that observed in chronic pyelo- and glomerulo-nephritis and of that occasionally encountered in the human being following infarction of the kidney. That the induction of hypertension, at least in its early stages, is mediated through the action on the kidney of a substance liberated from the infarcted kidney has been demonstrated by renal transplantation (KAWABE et al., 1972) and by studies on parabiotic rats (EBIHARA, 1972). The pressor agent responsible for the action has been designated as nephrotensin (GROLLMAN, 1970b).

V. Adrenal Regeneration Hypertension

SKELTON (1955) noted that hypertension may be produced in rats sensitized by unilateral nephrectomy and a high sodium intake (1% NaCl drinki ng solution) by removing one adrenal and enucleating the other by incising the capsule and expressing its medulla and most of the fascicular zone. The adrenal cortex regenerates from the remaining zona glomerulosa, and the animals develop an elevated blood pressure and the characteristic pathologic lesions of hypertension in the course of about 7 weeks. Periarteritis nodosa also develops but is less pronounced than that noted after the injection of desoxycorticosterone (DOCA) (CHART et al., 1957).

The development of adrenal regeneration hypertension has been attributed to an overproduction of aldosterone by the regenerated adrenal (GIROUD et al., 1956) or the abnormal electrolyte pattern induced by the operation (GROLLMAN, 1958). Since the concentration of DOCA in the peripheral plasma rises to 6 times that of controls at 3 weeks following enucleation, adrenal regeneration hypertension may be considered to be mediated by the same mechanism as that which operates following DOCA injections as described later. Since the plasma DOCA levels decline to normal levels at 7 weeks postoperatively, other factors are involved in its maintenance, as is also the case when DOCA injections are discontinued (BROWN et al., 1972).

VI. Miscellaneous Surgical Procedures

A variety of other surgical procedures have been described for inducing chronic diastolic hypertension but are now rarely used. The application of a capsule of silk, cellophane, collodion or cotton to compress the kidney has been used for eliciting hypertension in rats and dogs (KEMPF and PAGE, 1942; GROLLMAN and WILLIAMS, 1942). It was assumed that the development of hypertension was due to the formation of a perinephric fibro-collagenous hull around the kidney. The latter, however, is not essential for eliciting hypertension since a similar result can be more easily and better obtained by application of a figure-of-eight ligature. The latter method has, therefore, replaced the former for the induction of hypertension in laboratory animals.

ZBINDEN (1946) utilized a cellulose-acetone capsule to compress the kidney. Combined with contralateral nephrectomy this procedure results within 2 months in an elevation of the blood pressure to 200 to 400 mm Hg; the blood pressure remains elevated following removal of the applied capsule. Others have attempted to block the renal circulation by injecting a sclerosing agent (TAKATS et al., 1962), finely divided silica (MOSES et al., 1954), and other materials into the renal artery instead of occluding it externally. These and other exotic procedures have not been adopted by other investigators.

D. Non-Surgical Procedures for Inducing Experimental Chronic Diastolic Hypertension

Several well-established non-surgical methods are used as experimental models of chronic diastolic hypertension, and like those just described, they result in the induction of a disorder resembling in many respects that of essential hypertension. The hypertension so produced is accompanied usually by renovascular lesions and some degree, usually minor, of excretory renal deficiency. They are, therefore, not exact models of essential hypertension in the sense that spontaneous hypertension is, although the elevation in blood pressure is probably caused by the same basic defect in the kidney (GROLLMAN, 1966).

I. Salt-Induced Hypertension

The administration of sodium chloride to animals either admixed with their food or as a substitute for their drinking water in an amount in excess of the capacity of their kidneys to excrete same, results in a rise in blood pressure and cardiovascular lesions (SAPIRSTEIN et al., 1950). If the administration of the salt is continued for only a short period, the blood pressure returns to normal on withdrawal of the salt, but if continued, cardiovascular lesions are induced and a chronic elevation in blood pressure ensues (FREGLY, 1961). The resultant hypertension is a response to the toxic effects of the salt (MENEELY et al., 1953), mediated possibly by the action of the sodium ion on the contractile protein of arterial tissue (SHIBATA et al., 1972). It is enhanced by water restriction (COUSINEAU and BIRON, 1972) since the rat is unable to concentrate and excrete salt loads without an adequate water load. The intake of water as well as the amount of salt ingested will determine therefore the hypertension-producing effect of salt ingestion, and the addition of sucrose or glucose to the drinking water will enhance the development of salt-induced hypertension (HALL et al., 1972b). The amount of salt and water ingested will determine the severity of the induced hypertension. Failure to consider this factor accounts, in part, for the variation in the susceptibility of different stocks of rats to develop hypertension on salt feeding (MOLTENI and BROWNIE, 1972).

Another factor which probably accounts for the difference in response of different rats of the same strain and of different strains is the incidence of mild hypertension in various colonies. The last named factor explains the assumed genetic variation in sensitivity of different colonies as reported by DAHL et al. (1963) and by BEN-ISHAY et al. (1972). The salt-sensitive rats reported in both of these studies had a pretreatment pressure higher than those of the resistant animals, suggesting that the former had a greater propensity to spontaneous hypertension and hence responded more intensely, as is also the case with other stimuli such as unilateral nephrectomy (GROLLMAN, 1972).

In addition to the rat, chronic hypertension has been induced in the chicken (LENEL et al., 1948), the pouch opossum (GROLLMAN, 1970a) and in the offspring of pregnant rats (GROLLMAN and GROLLMAN, 1962) by excess salt administration. Due to its greater capacity to excrete exogenous salt, it is more difficult to produce salt-induced hypertension in the dog. VOGEL (1966), however, induced a 55% increase in the arterial blood pressure of dogs by increasing their dietary intake of NaCl to 2 g per kg of body weight per day and providing a 0.9% NaCl solution instead of tap water to drink for a period of 26 days. In the uninephrectomized rat it is only necessary to provide a 0.9% NaCl solution containing 2% sucrose or glucose as drinking water with a normal diet to induce hypertension.

Although vascular lesions resembling those observed in human essential hypertension are produced in salt-induced hypertension in rats (KOLETSKY, 1958), the two conditions are not comparable in several respects. Salt-induced hypertension is accompanied by edema (MENEELY et al., 1953), an increased serum cholesterol (DAHL, 1961), and a doubling of the total exchangeable body sodium (VOGEL, 1966). The condition also differs hemodynamically from that observed in essential hypertension, the salt-induced disorder being associated with a marked increase in blood volume and cardiac output without a change in peripheral resistance (GROLLMAN, 1962; VOGEL, 1966).

Spontaneously hypertensive rats develop hypertension in spite of a low sodium intake (AOKI et al., 1972), although various substrains may show some difference in sensitivity to salt ingestion. Genetic factors are accordingly predominant, the ingestion of salt playing only a minor role in inducing hypertension. Epidemiological studies in man support this conclusion (MADDOCKS, 1964).

II. DOCA-Induced Hypertension

The experimental induction of hypertension by desoxycorticosterone (DOCA), a salt-retaining hormone of the adrenal cortex, in rats (GROLLMAN et al., 1940) has been widely used for inducing chronic diastolic hypertension. SELYE et al. (1943) showed that the simultaneous administration of sodium chloride accelerated the development of hypertension and aggravated the lesions. He designated the condition as metacorticoid hypertension.

The susceptibility of rats to the pressor action of DOCA varies depending probably on the incidence and degree of genetic spontaneous hypertension present in different strains (MOLTENI and BROWNIE, 1972). GROSS (1950) obtained no clear-cut increase in hypertension with DOCA alone dissolved in peanut oil in doses of 5 mg/kg on alternate days, but others have induced hypertension by this means. HALL et al. (1972a) also noted that, in contrast to Sprague-Dawley rats, Long-Evans rats remained normotensive when given DOCA with saline solution to drink and attributed this finding to the fact that the former consumed less sodium chloride. An explanation for this difference may perhaps reside in the retention of salt by hypertensive rats (EBIHARA et al., 1970).

DOCA hypertension is generally induced by injecting the drug into uninephrectomized rats given a 0.9% NaCl solution containing 0.2% KCl (to counter the potassium losing effect of the DOCA) and 2% glucose to increase the intake of NaCl. The DOCA may be administered intramuscularly as a suspension or dissolved in oil, or in the form of pellets inserted subcutaneously. A dose of 5 mg per day is usually injected for about 8 weeks. DOCA trimethylacetate may also be used by intramuscular injection in doses of 12.5 mg 3 times weekly for 4 weeks followed by 6.25 mg twice weekly for the next 3 weeks. In 70% of rats weighing 190 to 220 g and receiving 50 mg per kilo of body weight of DOCA weekly, hypertension of over 180 mm Hg develops within 6 weeks (GROSS, 1950). The blood pressure remains high if the administration of DOCA is maintained for at least 2 to 3 months, but if the drug is withdrawn after 2 to 3 weeks, it usually declines to normal. Some self-sustaining mechanism thus replaces the initial stimulus of the DOCA.

ORMSBEE and RYAN (1973) induced hypertension within 3 weeks after implanting dimethylpolysiloxane impregnated with desoxycorticosterone in doses of 100 mg/kg into unilaterally nephrectomized rats given 1% NaCl instead of tap water. The drug was incorporated in unpolymerized silicone rubber in a methyl acrylate mold and a catalyst added to produce a solid cast.

Several theories have been offered to explain the action of DOCA on the blood pressure. Although its acute effects may be due to expansion of the extracellular fluid volume as a result of salt retention, this does not explain its sustained action following withdrawal of the drug. That DOCA acts on the kidney was first demonstrated by SELYE (1943) and is also suggested by its teratogenic action (GROLL-

MAN and GROLLMAN, 1962) and compensatory hypertrophy of the kidney which follows its administration (MALYUSZ et al., 1972).

Rats with post-DOCA hypertension show an increased arteriolar response to norepinephrine and 5-hydroxytryptamine, increased maximal contractile responses to norepinephrine, and increased resistance to flow under conditions of maximum vasodilation. These abnormalities have been attributed to thickening of the arteriolar wall (BEILIN and ZIAKAS, 1972) but are more likely due to the direct effect of DOCA on the vascular smooth muscle. The latter in turn may initiate an immune response which maintains the hypertension despite the withdrawal of the initiating stimulus (GIESE, 1971; OLSEN, 1971).

III. Hypertension Induced by Dietary Deficiencies

Animals on a choline or potassium deficient diet develop hemorrhagic lesions in the heart, liver and kidney (FOLLIS et al., 1942). In weanling rats the lesions appear within a few days but if restored to a normal diet, healing occurs and the animals ultimately develop hypertension as shown in the case of choline deficiency in rats by HARTROFT and BEST (1949). The development of hypertension is accelerated if the animals are sensitized by unilateral nephrectomy and the substitution of a 1% NaCl for their drinking water. This procedure offers a convenient method for obtaining a colony of hypertensive rats and dogs (GROLLMAN and WHITE, 1958). For this purpose the animals at the time of weaning are placed on the deficient diet for 2 to 3 weeks, but a shorter period suffices to induce hypertension in most of the animals. MOSES et al. (1950), for example, found that of 28 weanling rats surviving a 5-day choline-deficient diet and maintained on a normal diet thereafter, 20 showed an elevated arterial blood pressure 6 months later.

The effects of administering potassium- and choline-deficient diets to weanling rats are shown in Table 2. The potassium-free diet was obtained commercially and consisted of cornstarch (64.2%), casein (30.0%), butterfat (3.5%), calcium carbonate (1.3%) and sodium chloride (1.0%), plus complete vitamin supplements. The choline-deficient diet, prepared by the method of COPELAND and SALMON (1946), contained 30% alcohol-extracted peanut meal, 6% alcohol-extracted casein, 40% sucrose, 20% pure lard and 4% salt mixture. To each kilogram of diet was added 200 mg inositol, 10 mg calcium pantothenate, 50 mg α-tocopherol, 4 mg riboflavin, 2 mg thiamine, 4 mg carotene, 2 mg pyridoxine, and 0.125 mg calciferol.

Table 2. Systolic blood pressure of normal and unilaterally-nephrectomized rats on potassium and chloline-deficient diets. (After GROLLMAN and WHITE, 1958)

Experimental procedure	Age in months		
	2	6	12
Unilaterally nephrectomized with 1% NaCl in drinking water	80–120[a] (102)	92–130 (110)	100–135 (124)
K-deficiency	100–160 (130)	130–200 (158)	140–220 (170)
Choline-deficiency	90–140 (120)	120–170 (136)	140–190 (172)

[a] Range of blood pressure in mm Hg is given on the left; the average, in parentheses, on the right.

The development of hypertension on a deficient choline or potassium diet is believed to be due to the renal damage incurred by this procedure. During the acute stage of the process, electron microscopy of the kidney of rats rendered hypertensive by choline deficiency reveals swelling of the endothelial cytoplasmic lining of the glomeruli with fusion of the trabeculae and pedicles of the epithelial cells, focal widening of the slit pores between the pedicles and reduction of the intertrabecular spaces. Later, the basement membrane of the capillary wall in the glomeruli also becomes thickened (ASHWORTH and GROLLMAN, 1959).

Other forms of dietary restriction have also been described as inducing hypertension but are too difficult to apply and too ineffective for use in producing an hypertensive colony. CALDER (1942) for example, induced mild hypertension in rats on a vitamin deficient diet. WILHELMJ et al. (1956) produced it in a few dogs subjected to episodes of fasting and realimentation with a low-calorie diet of raw meat. Neither procedure has been used subsequently.

E. Induction of Special Forms of Hypertension

Although essential hypertension constitutes by far the most prevalent form of chronic hypertensive cardiovascular disease in man, other rare forms of chronic hypertension occur which differ pathogenetically and hemodynamically from it. Experimental models of these disorders are also available and will now be discussed.

I. Systolic Hypertension

The most commonly observed cause of an elevation in blood pressure in the human being is a hemodynamic response to generalized atherosclerosis; it is also observed in some laboratory animals. The gradual increase in blood pressure observed with age in man as well as in the experimental animal is a consequence of the loss of elasticity of the blood vessels due to atherosclerosis. Only in a few isolated aboriginal groups (*cf.* GROLLMAN, 1973b) is atherosclerosis absent, and in these the blood pressure does not increase with age but declines slightly as one would anticipate from the normal decrease in cardiovascular activity which accompanies the aging process. The hypertension secondary to atherosclerosis involves primarily the systolic blood pressure but when the smaller arteries are also affected the resultant elevation in blood pressure will also involve the diastolic level. When the arteriosclerotic process involves the kidney, one would anticipate that the two processes (arteriosclerosis and hypertensive disease) would combine to elevate the blood pressure and set up a vicious cycle in which each pathological process exacerbates the effect of the other (GROLLMAN, 1951).

Atherosclerosis occurs spontaneously and is particularly severe in the bird. In the chicken, atherosclerosis and hypertension are independent processes; both disorders are accentuated with age but are pathogenetically unrelated (GROLLMAN et al., 1963). Any procedure which accelerates the development of atherosclerosis (e.g. cholesterol feeding in the rabbit, thyroidectomy and the administration of thiouracil in the dog, *etc.*) will induce the development of atherosclerosis and systolic hypertension. Such preparations are experimental models of the disorder encountered in the human being (PARWARESCH et al., 1973).

For the induction of atherosclerosis experimentally in laboratory animals, procedures are used which raise the serum level of cholesterol, decrease the metabolic rate, or both (CLARKSON et al., 1970). Since its first use by ANITSCHKOW in 1913, the rabbit has been most widely used for this purpose. Atherosclerosis may be produced readily in this animal by feeding a protein-poor, fat-rich diet to which is added 3% cholesterol and administering orally 35 mg of cholic acid per kg of body weight daily. Within 50 days well-defined atherosclerosis is produced.

The susceptibility of most other laboratory animals to atherosclerosis is not great. Dogs, however, fed a cholesterol-rich diet for a year develop typical atherosclerotic plaques on the aorta. The rate of plaque formation may be accelerated by feeding thiouracil to depress thyroid function or by thyroidectomy (STEINER et al., 1949). Atherosclerosis has also been produced in dogs by administering 250 mg/kg of Triton, a non-ionic surface-active detergent, every fourth day (SCANU et al., 1961).

Miniature swine on a diet containing 20% solid or unsaturated fat and 20% cholesterol also develop atherosclerosis (GYÖRKEY and REISER, 1964). Atherosclerosis has also been produced in the rhesus monkey (CLARKSON et al., 1970), in the marmoset (DREIZEN et al., 1973), and in five diverse species of wild rodents (DIETRICH et al., 1973) by high-fat high-cholesterol diets.

Atherosclerosis, as already indicated, occurs spontaneously in the chicken but may be accelerated by adding cholesterol to the diet. Aortic atherosclerosis has also been induced in Japanese quail (*Coturnix coturnix japonica*) placed on diets high in saturated fat, fatty acids and sucrose to which cholesterol is added (SMITH and HILKER, 1973).

II. Hypertension Secondary to Nephritis and Nephrosclerosis

Hypertension commonly accompanies pyelonephritis and other forms of nephritis observed clinically. Models of the human disorder have been produced in the dog by the injection of streptococci (DICK, 1945) and in the rat by injection of coliform bacilli after injury of the kidney by vigorous massage (SHAPIRO and KOBERNICK, 1961). In the case of the chronic nephritides, an autoimmune reaction (AKAMATSU et al., 1962) serves as the mechanism whereby renal damage is established and gives rise to hypertension (WHITE and GROLLMAN, 1964a).

Mice and guinea pigs are subject to kidney infections. As is the case in the human being, such infections are accompanied by an elevation in blood pressure. Other rare disturbances observed in the dog such as kidney worms and hydronephrosis secondary to ureteral obstruction are also accompanied by hypertension as in the human being.

Certain strains of guinea pigs develop kidney lesions of unknown origin which resemble those of nephrosclerosis as observed in the human being. As in the case of the latter, these changes in the kidney are accompanied by the development of hypertension (TAKEDA and GROLLMAN, 1970).

III. Surgically Remediable Hypertension

So-called renovascular or surgically remediable hypertension is easily reproducible in the experimental animal by drastic constriction of the renal artery in the rat and dog and by infarction of a kidney in the rat. Like its human counterpart the hypertension is remediable by removal of the constriction or by nephrectomy. OGDEN et al. (1946) first noted a difference in the mechanism responsible for the elevation in blood pressure during the acute stage following application of a clamp to the renal artery and its subsequent chronic elevation, a difference ignored in earlier experimental studies.

Experimental analogues of surgically remediable hypertension are produced by the same procedures as have been described above for producing chronic diastolic pressure. In the dog it is only necessary to apply the clamp or other constriction of the renal artery to a greater degree in order to produce a more intense ischemia (EBIHARA and GROLLMAN, 1968) or in the case of the rat to produce a focal infarct of the kidney as described previously (GROLLMAN, 1970b). The pressure usually begins to rise within an hour following recovery from the anesthesia and continues to rise reaching a maximum within 3 or 4 days. In the dog this rise is maintained for about a week; in the rat after bilateral infarction of both kidneys, for as long as a month, after which it may subside only to rise again as chronic hypertension develops after removal of the contralateral kidney (SOKABE and GROLLMAN, 1963a).

The acute elevation in blood pressure observed in surgically remediable hypertension is mediated by the release of a pressor agent (nephrotensin) which may be demonstrated in the venous effluent of the involved kidney. After removal of the affected kidney or with the passage of time and the establishment of chronic hypertension, the pressor agent is no longer demonstrable in the circulating blood.

Hypertension mediated by the liberation from the kidney of a pressor agent may also be produced by completely occluding one or both renal arteries. On releasing the clamp or ligature the blood pressure rises to hypertensive levels.

IV. Renoprival Hypertension

The term "renoprival hypertension" is used generally to denote the rise in blood pressure that follows bilateral nephrectomy. In a broader sense, it is also applicable to hypertension resulting from partial and unilateral nephrectomy as well as to the hypertension accompanying the loss of renal tissue such as occurs in chronic nephritis. The use of the term "renoprival" on the assumption that one is dealing with a specific and unique form of hypertension, accordingly, is arbitrary and unjustified.

The earliest studies of the effects of bilateral nephrectomy on the blood pressure led to the erroneous conclusion that the maintenance of an elevated blood pressure requires the presence of renal tissue, since removal of the kidneys resulted in a decline in blood pressure in normal as well as in hypertensive animals. The fact that the elevated blood pressure was not maintained in hypertensive animals following nephrectomy was considered as evidence that hypertension was mediated by a circulating pressor agent of renal origin. The blood pressure observed in these early studies reflected the *pre-mortem* state of the animals (ALLBUTT, 1915). Some days must elapse and the subject must remain in good condition following bilateral nephrectomy before hypertension develops; failure to note a rise in blood pressure after only 3 or 4 days of survival is of no significance. Nephrectomy in cases of surgically remediable hypertension, as we have seen, will cause a decline in blood pressure rather than an increase, which it does in the absence of a circulating pressor agent. In malignant hypertension, also, bilateral nephrectomy causes a decline in blood pressure from its inordinately elevated level but not to normal unless one also induces a hypovolemic state or administers drugs (ganglionic blocking agents, guanethidine or other antipressor agents) which lower the blood pressure (GROLLMAN, 1973d).

Unilateral nephrectomy in the human being and in the experimental animal induces no appreciable effect on the blood pressure. This is not unexpected since removal of one kidney is followed by compensatory hypertrophy of the remaining organ which presumably takes over the function of both organs. If the contralateral kidney, however, is unable to maintain this function, or in the presence of an already existent hypertension, even of a minimal degree, unilateral nephrectomy results in a further rise in blood pressure (GROLLMAN, 1972). In the dog chronic hypertension ensues only rarely following removal of one kidney. In the rat, on the other hand, approximately 20% of the animals in some colonies develop mild hypertension following unilateral nephrectomy. The incidence of hypertension following unilateral nephrectomy is dependent on the status of the contralateral kidney at the time of operation and on the pre-operative level of the blood pressure (GROLLMAN, 1972). Since dogs, unlike rats, do not manifest an appreciable degree of spontaneous hypertension, their blood pressure will not rise if the animal is free of renal disease.

Removal of the kidneys in the frog, rat, dog, opposum and man results in the development of hypertension if the animal survives a sufficiently long time (4 to 6 days) and is maintained in good condition and in normal electrolyte-water balance. Despite the common observation that the blood pressure of the hypertensive human being and of the laboratory animal declines in the face of salt depletion, a decrease in the volume of the extracellular fluid, heart failure, adrenal insufficiency or other debilitating influences, the failure of human patients in a moribund condition to manifest an elevated blood pressure has been cited as evidence that man and the dog react differently to bilateral nephrectomy. The failure of the salt- or protein-depleted dog to maintain an elevated blood pressure has also been cited as evidence that overloading of the extracellular fluid is responsible for renoprival hypertension. If proper precautions are taken to maintain a normal electrolyte-water balance and no serious complications are present, the human patient or experimental animal will invariably become hypertensive following bilateral nephrectomy. Only in the case of surgically remediable and of malignant hypertension will nephrectomy result in a decline in blood pressure which is attributable to the removal of a source of circulating pressor agent (nephrotensin).

Renoprival hypertension has also been produced by removing the kidneys of one of a pair of rats in parabiotic union (JEFFERS et al., 1940; GROLLMAN and RULE, 1943). Only the nephrectomized parabiont develops hypertension. Following drastic occlusion of the renal artery or infarction of the kidney of one parabiont, the hypertension is transmitted to its partner since it is mediated by the release of nephrotensin, as already described (EBIHARA, 1972).

V. Neurogenic Hypertension

The nervous system is concerned with the regulation of the blood pressure, and it is not unexpected that nervous stimuli and certain procedures involving control of circulation by the central nervous system should induce an elevation in blood pressure. Neurogenic hypertension, as this elevation is designated, is observed in man as a focal neurologic sign indicative of a mass lesion in the posterior fossa. An increase in intracranial pressure (the Cushing response) evokes a hypertensive response after prepontine decerebration, transection of all cranial nerves and cerebellumectomy but is abolished by transection of the spinal cord at the first cervical segment (GRIMSON, 1945; REIS and DOBA, 1972). It can also be elicited by the rapid microinjection of 1 to 3 μl of artificial spinal fluid into the grey matter of the lower brainstem or by electrical stimulation of this area.

The neurogenic hypertension which accompanies an elevation in intracranial pressure is reproducible in the experimental animal (FOLKOW and RUBINSTEIN,

1966). Trephination of the skull and application of pressure to the dura or brain, for example, causes an immediate rise in blood pressure which persists as long as the elevated pressure is maintained (GOODMAN et al., 1972). The injection of colloidal kaolin intracranially, which produces an arachnoiditis (HIRAKAWA, 1959) and elevated intracranial pressure (GRIFFITH et al., 1935), also results in a variable elevation in blood pressure, as does ligation of the vessels in the neck or stimulation or ablation of the cortical and subcortical areas of the brain. The most commonly used procedure for inducing neurogenic hypertension has been sectioning of the moderator nerves (KOCH, 1931) and subjecting animals to audiogenic (YEAKEL et al., 1948) or other noxious stimuli (DYKMAN and GANTT, 1960).

HEYMANS and NEIL (1958) and DICKINSON (1965) found that bilateral section of the carotid sinus nerves, leaving the nerves from the aortic and other baroreceptors intact, did not lead to sustained hypertension. Dogs subjected to such a procedure either become hypertensive for some days or weeks after which the blood pressure returns to normal or exhibit elevated blood pressure during periods of excitement when acute pressor influences are presumably inadequately buffered by the remaining intact baroreceptor reflexes.

DEROM (1958), using an intrathoracic approach to the cardioaortic nerves, reduced the mortality of carotid sinus and aortic denervation from 40 to 60 to 20% and induced a sustained hypertension in all cases. His procedure consisted of cutting all the fibers of the left cardio-aortic depressor and recurrent nerves, leaving the main vagal nerve intact. At a subsequent operation, the right cardio-aortic and vagus nerves were cut below the origin of the recurrent nerve and the carotid sinus was denervated bilaterally.

BURSTYN et al. (1972) have also induced chronic hypertension in rabbits by bilateral placement of rigid casts around the carotid sinus area. For this purpose they occluded the carotid artery and covered the carotid sinuses with a rapidly setting dental cement cast. When the latter had hardened, the clamp on the carotid artery was removed and the process repeated on the opposite side. After 50 days animals manifesting intact sinus reflexes maintained a sustained average rise in blood pressure of 37.6% $\pm$ 2.3 SEM. They concluded that primary interference with baroreceptor function can lead to a sustained rise in blood pressure.

Neurogenic hypertension differs hemodynamically from the hypertension induced by manipulation of the kidney, spontaneous hypertension in the rat, and essential, and other forms of hypertensive cardiovascular disease observed in the human being. The latter conditions are accompanied by an increase in peripheral resistance, the cardiac output remaining normal. In neurogenic hypertension, on the other hand, the cardiac output is increased and the blood pressure is exceedingly labile. In the dog, for example, it tends to return to normal with exercise and rest. Of particular significance is the long survival and absence of cardiac hypertrophy and arteriolosclerosis in dogs rendered hypertensive by carotid sinus denervation. DAMMIN et al. (1956), on the other hand, reported that neurogenic hypertension induced by section of the moderator nerves bilaterally in dogs, induced arteriosclerosis after 2 to $3^1/_2$ years which resembled the lesion seen in hypertension of the human being. They, therefore, regard neurogenic hypertension as an experimental counterpart of essential hypertension in man.

Although the blood pressure may remain elevated for a time after the cessation of a stressful stimulus (LAMPRECHT et al., 1973), it is questionable if this rise has any relationship to hypertensive cardiovascular disease. It would be less misleading to refer to the condition as "an elevation in blood pressure" rather than as "hypertension". The elevation in blood pressure observed in individuals manifesting so-called "labile" or "hyperkinetic" hypertension also probably reflects the instability of the blood pressure in these individuals rather than an early stage of hypertensive disease as has often been assumed.

VI. Malignant Hypertension

Malignant hypertension may be defined as a syndrome characterized by an inordinate rise in arterial pressure, focal fibrinoid arteriolar necroses (particularly in the kidneys) and retinal vascular lesions usually accompanied by papilledema. Neither the fibrinoid arteriolar necrosis nor the papilledema is, however, specific for severe hypertension. The former may occur without hypertension in polyarteriitis nodosa, at the edges of infarcts or of areas of intense vasoconstriction, and in a variety of experimental conditions (Muirhead et al., 1950). Vascular necrosis is a relatively non-specific lesion and its presence is therefore no indication that malignant hypertension has been induced by a given procedure, as is often assumed.

Goldblatt (1938) induced vascular necrosis in dogs when the renal artery was occluded to a degree sufficient to induce uremia and suggested, therefore, that malignant hypertension was due to a rise in blood pressure complicated by severe renal insufficiency. Selye (1943) considered malignant hypertension and nephrosclerosis as part of the "general adaptation syndrome". Masson et al. (1962) produced occlusive glomerular lesions, renal failure, edema and acute vascular lesions by the injection of renin preparations into rats pretreated with aldosterone and salt and suggested that high blood levels of renin and aldosterone were of pathogenetic significance in the induction of malignant hypertension. Since high levels of nephrotensin are present in the circulating blood in the malignant phase of hypertension and the lesions characteristic of the disorder can be induced by the injection of this pressor agent, Grollman (1973a) has suggested that this agent liberated from focal areas of ischemia of the kidney is responsible for the appearance of this form of hypertension.

F. Other Procedures for Inducing Experimental Hypertension

A number of other procedures have been used for inducing hypertension in laboratory animals. Since these do not represent clear-cut models of specific clinical conditions, they are being considered separately here. It is highly probable, however, that they are related pathogenetically to forms of hypertension observed in the human being and hence are of interest in elucidating the latter conditions (Selye and Stone, 1946; Skelton, 1953; Saruta et al., 1972).

I. Induction of Hypertension by Steroids and Other Hormones

Patients suffering from Cushing's disease (Gotzen et al., 1971) or other disorders of the adrenal, and those receiving adrenal steroids, androgens or estrogen-progestogen preparations as contraceptives often manifest marked elevations in blood pressure. Grollman et al. (1940) demonstrated that these steroids when administered in large doses to rats also caused an elevation in blood pressure. As shown by Selye (1943), the hypertension was accentuated by the simultaneous administration of salt.

1. Adrenal Cortical Hormones

Of the adrenal cortical steroids, DOCA as described in an earlier section, is by far the most consistent and effective pressor agent when administered with sodium chloride in the uninephrectomized animal. Aldosterone, a potent salt-retaining hormone, is believed to mediate the rise in blood pressure observed in primary aldosteronism. When injected in doses of 0.5 to 1.0 μg every 48 h for several months, it was reported to produce hypertension in sensitized rats (KUMAR et al., 1956); but GAUNT et al. (1957) and GROSS et al. (1957) failed to produce any signs of hypertensive disease or pathological lesions when this hormone was administered in doses of 40 μg/day for 32 days or 0.5 μg/day for 6 days per week for 7 months, respectively. The reason for this discrepancy remains unknown.

Crude preparations of the pituitary, presumably through their ACTH content, as well as ACTH itself also cause an elevation in blood pressure which is presumed to be secondary to their stimulting action on the adrenal cortex (PRADO, 1950).

The glucocorticoids (cortisone, cortisol, etc.), although exhibiting less sodium-retaining action than the mineralocorticoids, also cause an elevation in blood pressure (GROSS, 1960) which is probably secondary to their action on the kidney and blood vessels.

2. Sex Hormones

Other steroids, particularly the sex hormones, induce hypertension in the human being as well as in the experimental animal. This action is of practical importance particularly in their therapeutic use as contraceptive agents (FREGLEY, 1973).

MOLTENI et al. (1972) induced severe hypertension with extensive renal and cardiovascular damage in uninephrectomized female Sprague-Dawley rats receiving 1% NaCl as drinking water by the injection of 10 mg of methylandrostenediol for 10 weeks. This action is believed to be the result of an increased production of DOCA. Hypertensive vascular disease was also induced in rats by the injection of methyltestosterone (MOLTENI et al., 1972).

The demonstration that progesterone when administered over a long period to rabbits causes an elevation in blood pressure led HORROBIN (1968) to postulate that this steroid may play a pathogenetic role in the induction of eclampsia, which is also accompanied by hypertension. OKUDA and GROLLMAN (1966), on the other hand, have shown that a better model of this disease is reproducible in the rat by sensitization with placental tissue.

3. Other Hormones

BLACKET et al. (1950) reported the induction of hypertension in rabbits by the infusion of renin for periods up to 23 days. MASSON et al. (1962) reported similar effects in rats by intermittent injections of purified renin. It is doubtful if renin is concerned in these actions (WHITE and GROLLMAN, 1964a).

II. Induction of Hypertension by Other Drugs and Poisons

Hypertension is a common complication of the administration of a number of drugs and poisons, presumably as a result of injury to the kidney and blood vessels. Lead poisoning, for example, induces hypertension and obvious renal damage (GALLÉ and MOREL-MAROGER, 1965). When salts of lead or other nephrotoxic agents are incorporated in the food of rats, hypertension and renal lesions develop in a large percentage of animals, but the high mortality and morbidity attending such poisoning renders this procedure of no value as a means of inducing hypertension for experimental studies.

SCHROEDER (1964) reported the development of hypertension in rats receiving 5 parts per million of cadmium in their drinking water which was reversed by the administration of a chelate of zinc. THIND et al. (1973), on the other hand, observed only slight increases in the blood pressure of dogs injected intraperitoneally with 2 mg/kg of cadmium daily for 9 months. One week following the last injection, the cardiac output, peripheral resistance and blood pressure were unaltered from their pretreatment levels, but 3 to 5 weeks later, four of the dogs manifested a slight systolic hypertension and bradycardia. PERRY (1972) in a review of the literature found no evidence to indicate that the geochemical environment contributed to the development of hypertension.

Thyroxine, triiodothyronine and dinitrophenol accelerate the production of a sustained salt hypertension in rats, the last-named substance acting only in sexually immature animals. The observed elevation in blood pressure in animals receiving these drugs is attributable to the increased metabolism induced by the drugs and is thus comparable to the systolic hypertension noted in severe hyperthyroidism.

KELLER and ANDERSON (1972) reported that 3 separate injections of 2 mg of 7.12-dimethylbenz(α)anthracene, a potent carcinogen, produced hypertension in over 50% of rats, which persisted during the 5 months of observation. This rise in pressure which they attributed to damage of the adrenal was, however, only slight, 139 mm Hg compared to 125 mm Hg in their controls.

One would anticipate that any poison acting on the kidney, blood vessels or on the nervous system, all of which are concerned in the regulation of the blood pressure, would affect this parameter of the circulation. As in the case of the metal poisons, however, the high mortality and poor yield of hypertensive animals renders the available procedures of no value for the production of animal models of the human disorder. Unless the exact mechanism of action of these procedures is established, the demonstration of an elevation in blood pressure is of little significance in elucidating the pathogenesis of hypertension.

III. Induction of Hypertension by Activation of the Immune Mechanism

There is evidence available to indicate that the experimental induction of hypertension as well as its occurrence clinically is attributable in many cases to an activation of the immune mechanism. For example, daily injections of renal tissue for ten days, either alone or with Freund's complete adjuvant, induce irreversible hypertension in the rat (WHITE and GROLLMAN, 1962). The serum of such rats and that of animals following infarction of the kidney gives a precipitin reaction against trypsinized digests of isologous kidney and arterial tissues, and fluorescein-conjugated globulins are bound to the glomerular and basement membranes and arterial components of normal rat kidneys. Suppressants of antibody reactions (cortisone or 6-mercaptopurine) inhibit the development of hypertension following infarction (WHITE and GROLLMAN, 1964a).

Hypertension similar to that observed in the rat has also been noted in the human being following infarction of the kidney. The fact that blood sera of certain patients with hypertension and renal disease contain anti-kidney components (WHITE and GROLLMAN, 1964a) suggests that the continued destruction of the kidney and the hypertension which occurs in such renal disorders as pyelonephritis and certain other forms of chronic nephritis may be the result of an antigen-antibody response analogous to that observed in postinfarction hypertension in the rat.

OKUDA and GROLLMAN (1966) demonstrated that hypertension induced by infarction of the kidney of rats could be transferred by viable lymph node cells into rats rendered immunologically tolerant by treatment neonatally with normal rat spleen cells. OLSEN (1971) and SVENDSEN (1973) have also shown that the cellular reaction in the arterioles of rats with acute hypertension induced by angiotensin is altered by repeating the injection after a week, and by injection of thoracic duct lymphocytes from donor rats treated with angiotensin.

In view of the foregoing observations, it is probable that activation of the immune mechanism either as a result of a direct action on the kidney or on the vascular system generally (WHITE and GROLLMAN, 1964b) may be responsible for the continued development of hypertension after preliminary injections of DOCA and other steroids, following the administration of large doses of salt, etc. and the failure of patients with primary hyperaldosteronism, Cushing's syndrome, pheochromocytoma, etc. to respond to surgical intervention. In these cases, initial injury of the blood vessels may institute, through vascular damage, an autoimmune process which is maintained after withdrawal of the initial causative agent (IRINO et al., 1967; SVENDSEN, 1973).

G. Conclusion

It is obvious from the preceding discussion that a variety of procedures are available for producing hypertension in laboratory animals. In many cases the resultant disorder mimics the corresponding disorder of the human being so closely as to leave little doubt that we are dealing with the same disease. Such laboratory preparations may be used for a study of the disorder observed in man and have served to elucidate the latter disorder.

The different methods used for inducing hypertensive cardiovascular disease have in common the fact that they all appear to act on the kidney directly or on its arterial blood supply. In the rare cases of surgically remediable hypertension, in infarction of the kidney and in malignant hypertension, a pressor agent is demonstrable which mediates the rise of blood pressure. In the vast majority of cases, however, no pressor agent is demonstrable. It has been suggested, therefore, that the kidney's role in hypertension is mediated through a failure of its normal function in maintaining constancy of the internal environment. However, this seems improbable since no aberration of this function is demonstrable in essential hypertension, while in many cases where such dysfunction exists (*e.g.* some cases of amyloidosis of the kidney or cystic disease of the renal medulla), hypertension is absent. An alternative hypothesis, *viz.*, that the kidney subserves a hormonal function concerned with the maintenance of the normotensive state, would appear to be most consistent with the available facts.

References

AKAMATSU, T., IRINO, T., HAMAMOTO, Y.: Studies on the antigen-antibody reaction in the kidney. Bull. Osaka med. Sch. 8, 80–93 (1962).

ALEXANDER, N., HENSHAW, L. B., DRURY, D. R.: Further observations on development of a colony of spontaneously hypertensive rabbits. Proc. Soc. exp. Biol. (N.Y.) **86**, 855–858 (1959).

ALLBUTT, C.: Diseases of the arteries, including angina pectoris. London: Macmillan & Co. 1915.
ANITSCHKOW, N.: Ueber die Veränderung der Kaninchenaorta bei experimenteller Cholesterinsteatose. Beitr. path. Anat. **56**, 379–404 (1913).
AOKI, K., YAMORI, Y., OOSHIMA, A., OKAMOTO, K.: Effects of high or low sodium intake in spontaneously hypertensive rats. Jap. Circulat. J. (En.) **36**, 539–545 (1972).
ASHWORTH, C. T., GROLLMAN, A.: Electron microscopy in experimental hypertension. Glomerular changes in choline-deficiency-induced hypertension in the rat. Arch. Path. **68**, 148–153 (1959).
BEILIN, L. J., ZIAKAS, G.: Vascular reactivity in post-desoxycorticosterone hypertension in rats and its relation to irreversible hypertension in man. Clin. Sci. **42**, 579–590 (1972).
BEN-ISHAY, D., SALITERNIK, R., WELNER, A.: Separation of two strains of rats with inbred dissimilar sensitivity to DOCA-salt hypertension. Experientia (Basel) **28**, 1321–1322 (1972).
BLACKET, R. B., DEPOORTER, A., PICKERING, G. W., SELLERS, A. L., WILSON, G. M.: Hypertension produced in the rabbit by long continued infusions of renin. Clin. Sci. **9**, 223–245 (1950).
BRAUN-MENÉNDEZ, E., COVIAN, M. R.: Mechanismo de las hipertension de las ratas totalmente nefrectomizadas. Rev. Soc. argent. Biol. **24**, 130–133 (1948).
BROOKS, B., BROWN, G. B., MUIRHEAD, E. E.: Rectangular renal artery clip for standardized hypertension in the rat. Arch. Path. **93**, 116–117 (1972).
BROWN, R. D., GAUNT, R., GISOLDI, E., SMITH, N.: The role of deoxycorticosterone in adrenal regeneration hypertension. Endocrinology **91**, 921–924 (1972).
BURSTYN, P. G., HORROBIN, D. F., LLOYD, I. J.: Chronic hypertension in rabbits induced by bilateral placement of rigid casts around the carotid sinus regions. Cardiovasc. Res. **6**, 54–56 (1972).
CALDER, R. M.: Nutritional deficiencies as a cause of elevated blood pressure in rats (with especial reference to the Vitamin B_2 complex). J. exp. Med. **76**, 1–14 (1942).
CHANUTIN, A., FERRIS, E. B.: Experimental renal insufficiency produced by partial nephrectomy. Arch. intern. Med. **49**, 767–787 (1932).
CHART, J. J., ULSAMER, G., QUINN, L., HOWIE, N., SULLIVAN, B., GAUNT, R.: Adrenal regeneration hypertension. Endocrinology **61**, 692–700 (1957).
CLARKSON, T. B., PRICHARD, R. W., BULLOCK, B. C., LEHNER, N. D. M., LOFLAND, H. B., ST. CLAIR, R. W.: Animal models of atherosclerosis. In: Animal Models for Biomedical Research, National Academy of Sciences, 1970. Washington, D.C. **3**, 22–42 (1970).
COPELAND, D. H., SALMON, W. D.: The occurrence of neoplasms on the liver, lungs, and other tissues of rats as a result of prolonged choline deficiency. Amer. J. Path. **22**, 1059–1079 (1946).
COUSINEAU, E., BIRON, P.: Water intake: influence on development of rat saline hypertension. Experientia (Basel) **28**, 282 (1972).
DAHL, L. K., Effects of chronic excess salt feeding. Induction of self-sustaining hypertension in rats. J. exp. Med. **114**, 231–236 (1961).
DAHL, L. K., HEINE, M., TASSINARI, L.: Effects of chronic excess salt ingestion. Role of genetic factors in both DOCA-salt and renal hypertension. J. exp. Med. **118**, 605–617 (1963).
DAMMIN, G. J., GOLDMAN, M. L., SCHROEDER, H. A., PACE, M. G.: Arterial hypertension in dogs. II. The effects of neurogenic hypertension with a study of periodic renal biopsies over a seven-year period. Lab. Invest. **5**, 72–96 (1956).
DEROM, F. E.: Methode d'hypertension chronique neurogene chez le chien. Arch. int. pharmacodyn. **116**, 237–244 (1958).
DICK, G. F.: Experimental hypertension: its production in dogs by intravenous injection of streptococci. Arch. Path. **39**, 81–88 (1945).
DICKINSON, C. J.: Neurogenic hypertension. Oxford: Blackwell Scientific Publications 1965.
DIETRICH, R. A., PELT, R. W. VAN, GALSTER, W. A.: Diet-induced cholesterolemia and atherosclerosis in wild rodents. Atherosclerosis **17**, 345–352 (1973).
DREIZEN, S., LEVY, B. M., BERNICK, S.: Diet-induced atherosclerosis in the marmoset. Proc. Soc. exp. Biol. (N.Y.) **143**, 1218–1223 (1973).
DRURY, D. R.: Production by new method of renal insufficiency and hypertension in rabbit. J. exp. Med. **68**, 693–701 (1938).
DYKMAN, R. A., GANTT, H.: Experimental psychogenic hypertension: blood pressure changes conditioned to painful stimuli (schizokinesis). Bull. Johns Hopk. Hosp. **107**, 72–89 (1960).
EBIHARA, A.: Studies on the pathogenesis of experimental hypertension in rats. Jap. Circulat. J. (En.) **36**, 603–605 (1972).
EBIHARA, A., GROLLMAN, A.: Pressor activity of renal venous effluent following constriction of the renal artery in dogs. Amer. J. Physiol. **214**, 1–5 (1968).
EBIHARA, A., MARTZ, B. L., GROLLMAN, A.: Effect of withdrawal of dietary sodium in hypertensive and normotensive rats. Jap. Heart J. **11**, 365–372 (1970).

Floyer, M. A.: Further studies on mechanism of experimental hypertension in rat. Clin. Sci. **14**, 163–181 (1955).
Folkow, B., Rubinstein, E. H.: Cardiovascular effects of acute and chronic stimulation of the hypothalamic defence area in the rat. Acta physiol. scand. **68**, 48–57 (1966).
Follis, R. H., Orent-Keiles, E., McCallum, E. V.: The production of cardiac and renal lesions in rats by a diet extremely deficient in potassium. Amer. J. Path. **18**, 29–40 (1942).
Fregly, M. J.: Seminar on the role of salt in cardiovascular hypertension. Amer. J. Cardiol. **8**, 526–602, 684–756, 863–912 (1961).
Fregly, M. J.: Oral contraceptives and high blood pressure. Gainesville, Florida: Dolphin Press 1973.
Funder, J. W., Blair-West, J. R., Cain, M. C., Catt, K. J., Coghlan, J. P., Denton, D. A., Nelson, J. F., Scoggins, B. A., Wright, R. D.: Circulatory and humoral changes in the reversal of renovascular hypertension in sheep by unclipping the renal artery. Circulat. Res. **27**, 249–258 (1970).
Gallé, P., Morel-Maroger, L.: Les lésions rénales du saturnisme humain et experimental. Nephron **2**, 273–286 (1965).
Gaunt, R., Ulsamer, G. J., Chart, J. J.: Aldosterone and hypertension. Arch. int. pharmacodyn. **110**, 114–118 (1957).
Giese, J.: The pathogenesis of hypertensive vascular disease. Copenhagen: Munksgaard 1971.
Giroud, C. J. P., Stachenko, J., Venning, E. H.: Secretion of aldosterone by the zona glomerulosa of rat adrenal glands incubated *in vitro*. Proc. Soc. exp. Biol. (N.Y.) **92**, 154–158 (1956).
Goldblatt, H.: The production of persistent hypertension in monkeys (Macaque) by renal ischemia. J. exp. Med. **65**, 671–675 (1937).
Goldblatt, H.: The production of the malignant phase of hypertension. J. exp. Med. **67**, 809–826 (1938).
Goldblatt, H., Kahn, J. R., Hanzal, R. F.: The effect on blood pressure of constriction of the abdominal aorta above and below the site of origin of both main renal arteries. J. exp. Med. **69**, 649–674 (1939).
Goldblatt, H., Kahn, J. R., Lewis, H. A.: Studies on experimental hypertension. XIX. The production of persistent hypertension in sheep and goats. J. exp. Med. **77**, 297–307 (1943).
Goldblatt, H., Lynch, J., Hanzal, R. F., Summerville, W. W.: Studies on experimental hypertension: I. The production of persistent elevation of systolic blood pressure by means of renal ischemia. J. exp. Med. **59**, 347–379 (1934).
Goodman, S. J., Becker, D. P., Seelig, J.: The effects of mass-induced intracranial pressures on arterial hypertension and survival in awake cats. J. Neurosurg. **37**, 514–527 (1972).
Gotzen, R., Dissmann, T., Lohmann, F. W., Molzahn, M., Kalinke, J.: Blutvolumen und Kreislaufmechanik bei der arteriellen Hypertonie des Cushing-Syndroms. Klin. Wschr. **49**, 19–23 (1971).
Griffith, J. Q., Jr., Jeffers, W. A., Lindauer, M. A.: A study of the mechanism of hypertension following intracranial kaolin injection in rats; leucocytic reaction and effect on lymphatic absorption. Amer. J. Physiol. **113**, 285–290 (1935).
Grimson, K. S.: Blood pressure of renal and of early and late neurogenic hypertension dogs after low cervical cord section. Ann. Surg. **122**, 990–995 (1945).
Grollman, A.: A simplified procedure for inducing chronic renal hypertension in the mammal. Proc. Soc. exp. Biol. (N.Y.) **57**, 102–104 (1944a).
Grollman, A.: Experimental chronic hypertension in the rabbit. Amer. J. Physiol. **142**, 666–670 (1944b).
Grollman, A.: Experimental hypertension in the dog. Amer. J. Physiol. **147**, 647–653 (1946).
Grollman, A.: The relation of arteriolarsclerosis to hypertension as elucidated by studies on the nephrectomized dog. J. Geront. **6**, 96 (1951).
Grollman, A.: The pathogenesis and treatment of hypertension. J. Amer. Geriat. Soc. **1** 223–232 (1953).
Grollman, A.: The pathogenesis of adrenal regeneration hypertension. Endocrinology **63**, 460–463 (1958).
Grollman, A.: A unitary concept of experimental and clinical hypertensive cardiovascular disease. Perspect. Biol. Med. **2**, 208–220 (1959).
Grollman, A.: The relationship of salt and diet to diastolic hypertension. Amer. J. Cardiol. **9**, 700–703 (1962).
Grollman, A.: The humoral role of the kidney in hypertension. In: International Club on Arterial Hypertension. Paris: L'expansion scientifique francaise 1966.
Grollman, A.: Pathogenesis of hypertension and implications for its therapeutic management. Clin. Pharmacol. Ther. **10**, 755–764 (1969).
Grollman, A.: Hypertension in the opossum (Didelphis virginiana). Amer. J. Physiol. **218**, 82–85 (1970a).

Grollman, A.: Pressor activity of circulating blood after focal infarction of the kidney in the rat. Proc. Soc. exp. Biol. (N.Y.) **134**, 1120–1122 (1970b).
Grollman, A.: The spontaneous hypertensive rat: an experimental analogue of essential hypertension in the human being. In: Spontaneous hypertension—its pathogenesis and complications. Tokyo: Igaku Shoin Ltd. 1972.
Grollman, A.: The pathogenesis of malignant hypertension. IRCS. **1**, 16 (1973a).
Grollman, A.: Epidemiology of essential hypertension. In: Hahnemann symposium on hypertension. New York: Grune & Stratton 1973b.
Grollman, A.: A survey of experimental studies of renal hypertension. In: Hahnemann symposium on hypertension. New York: Grune & Stratton 1973c.
Grollman, A.: Renoprival hypertension. In: Hahnemann symposium on hypertension. New York: Grune & Stratton 1973d.
Grollman, A., Ashworth, C., Suki, W.: Atherosclerosis in the chicken. Arch. Path. **75**, 618–626 (1963).
Grollman, A., Ebihara, A.: Comparison of the pressor activity and the renin content of the renal venous effluent in patients suspected of suffering from surgically remediable hypertension. Tex. Rep. Biol. Med. **26**, 313–319 (1968).
Grollman, A., Grollman, E. F.: The teratogenic induction of hypertension. J. clin. Invest. **41**, 710–714 (1962).
Grollman, A., Harrison, T. R., Williams, J. R., Jr.: The effect of various sterol derivatives on the blood pressure of the rat. J. Pharmacol. exp. Ther. **69**, 149–155 (1940).
Grollman, A., Krishnamurty, V. S. R.: A new pressor agent of renal origin: its differentiation from renin and angiotensin. Amer. J. Physiol. **221**, 1499–1506 (1971).
Grollman, A., Muirhead, E. E., Vanatta, J.: Role of the kidney in pathogenesis of hypertension as determined by a study of the effects of bilateral nephrectomy and other experimental procedures on the blood pressure of the dog. Amer. J. Physiol. **157**, 21–30 (1949).
Grollman, A., Rule, C.: Experimentally induced hypertension in parabiotic rats. Amer. J. Physiol. **138**, 587–592 (1943).
Grollman, A., White, F. N.: Induction of renal hypertension in rats and dogs by potassium or choline deficiency. Amer. J. Physiol. **193**, 144–146 (1958).
Grollman, A., Williams, J. R., Jr.: Experimental chronic hypertension in the rat. Amer. J. Med. Sci. **204**, 73–79 (1942).
Grollman, E. F., Grollman, A.: Induction of hypertension in the frog by bilateral nephrectomy. Amer. J. Physiol. **199**, 19–21 (1960).
Gross, F.: Die Wirkung von Desoxycorticosteroneacetat und Kochsalz auf den experimentellen Hochdruck der Ratte. Arch. int. Pharmacodyn. **81**, 211–221 (1950).
Gross, F.: Adrenocortical function and renal pressor mechanism in experimental hypertension. In: Essential hypertension, an international symposium. Berlin-Göttingen-Heidelberg: Springer 1960.
Gross, F., Loustalot, P., Meier, R.: Production of experimental hypertension by aldosterone. Acta endocr. (Kbh.) **26**, 417–423 (1957).
Györkey, F., Reiser, R.: Experimental dietary arteriosclerosis in young swine. Acta morph. Acad. Sci. hung. **12**, 415–427 (1964).
Hall, C. E., Ayachi, S., Hall, O.: Salt appetite and hypertensive response to salt and to deoxycorticosterone in Sprague-Dawley and Long-Evans rats. Tex. Rep. Biol. Med. **30**, 143–153 (1972a).
Hall, C. E., Ayachi, S., Hall, O.: Salt hypertension produced by sucrose facilitation of saline consumption in Long-Evans rats. Tex. Rep. Biol. Med. **30**, 155–162 (1972b).
Hartroft, W. S., Best, C. H.: Hypertension of renal origin in rats following less than one week of choline deficiency. Brit. med. J. **1**, 423–426 (1949).
Heymans, C., Neil, E.: Reflexogenic areas of the cardiovascular system. London: Churchill 1958.
Hirakawa, A.: Experimental chronic neurogenic hypertension in dogs with piarachnitis adhesiva thoracolumbalis spinalis. Jap. Circulat. J. (En.) **23**, 1–24 (1959).
Horrobin, D. F.: Some effects of long-term progesterone treatment in rabbits and their relevance to pre-eclampsia. Lancet **1**, 170–173 (1968).
Irino, T., Okuda, T., Grollman, A.: Changes induced in the glomeruli of the kidney of rats by placental extracts as observed with the electron microscope. Amer. J. Path. **50**, 421–433 (1967).
Jeffers, W. A., Lindauer, M. A., Twaddle, P. H., Wolferth, C. C.: Experimental hypertension in nephrectomized parabiotic rats. Amer. J. med. Sci. **199**, 815–818 (1940).
Kawabe, K., Merrill, J. P., Oken, D. E.: Role of the kidney in hypertension due to renal infarction in the rat, determined by renal transplantation. Jap. Circulat. J. (En.) **36**, 607–610 (1972).

KELLER, J. A., ANDERSON, K. M.: Hypertension in Sprague-Dawley rats after single or multiple challenge with DMBA. Res. Commun. Chem. Pathol. Pharmacol. **3**, 123–128 (1972).
KEMPF, G. F., PAGE, I. H.: Production of experimental hypertension and the indirect determination of systolic arterial pressure in rats. J. Lab. clin. Med. **27**, 1192–1196 (1942).
KOCH, E.: Die reflektorische Selbststeuerung des Kreislaufes. Leipzig: Steinkopf 1931.
KOLETSKY, S.: Hypertensive vascular disease produced by salt. Lab. Invest. **7**, 377–386 (1958).
KUMAR, D., ANDERSON, W., GORNALL, A. G.: Postmortem study of rats made hypertensive by aldosterone. J. Clin. Endocr. **16**, 918 (1956).
LAMPRECHT, F., WILLIAMS, R. B., KOPIN, I. J.: Serum dopamine-beta-hydroxylase during development of immobilization-induced hypertension. Endocrinology **92**, 953–956 (1973).
LEDINGHAM, J. M.: Extrarenal factors in the pathogenesis of hypertension. In: Hypotensive drugs. London: Pergamon Press 1956.
LENEL, R., KATZ, L. M., RODBARD, S.: Arterial hypertension in the chicken. Amer. J. Physiol. **152**, 557–562 (1948).
LOOMIS, D.: Hypertension and necrotizing arteritis in the rat following renal infarction. Arch. Path. **41**, 231–268 (1946).
MADDOCKS, I.: Dietary factors in the genesis of hypertension. In: Nutrition. Proceedings of the Sixth International Congress Edinburgh: Livingstone 1964.
MALYUSZ, O., MENDOZA-OSORIO, V., OCHWADT, B.: Nierenfunktion bei Ratten mit experimentellem DOCA-Hochdruck. Pflügers Arch. ges. Physiol. **332**, 28–39 (1972).
MASSON, T. M. C., MIKASA, A., YASUDA, H.: Experimental vascular disease elicited by aldosterone and renin. Endocrinology **71**, 505–512 (1962).
MENEELY, G. R., TUCKER, R. G., DARBY, W. J., AUERBACH, S. H.: Chronic sodium chloride toxicity: hypertension, renal and vascular lesions. Ann. intern. Med. **39**, 991–998 (1953).
MOLTENI, A., BROWNIE, A. C.: Incidence of salt-induced hypertension in rats from different stocks. J. Med. (Basel) **3**, 193–198 (1972).
MOLTENI, A., BROWNIE, A. C., NICKERSON, P. A., SKELTON, F. R.: Irreversibility of methylandrostenediol-induced hypertension in the rat after suspension of the androgen treatment. Amer. J. Path. **69**, 179–193 (1972).
MOLTENI, A., BROWNIE, A. C., SKELTON, F. R.: Production of hypertensive vascular disease in the rat by methyltestosterone. Lab. Invest. **21**, 129–137 (1969).
MOSES, C.: Production of renal hypertension by injection of finely divided silica into the renal artery. Proc. Soc. exp. Biol. (N.Y.) **85**, 590–592 (1954).
MOSES, C., LONGABAUGH, G. M., GEORGE, R. S.: Production of hypertension following choline deficiency in weanling rats. Proc. Soc. exp. Biol. (N.Y.) **75**, 660–661 (1950).
MUIRHEAD, E. E., GROLLMAN, A., VANATTA, J.: Hypertensive cardiovascular disease ("malignant hypertension"). Changes in canine tissues induced by various manipulations of the kidney, with special reference to vascular and myocardial lesions. Arch. Path. **50**, 137–150 (1950).
OGDEN, E., COLLINGS, W. D., SAPIRSTEIN, L. A.: A change of mechanism in the course of hypertension of renal origin. Special Publications N.Y. Acad. Sci. **3**, 153–167 (1946).
OKAMOTO, K. (ed.): Spontaneous hypertension—its pathogenesis and complications. Tokyo: Igaku Shoin Ltd. 1972.
OKAMOTO, K., AOKI, K.: Development of a strain of spontaneously hypertensive rats. Jap. Circulat. J. (En.) **27**, 282–293 (1963).
OKUDA, T., GROLLMAN, A.: Renal lesions in rats following injection of placental extracts. Arch. Path. **82**, 246–258 (1966).
OLSEN, F.: Inflammatory cellular reaction in hypertensive vascular disease. Copenhagen: Munksgaard 1971.
ORMSBEE, H. S., RYAN, C. F.: Production of hypertension with desoxycorticosterone acetate-impregnated silicone rubber implants. J. pharm. Sci. **62**, 255–257 (1973).
PARWARESCH, M. R., MADER, C., HILL, W., WISWEDEL, K.: Ein kombiniertes Verfahren zur Erzeugung von Arteriosklerose bei Kaninchen. Z. ges. exp. Med. **160**, 269–291 (1973).
PERRY, H. M., JR.: Hypertension and the geochemical environment. Ann. N.Y. Acad. Sci. **199**, 202–216 (1972).
PLATT, R.: Das Wesen der essentiellen Hypertonie. In: Essentielle Hypertonie, ein internationales Symposium. Berlin-Göttingen-Heidelberg: Springer 1960.
PRADO, J. L.: Estudos Sobre Hipertensao Hormonal Experimental. Thesis, Sao Paulo 1950.
REIS, D. J., DOBA, N.: Hypertension as a localizing sign of mass lesions of brainstem. New Engl. J. Med. **287**, 1355–1356 (1972).
SAPIRSTEIN, L. A., BRANDT, W. L., DRURY, D. H.: Production of hypertension in the rat by substituting hypertonic sodium chloride for drinking water. Proc. Soc. exp. Biol. (N.Y.) **73**, 82–85 (1950).

SARUTA, T., OZAWA, Y., SEIICHI, A.: The mechanism of estrogen hypertension. Jap. Circulat. J. (En.) **36**, 611–616 (1972).
SCANU, A., ORIENTE, P., SZAJEWSKI, J. M., MCCORMACK, L. J., PAGE, I. H.: Triton hyperlipemia in dogs. J. exp. Med. **114**, 279–294 (1961).
SCHROEDER, H. A.: Cadmium hypertension in rats. Amer. J. Physiol. **207**, 62–66 (1964).
SELYE, H.: On the production of malignant hypertension by chronic exposure to various damaging agents. Rev. canad. Biol. **2**, 501–505 (1943).
SELYE, H., HALL, C. E., ROWLEY, E. M.: Malignant hypertension produced by treatment with desoxycorticosterone acetate and sodium chloride. Canad. med. Ass. J. **49**, 88–92 (1943).
SELYE, H., STONE, H.: Pathogenesis of the cardiovascular and renal changes which usually accompany malignant hypertension. J. Urol. (Baltimore) **56**, 399–419 (1946).
SHAPIRO, A. P., KOBERNICK, J. L.: Susceptibility of rats with renal hypertension to pyelonephritis and predisposition of rats with chronic pyelonephritis to hormonal hypertension. Circulat. Res. **9**, 869–880 (1961).
SHIBATA, N., YAMAGAMI, T., YONEDA, H., AKAGAMI, H.: A consideration of a mechanism of hypertension through effects of ions upon the contractility of arterial tissue and its contractile protein. Jap. Circulat. J. (En.) **36**, 575–581 (1972).
SKELTON, F. R.: The production of hypertension, nephrosclerosis and cardiac lesions by methylandrostenediol treatment in the rat. Endocrinology **53**, 492–505 (1953).
SKELTON, F. R.: Development of hypertension and cardiovascular renal lesions during adrenal regeneration in the rat. Proc. Soc. exp. Biol. (N.Y.) **90**, 342–346 (1955).
SMIRK, F. H., HALL, W. H.: Inherited hypertension in rats. Nature (Lond.) **182**, 727–728 (1958).
SMITH, R. L., HILKER, D. M.: Experimental dietary production of aortic atherosclerosis in Japanese quail. Atherosclerosis **17**, 63–70 (1973).
SOKABE, H.: Experimental Hypertension: an Introductory Textbook. Tokyo: Eikodo 1968.
SOKABE, H., GROLLMAN, A.: Pressor activity of renal venous effluent of normal and hypertensive rats. Amer. J. Physiol. **205**, 264–266 (1963a).
SOKABE, H., GROLLMAN, A.: A study of hypertension in the rat induced by infarction of the kidney. Tex. Rep. Biol. Med. **21**, 93–100 (1963b).
STEINER, A., KENDALL, F. E., BEVANS, M.: Production of arteriosclerosis in dogs by cholesterol and thiouracil feeding. Amer. Heart J. **38**, 34–42 (1949).
STROIA, L. N., BOHR, D. F., VOCKE, L.: Experimental hypertension in the hamster. Amer. J. Physiol. **179**, 154–158 (1954).
SVENDSEN, V. G.: Increased cellular reaction to damage caused by angiotensin in arterioles or normal recipient rats after transfer of lymphocytes from hypertensive rats. Acta path. microbiol. scand. **81**, 241–246 (1973).
TAKATS, G. DE, LINDSTROM, B. L., MEDGYESY, S. L., WIBIN, E. L.: Experimental production of renal hypertension. Ann. Surg. **156**, 292–326 (1962).
TAKEDA, T., GROLLMAN, A.: Spontaneously occurring renal disease in the guinea pig. Amer. J. Path. **60**, 103–118 (1970).
THIND, G. S., BIERY, D. N., BOVEE, K. C.: Production of arterial hypertension by cadmium in the dog. J. Lab. clin. Med. **81**, 549–556 (1973).
VOGEL, J. A.: Salt-induced hypertension in the dog. Amer. J. Physiol. **210**, 186–190 (1966).
WHITE, F. N., GROLLMAN, A.: Autoimmune factors associated with infarction of the kidney. Nephron **1**, 93–102 (1964a).
WHITE, F. N., GROLLMAN, A.: Experimental periarteritis nodosa in the rat. Arch. Path. **78**, 31–36 (1964b).
WILHELMJ, C. M., SHUPUT-MEYERS, D., MCCARTHY, H. H.: Prolonged diastolic hypertension of dietary origin. Exp. Med. Surg. **14**, 286–298 (1956).
YEAKEL, E. H., SHENKIN, H. A., ROTHBALLER, A. B., MCCANN, S. M.: Blood pressures of rats subjected to auditory stimulation. Amer. J. Physiol. **155**, 118–127 (1948).
ZBINDEN, F.: Neues Verfahren zur experimentellen Erzeugung permanenten bzw. reversiblen Hochdruckes durch standardisierte Kompression der Niere. Helv. physiol. pharmacol. Acta **4**, 513–530 (1946).

Experimental Production of Atherosclerosis: Nutritional Influences[1]

S. Heyden

With 4 Figures

A. Introduction

In an equally elegant and confusing editorial—confusing because of the multitude of contradictory findings in a few animals of several different species—Professor Vastesaeger (1968) reached the following conclusion: "*In the present state of knowledge, the contribution of comparative arterial pathology to the understanding of human atherosclerosis is not very great* ... Further research work is needed to shed light on the actual causes of the specific differences in vulnerability to spontaneous atherosclerosis before definite conclusions may be drawn ... Well established specific differences must be kept in mind. They emphasize the danger of transposing facts of experimental atherosclerosis from one species to another."

Inspite of many well-recognized limitations on the applicability of results derived from animal experiments to the human atherosclerotic process, this writer has been impressed by two distinct pointers from experimental work; one, the role of arterial tissue susceptibility in atherogenesis (Haimovici and Maier, 1971) and two, variations in atherogenic reactions to the same stimuli in different vascular beds. Both of these pointers may in time help to explain still puzzling epidemiological observations, regional differences as well as so-called "racial" differences, the differing roles of hypertension and cigarette smoking in cerebrovascular disease versus peripheral vascular disease, or the influence of hypercholesterolemia in ischemic heart disease and the apparent lack of any influence on intracerebral vascular disease, the role of diabetes in atherogenesis in industrialized nations versus developing countries, to name but a few of many unsolved problems. From a literature which counts legions, the two experimental results mentioned (vide supra) will be described briefly before evaluating a selection of a few important studies of recent years.

The nature of the vessel wall may be a determinant in the differential rates of atherogenesis. This was suggested by experimental studies in which surgically transposed aortic and pulmonary artery segments maintained the atherosclerotic propensities characteristic of their original locations.

Haimovici and Maier summarized in 1964 their animal experiments which were based on the well-recognized fact of a predilection of the human abdominal aorta for developing atherosclerosis in contrast to the thoracic segment. "Fresh thoracic and abdominal aortic homografts were implanted into the abdominal aorta of dogs subsequently subjected to a chronic atherogenic regimen. The thoracic implants exhibited minimal or no atheromatous changes in contrast to

[1] From the Department of Community Health Sciences, Duke University Medical Center, Durham, North Carolina (USA) 27710.

the abdominal implants which always developed marked lesions." In another experiment, thoracic and abdominal homografts were implanted into the thoracic aorta. While the thoracic implants, again, were only mildly affected by the same degree and duration of hypercholesterolemia, the abdominal implants were markedly involved by the atherosclerotic process and thus demonstrated the high susceptibility to induced hypercholesterolemia. This suggests "that susceptibility of the arterial tissue itself rather than its location in the aorta may determine the development and degree of atherosclerosis". WOYDA et al. (1960) exchanged autografts of the abdominal aorta and pulmonary artery. The aortic graft segment in the pulmonary circulation developed gross atheromatous plaques in contradistinction to the absence of lesions in the transposed pulmonary artery segment in the abdominal aorta. HAIMOVICI and MAIER concluded: "The biologic dissimilarity between the abdominal and thoracic aortic segments is most likely only a difference in degree of susceptibility of atherosclerosis. High levels of hypercholesterolemia for prolonged periods may occasionally narrow or obscure the differences between the two segments."

Many years ago, STAMLER and co-workers (1963) observed marked discrepancies in the experimental production of atherosclerosis between the aorta and coronary arteries of cockerels fed an atherogenic diet, one group, however, being simultaneously treated with estrogens. "After several weeks of this experimental regimen the two groups of birds were sacrificed and studied histologically. Gross examination quickly revealed the presence of marked atherogenesis in the aortas of both groups. The estrogen-treated birds had at least as much aortic atherosclerosis as did the controls, similarly fed cholesterol-fat but receiving no hormone. In subsequent detailed histological studies, however, it became apparent that the estrogen-treated birds—in marked contrast to the controls—were practically free of lesions in the coronary arterial tree. Thus, segmental differences in atherogenesis were demonstrated, indicating that both systemic metabolic factors and local factors influence the process of atherogenesis. Thus, it remains a puzzle why—if a systemic lipid metabolic factor is the key—the outcome is different in aorta versus coronary arteries."

Another dimension to this aspect of segmental differences in atherogenesis has been added with the time factor (MANNING and CLARKSON, 1972). Experiments with rhesus monkeys placed on an atherogenic diet revealed fatty streaks in the aorta and coronary arteries after 4 to 6 months. Plaque formation was seen in only a few animals at this point. After 18 months on the same diet, fatty streaks became visible in the common carotid, renal, mesenteric and common iliac arteries. Almost all monkeys had developed severe extensive atherosclerosis of the abdominal aorta (not the thoracic aorta!), but plaque formation was also common in the aortic arch and near the origin of the major branches of the thoracic aorta. The cholesterol content of the aortic tissue increased with the time the atherogenic diet was fed. Early and advanced lesions appeared, morphologically like those of man, even in the same time sequences for different vascular beds. The generalized lipidosis, which occurs frequently in rabbits, did not occur in the monkeys.

B. The Peanut Oil Problem

During the past 60 years, atherogenesis has been produced innumerable times in experimental animals by means of dietary changes. ANITSCHKOW, in 1913, was the first to demonstrate a causal relationship between a high saturated fatty acid diet and severe degrees of atherosclerosis. My objective is not to review the methods and results of animal experiments of the past six decades but to examine some of the more recent significant experiments.—It is of great practical value, e.g. to find that peanut oil, which was generally regarded as one of the more "desirable" oils in modern nutrition, may not be desirable after all. It was in general use until recently because of its relatively low saturation, containing 31% polyunsaturated fatty acids. According to HOWARD (1972), it is experimentally very easy to produce fatty streaks in animals, whereas fibrous plaques are rarely seen. However, by feeding peanut oil, fibrous plaques can be induced readily in rats, rabbits, dogs and monkeys. WISSLER et al. (1967) found that peanut oil when fed to rats on a high-cholesterol diet causes atherosclerosis. Peanut oil seemed even more atherogenic than either butter or corn oil when rhesus monkeys were fed a diet containing 2% cholesterol and 25% fat for a year. The next step in the clarification of an adverse effect of peanut oil was the finding by KRITCHEVSKY et al. (1971) that the structure of fats is decisive in atherogenesis. First, he showed that the atherogenic effect of peanut oil was similar to that of coconut oil and that both were considerably more atherogenic than corn oil or an artificial oil (peanut oil from which arachidic and behenic acids were removed). As expected, atherosclerosis in rabbits fed corn oil was less apparent than in those fed the artificial oil. Visualized grossly, the character of the lesions seemed different: In animals on peanut oil the lesions were raised and sometimes very thick, while in the animals fed coconut oil the lesions were pale yellow and relatively flat. Although animals fed corn oil had lesions, these were small, pale and only slightly elevated. The lesions of the animals on the artificial oil diet (peanut oil minus the 2 long-chained saturated fatty acids, arachidic and behenic acids) were similar in appearance, but less severe than those in the group fed peanut oil. The practical value of this experimental finding is significant: In a country like the United States whole generations of children are being raised on peanut butter, simultaneously with a high cholesterol diet!

C. Dietary-Induced Cerebral Atherosclerosis

Most investigators would agree with STUDER and REBER (1963) that "experimental atherosclerosis" as a concept for clarification of etiology, early detection, prevention or intervention "is a promise that cannot be kept". However, there are pointers from experimental research and from experimentally induced atherogenesis which are of great importance such as the recently reported experimental cerebro-atherosclerosis in dogs and pigs.

As SUZUKI (1972) has demonstrated, prolonged feeding with an atherogenic diet can induce occlusive disease of the intracranial arteries and cerebral infarction in dogs. The morphologic findings suggest that separation of the internal elastic lamina from the endothelial basement membrane is a consistent change and probably an initiating mechanism in the pathogenesis of atherosclerosis of the cerebral arteries. There is no evidence at the present time from prospective epidemiologic studies (Framingham, Evans County, Los Angeles and others) that factors of human nutrition are involved in the atherogenesis of the *intra*cerebral arteries. There is, however, indirect evidence for the development in *extra*cranial major arteries in man, of severe stenosing lesions parallel to the lesions seen in coronary arteries of man. Atherosclerosis apparently also can be produced readily in the extracranial major arteries by dietary means in various mammals. On the other hand, the problem of intracerebral atherosclerosis and intracerebral infarction (without embolization) is still a subject of discussion in regard to etiology.

It is therefore most important to encourage at this point animal experimentators to continue their work with cerebral atherosclerosis particularly in dogs, monkeys and swine. RATCLIFFE et al. (1970) have convincingly shown that swine can be highly valuable experimental models for studies of coronary *and* cerebral atherosclerosis. They develop significant lesions of both arterial systems within 1 year without the dietary manipulations that have so long been necessary in the experimental study of atherosclerosis. Swine are readily available at reasonable costs from established breeding lines. In their study, extramural coronary, aortic and intracranial atherosclerosis was most advanced in swine that were fed garbage. Cerebral infarction was most advanced in the garbage-fed swine, but it also developed in swine of younger age groups, in which it was associated with atherosclerosis of small intracranial extracerebral arteries. The authors found that the morphologic changes were identical with those in the corresponding stages of human atherosclerosis in all 3 arterial systems: aorta, coronary and cerebral arteries.

D. Recent Atherosclerosis-Regression Studies (Aorta and Coronary Artery Only)

DAYTON et al.[2] (1969) remarked that since regression of atherosclerotic lesions in man could hardly be proved, it would be satisfactory to stop the development of a progressively worsening disease of the coronary arteries by means of dietary intervention. In several species of animals reversibility of atherosclerosis has been demonstrated. Even ANITSCHKOW (1933) claimed that arterial lesions of rabbits regressed when the serum cholesterol level returned to normal and that this process took an extremely long time. ANITSCHKOW described *loss of visible lipid* from lesions in the rabbit in regression studies. He studied *aortic lesions only*. HORLICK and KATZ (1949) described partial reversibility of intimal lesions in the *coronary arteries* of chicken in a pioneering dietary regression study! BORTZ (1968) concluded from his own experiments in rabbits that even significant lesions in the aortas after short-term cholesterol feeding decreased markedly some weeks after the serum cholesterol had returned to normal levels (that is, after appropriate dietary changes). He also referred to isotope experiments which demonstrated that there is an exchange of arterial and blood cholesterol, indicating potentiality of retrogression of the lesions. More important, ARMSTRONG et al. (1970) demonstrated unequivocally that uncomplicated (non-ulcerated) coronary atheromas can regress *in primates* under appropriate dietary changes. (More importantly, because investigations were not limited to the aorta but were extended to the coronary arteries and were done over a period of 17 months.) In the result section of this paper, the morphologic findings were most interesting: the average luminal narrowing in the control group (not on a regression diet) was 58%. In the regression groups, over-all narrowing was 22% in one group fed corn oil and 18% in the group fed a low-fat diet. It must be mentioned, however, that both so-called regression diets were cholesterol-free. As the authors pointed out, a critical question was whether the mass of intimal tissue found in regression animals was in fact less or whether the cross-sectional dimensions of the arteries of animals studied after regression diets were greater than those studied without any intervention. "The absolute mean intimal area was more than 3 times greater in the

[2] "There is every logical and pathophysiological reason to believe that stabilization of the degree of atherosclerosis would alone be sufficient to achieve all the goals of primary prevention, and that even reduction in the rate of growth of atheromata could yield major benefits."

untouched group than in the regression diet groups. Furthermore the total lumen-intima-media areas show that dilatation could not be detected by significant differences in average total transverse area among the groups." To the authors the most notable evidence *in favor of regression through diet* was found in the histologic differences of the coronary sections in the regression groups compared to the control group (not treated by diet).

It was concluded that the regression diets (cholesterol-free and either low in fat or enriched with corn oil) were approximately equal in effect as judged by the residual intimal narrowing of the lumen. However, the relatively small numbers of monkeys assigned to each of the regression diets prevented more than tentative assessments of their comparative merit. Within 60 days after the 2 regression diets were started, the serum cholesterol of the hypercholesterolemic animals had returned to the levels observed at the start of the study with little subsequent change. The study practically confirmed an earlier study by MARUFFO and PORTMAN (1968) in which squirrel monkeys on a butter-containing diet developed coronary atherosclerosis—a corn oil-containing control diet stopped or partially inhibited the process!

ARMSTRONG and co-workers (1970) were concerned about one point in their study, that they had to deal with *uncomplicated coronary atheromas. No ulceration was found* in any lesion in these studies. Interestingly, a morphologic study showed a condensation rather than a decrease in the *intimal connective tissue* after regression. But at the same time there was strong evidence that the diets caused a large loss of lipid in the atheromatous tissue under study. The problem in human beings with advanced atherosclerotic disease remains open, i.e. how lesions significantly complicated by hemorrhage, ulceration, massive accretion of scleroproteins, necrosis and calcium formation might respond in comparable dietary settings.

DEPALMA et al. (1970) pointed out that hyperlipidemia plays a dominant role in initiating the atherosclerotic lesion in the experimental dog. They also found that regression of atheromas can occur under conditions favoring reabsorption of cholesterol from the lesion, such as reduction of the serum cholesterol level. Their animal experiment was complicated by the fact that all dogs were thyroidectomized. The advantage of this study was that each dog served as his own control and that the changes in individual lesions were judged in relation to their previously observed morphologic appearance. The severity of lesions in the inferior mesenteric artery was estimated to parallel the degree of involvement with the aorta and coronary arteries. While in the hypothyroid dogs the return to a normal regression diet alone did not result in effective reduction of hypercholesterolemia or in a decrease in plaque formation in the inferior mesenteric artery, the authors stated that "progression and regression is the function of the concentration of serum cholesterol and the duration of hypercholesterolemia. Weight loss was not a factor in inducing regression, as several actually gained weight while the lesions were regressing after the atherogenic regimen was discontinued and internal biliary diversion established."

TUCKER et al. (1971) also reported that early uncomplicated cholesterol-induced aortic lesions in rhesus monkeys were definitely reversible and that qualitative changes in the lesions occurred 16 weeks after withdrawal from the diet. "From this study, it appears that lipid moves from an intracellular to an extracellular position when the high-cholesterol stimulus is removed ... If the fate of all or many of the monocytes in the progression animals is degeneration and liberation of their contents, then this may be the source of the increased extracellular lipid seen in the regression lesions."

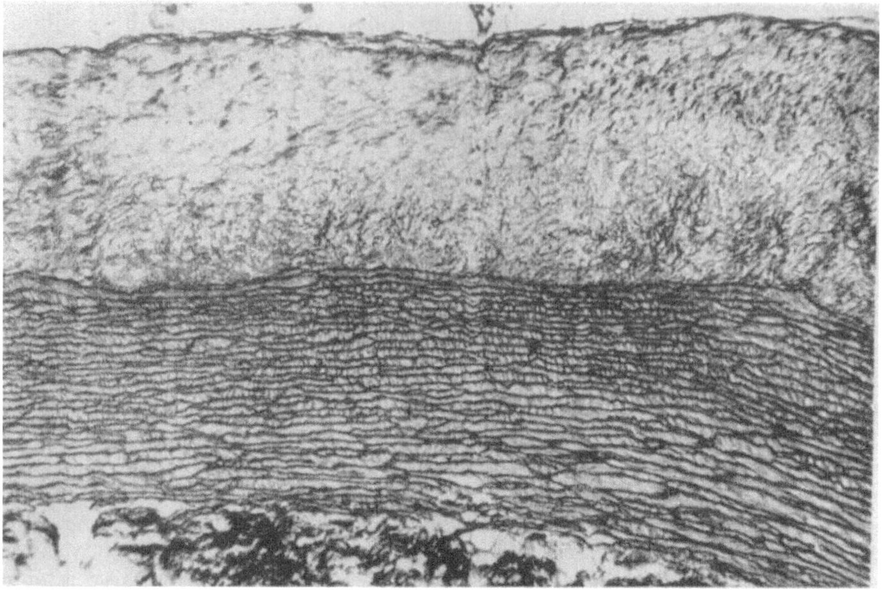

Fig. 1. Organized plaque and absence of foam cells in the aorta of an animal of the *soybean oil-fed group*. (With kind permission of the authors BULLER and VLES)

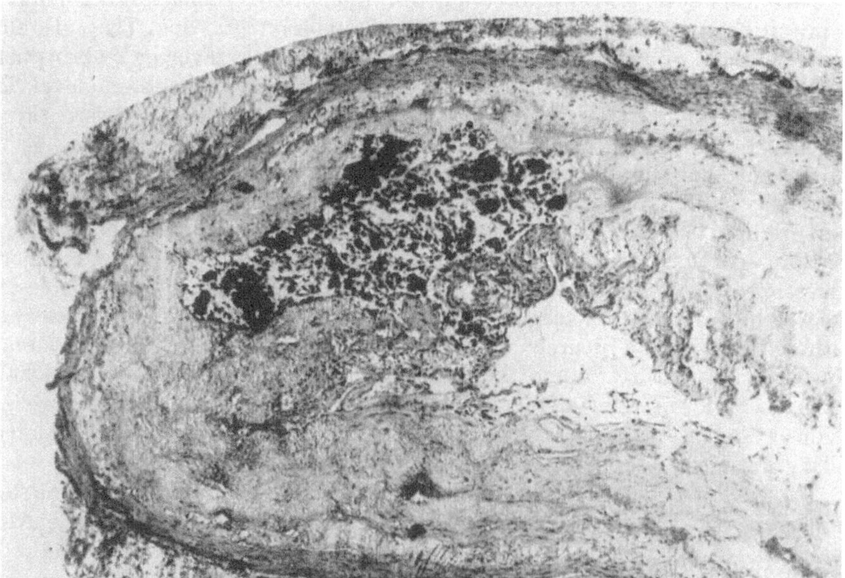

Fig. 2. The atheromatous mass in the aortic plaque of an animal of the *coconut oil group* is calcified and protrudes into the lumen. There is no subendothelial fibrosis on that site. Narrowing and even disappearance of the media. (With kind permission of the authors BULLER and VLES)

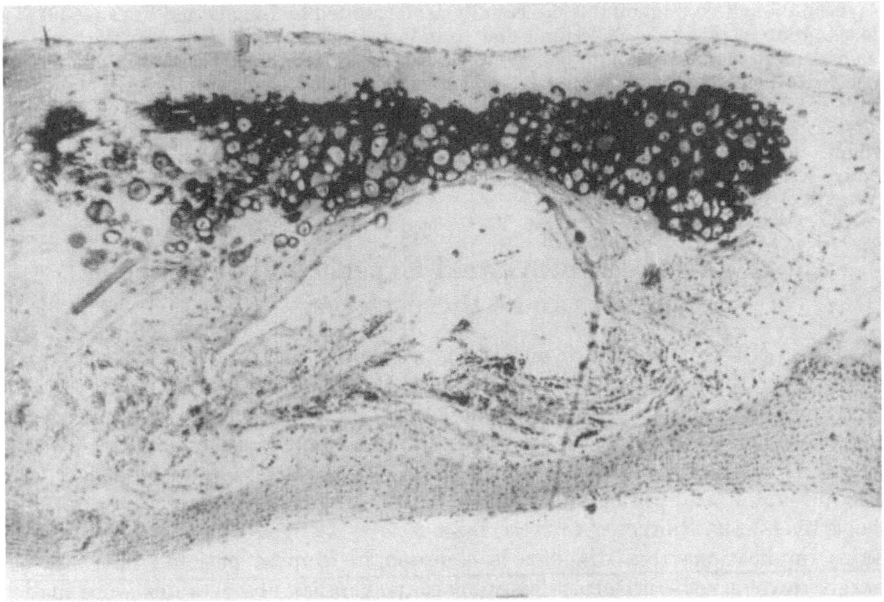

Fig. 3. Cartilage formation in a calcified mass of an animal of the *coconut oil group*. Narrowing of the media. The cavern was probably filled with fatty material with slight calcium deposit on the medial side. (With kind permission of the authors BULLER and VLES)

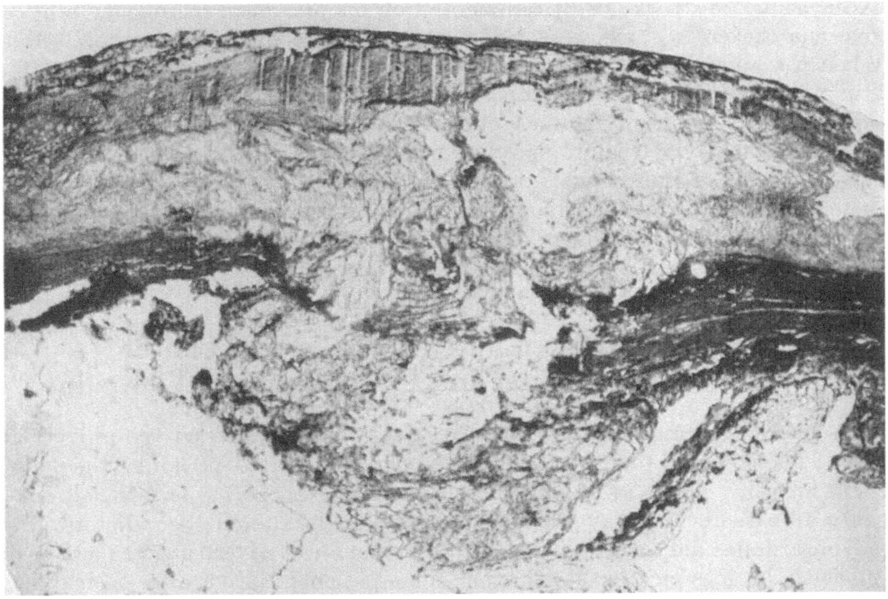

Fig. 4. Intimal capsule of collagen fibers in an animal of the *coconut oil group*. The media is locally ruptured. The atheromatous mass penetrates into the adventitia. (With kind permission of the authors BULLER and VLES)

One of the earlier attempts to show differences in the reaction of the aorta in rabbits to soybean oil and coconut oil was successfully demonstrated by BÜLLER and VLES (1966). They fed a group of rabbits a cholesterol diet to induce atheromatous plaques in the aorta. The animals were then divided into one group fed saturated fatty acids (coconut oil) and another one fed a highly polyunsaturated fatty acid-containing oil (soybean oil). In this long-term experiment the investigators demonstrated convincingly that the feeding of *soybean oil retarded the further development of a cholesterol-induced lesion:* The histological picture showed fibrotic changes with even a reparative tendency (Fig. 1). In contrast, coconut oil caused active lesions with much cellularity, ulceration, calcification, medial damage and sometimes aneurysm (Figs. 2, 3, 4).

E. Lessons from Animal Experiments in Diabetes and Atherosclerosis

KEEN (1972) concluded from his studies that diabetics are not "condemned" to develop atherosclerotic disease. He quoted a Japanese-American autopsy study in which only 5% of 865 Japanese diabetics died from ischemic heart disease. On the other hand 54% of 1283 American diabetics died of ischemic heart disease—a difference which was so large that it could not be accounted for by differences in the method of autopsy or in differences of criteria or definitions. The remarkable book by ISRAEL SNAPPER, *Chinese Lessons to Western Medicine (1941)*, also contains implications that diabetes is common in Chinese patients but that they rarely develop atherosclerotic complications. Similar observations were made in Ceylon. BRUNNER (1972) drew attention to the relative absence of vascular disease, including coronary artery disease, in Yemenite Jews who suffered from diabetes. In 76 diabetic Yemenites 50% needed more than 30 units insulin per day and 50% suffered from clinical diabetes for more than 5 years. Only 1 man had a myocardial infarction. No pathological electrocardiographic changes were detected in the other 75. There were no cases of cerebrovascular or peripheral vascular disease. In view of these epidemiologic findings, it was interesting to review animal experiments. STAMLER (1972) commented on his previous experiments in hyperglycemic cockerels which were made atherosclerotic by cholesterol-fat feeding. When the animals were taken off their atherogenic diet, it was observed that insulin delayed regression of lesions, in other words, insulin did not aid in resolution of atherosclerosis (STAMLER et al., 1960). Dr. STAMLER (1972) remarked: "Given the ability of insulin to produce hypoglycemia, the consequent outpouring of catecholamines and corticoid, and the interplay between high serum lipids and these factors (and their effects on blood pressure for example), it is not hard to conceive that these treatment regimens for diabetes, *high animal fat diet plus insulin*, may aggravate atherogenesis."

F. "Polyunsaturated Fatty Acid Diet and Cancer" — From the Experimental and Epidemiological Viewpoint

A recent editorial in the American Heart Journal carried the provocative title: "The potential toxicity of excessive polyunsaturates—do not let the patient harm himself" (PINCKNEY, 1973). After lamenting about the fact that 9 out of every 10 patients who say they have intentionally altered their diet to stress polyunsaturates did so as a direct result of commercial advertising or news media publicity, he goes on to complain that these patients did not alter their dietary intake on the advice of or even with the knowledge of their personal physician. Of course, this could easily be interpreted as a *lack of information* on the part *of the physician* who has not taken the time to keep up with the latest developments in nutritional physiology. Dr. PINCKNEY goes on to warn that patients may harm themselves by adhering to a high polyunsaturated fatty acid diet. His reasoning: "There have been innumerable reports that show that an excess of polyunsaturates in the diet do seem to have a number of serious side effects (including death); more so in animals, to be sure, but also in humans ... and there is certainly a reasonable epidemiological association between a diet high in polyunsaturates and the increased incidence of cancer (especially gastric) in humans." The evidence is, by no means, as Dr. PINCKNEY likes to think, convincing that polyunsaturated fatty acid diets are carcinogenic or in any way harmful. The question of undesirable side effects from the long-term use of a low cholesterol diet with emphasis on polyunsaturated fatty acids briefly developed into a major public concern after the publication of an article by Drs. PEARCE and DAYTON (1971): "Incidence of Cancer in Men on a Diet High on Polyunsaturated Fat." In their 8-year-controlled clinical trial of a diet high in polyunsaturated vegetable oils and low in saturated fat and cholesterol, 174 deaths were noted in the experimental group and 178 deaths in the control group. Thirty-one of the 174 deaths in the experimental group were due to cancer as opposed to 17 of 178 deaths in the control group. The authors, unfortunately, concluded from their findings that it is "premature to make a blanket prescription of a diet high in polyunsaturated fat for the entire population", implying that their data could mean that the polyunsaturated fatty acid diet might have had a co-carcinogenic effect in the experimental group. However, a review of the table showing adherence to diet in patients with fatal carcinomas during the diet phase clarifies the situation and removes any doubt that the diet high in polyunsaturated fatty acids and low in cholesterol might have had anything to do with carcinogenesis or co-carcinogenesis: not less than 12 cases of fatal carcinoma were found in persons who adhered less than 20% of the time to the experimental diet.

Table 1. Adherence to diet in patients with fatal carcinoma during the diet phase. Adherence, calculated from attendance records, is expressed as a percentage of the maximum number of meals which could have been taken in the study dining-hall. (From PEARCE and DAYTON, 1971)

Adherence (%)	Control group	Experimental group	Adherence (%)	Control group	Experimental group
0–10	2	10	50– 60	3	3
10–20	1	2	60– 70	0	4
20–30	1	3	70– 80	2	2
30–40	0	0	80– 90	4	1
40–50	3	3	90–100	1	3

Only 19 persons from the experimental group, thus, died with cancer and adhered to the prescribed diet between 20 and 100% during the 8-year-observation period. Therefore, any statistical significance is automatically removed between the control and the experimental group since people in the experimental group who did not adhere to the diet can hardly be called dieters. It was, therefore, not surprising that another group of *4 investigators* (EDERER et al., 1971) found that the *results of their studies* "are consistent with the hypothesis that the *cholesterol-lowering diets do not influence cancer risk*".

The problem, then, has been solved in prospective epidemiological observations. But where did the idea—the idea that polyunsaturated fatty acids might be harmful and even carcinogenic—originate? We have reviewed the literature on the most frequently quoted allegations of an association of dietary fat intake and gastric cancer. At present it is safe to state that thus far, evidence from animal experiments and a few retrospective studies of human cancer patients, concerning cancer induction with dietary fats, has had an academic interest only.

O'GARA et al. (1969) concluded from *animal studies* that "corn oil appears to contain either more of the carcinogen or a more potent one than hydrogenated fat" and, therefore, suggested that it would be "advisable to avoid the excessive reuse of cooking fats in the preparation of foods for human consumption". Two retrospective studies of *human stomach cancer patients* and controls *did not show* any difference in the use of fat. GRAHAM et al. (1967) used the questionnaire method on 188 males with cancer of the stomach and 800 control patients without neoplastic disease and found no significant differences in the type of fats used for frying. HIGGINSON (1966) stated that gastric cancer patients showed a dietary pattern indicating an increased use of animal fats, cooked fats, fried foods, bacon and a decreased use of dairy produce in comparison to control persons. However, the differences between patients and controls were not statistically significant. Gastric cancer patients showed a *slight* increase in daily use of pork, sausage and bacon. They also had a slightly increased use of fried potatoes, fried foods for breakfast and fried meats. Furthermore, the gastric cancer patients showed a slightly increased use of lard, collected fats, and they used predominantly animal fat in cooking as compared to the controls. A higher proportion also reused cooking fats, but the answers were open to doubt because a social stigma is attached to reuse of fat. Higginson concluded that the degree of increased use of homemade lard, bacon drippings, collected fats and/or of reduced use of refrigeration among the gastric cancer patients was insufficient to support a causal relationship between fat and gastric cancer. "Thus, while heated or animal fats would appear unlikely as major carcinogenic or co-carcinogenic agents in gastric carcinoma, our findings would suggest that they cannot be completely excluded as of etiological significance, since they are widespread dietary items in many communities with a high frequency of gastric carcinoma."

Even more important are the rapidly changing age-standardized rates of mortality from gastric cancer in Japanese men and women moving to Hawaii and the West Coast of the United States. Stomach cancer mortality decreases almost by half in the foreign born Japanese living in Hawaii and on the West Coast of the United States, and a further decline occurs in US born Japanese, approximating the rates of the host country, keeping in mind that the traditional Japanese diet is low in saturad fats and, if anything, relatively higher in PUFA than the American diet.

There are occasional flare-ups on the dietary fat-cancer issue, lately particularly in regard to breast cancer.

In considering dietary fat intake and breast cancer, we are probably not even dealing tangentially with a causal relationship. *Animal experiments* in rats in the hands of one group of investigators (CARROLL and KHOR, 1971) showed that semisynthetic diets containing 10% and 20% by weight of corn oil produced more mammary adenocarcinomas after treatment with a single oral dose of DMBA than did diets containing only 0.5% or 5% corn oil. The same investigators reported that experiments with 10 different fats and oils fed at the 20% level indicated that unsaturated fats enhance the yield of adenocarcinomas more than saturated fats. In addition, it was found that the high corn oil diet enhanced the tumor yield when it was fed only after administration of the carcinogen but not when it was fed only before. This finding suggested to these authors that the effect was related to development of the tumors rather than to distribution and metabolism of the carcinogen or other factors concerned with tumor initiation. Reviewing other animal studies[3], it appears that edible oils such as olive oil, Crisco and lard can enhance mammary carcinogenesis in the rat. The incidence of spontaneously occurring mammary tumors in rats was independent whether the fats were heat treated or untreated. The level of alpha-tocopherol was increased in another rat experiment containing 20% corn oil, and the result was a decrease in tumor yield in rats treated with DMBA.

CARROLL and co-workers (1968) admitted that their findings with *corn oil* in animals did not support the *epidemiologic observations* by LEA in the last few years, who suggested that there was a positive correlation between consumption of fats and oils and death rates from malignant neoplasm of the breast, which he related to the *cholesterol and cholesterogenic content of these dietary constituents.* The example of the American black female with a definitely lower breast cancer incidence in comparison to the white counterpart in the United States provides a good example of the *irrelevance of this fat hypothesis in carcinogenesis of the breast.* Black females are known to have used in the past and are still using at the present time more *animal fats* in their diets than white females. There are more powerful environmental and sociological influences involved in the development of breast cancer than dietary factors, among others the age at first pregnancy, the number of pregnancies, breast feeding vs. non-breast feeding, the age at menarche, the age at menopause and artificial menopause, family history of mamma ca, the presence or absence of benign cystic disease or treatment with estrogen-containing hormones. For each one of the factors cited, one, can show large differences between white and black females and between Japanese women and US white females. The mortality from breast cancer is believed to be nine times higher among US whites compared to Japanese women. However, environmental and sociological factors change drastically in Japanese immigrating to the United States West Coast and Hawaii, and with these changes there are indeed increases in breast cancer reported among first and second generation Japanese women.

Disregarding for the moment the isolated experimental finding of corn oil as co-carcinogenic in breast cancer development, one is more impressed by the several laboratory studies revealing that increasing the level of fat in general in the diet increases the yield of mammary tumors in laboratory animals. The higher incidence of spontaneous breast carcinoma in mice fed a high fat diet has been reported as early as 1945. Other workers observed that rats develop more mammary fibroadenomas when fed on high fat diets regardless of the type of fat used. On the other hand, there is ample evidence from animal experiments that underfeeding and caloric restriction decrease the incidence of a variety of tumors, including breast tumors. The literature on this subject has been summarized by TANNENBAUM (1959). But even this finding of an increase in breast cancer in overfed animals cannot be confirmed from human experiences. Body weight and cancer incidence of the breast cannot be correlated in most studies. The topic has been well reviewed in the German literature by BORNEFF and FABIAN (1966) and by SCHETTLER and WAGENER (1965).

G. The Soft and Hard Water Hypothesis in Atherogenesis — From the Combined Experimental-Epidemiological Viewpoint

For over a decade, different medical journals all over the world have been carrying alarming stories on the alleged relationship between soft drinking water and cardiovascular mortality. Ever since SCHROEDER (1966) published his purely

[3] For lit. see article by CARROLL and KHOR, 1971.

statistical observations, articles have appeared which commonly start as follows: "It is well known that there is a negative correlation between atherosclerotic heart disease and hardness of the finished drinking-water" (VOORS, 1969); or: "It is now established that there is a statistical association between mortality, in particular from cardiovascular disease, and the hardness of drinking water—the harder the water, the lower the local death-rates" (CRAWFORD et al., 1971). Similar associations were described from Sweden, the United States, Scotland, and England.

What was the next step? Well-known, established risk factors for ischemic heart disease, in particular hypercholesterolemia, were searched for in hard water and soft water communities. Two recent reports are obviously contradictory. Whereas the British group comparing 244 civil servants living in 6 hard water towns found lower cholesterol levels (237 mg-%) than in 245 civil servants living in 6 soft water towns (245 mg-%) (STITT et al., 1973), an American group found the opposite to be true. BIERENBAUM et al. (1973) showed that serum cholesterol levels were diet-related. The higher cholesterol levels were found in Omaha (241 mg-%) and London (230 mg-%) with their hard water supply and lower in their soft water counterparts, Winston-Salem (228 mg-%) and Glasgow (216 mg-%).

Meanwhile, several animal experiments were undertaken, all with negative results. HOWARD et al. (1967) were unable to demonstrate any difference in atherosclerosis between 2 pig populations raised on different drinking water (hard water versus soft water). PÜSCHNER et al. (1969) kept 2 groups of pigs under identical environmental conditions with the exception of differences in the water hardness. The arteriosclerotic lesions were studied, using histologic and planimetric methods, and serum lipids were measured. The results of these determinations confirmed the findings of HOWARD and co-workers, that the mineral content of drinking water does not influence the formation of early arteriosclerotic lesions in pigs, The authors also quote a *personal communication* of GRÜNBERG and KAISER, who found no difference in atherogenesis among chicks raised under identical conditions with different kinds of water consumption (one group with hard water, one group with soft water supply).

These animal experiments cannot be called essential as far as the solution of the problem is concerned; however, they contributed some valuable information. In the meantime, several other epidemiological observations have pointed in the same direction as the animal experiments. COMSTOCK (1970) concluded from a very detailed study in Washington County, Maryland: "No significant association of atherosclerotic and degenerative heart disease deaths could be found with water hardness." The International Atherosclerosis Project (STRONG et al., 1968), deriving data from autopsied cases, summarized their findings: "The prevalence and extent of atherosclerotic lesions in 18 geographic and ethnic groups did not appear to be associated with water hardness or the concentration of common minerals. The results suggest that variations of water hardness do not materially contribute to the explanation of major differences in the extent of arterial atherosclerosis among cases from these different geographic locations." HANKIN et al. (1970) thoroughly examined the dietary habits of people living in a hard water area. These investigators found that residence in a hard water area did not insure intake of only hard water. Approximately half of their subjects drank softened or treated water at home, a fact which has been completely overlooked by all the previous statistical analyses. The participants of this study were highly mobile, and several reported drinking water or coffee in 6 or 7 different localities during the week. This suggested to the authors that other factors, such as the use of home water softeners, place and kind of employment, and location of restaurants may be as important as the reported hardness of the municipal water supply. Thus no convincing evidence exists to associate water hardness with coronary artery stenosis!

H. The Issue of Coffee-Caffeine Administration and Atherogenesis of the Aorta and the Coronary Arteries

Approximately 90 substances or procedures have been examined in regard to their influences on the nutritionally induced atheromatosis in various animals—with the exception of caffeine. STUDER and REBER (1963) have shown this in a very extensive review paper. A Polish group at the University of Lublin had indeed explored this problem—however, the Polish medical literature had not been translated into any of the Western languages. In view of the lack of any clear information aside from some contradictory statements in the medical literature, we felt it necessary to conduct our own experiments (HEYDEN and RÜTTNER, 1966; HEYDEN et al., 1969).

Recent reports have dealt with the possible lipid-elevating effect of coffee or caffeine. One group's (LITTLE et al., 1966) conclusions were as follows: "The data suggest that coffee contains a substance which elevates serum-lipids in susceptible persons and that such persons may be liable to coronary heart disease." These authors, however, noted that "it has yet to be shown that other serum lipid fractions (besides plasma non-esterified fatty acids) will become elevated with long-term drinking of coffee or that increased atherosclerosis results". Another study (BELLET et al., 1964) revealed a rise of free fatty acids in human subjects after drinking two cups of coffee. Since de-caffeinated coffee showed no effect, it was suggested (BELLET et al., 1966) that caffeine is the lipolytic ingredient of coffee and further—"These findings are of interest in view of the relationship of free fatty acid elevation to that of other lipid fractions, notably triglycerides and cholesterol." In contrast to these assumptions, other authors (CZOCHRA-LYSANOWICZ et al., 1959; KEDRA, 1960) observed in animal experiments that caffeine did not have a cholesterol-increasing effect in cholesterol-fed rabbits and that these rabbits did not show more aortic atherogenesis than the control animals. Confirmation of these results was reported by us in 1966 and 1969.

It is interesting to note that ZELLER and AMMON (1967) were unable to change the cholesterol level or the level of esterified fatty acids in the serum of 52 patients with liver disease, as well as 41 healthy control persons after injections of caffeine or oral ingestion of coffee. These results were obtained in six laboratory determinations on each subject over a period of 3 h after intravenous application of 250 mg of caffeine or consumption of 225 mg of caffeine. However, as expected, they saw a marked elevation of free fatty acids in healthy persons with a peak serum level 2 h after caffeine administration and a peak serum level 1–6 h after caffeine administration in patients with liver disease. It is known that caffeine stimulates an increased level of urinary and plasma catecholamines and exerts a very significant effect on adrenaline excretion and to a lesser extent on noradrenaline excretion into the urine (LEVI, 1967). To assume that this would have an effect on the cholesterol metabolism because of the obvious catecholamine induced effect on free fatty acids, seems unjustified.

We administered caffeine in 2 forms, orally (50 mg of instant coffee added to the drinking water) and subcutaneously (0.22 cm^3 caffeine benzoate daily) in addition to an atherogenic diet, containing 1 g of cholesterol per day in 2 different sets of experiments (1966, 1969). We interpreted the findings of slightly lower cholesterol levels in the caffeine-treated group in comparison to the control animals as signifying that the administration of caffeine—if it has any effect in rabbits—has no hypercholesterolemia enhancing effect. The observation of higher individual cholesterol levels as well as higher mean cholesterol levels in the *control* group and not in the caffeine-treated group has to be weighed in the light of the following:

a) The rabbit is known to have a species specific susceptibility for hypercholesterolemia and its sequelae. If caffeine would indeed have a hypercholesterolemia enhancing effect as proposed in the recent statements mentioned, we would have expected a higher mean cholesterol level in the caffeine-treated group than in the control group.

b) The dosage of the daily caffeine injections for rabbits can be compared with a very high coffee consumption in man.

At the onset the rabbits weighed 1.5–2 kg, therefore the daily caffeine dosage on a body weight basis was 12.5–16.7 mg. The average cup of coffee probably contains about 100 mg of caffeine and in a 70 kg man this is about 1.4 mg of caffeine per kg of body weight. Assuming no differences in species sensitivity, this translated the rabbit dose to a daily human coffee intake equivalent of 9–12 cups. Although it could be argued that such an intake is "excessive", it is certainly not out of the realm of reality. Furthermore our concern, if any, would probably be with individuals who do consume coffee at these levels.

The results reported in our caffeine-benzoate injection group are similar to those reported by KEDRA et al. (1967), who administered caffeine-benzoate by mouth. They summarized their second 3-months' experiment which involved 18 rabbits receiving 1 g of cholesterol plus 80 mg of caffeine-benzoate in water per day and 17 control animals receiving the same amount of cholesterol without caffeine as follows: "This study showed that atherosclerosis is more extensive in cholesterol-fed rabbits (mean index 2.32) than in those simultaneously treated with cholesterol and caffeine (mean index 1.61). However, the difference is not statistically significant ... It is a fact that the rabbits of this group (cholesterol and caffeine) exhibited a lower level of total lipids, cholesterol and lipoproteins than those of the control group. Again, the differences are statistically insignificant."

Interpretation of these combined results led us to state that in spite of administration of 25 mg of caffeine for a considerable length of time and in spite of the well-known high susceptibility of rabbits for the development of hypercholesterolemia and atherosclerosis, the proposed cholesterol-elevating effect of coffee was not observed.

With our last experiment (HEYDEN et al., 1969) we were able, however, to answer a much more important question, i.e. the influence of caffeine on atherogenesis in the coronary arteries.

At the termination of the experiment, after 84 days, all animals were sacrificed and the hearts and aortas removed. The grading of aortic atherosclerosis was done by three observers independently without prior knowledge concerning the group to which the aortas belonged. No ulcerating lesion was seen. In cases of disagreement between the three observers, the aortas were rearranged and reviewed until two observers agreed. Each heart was sectioned transversely at 2 mm intervals from base to apex and fixed in 10% formalin. The first three transverse sections from each heart were submitted for paraffin blocks. A hematoxylin and eosin section was cut from each block. The degree of coronary atherosclerosis was evaluated microscopically in three ways. In the three hematoxylin and eosin sections from each heart, all arterial sections were studied and counted. An estimate of the extent of arterial disease was obtained from the ratio of diseased arterial sections to total arterial sections counted. As a second parameter for evaluating coronary arterial disease the arterial sections were graded for degree of arterial occlusion. As a third parameter for evaluating coronary artery disease, the major epicardial branches of the left and right coronary arteries were studied for degree of atherosclerotic occlusion using the same grading system.

First of all, there was no significant difference in the degree of atherosclerosis of the aorta between the caffeine group and the control group, with only a few more control animals showing rather extensive atherosclerosis of the aorta.

Microscopic examination of the coronary arteries showed atherosclerotic changes which are characteristic for rabbits fed a diet rich in cholesterol. There was a generalized involvement of the coronary arterial tree with lipid deposits lying both free in the tissues and in macrophages. In some vessels, the lesions were limited to the intima and were characterized by aggregations of lipid-filled macrophages forming a plaque. In other vessels, the lesions were much more extensive and involved the entire thickness of the arterial wall. Heavy concentrations of lipids were also observed in the sub-endocardial tissues and myocardium. Extent and severity of lipid involvement increased as vessel size decreased.

Careful analysis revealed that the percentage of arterial sections in each animal heart showing atherosclerosis varied from animal to animal both within the caffeine-treated group and the control rabbits. Thus, atherosclerosis of coronary arteries averaged 71% in the caffeine-treated rabbits and 76% in the control rabbits. The differences between the animal groups were not statistically significant. Likewise, marked fluctuations between animals in each group in the severity of arterial occlusion were observed. Again, the differences between the caffeine-treated rabbits and the control rabbits were not statistically significant.

One year later another group of investigators (Poleszak and Rucinski, 1970) examined the influence of caffeine on the development of atheromatosis in 34 pigs receiving caffeine-benzoate orally. The cholesterol level was very similar in the experimental group and in the control group consisting of 32 pigs of the same age. The degree of the atherosclerotic changes of the aorta did not show any significant difference in the 2 groups.

This does not prove anything as far as the human atherogenetic process is concerned but is certainly an important piece of information which confirms the prevailing epidemiologic viewpoint disproving any association between coffee consumption and myocardial infarction in humans. The topic is rather relevant at the present time, because the so-called *Boston Collaborative Drug Surveillance Program* published 2 articles in *December 1972* and *July 1973* which indicate "a positive association between coffee consumption and acute myocardial infarction. As compared with those who drink no coffee, the risks of infarction among those drinking 1–5 and 6 or more cups of coffee per day are estimated to be increased by 60 + 120% respectively". In contrast to this epidemiologic, retrospective study, the Evans County Study (Heyden et al., 1972), the Framingham Study (Kannel and Dawber, 1973) and the Chicago Study by Paul (1968) have all failed to provide any evidence of an association between coffee intake and myocardial infarction.

I. Pointers from Animal Experiments on Vitamin D Toxicity

Taylor et al. (1972) reported, as they called it, on "exciting" and equally "shocking" experimental studies in rabbits, demonstrating unexpected effects of the combination of nicotine and small doses of vitamin D in addition to a hypercholesterolemic diet (Hass et al., 1966). Similar observations were made in monkeys (Liu and Taylor, 1969). Within a few months, those animals developed progressive degrees of arteriosclerosis, arteriitis and thrombosis. "Obviously, cigarettes are the main culprit in the deliverance of the nicotine, toxic to the vessel wall." In regard to the excessive amounts of vitamin D, the authors feel that politicians and other people concerned with mercury pollution of fish and in rivers, should better be concerned about the problem of "operation over-kill"—the addition of vitamin D to almost anything and everything with the exception of cigars. According to these authors (TAYLOR and co-workers), this particular superaction with the inclusion of vitamin D could possibly add to one of the "most important pathogenetic factors of human atherosclerosis". The investigators claim that the population of the United States could possibly have been fooled by the so-called Madison-Avenue advertising, the nutrition industry and the dieticians who did not even suspect anything and the physicians who never would take any positions—however, excessive amounts of vitamin D are being added to a multiplicity of different food items. Indeed, vitamin D can be easily synthesized by the body, even if only a small part of the skin is exposed to sun light. In our nomenclature vitamin D is not correctly classified as a vitamin. It should rather be declared a very potent and toxic hormone which (when given in excess) is able to damage the arterial system and the kidneys. It was also pointed out that it is rather difficult for the body to get rid of vitamin D excesses resulting from prolonged and excessive intake of vitamin D.

J. Disturbance of Lipid Metabolism in Animals with Brominated Vegetable Oils

Recently, concern has been expressed about the use of brominated vegetable oils (BVO), used as "stabilizers" in soft drinks and citrus-flavored beverages, in ice cream and ices and in bakery products. Apparently the addition of BVO, as high-density oils, acts to increase the specific gravity of low-density essential oil components in soft drinks and in some foods. The effect is to prevent the formation of rings of essential oil at the necks of bottles where the oil would, in time, oxidize and give off rancid odors and flavors. To produce BVO, the chemists saturate some or all of the chemical double bonds of edible oils with bromine, a highly toxic element. It has been demonstrated in experiments with rats that *low levels (0.5%) of BVO in the diet interfered with their normal metabolism of fat.* Attention was directed to the problem in the Report of the 1969 Joint Meeting of the FAO Working Party of Experts on Pesticide Residues and the WHO Expert Group. Data regarding the tissue storage of bromine in animals treated with BVO were considered particularly significant. It was reported by the British Industrial Biological Research Association (BIBRA) that in rats which had been fed BVO in their diet, bromine was found in the tissue bound to the fat molecules in proportion to the dosages given. Fatty infiltration of liver occurred at all dietary levels. At high dietary levels, fat deposits were noted in the kidney and heart. Pigs fed BVO in their diets stored bromine bound to fat in all of the organs examined. The highest concentration of fat was found in and extracted from the spleen. Fat was also found in high concentrations in the pancreas, lung, aorta, liver, skeletal muscles and heart.

The Canadian Food and Drug Directorate (CFDD) studies showed extensive biochemical and pathological changes in rats consuming feed containing BVO for a period of 80 days. Among the adverse effects noted at the 0.5% level were enlargement of the heart and growth retardation; at the 2.5% level again enlargement of the heart and liver. All BVO-treated animals showed thyroid abnormalities and inflammation of the myocardium. Canadian studies apparently have also shown the presence of fat-bound bromine in human tissues after humans have ingested BVO-treated foods and beverages. At this point in time no report has come out associating BVO use and development of atherogenesis in animals. However, any disturbance of a normal fat metabolism must be viewed as a potential threat to atherogenesis. The American Food and Drug Administration has not taken a final position in the presently ongoing discussion but apparently will come up with a conclusive decision. A detailed report was given by B. HUNTER in the magazine "Consumer's Research" of July 1973.

References

ANITSCHKOW, N.: Experimental atherosclerosis in animals. In: Arteriosclerosis: Review of problem. New York: Macmillan 1933.

ARMSTRONG, M. L., WARNER, E. D., CONNOR, W. E.: Regression of coronary atheromatosis in rhesus monkeys. Circulat. Res. **27**, 59 (1970).

BELLET, S., ASPE, J., KERSHBAUM, A., ZANUTTINI, D.: Effect of caffeine on free fatty acids. Circulation **29–30**, 45 (1964).

BELLET, S., KERSHBAUM, A., FINCK, E. M.: Effect of caffeine on free fatty acids: Mechanism of effect. Circulation **33–34**, 53 (1966).

BIERENBAUM, M. L., FLEISCHMAN, A. I., DUNN, J. P., HAYTON, T., PATTISON, D. C., WATSON, P. B.: Serum parameters in hard and soft water communities. Amer. J. publ. Hlth **63**, 169 (1973).

BORNEFF, J., FABIAN, B.: Kanzerogene Substanzen in Speisefett und -oel. Arch. Hyg. (Berl.) **150**, 485 (1966).

BORTZ, W. M.: Reversibility of atherosclerosis in cholesterol-fed rabbits. Circulation **22**, 135 (1968).

Boston Collaborative Drug Surveillance Program: Coffee drinking and acute myocardial infarction. Lancet **1972II**, 1278.

Boston Collaborative Drug Surveillance Program: JICK, H., MIETTINEN, O. S., NEFF, R. K., SHAPIRO, S., HEINONEN, O. P., SLONE, D.: Coffee and myocardial infarction. New Engl. J. Med. **289**, 63 (1973).

BRUNNER, D.: Discussion. In: The artery and the process of arteriosclerosis. Measurement and modification. Advances in experimental medicine and biology, vol. 16. New York: Plenum Press 1972.

BÜLLER, J., VLES, R. O.: Dietary fats and atherosclerosis in the rabbit. Voeding **27**, 223 (1966).

CARROLL, K. K., GAMMAL, E. B., PLUNKETT, E. R.: Dietary fat and mammary cancer. Canad. med. Ass. J. **98**, 590 (1968).

CARROLL, K. K., KHOR, H. T.: Effects of level and type of dietary fat on incidence of mammary tumors induced in female Sprague Dawley Rats by 7,12-dimethylbenz anthracene. Lipids **6**, 415 (1971).

COMSTOCK, G. W.: Fatal arteriosclerotic heart disease, water hardness at home, and socioeconomic characteristics. Amer. J. Epidem. **94**, 1 (1970).

CRAWFORD, M. D., GARDNER, M. J., MORRIS, J. N.: Changes in water hardness and local death-rates. Lancet **1971**, 327.

CZOCHRA-LYSANOWICZ, A., GORSKI, M., KEDRA, M.: The effect of nicotine and caffeine on the development of arteriosclerosis in rabbits. Ann. Univ. M. Curie-Sklodowska **14**, 181 (1959).

DAYTON, S., PEARCE, M. L., HASHIMOTO, S., DIXON, W. J., TOMIYASU, U.: A controlled clinical trial of a diet high in unsaturated fat—In: Preventing complications of atherosclerosis. Amer. Heart Ass. Monograph **25**, 1 (1969).

DEPALMA, R. G., HUBAY, C. A., INSULL, W., JR., ROBINSON, A. V., HARTMAN, P. H.: Progression and regression of experimental atherosclerosis. Surg. Gynec. Obstet. **131**, 633 (1970).

EDERER, F., LEREN, P., TURPEINEN, O., FRANTZ, I. D., JR.: Cancer among men on cholesterol-lowering diets, experience from 5 clinical trials. Lancet **1971**, 203.

GRAHAM, S., LILIENFELD, M., TIDINGS, J. E.: Dietary and purgation factors in the epidemiology of gastric cancer. Cancer (Philad.) **20**, 2224 (1967).

HAIMOVICI, H., MAIER, N.: Fate of aortic homografts in canine atherosclerosis. Arch. Surg. **89**, 961 (1964).

HAIMOVICI, H., MAIER, N.: Experimental canine atherosclerosis in autogenous abdominal aortic grafts implanted into the jugular vein. Atherosclerosis **13**, 375 (1971).
HANKIN, J. H., MARGEN, S., GOLDSMITH, N. F.: Contribution of hard water to calcium and magnesium intakes of adults. J. Amer. diet. Ass. **56**, 212 (1970).
HASS, G. M., LANDERHOLM, W., HEMMENS, A.: Production of athero-arteriosclerosis and thromboarteriitis with nicotine, vitamin D and dietary cholesterol. Amer. J. Path. **49**, 739 (1966).
HEYDEN, S., BARTEL, A., CASSEL, J. C., HAMES, C. G., TYROLER, H. A., MEIER, R.: Kaffeekonsum, Gefäßerkrankungen und Risikofaktoren in der Evans County/Georgia-Studie. Z. Ernährungsw. **14**, 1–10 (1972).
HEYDEN, S., DEMARIA, W., JOHNSTON, W. W., O'FALLON, W. M.: Caffeine effects on cholesterol and development of aortic and coronary atherosclerosis in rabbits. J. chron. Dis. **21**, 677 (1969).
HEYDEN, S., RÜTTNER, J.: Die Beeinflussung des Cholesterinspiegels durch Coffein im Tierversuch. Path. et Microbiol. (Basel) **29**, 291 (1966).
HIGGINSON, J.: Etiological factors in gastrointestinal cancer in man. J. nat. Cancer Inst. **37**, 527 (1966).
HORLICK, L., KATZ, L. N.: Retrogression of atherosclerotic lesions on cessation of cholesterol feeding in the chick. J. Lab. clin. Med. **34**, 1427 (1949).
HOWARD, A. N.: Discussion. In: The artery and the process of arteriosclerosis. Measurement and modification. Advances in experimental medicine and biology, vol. 16. New York: Plenum Press 1972.
HOWARD, A. N., JENNINGS, I. W., GRESHAM, G. A.: Atherosclerosis in pigs obtained from two centers in hardness of water supply. Path. et Microbiol. (Basel) **30**, 676 (1967).
KANNEL, W. B., DAWBER, T. R.: Coffee and coronary disease. Editorial, New Engl. J. Med. **289**, 100 (1973).
KEDRA, M.: Influence of caffeine and nicotine on the development of arteriosclerosis in rabbits. Pol. Arch. Med. wewnęt **30**, 1004 (1960).
KEDRA, M., CHIBOWSKI, D., POLESZAK, J.: Effect of caffeine on the development of atherosclerosis in cholesterol-fed rabbits. Pol. med. J. **6**, 352 (1967).
KEEN, H.: Glucose tolerance, plasma lipids and atherosclerosis. Proc. Nutr. Soc. **31**, 339 (1972).
KRITCHEVSKY, D., TEPPER, S. A., VESSELINOVITCH, D., WISSLER, R. W.: Cholesterol vehicle in experimental atherosclerosis, part 11. Peanut oil. Atherosclerosis **14**, 53 (1971).
LEVI, L.: The effect of coffee on the function of the sympathoadrenomedullary system in man. Acta med. scand. **181**, 431 (1967).
LITTLE, J. A., SHANOFF, H. M., CSIMA, A., YANO, R.: Coffee and serum-lipids in coronary heart disease. Lancet **1966 I**, 732.
LIU, L. B., TAYLOR, C. B.: Effect of nicotine and vitamin D on the genesis of dietary hypercholesterolemia and experimental arteriosclerosis in rhesus monkeys. Circulation **40**, (Suppl. 3), 16 (1969).
MANNING, P. J., CLARKSON, T. B.: Nutrition and the pathology of atherosclerosis in monkeys. Exp. molec. Path. **17**, 38 (1972). Reviewed in: Nutr. Rev. **31**, 100 (1973).
MARUFFO, C. A., PORTMAN, O. W.: Nutritional control of coronary artery atherosclerosis in the squirrel monkey. J. Atheroscler. Res. 8, 237 (1968).
O'GARA, R. W., STEWART, L., BROWN, J., HUEPER, W. C.: Carcinogenicity of heated fats and fat fractions. J. nat. Cancer Inst. **42**, 275 (1969).
PAUL, O.: Stimulants and coronaries. Postgrad. Med. **44**, 196 (1968).
PEARCE, M. L., DAYTON, S.: Incidence of cancer in man on a diet high in polyunsaturated fat. Lancet **1971**, 464.
PINCKNEY, E. R.: The potential toxicity of excessive polyunsaturates (Do not let the patient harm himself). Amer. Heart J. **85**, 723 (1973).
POLESZAK, J., RUCINSKI, T.: The influence of caffeine on the development of atheromatosis in pigs. Pol. Tyg. lek. **25**, 1567 (1970).
PÜSCHNER, H., DAHME, E., ZÖLLNER, N., WOLFRAM, G., KALICH, J.: Der Einfluß weichen und harten Trinkwassers auf die Ausbildung arteriosklerotischer Frühveränderungen und die Plasmalipoide beim Hausschwein. J. Atheroscler. Res. **9**, 17 (1969).
RATCLIFFE, H. L., LUGINBÜHL, H., PIVNIK, L.: Coronary, aortic and cerebral atherosclerosis in swine of 3 age-groups: Implications. Bull. Wld Hlth Org. **42**, 225 (1970).
SCHETTLER, G., WAGENER, H.: Krebs und Fettstoffwechsel. Med. Welt (Berl.) **38**, 2135 (1965).
SCHROEDER, H. A.: Municipal drinking water and cardiovascular death rates. J. Amer. med. Ass. **195**, 81 (1966).
SNAPPER, I.: Chinese lessons to Western medicine, 1st ed. New York: Interscience Publishers 1941.

STAMLER, J.: Sex and gonadal hormones. In: Atherosclerosis and its origin. New York: Academic Press 1963.

STAMLER, J.: Discussion. In: The artery and the process of arteriosclerosis. Measurement and modification. Advances in experimental medicine and biology, vol. 16. New York: Plenum Press 1972.

STAMLER, J., PICK, R., KATZ, L. N.: Effects of insulin in the induction and regression of atherosclerosis in the chick. Circulat. Res. **8**, 572 (1960).

STITT, F. W., CRAWFORD, M. D., CLAYTON, D. G., MORRIS, J. N.: Clinical and biochemical indicators of cardiovascular disease among men living in hard and soft water areas. Lancet **1973**, 122.

STRONG, J. P., CORREA, P., SOLBERG, L. A.: Water hardness and atherosclerosis. Lab. Invest. **18**, 160 (1968).

STUDER, A., REBER, K.: Der Tierversuch in der Arterioskleroseforschung. Ergebn. allg. Path. path. Anat. Berlin-Göttingen-Heidelberg: Springer 1963.

SUZUKI, M.: Experimental cerebral atherosclerosis in the dog.—I. A morphologic study. Amer. J. Path. **67**, 387 (1972).

TANNENBAUM, A.: Nutrition and cancer. In: The physiopathology of cancer, 2nd ed. New York: Paul B. Hoeber, Inc. 1959.

TAYLOR, C. B., HASS, G. M., LIU, L. B., HO, K. J.: Risk factors in the pathogenesis of atherosclerotic heart disease and generalized atherosclerosis. Ann. Clin. Lab. Sci. **2**, 239 (1972).

TUCKER, C. F., CATSULIS, C., STRONG, J. P., EGGEN, D. A.: Regression of early cholesterol-induced aortic lesions in rhesus monkeys. Amer. J. Path. **65**, 493 (1971).

VASTESAEGER, M. M.: The contribution of comparative atherosclerosis to the understanding of human atherosclerosis. J. Atheroscl. Res. **8**, 377 (1968).

VOORS, A. W.: Does lithium depletion cause atherosclerotic heart disease? Lancet **1969**, 1337.

WISSLER, R. W., VESSELINOVITCH, D., GETZ, G. S., HUGHES, R. H.: Aortic lesions and blood lipids in rhesus monkeys fed three different food fats. Fed. Proc. **26**, 371 (1967).

WOYDA, W. C., BERKAS, E. M., FERGUSON, D. J.: Atherosclerosis of aortic and pulmonary artery exchange autografts. Surg. Forum **11**, 174 (1960).

ZELLER, W., AMMON, H. P. T.: Der Einfluß von Koffein auf den Fettstoffwechsel bei Lebererkrankungen. Z. Gastroent. **5**, 84 (1967).

Production of Myocardial Infarcts in Animal Experiments[1]

H. Tillmanns, S. Ikeda, and R. J. Bing

A. Historical Background

Early attempts to produce myocardial necrosis were the outgrowth of efforts to investigate the effect of interruption of the coronary circulation on cardiac function. One of the first to study the effect of ligation of the coronary arteries was Pierre Chirac. In 1698 he noted that ligation resulted in cardiac standstill. In 1842, Erichsen ligated the coronary vessels of dogs and observed that the average duration of the ventricular action after ligation of these vessels was 23.5 min.

Other early studies have been primarily performed in Germany as the outgrowth of the flowering of experimental pathology in the second half of the nineteenth century, spearheaded by such giants as Rokitansky in Vienna and Virchow in Berlin. Much of this early work was influenced by Virchow's paper in 1856 on Thrombosis and Embolism, which laid the foundation for the later studies of his pupils, particularly of Cohnheim. In 1867, von Bezold and Breymann ligated the coronary arteries of rabbits and studied the effect of this procedure on cardiac movement. In 1880, Samuelson ligated the left anterior descending coronary artery in rabbits for a period of 30–40 min. It was Cohnheim and von Schulthess-Rechberg who studied the effect of coronary artery ligation on the dog heart. Cohnheim was the recognized master of experimental pathology of his time, and his studies must be considered the first on the coronary circulation in which careful physiological measurements were made. On the basis of this work, Cohnheim propounded his well-known hypothesis that the coronary arteries are normally end-arteries, that is vessels without anastomoses. He ligated the circumflex coronary artery, the right descending as well as the left anterior descending coronary arteries. Both arteries and accompanying veins were ligated together. Cohnheim quotes Panum, who in 1862 embolized the coronary arteries by means of injection of powder, wax, oil, and India ink. Similarly in 1893 Kolster placed a ligature around the branches of the left coronary artery. Michaelis noted in 1894 that ligation of smaller branches of coronary arteries prior to tying the major branches prevented cardiac standstill, which otherwise occurred 2 min after ligation of the major branches. Baumgarten in 1899 described ligation of the circumflex, descending, and septal branches of the left coronary artery as well as the trunk of the right coronary artery. In 1941 Blumgart employed ligation of various branches of the coronary artery in his study on the effect of temporary occlusion of these vessels.

---

[1] From the Huntington Memorial Hospital, Pasadena, California; the University of Southern California, Los Angeles, California and the California Institute of Technology, Pasadena, California.

Since that time, many investigators have studied the effect of ligation of the coronary arteries (ORIAS, 1932; JOHNSTON et al., 1935; GROSS et al., 1937; MENDLOWITZ et al., 1937; MANNING et al., 1939; CORDAY et al., 1949; BLUMGART et al., 1950; KUPFER, 1951; WEGRIA et al., 1954).

Occlusion of the coronary arteries by embolization was first attempted in 1926 by HAMBURGER and associates, who used lycopodium spores. HERRMANN and DECHERD (1934) introduced metallic mercury into the coronary ostia through the carotid artery, but it was ROOS and SMITH in 1948 who first produced "coronary shock" by injecting a 3% starch suspension into the left ventricle of the open-chest dog while manually occluding the aorta.

It is the purpose of this chapter to describe various methods of occlusion of coronary arteries. Emphasis will be placed on techniques, since other chapters will deal with the physiological and pathological effects of these procedures.

B. Methods for Production of Complete or Partial Obstruction of Coronary Arteries

I. Ligation of Coronary Arteries

This procedure could only be carried out in the open-chest dog although many investigators ligated the coronary arteries to produce chronic preparations following closure of the chest (LE ROY et al., 1942; HARRIS, 1950; HAHN and BECK, 1952; BECK and LEIGHNINGER, 1955; CHARDACK et al., 1955; LUMB et al., 1960; PATT et al., 1960; ELLIS et al., 1964; GUDBJARNASON et al., 1964; KRUG, 1965, 1970; REES and REDDING, 1967; HOOD et al., 1967; BING et al., 1969; HOOD, 1970; ALLENBERG et al., 1971; MAROKO et al., 1972; MOORE and PARRATT, 1973; MARSHALL et al., 1974). Investigations included morphological and histopathological observations, mortality studies in animals with coronary artery constriction, the action of counterpulsation and other procedures on cardiogenic shock, production of myocardial failure, and the effect of temporary occlusion and varying periods of ischemia on myocardial function. Several investigators were interested in intercoronary reflexes and the effect of coronary vasodilators on cardiac function and rhythm.

In most experiments ligation was carried out with silk. The coronary arteries were either completely ligated (LE ROY et al., 1942; BECK and LEIGHNINGER, 1955; CHARDACK et al., 1955; PATT et al., 1960; ELLIS et al., 1964, 1965; GUDBJARNASON et al., 1964; GOLDFARB et al., 1966; GALLO et al., 1966; MAROKO et al., 1972; MARSHALL et al., 1974) or, if only partial narrowing was desired, a hypodermic needle or a stilet of varying caliber was positioned alongside the artery, a ligature was tightened around both artery and needle, and the needle was then withdrawn (HARRIS, 1950; HAHN and BECK, 1952; LUMB et al., 1960). This constricted the lumen of the artery to the diameter of the needle.

In most cases major branches of the coronary arteries were ligated in one stage. LE ROY and coworkers (1942) placed a linen ligature around the circumflex branch of the left coronary artery 1.0–2.0 cm distal to its origin. GOLDFARB in his study on cardiogenic shock also ligated the left circumflex coronary artery (GOLDFARB et al., 1966). OPDYKE in his study of intercoronary reflexes placed ligatures around the left anterior descendens or right coronary artery (OPDYKE and SELKURT, 1948), and MAROKO and coworkers (1972) placed silk ligatures around the anterior descending coronary artery and its major branches. Similar procedures were performed by HAHN and BECK (1952), BECK and LEIGHNINGER (1955), CHARDACK et al. (1955), YABUKI et al. (1959), LUMB et al. (1960), PATT et al. (1960), FINEBERG et al. (1962), KRUG (1965, 1970), REES and REDDING (1967), ENDERLE et al. (1969), OWEN et al. (1970), PARRATT et al. (1973), MOORE and PARRATT (1973), and by MARSHALL et al. (1974). The literature quotes of mortality rate following ligation of the anterior descending artery vary between 10 and 100% (dependent on the location of the ligature), most results lying between 70 and 90%. HAHN and BECK (1952) stated that infarcts are obtained in all dogs that survive ligation of the anterior descending coronary artery directly at its origin. More than 50% of these infarctions were larger than 4 cm in diameter and involved all muscle layers, while the minority was smaller and limited to the subendocardial layer. The operative mortality consistently amounted to 70%. After acute ligation of the anterior descending branch of the left coronary artery, ALLENBERG and coworkers (1971) demonstrated an average survival rate of 7.7–9.1%; after pretreatment with coronary vasodilators, such as Intensain, Persantin, or Carduben, the survival rate increased considerably.

Ligation of a single large coronary artery often fails to produce an infarct in the experimental animal because of the extensive collateral circulation occurring through the remaining vessels. Therefore, techniques have been developed in which all major arteries supplying a specific area of the heart are interrupted by suture ligatures so as to produce a circumscript infarction. ELLIS et al. (1964, 1965), interrupted all vessels supplying the apex by suture ligatures. Additional ligatures were placed around the anterior descending coronary artery (1 cm below its origin to avoid the septal branch) and its branches to interrupt collateral flow. GALLO et al. (1966) used the same method in order to study the influence of counterpulsation on experimental acute cardiac failure. GUDBJARNASON and coworkers (1964) and BING et al. (1969) chose an area of the left ventricle which was supplied by various branches of the anterior or posterior descending coronary artery. An infarcted area, 2 to 3 cm in diameter, was obtained by ligation of the branches of the arteries and accompanying veins with silk thread. A similar technique was employed by BECKER and coworkers (1973) who passed silk ligatures around all of the major free wall diagonal branches of the left anterior descending coronary artery in order to map left ventricular blood flow with radioactive microspheres.

To avoid the early development of ectopic ventricular discharges and ventricular fibrillation, which often follows the experimental abrupt occlusion of a large coronary artery in the dog, HARRIS (1950) introduced a two-stage occlusion of the anterior descending artery: Two ligatures were passed under the freed artery; the first ligature was drawn snugly but tightly around the artery together with a 20-gauge hypodermic needle. The needle was withdrawn immediately, leaving the artery constricted but still permitting some blood to pass. The second ligature was tightened 30–60 min after the first in order to completely and permanently close the artery. HOOD and coworkers (1967, 1970) employed the same technique in their studies on myocardial infarction following coronary ligation in dogs.

II. Methods of Producing Complete or Partial Occlusion by Means of Clips, Cuffs, Balloons, Screw Forceps, Snares, and Intracranial Arterial Clamps

Some of these procedures permit restriction of coronary flow without thoracotomy. For example, HOOD in his study of the production of left ventricular failure by gradual coronary occlusion in the intact conscious dog, implanted coronary occlusion balloons as well as monitoring catheters (HOOD et al., 1970a). The site of the balloon placement was approximately 1 cm from the vessel's origin, and the balloon could be inflated by saline. Inflation was maintained for a period of approximately one minute, and changes in ECG confirmed that the balloon was intact and the system was operational. This investigator also produced gradual occlusion of the artery by slow inflation of the cuff by means of a microflow-infusion pump. The procedure made possible occlusion of the coronary artery for longer periods of time. A similar procedure was followed by KHOURI et al. (1968), who used pneumatic occlusive cuffs. The cuffs were adjustable hydraulic occlusive devices which were placed around the circumflex branch of the left coronary artery and then filled with air. The inflatable portion is completely enclosed in a tight-fitting silver capsule so that expansion of the cuff occludes only the vessel which it surrounds. The external end is attached to a stainless steel micrometer piston. The whole system is filled with mercury. Both of these devices permit long-range observation of animals and are thus helpful in the study of experimental coronary insufficiency in unanesthetized dogs.

DRISCOL and ECKSTEIN (1967) occluded coronary arteries by polyethylene snares. This necessitated open-chest preparations in order to place the device, but the chest could subsequently be closed. They used this technique primarily for acute experiments in order to study the effect of occlusion on arterial inflow, venous outflow, and oxygen saturation of coronary venous blood from the non-ischemic portions. HILL and coworkers in 1973 placed a nylon filament snare around the left anterior descending coronary artery of rhesus monkeys 2 or 3 mm distal to the origin of the circumflex branch. A polyvinyl tube was passed through the left 6th intercostal space, and the ends of the nylon snare were passed through the tube. After closing the thorax and allowing the animals to recover for 3 to 5 days, a myocardial infarction was produced in the unanesthetized monkey by tightening the snare. GRAYSON et al. (1973) employed a similar technique in their heat clearance and heat production studies after acute experimental coronary occlusion. JENNINGS and coworkers (1960) used temporary occlusion (5–60 min) of the circumflex branch of the left coronary artery in an attempt to determine the minimal period of ischemia sufficient to produce necrosis of myocardial cells. They used three procedures: 1. clamping of the coronary artery with a bulldog clamp or hemostat applied over a strip of umbilical tape that had previously been placed around the artery; 2. traction of the ends of the umbilical tape instead of clamping it, and 3. occluding the coronary artery by means of a Goldblatt clamp; with this device the occlusion could be maintained with less trauma to the vessel, and the rate of release could be easily controlled.

FISCHER and EDWARDS in 1963, produced coronary occlusion by passing a small #90 polyethylene tube around a dissected portion of the artery. Both ends of this small tube were passed through a large, soft polyethylene tube; the ends of the smaller tube could then be pulled to afford an adequate method of occluding circulation without producing any significant damage. RUSHMER and coworkers in 1963 accomplished abrupt occlusion of a major coronary artery by encircling the left anterior descending or circumflex artery with a loop of nylon suture, passed through a length of polyethylene tubing extending to a point just under the skin. Tension on the suture with counterpressure on the polyethylene tubing produced complete occlusion of the artery, but could be instantly released if the animal displayed evidence of discomfort. A similar procedure was employed by SEDEK and LEWARTOWSKI in 1973 to study the mechanism of changes in left ventricular function after acute experimental coronary occlusion.

The Schwartz device (intracranial artery clamps) has been primarily used by MAROKO et al. (1971) and by GINKS et al. (1972). They were interested in the effect of both temporary and chronic occlusion on the size of the infarct. In one paper (GINKS et al., 1972) coronary artery reperfusion was carried out in order to investigate whether or not the size of the myocardial infarct could be effectively reduced. The Schwartz clamp, originally devised for ligation of cerebral vessels, fits squarely around the origin of the vessel. The use of this clamp avoids traumatizing the vessel. KJEKSHUS (1974) occluded either the left anterior descending or circumflex coronary artery by applying a releasable Schwartz intracranial clip in his investigation of the effect of inhibition of lipolysis on heart failure following acute coronary occlusion in the dog.

Gradual occlusion of one of the coronary arteries was also attempted by means of screw forceps with a small foot resting on the epicardium beneath the isolated coronary ramus and between its accompanying veins. The screw of the forceps could be adjusted to produce sudden occlusion or gradual narrowing with subsequent prompt release of the vessel. According to SAYEN and coworkers (1958), the method avoids undesirable effects of traction on a coronary ligature. Screw clamps were also used by GREGG and his associates (1939), who were primarily interested in the collateral circulation as measured by retrograde flow. BORER et al. (1974) clamped the left anterior descending and septal coronary arteries simultaneously at their origins; the clamp was suspended by sutures from an overriding cross bar so that traction on the coronary arteries was relatively constant despite respiratory movements.

BURCHELL in 1940 used a constricting metal collar with an internal diameter of 1.5 to 2.5 mm and a length of 6 to 8 mm around all three main coronary vessels in two operations about two weeks apart.

Mention also should be made of a closed-chest model of intracoronary occlusion, introduced by CORDAY and associates (1974). In one of these procedures, a double lumen catheter is used, one lumen terminating in an inflatable balloon, the other lumen permitting sampling of blood distal to the occlusion. The intracoronary catheter is maneuvered under fluoroscopic control through an angiographic cannula positioned in the left coronary artery. Using this procedure, blood from the great cardiac veins and the coronary sinus can be sampled simultaneously with blood from the distal end of the occluded segment of the coronary artery. The procedure has the advantage that it can be carried out in closed-chest animals and that temporary occlusion and reperfusion are feasible (LANG et al., 1974).

III. Occlusion by Means of Embolization and Thrombosis

In order to simulate closely the human condition in which, superimposed on arteriosclerotic disease, thrombosis within the coronary vessel can produce a gradual narrowing of the lumen, and finally obstruction, gradual occlusion by thrombogenesis in one of the coronary arteries was accomplished in closed-chest dogs. It can be carried out without thoracotomy and lends itself to prolonged observations. In most of these procedures, hastening of the clotting process is accomplished by the introduction of a foreign body or by an electrical current, as employed by SALAZAR (1961) and WEISSE and coworkers (1969, 1970, 1973). Under fluoroscopic guidance, SALAZAR advanced a Teflon-coated stainless steel electrode exposed at its tip for about 3 mm through a catheter to the desired location in a major trunk of a coronary artery. The intraluminal electrode is connected to the positive side of a circuit with the negative electrode located on the chest wall.

The intensity of the current can be regulated by a potentiometer. The intensity is increased until the electrocardiogram shows definite changes. Postmortem studies of these hearts showed thrombi present distal to the electrode. Diffuse myocardial necrosis can also be observed several days later. WEISSE et al. (1969, 1970, 1973) produced myocardial infarction by a slight modification of Salazar's method in which a thrombus was produced by means of an electrode catheter introduced through the left common carotid artery into either the circumflex or anterior descending branch of the left main coronary artery.

In other techniques designed to produce intravascular thrombosis, foreign objects are employed. The thrombogenic properties of wires inserted into the arterial lumen were first recognized by STONE and LORD in 1951, who found an alloy of 98% magnesium and 2% aluminum to be highly thrombogenic. In 1956 GAGE and associates inserted sharpened wires into the lumen of the anterior descending and the circumflex branch of the left coronary artery at the level of bifurcation. Both wires were pushed down into the arterial lumen approximately 1 to 2 cm. A similar method was used by MALM and coworkers (1960) in their study on experimental thrombosis in the dog. They modified Gage's method by bending the distal end of the needle to prevent it from slipping out of position. It was also covered with a small piece of gel foam sutured with atraumatic silk to the myocardium on both sides of the coronary artery. BLAIR and associates (1964) induced thrombogenesis in a desired coronary artery branch by inserting a spiral wire with a sharpened end fashioned from aluminum-magnesium alloy. SEWELL and KOTH (1955) inserted small pieces of polyethylene tubing into the anterior descending artery of dogs; these tubes result in the formation of a clot over a period of about 24 h.

Whereas the aforementioned techniques necessitate thoracotomy, other investigators (NAKHJAVAN et al., 1968; JOHNSRUDE and GOODRICH, 1969; KORDENAT et al., 1972) produced narrowing of a coronary artery and its subsequent occlusion by thrombogenesis in closed-chest animals. NAKHJAVAN et al. (1968) advanced stainless steel cylinders (4 mm in length, 3.25 mm in external diameter, and 2 mm in internal diameter) into the desired position in the coronary artery by means of a $7^1/_2$ F radiopaque J-shaped polyethylene catheter and a Teflon-coated guide wire inserted into the left carotid artery. JOHNSRUDE and GOODRICH (1969) used a partial occluding device (P.O.D.) consisting of a small strip of lead foil, encased in heat-shrinkable plastic tubing, which was positioned in the coronary artery by an assembled catheter. Use of this device results in a stenosis, followed by a gradual occlusion by thrombogenesis. A similar technique was employed by KORDENAT and associates (1972) who placed a helically shaped thrombogenic device, made of copper or magnesium alloy, into the lumen of the circumflex or anterior descending branch of the left coronary artery. ELZINGA precipitated coronary thrombosis in dogs by first placing a magnet around a coronary artery; the chest was then closed. Several days later blood iron particles (4 μm in diameter) were injected peripherally. These particles accumulated at the site of the activated magnet, resulting in thrombosis.

Embolization of coronary arteries was used in an effort to produce coronary occlusion within the closed-chest dog. First the method was established in the open-chest dog by AGRESS and coworkers (1951) who, in order to produce cardiogenic shock, injected 3% starch particles and plastic beads through a polyvinyl catheter inserted through the left carotid artery and positioned just cephalic to the aortic valves, while the aorta was occluded distal to this point by manual finger pressure. MUNRO et al. (1956) injected styrene divinyl-benzene spheres kept in suspension with 15% acacia, through a polyethylene catheter advanced to the level of the coronary ostia; the aortic arch, the left subclavian and brachiocephalic arteries were occluded for 20 sec. A slightly modified technique was used by MARCUS and coworkers (1958) who suspended the beads in saline. WEBER et al. (1972) produced myocardial ischemia and infarction in unanesthetized calves by intracoronary injection of microspheres through a flared coronary arterial catheter (Teflon) inserted into the left main coronary artery.

AGRESS and associates in 1952 modified their own procedure to produce coronary embolization in the closed-chest dog. They injected graded plastic microspheres (190, 325, and 450 μm in diameter) through a specially devised double-lumen steel catheter equipped with an inflatable rubber balloon attached near the tip of the catheter to arrest flow through the aorta during the time of injection. The same procedure was also used in animals by BING and associates (1956) to study the progression of circulatory, biochemical, and histologic changes resulting from myocardial infarction. In the dog, the catheter is usually introduced into the external carotid artery until the catheter tip makes contact with the aortic valve. The catheter is then slightly withdrawn (about 1 cm), the balloon is inflated, and the spheres are injected. Immediately following this the balloon is deflated. In early experiments following AGRESS' example, BING and associates (1956) suspended the spheres in gum acacia. However, gum acacia without the addition of the spheres produced many dynamic and biochemical effects of coronary occlusion. Consequently, in the later experiments the spheres were suspended in human albumin or in the dog's own plasma. Using essentially the same method, KUHN et al. (1960) performed coronary embolization with a nylon plastic cardiac catheter instead of a metal cannula inserted via a femoral or carotid artery and positioned fluoroscopically just above the aortic valve.

A metal catheter for selective coronary artery catheterization and embolization was used by WEST and associates (1958, 1959, 1962) who injected lycopodium spores suspended in saline. GUZMAN and coworkers (1962, 1962a) catheterized the anterior descending or the circumflex branch of the left coronary artery under fluoroscopic guidance with the same metal catheter described by WEST, and produced coronary embolization by means of lycopodium spores or glass microspheres (30–40 μm in diameter).

The use of flexible catheters to selectively occlude coronary arteries was introduced by RIBEILIMA, by GENSINI, and by TILLMANNS and coworkers. RIBEILIMA in 1964 injected steel ball bearings (1.1 mm in diameter) into the circumflex branch of the left coronary artery through a #7 aortographic catheter under fluoroscopic control. GENSINI and associates in 1966 performed a selective catheterization of the left coronary artery by means of a Sones catheter introduced through the carotid artery; a radiopaque sphere of appropriate diameter was placed in the initial segment of the anterior descending coronary artery of dogs (3 to 7 mm distal to the take-off of the first septal branch). TILLMANNS et al. (1974) catheterized the anterior descending or circumflex branch of the left coronary artery by means of a Judkins catheter introduced through the femoral artery (Seldinger technique). Once the catheter is in place, renografin is injected to confirm its position; this is followed by the injection of 0.4 g of clots from the dog's own blood. Renografin is injected again to verify the occluded region. In other experiments the clots were labelled with chromium-51 to delineate the size of the infarct at autopsy.

Mercury has also been used for embolization of coronary arteries, primarily to develop a suitable model of cardiogenic shock in animals. It was injected either at the origins of the coronary arteries (HERRMANN and DECHERD, 1934) or directly into them (PISA and HAMMER, 1961). LLUCH and associates (1969) produced cardiogenic shock in intact unanesthetized dogs by embolization of the circumflex branch of the left coronary artery with a single, minute dose (0.2 ml) of metallic mercury. The metal was injected through a Ducor catheter (#8) introduced into the left circumflex artery by way of the right carotid artery. This procedure results in a shock-like state in the dog, leading to death of the animal in 5 to 48 h. Using the same technique, CHANDRARATNA et al. (1973) concluded that embolization of the coronary arteries with mercury consistently results in hemodynamic deterioration but rarely in cardiogenic shock. FALICOV and coworkers (1973) performed a selective embolization of the left coronary arterial system by a slight modification of the method of Lluch and associates: instead of one single dose, 2 doses of mercury (0.12 and 0.08 ml) were injected a few minutes apart in the left coronary arterial bed, because two smaller injections of mercury were found to produce less serious ventricular dysrhythmias than a single larger bolus. These techniques are adequate for acute experiments whereby a number of vessels of smaller caliber are blocked.

Clinical myocardial infarction usually is the result of blockage of the larger vessels. In order to produce isolated gradual occlusion of a main branch of a coronary artery in closed-chest dogs, HAMMER and PISA (1962) employed an assembled Oedman (Kifa) catheter with a detachable tip, which is introduced under fluoroscopic control into the left coronary artery by way of the carotid artery. By this method, the coronary lumen is actually narrowed internally to simulate an atherosclerotic plaque, and is then gradually closed by thrombosis. Similar procedures were employed by SZAMOSI (1972) as well as COHEN and ELDH (1973) who produced delayed occlusion of the coronary arteries with plastic cones and hollow plugs respectively. These methods make it possible to produce a model of coronary occlusion and to study medical and surgical procedures intended to improve revascularization without the complication of a previous thoracotomy.

IV. Progressive Obstruction Resulting from Application of Ameroid Clamps

This method was introduced by BERMAN and coworkers in 1956. These workers used various substances which resulted in gradual occlusion of coronary arteries through their hygroscopic properties. Employed were reactive polythene film tied with silk ligatures around cylinders of different sizes, sodium dicetyl phosphate powder, silk dusted with dicetyl phosphate, silk bands dusted with sulfathiazole powder, and finally Ameroid cylinders or rings encased in a rigid capsule or shell of silver or stainless steel. This material has found widespread recognition and is still used extensively. The hygroscopic material is a casein derivative which absorbs water slowly. It narrows the vessel of the dog if it is encased in a capsule or shell sufficiently rigid to withstand peripheral expansion. BERMAN found that the Ameroid constrictor was well tolerated by the tissue, producing a minimal amount of foreign-body reaction. The procedure was popularized by LITVAK and his associates in 1957. They produced Ameroids of compressed casein, cured in formalin for purposes of hardening. In essence, the procedure is identical to that described by BERMAN. The Ameroid constrictors can be manufactured to fit arteries of varying diameters. The rate of absorption of plain Ameroid was found to be too rapid for long-term survival; the plastic was therefore coated with various substances in order to slow down the rate of water absorption. DUCHESNE and VINEBERG (1958) stated that the most suitable coating appeared to be melted Vaseline in which the Ameroid was soaked for a period of 30 min after sterilization with benzalkonium chloride. In order to obtain uniform Vaseline impregnation of the Ameroid material, a procedure which is necessary to result in gradual long-term obstruction of the vessel, it has been recommended that the jar containing Vaseline and Ameroids be placed in a hot-water bath for one hour (VINEBERG et al., 1960).

The Ameroid constrictors have been used for a variety of physiological studies. TSCHOPP and coworkers (1968) investigated the revascularization of the heart after a Vineberg implantation; others have used it to study the collateral circulation. Within recent years, SCHAPER (1973) has employed it to examine "coronary steal" following application of coronary vasodilator drugs.

The advantage of Ameroid constrictors is that they closely mimic atherosclerotic obstruction of the coronary arteries. One is able to adjust the time period of vascular obstruction. The procedure can be carried out in chronic preparations after initial thoracotomy for placement of the constrictors. However, one cannot always predict the degree of constriction. As a result, complete occlusion may be produced in a few days, leading to early death of the animal.

V. Experimental Production of Atherosclerosis through Diet

In 1946 STEINER and KENDALL produced atherosclerosis in dogs following ingestion of cholesterol and chemical ablation of the thyroid with thiouracil. Dogs were fed 0.5 g of thiouracil daily for the first month; the dose was then increased to 0.8 g during the second and third month until a final dosage of 1.2 g was administered. At the same time 10 g of crystalline cholesterol mixed in 40 ml of cottonseed oil were added daily to the diet. This resulted in gross changes in the aorta as well as in the coronary arteries. Lesions in the latter vessels and their branches measured up to 2 cm in length and seemed to occlude the lumen. In 1949, the same authors again produced arteriosclerosis in dogs by a slightly varied procedure. There was evidence of severe coronary artery narrowing, including hemorrhages and calcifications in coronary arteries.

In 1954, WISSLER and coworkers produced lipomatous and atheromatous arterial lesions in the albino rat by means of fat, choline, cholesterol and thiouracil. The most noteworthy finding was the presence of lipids in many of the coronary arteries. The atheromatous coronary lesions were usually accompanied by lipomatous changes in nearby arteries. Hypertensive animals had a much higher incidence of coronary lesions. Experimental coronary atherosclerosis in rabbits was described by Besterman, who fed cholesterol intermittently to mature rabbits for periods of 6 to 30 months and saw lesions of the main coronary arteries apparently similar to those found in man. FLAHERTY in 1972, summarized experimental studies on the production of atherosclerosis in animals. He discussed the topography of these lesions as well as species characteristics.

References

AGRESS, C. M., ROSENBERG, M. J., BINDER, M. J., SCHNEIDERMAN, A., CLARK, W. G.: Blood volume changes in protracted shock resulting from experimental myocardial infarction. Amer. J. Physiol. **166**, 603–609 (1951).

AGRESS, C. M., ROSENBURG, M. J., JACOBS, H. I., BINDER, M. J., SCHNEIDERMAN, A., CLARK, W. G.: Protracted shock in the closed-chest dog following coronary embolization with graded microspheres. Amer. J. Physiol. **170**, 536–549 (1952).

ALLENBERG, J. R., GERSTENBERGK, L. VON, MAST, G. J., MEHMEL, H., MITTMANN, U., NEELEY, R., SCHMIDT, H. D., SCHMIER, J.: Mortality after high ligation of the anterior descending branch of the left coronary artery in dogs; effects of various pharmacological agents. Klin. Wschr. **49**, 1088–1090 (1971).

BAUMGARTEN, W.: Infarction in the heart. Amer. J. Physiol. **2**, 243–265 (1899).

BECK, C. S., LEIGHNINGER, D. S.: Operations for coronary artery disease. Ann. Surg. **141**, 24–37 (1955).

BECKER, L. G., FERREIRA, R., THOMAS, M.: Mapping of left ventricular blood flow with radioactive microspheres in experimental coronary artery occlusion. Cardiovasc. Res. **7**, 391–400 (1973).

BERMAN, J. K., FIELDS, D. C., JUDY, H., MORI, V., PARKER, R. J.: Gradual vascular occlusion. Surgery **39**, 399–410 (1956).

BESTERMAN, E. M. M.: Experimental coronary atherosclerosis in rabbits. Atherosclerosis **12**, 75–83 (1970).

BEZOLD, A. VON, BREYMANN, E.: Von den Veränderungen des Herzschlages nach dem Verschlusse der Coronarnerven. Untersuchungen aus dem physiol. Lab. Würzburg 1. Heft, 288–313 (1867).

BING, R. J., CASTELLANOS, A., GRADEL, E., SIEGEL, A., LUPTON, C.: Enzymatic, metabolic, circulatory and pathologic studies in myocardial infarction. Trans. Ass. Amer. Phycns **69**, 170–186 (1956).

BING, R. J., GUDBJARNASON, S., TSCHOPP, H., BRAASCH, W.: Molecular changes in myocardial infarction in heart muscle. Ann. N.Y. Acad. Sci. **156**, 583–593 (1969).

BLAIR, E., NYGREN, E., COWLEY, R. A.: A spiral wire technique for producing gradually occlusive coronary thrombosis. J. thorac. cardiovasc. Surg. **48**, 476–485 (1964).

BLUMGART, H. L., GILLIGAN, D. R., SCHLESINGER, M. J.: Experimental studies on the effect of temporary occlusion of coronary arteries. II. The production of myocardial infarction. Amer. Heart J. **22**, 374–389 (1941).

BLUMGART, H. L., ZOLL, P. M., FREEDBERG, A. S., GILLIGAN, D. R.: The experimental production of intercoronary arterial anastomoses and their functional significance. Circulation **1**, 10–27 (1950).

BORER, J. S., KENT, K. M., GOLDSTEIN, R. E., EPSTEIN, S. E.: Nitroglycerin-induced reduction in the incidence of spontaneous ventricular fibrillation during coronary occlusion in dogs. Amer. J. Cardiol. **33**, 517–520 (1974).

BURCHELL, H. B.: Adjustments in coronary circulation after experimental coronary occlusion. Arch. intern. Med. **65**, 240–262 (1940).

CHANDRARATNA, P. A. N., OLEKSYN, T. W., SCHENK, E. A., COHEN, J.: Coronary embolization with metallic mercury. A pathophysiological assessment of the lesion as a model of cardiogenic shock. Cardiovasc. Res. **7**, 614–622 (1973).

CHARDACK, W. M., BOLGAN, F. J., OLSON, K. C., GAGE, A. A., FARNSWORTH, W. E.: The mortality following ligation of the anterior descending branch of the left coronary artery in dogs. Ann. Surg. **141**, 443–450 (1955).

CHIRAC, P.: De motu cordis adversaria analytica. Monspelii, Martel (1698).

COHEN, M. V., ELDH, P.: Experimental myocardial infarction in the closed-chest dog: Controlled production of large or small areas of necrosis. Amer. Heart J. **86**, 798–804 (1973).

COHNHEIM, J., SCHULTHESS-RECHBERG, A. VON: Über die Folgen der Kranzarterienverschließung für das Herz. Virchows Arch. path. Anat. **85**, 503–537 (1881).

CORDAY, E., BERGMAN, H. C., SCHWARTZ, L. L., SPRITZLER, R. J., PRINZMETAL, M.: Studies on the coronary circulation. IV. The effect of shock on the heart and its treatment. Amer. Heart J. **37**, 560–581 (1949).

CORDAY, E., LANG, T.-W., MEERBAUM, S., GOLD, H., HIROSE, S., RUBINS, S., DALMASTRO, M.: Closed chest model of intracoronary occlusion for study of regional cardiac function. Amer. J. Cardiol. **33**, 49–59 (1974).

DRISCOL, T. E., ECKSTEIN, R. W.: Coronary inflow and outflow responses to coronary artery occlusion. Circulat. Res. **20**, 485–495 (1967).

DUCHESNE, E. R., VINEBERG, A.: An experimental study of the effect of mechanically induced ischemia upon the mammary coronary anastomoses. Surgery **43**, 837–848 (1958).

ELLIS, P. R., JR., BAILAS, N. J., VISKOS, J. D., WONG, S. H., HYLAND, J. W.: Experimental heart failure in dogs. Arch. Surg. **89**, 299–306 (1964).

ELLIS, P. R., JR., LEE, C., WONG, S. H., DEL ROSARIO, V. C., HYLAND, J. W., PRATOR, G.: Assisted circulation in treatment of experimental heart failure. Arch. Surg. **90**, 879–889 (1965).

ELZINGA, W., KAUFMAN, W., UPRIGHT, D., POWELL, D.: A new animal model myocardial infarction. In: Artificial heart program conference (HEGYELI, R. J., Ed.). National Heart Institute Artificial Heart Program, p. 689–699 (1969).

ENDERLE, A., KORB, G., KRUG, A.: Tierexperimentelle Untersuchungen zur Beeinflussung der Folgen eines temporären Koronararterienverschlusses auf das Myokard. Z. Kreisl.-Forsch. **58**, 465–472 (1969).

ERICHSEN, J. E.: On the influence of the coronary circulation on the action of the heart. Med. Gazette, n.s. **30**, 561–564 (1842).

Falicov, R. E., Lipp, H., Resnekov, L., King, S.: Haemodynamic effects of low-dose isoproterenol and aminophylline after coronary embolization in dogs. Cardiovasc. Res. **7**, 63–68 (1973).

Fineberg, C., Foris, N., Camishion, R. C.: Revascularization of the dog myocardium. II. Acute ligation of the left circumflex coronary artery with and without hypothermia. Arch. Surg. **85**, 37–39 (1962).

Fischer III, S., Edwards, W. S.: Tissue necrosis after temporary coronary artery occlusion. Amer. Surg. **29**, 617–619 (1963).

Flaherty, J. T., Ferrans, V. J., Pierce, J. E., Carew, T. E., Fry, D. L.: Localizing factors in experimental atherosclerosis. In: Atherosclerosis and coronary heart disease. The twenty-fourth Hahnemann Symposium, ed. by Likoff, W., Segal, B. L., Insull, W., Jr., Moyer, J. H., p. 40–83. New York and London: Grune & Stratton 1972.

Gage, A. A., Olson, K. C., Chardack, W. M.: Experimental coronary thrombosis in the dog. Description of a method. Ann. Surg. **143**, 535–543 (1956).

Gallo, E., Eichelter, P., Schenk, W. G., Jr.: Influence of counterpulsation on experimental acute cardiac failure. J. thorac. cardiovasc. Surg. **52**, 745–754 (1966).

Gensini, G. G., Palacio, A., Buonanno, C., Kelly, A. E., Muller, W. F.: Superselective coronary occlusion under cinefluorographic control in experimental animals: Technique and Results. Circulation **33–34**, Suppl. III, 108–109 (1966).

Ginks, W. R., Sybers, H. D., Maroko, P. R., Covell, J. W., Sobel, B. E., Ross, J., Jr.: Coronary artery reperfusion. II. Reduction of myocardial infarct size at one week after the coronary occlusion. J. clin. Invest. **51**, 2717–2723 (1972).

Goldfarb, D., Conti, C. R., Brown, B. G., Gott, V. L.: Treatment of severe cardiogenic shock by diastolic augmentation after ligation and division of the left circumflex coronary artery in dogs. J. thorac. cardiovasc. Surg. **51**, 783–796 (1966).

Grayson, J., Robertson, M., Scott, C.: Heat clearance and heat production studies in acute experimental coronary occlusion. Cardiovasc. Res. **7**, 220–225 (1973).

Gregg, D. E., Thornton, J. J., Mautz, F. R.: The magnitude, adequacy and source of the collateral blood flow and pressure in chronically occluded coronary arteries. Amer. J. Physiol. **127**, 161–175 (1939).

Gross, L., Mendlowitz, M., Schauer, G.: Hemodynamic studies in experimental coronary occlusion; open chest experiments. Amer. Heart J. **13**, 647–663 (1937).

Gudbjarnason, S., Schryver, C. de, Chiba, C., Yamanaka, J., Bing, R. J.: Protein and nucleic acid synthesis during the reparative processes following myocardial infarction. Circulat. Res. **15**, 320–326 (1964).

Guzman, S. V., Swenson, E., Jones, M.: Intercoronary reflexes. Demonstration by coronary angiography. Circulat. Res. **10**, 739–745 (1962).

Guzman, S. V., Swenson, E., Mitchell, R.: Mechanism of cardiogenic shock. Circulat. Res. **10**, 746–752 (1962a).

Hahn, R. S., Beck, C. S.: Revascularization of the heart. A study of mortality and infarcts following multiple coronary artery ligation. Circulation **5**, 801–809 (1952).

Hamburger, W. W., Priest, W. S., Bettman, R. B.: Experimental coronary embolism. Amer. J. med. Sci. **171**, 168–185 (1926).

Hammer, J., Pisa, Z.: A method of isolated, gradual occlusion of a main branch of a coronary artery in closed-chest dogs. Amer. Heart J. **64**, 67–70 (1962).

Harris, S.: Delayed development of ventricular ectopic rhythms following experimental coronary occlusion. Circulation **1**, 1318–1327 (1950).

Herrmann, G., Decherd, G.: Creatine mobilization in myocardial damage. Proc. Soc. exp. Biol. (N.Y.) **32**, 477–478 (1934).

Hill, J. D., Lees, M. H., Malinow, M. R., Ochsner III, A. J., Thomas, C.: Regional blood flows in unanaesthetized rhesus monkeys during myocardial infarction. Cardiovasc. Res. **7**, 375–382 (1973).

Hood, W. B., Jr.: Experimental myocardial infarction. III. Recovery of left ventricular function in the healing phase. Contribution of increased fiber shortening in noninfarcted myocardium. Amer. Heart J. **79**, 531–538 (1970).

Hood, W. B., Jr., Joison, J., Kumar, R., Katayama, I., Neiman, R. S., Norman, J. C.: Experimental myocardial infarction. I. Production of left ventricular failure by gradual coronary occlusion in intact conscious dogs. Cardiovasc. Res. **4**, 73–83 (1970a).

Hood, W. B., Jr., McCarthy, B., Lown, B.: Myocardial infarction following coronary ligation in dogs. Hemodynamic effects of isoproterenol and acetyl-strophanthidin. Circulat. Res. **21**, 191–199 (1967).

Jennings, R. B., Sommers, H. M., Smyth, G. A., Flack, H. A., Linn, H.: Myocardial necrosis induced by temporary occlusion of a coronary artery in the dog. Arch. Path. **70**, 82–92 (1960).

JOHNSRUDE, I. S., GOODRICH, J. K.: An experimental partial occlusive device for vessels delivered by arterial catheter. Amer. Heart J. **77**, 805–808 (1969).
JOHNSTON, F. D., HILL, I. G. W., WILSON, F. N.: Form of electrocardiogram in experimental myocardial infarction: early effects produced by ligation of anterior descending branch of left coronary artery. Amer. Heart J. **10**, 889–902 (1935).
KHOURI, E. M., GREGG, D. E., LOWENSOHN, H. S.: Flow in the major branches of the left coronary artery during experimental coronary insufficiency in the unanesthetized dog. Circulat. Res. **23**, 99–109 (1968).
KJEKSHUS, J. K.: Effect of inhibition of lipolysis on heart failure following acute coronary occlusion in the dog. Cardiovasc. Res. **8**, 73–80 (1974).
KOLSTER, R.: Experimentelle Beiträge zur Kenntnis der Myomalacia cordis. Scand. Arch. Physiol. **4**, 1–45 (1893).
KORDENAT, R. K., KEZDI, P., STANLEY, E. L.: A new catheter technique for producing experimental coronary thrombosis and selective coronary visualization. Amer. Heart J. **83**, 360–364 (1972).
KRUG, A.: Untersuchungen am Katzenherzen nach temporärer Unterbindung einer Koronararterie. Z. Kreisl.-Forsch. **54**, 510–516 (1965).
KRUG, A.: The extent of ischemic damage in the myocardium of the cat after permanent and temporary coronary occlusion. J. thorac. cardiovasc. Surg. **60**, 242–247 (1970).
KUHN, L. A., GRUBER, F. L., FRANKEL, A., KUPFER, S.: Hemodynamic effects of extracorporeal circulation. In closed-chest normal animals and in those with myocardial infarction with shock. Circulat. Res. **8**, 199–206 (1960).
KUPFER, S.: Can experimental shock be induced by coronary occlusion? Proc. Soc. exp. Biol. (N.Y.) **76**, 134–140 (1951).
LANG, T.-W., CORDAY, E., GOLD, H., MEERBAUM, S., RUBINS, S., COSTANTINI, C., HIROSE, S., OSHER, J., ROSEN, V.: Consequences of reperfusion after coronary occlusion. Effects on hemodynamic and regional myocardial metabolic function. Amer. J. Cardiol. **33**, 69–81 (1974).
LE ROY, G. V., FENN, G. K., GILBERT, N. C.: The influence of xanthine drugs and atropine on the mortality rate after experimental occlusion of a coronary artery. Amer. Heart J. **23**, 637–643 (1942).
LITVAK, J., SIDERIDES, L. E., VINEBERG, A. M.: The experimental production of coronary artery insufficiency and occlusion. Amer. Heart J. **53**, 505–518 (1957).
LLUCH, S., MOGUILEVSKY, H. C., PIETRA, G., SHAFFER, A. B., HIRSCH, L. J., FISHMAN, A. P.: A reproducible model of cardiogenic shock in the dog. Circulation **39**, 205–218 (1969).
LUMB, G., SHACKLETT, R. S., COOK III, J. B.: The results of varying degrees of narrowing in the left circumflex coronary artery in dogs. Amer. J. Path. **36**, 113–123 (1960).
MALM, A., OHLSSON, N. M., SJÖSTRÖM, B., STERNBY, N. H., WEHLIN, L., JOHANSSON, B.: Experimental coronary thrombosis. An electrocardiographic, coronary arteriographic, and histopathologic study in the dog. Acta chir. scand. **120**, 36–46 (1960).
MANNING, G. W., MCEACHERN, C. G., HALL, G. E.: Reflex coronary artery spasm following sudden occlusion of other coronary branches. Arch. intern. Med. **64**, 661–674 (1939).
MARCUS, E., KATZ, L. N., PICK, R., STAMLER, J. In cooperation with DOMINGUEZ, P., GLASSBERG, J. E., HASBROUCK, E. E., LICHTON, I. J., WONG, S.: The production of myocardial infarction, chronic coronary insufficiency and chronic coronary heart disease in the dog. Acta cardiol. (Stockh.) **13**, 190–198 (1958).
MAROKO, P. R., KJEKSHUS, J. K., SOBEL, B. E., WATANABE, T., COVELL, J. W., ROSS, J., JR., BRAUNWALD, E.: Factors influencing infarct size following experimental coronary artery occlusions. Circulation **43**, 67–82 (1971).
MAROKO, P. R., LIBBY, P., GINKS, W. R., BLOOR, C. M., SHELL, W. E., SOBEL, B. E., ROSS, J., JR.: Coronary artery reperfusion. J. clin. Invest. **51**, 2710–2716 (1972).
MARSHALL, R. J., PARRATT, J. R., LEDINGHAM, I. MCA.: Changes in blood flow and oxygen consumption in normal and ischemic regions of the myocardium following acute coronary artery ligation. Cardiovasc. Res. **8**, 204–215 (1974).
MENDLOWITZ, M., SCHAUER, G., GROSS, L.: Hemodynamic studies in experimental coronary occlusion; closed chest experiments. Amer. Heart J. **13**, 664–674 (1937).
MICHAELIS, M.: Über einige Ergebnisse der Ligatur der Kranzarterien des Herzens. Z. klin. Med. **24**, 270–294 (1894).
MOORE, G. E., PARRATT, J. R.: Effect of noradrenaline and isoprenaline on blood flow in the acutely ischemic myocardium. Cardiovasc. Res. **7**, 446–457 (1973).
MUNRO, G., BALCHUM, O. J., OWENS, J. C., SWAN, H.: Experimental chronic myocardial insufficiency produced by coronary artery embolization. Proceedings of the Surgical Forum, 41st American College of Surgeons. Clinical Congress, Nov. 1955, vol. 6, p. 204–207 (1956).

NAKHJAVAN, F. K., SHEDROVILZKY, H., GOLDBERG, H.: Experimental myocardial infarction in dogs. Description of a closed chest technique. Circulation **38**, 777–782 (1968).

OPDYKE, D. F., SELKURT, E. E.: A study of alleged intercoronary reflexes following coronary occlusion. Amer. Heart J. **36**, 73–88 (1948).

ORIAS, O.: Dynamic changes in ventricles following ligation of ramus descendens anterior. Amer. J. Physiol. **100**, 629–641 (1932).

OWEN, P., THOMAS, M., YOUNG, V., OPIE, L.: Comparison between metabolic changes in local venous and coronary sinus blood after acute experimental coronary arterial occlusion. Amer. J. Cardiol. **25**, 562–570 (1970).

PANUM, P. L.: Experimentelle Beiträge zur Lehre von der Embolie. Virchows Arch. path. Anat. **25**, 308–338 (1862).

PARRATT, J. R., LEDINGHAM, I. MCA., MCARDLE, C. S.: Effect of a coronary vasodilator drug (carbochromen) on blood flow and oxygen extraction in acute myocardial infarction. Cardiovasc. Res. **7**, 401–407 (1973).

PATT, H. H., CLIFT, J. V., LOH, P. B., ROA, J. C., WEXLER, J., SELIGMAN, A. M.: Veno-arterial pumping in normal dogs and dogs with coronary occlusion. J. thorac. cardiovasc. Surg. **39**, 464–467 (1960).

PISA, Z., HAMMER, J.: Experimental myocardial infarction in closed-chest dogs with selective embolization of the coronary vascular bed. Exp. Med. Surg. **19**, 1–8 (1961).

REES, J. R., REDDING, V. J.: Anastomotic blood flow in experimental myocardial infarction. Cardiovasc. Res. **1**, 169–178 (1967).

RIBEILIMA, J. (introduced by BING, R. J.): Selective embolization of the coronary arteries. A hemodynamic, metabolic and radiologic study. Proc. Soc. exp. Biol. (N.Y.) **117**, 367–369 (1964).

ROOS, A., SMITH, J. R.: Production of experimental heart failure in dogs with intact circulation. Amer. J. Physiol. **153**, 558–566 (1948).

RUSHMER, R. F., WATSON, N., HARDING, D., BAKER, D.: Effects of acute coronary occlusion on performance of right and left ventricles in intact unanesthetized dogs. Amer. Heart J. **66**, 522–531 (1963).

SALAZAR, A. E.: Experimental myocardial infarction. Induction of coronary thrombosis in the intact closed-chest dog. Circulat. Res. **9**, 1351–1356 (1961).

SAMUELSON, B.: Über den Einfluß der Kranzarterienverschließung auf die Herzaktion. Centralblatt für med. Wissenschaften **18**, 209–211 (1880).

SAYEN, J. J., SHELDON, W. F., PEIRCE, G., KUO, P. T.: Polarographic oxygen, the epicardial electrocardiogram and muscle contraction in experimental acute regional ischemia of the left ventricle. Circulat. Res. **6**, 779–798 (1958).

SCHAPER, W., LEWI, P., FLAMENG, W., GIJPEN, L.: Myocardial steal produced by coronary vasodilation in chronic coronary artery occlusion. Basic Res. Cardiol. **68**, 3–20 (1973).

SEDEK, G., LEWARTOWSKI, B.: Mechanism of changes in left ventricular function after acute experimental coronary occlusion. Cardiovasc. Res. **7**, 313–321 (1973).

SEWELL, W. H., KOTH, D. R.: Experimental coronary occlusion using a polyethylene tube: A preliminary report. Yale J. Biol. Med. **13**, 259–270 (1955).

STEINER, A., KENDALL, F. E.: Atherosclerosis and arteriosclerosis in dogs following ingestion of cholesterol and thiouracil. Arch. Path. **42**, 433–444 (1946).

STEINER, A., KENDALL, F. E., BEVANS, M.: Production of arteriosclerosis in dogs by cholesterol and thiouracil feeding. Amer. Heart J. **38**, 34–42 (1949).

STONE, P., LORD, J. W., JR.: An experimental study of the thrombogenic properties of magnesium and magnesium-aluminum wire in the dog's aorta. Surgery **30**, 987–993 (1951).

SZAMOSI, A.: Experimental occlusion of the coronary arteries in the closed-chest dog. A selective method. Acta radiol. Diagn. **12**, 545–553 (1972).

TILLMANNS, H., FAUVEL, J.-M., IKEDA, S., BING, R. J.: Selective coronary embolization in the closed-chest dog (in preparation).

TSCHOPP, H. M., RAKUSAN, K., GUDBJARNASON, S., BING, R. J.: Physiologic studies on revascularization of the dog heart. J. thorac. cardiovasc. Surg. **55**, 466–478 (1968).

VINEBERG, A., MAHANTI, B., LITVAK, J.: Experimental gradual coronary artery constriction by ameroid constrictors. Surgery **47**, 765–771 (1960).

VIRCHOW, R.: Thrombose und Embolie, Gefäßentzündung und septische Infektion. In his gesammelte Abhandlungen zur wissenschaftlichen Medizin. Frankfurt: Meidinger 1856.

WEBER, K. T., MALININ, T. I., DENNISON, B. H., FUQUA, J. M., JR., SPEAKER, D. M., HASTINGS, F. W.: Experimental myocardial ischemia and infarction. Production of diffuse myocardial lesions in unanesthetized calves. Amer. J. Cardiol. **29**, 793–802 (1972).

WEGRIA, R., FRANK, C. W., MISRAHY, G. A., WANG, H.-H., MILLER, R., CASE, R. B.: Immediate hemodynamic effects of acute coronary artery occlusion. Amer. J. Physiol. **177**, 123–127 (1954).

WEISSE, A. B., LEHAN, P. H., ETTINGER, P. O., MOSCHOS, C. B., REGAN, T. J.: The fate of experimentally induced coronary artery thrombosis. Amer. J. Cardiol. **23**, 229–237 (1969).
WEISSE, A. B., NARANG, R., HAIDER, B., REGAN, T. J.: Right and left heart pressures in acute myocardial infarction. Cardiovasc. Res. **7**, 251–260 (1973).
WEISSE, A. B., SAFFA, R. S., LEVINSON, G. E., JACOBSON, W. W., JR., REGAN, T. J.: Left ventricular function during the early and late stages of scar formation following experimental myocardial infarction. Amer. Heart J. **79**, 370–383 (1970).
WEST, J. W., GUZMAN, S. V.: Coronary dilation and constriction visualized by selective arteriography. Circulat. Res. **7**, 527–536 (1959).
WEST, J. W., KOBAYASHI, T., ANDERSON, F. S.: Effects of selective coronary embolization on coronary blood flow and coronary sinus venous blood oxygen saturation in dogs. With special reference to coronary reflexes. Circulat. Res. **10**, 722–738 (1962).
WEST, J. W., KOBAYASHI, T., GUZMAN, S. V.: Coronary catheterization in the intact dog. Circulat. Res. **6**, 383–388 (1958).
WISSLER, R. W., EILERT, M. L., SCHROEDER, M. A., COHEN, L.: Production of lipomatous and atheromatous arterial lesions in the albino rat. Arch. Path. **57**, 333–351 (1954).
YABUKI, S., BLANCO, G., IMBRIGLIA, J. E., BENTIVOGLIO, L., BAILEY, C. P.: Time studies of acute, reversible coronary occlusions in dogs. J. thorac. cardiovasc. Surg. **38**, 40–45 (1959).

Experimental Cardiac Arrhythmias

L. Szekeres and J. Gy. Papp

With 10 Figures

A. Introduction

The importance of producing model arrhythmias in experimental animals, if possible, similar to the pathologic phenomena observed in patients, lies in the following facts:

1. A deeper insight into the basic phenomena underlying the pathomechanism of the type of arrhythmia in question may be achieved by analyzing the method utilized in producing the heart rhythm disturbance; furthermore, the experimental approach in animals is much less limited than in the patient suffering from arrhythmia.

2. Experimental arrhythmias may serve as a basis for the quantitative assay of antiarrhythmic drugs and may represent a useful tool in the search for effective new agents capable of preventing or suppressing heart rhythm disturbances. It must be born in mind that the collective term arrhythmia includes a number of heart rhythm disturbances of various types which differ considerably from each other in etiology as well in the pathomechanism. Accordingly, for each type of arrhythmia occurring in patients, elaboration of a corresponding experimental arrhythmia seems justified. However, this demand is by no means fulfilled at present, and we must be aware of the fact that the majority of the experimental arrhythmias hitherto produced do not correspond to the pathological phenomena observed in the patient. These models were developed under the assumption that if one or more symptoms, objectively measurable parameters of the human heart rhythm disturbance in question, could be reproduced, the mode and site of action of the measures evoking these disturbances could be related to the pathologic changes which underlie the arrhythmia occurring in man. This is, of course, not valid for all cases, but as a working hypothesis it proved quite useful, especially in the search for new antiarrhythmic drugs.

The most adequate arrhythmic models are those produced by toxic doses of certain drugs having a widespread use in clinical practice, e.g. the various arrhythmias due to an overdose of cardiac glycosides. Furthermore, adequate, but fairly special model arrhythmias occurring not infrequently in patients can be produced by the arrhythmogenic interaction of various drugs, e.g. that of hydrocarbon anesthetics and catecholamines. Usually our attention is drawn to the possibility of such interactions only by the occasional clinical reports of fatal cases. However, as the incidence of these interactions steadily increases as a consequence of the increased tendency to administer simultaneously a legion of drugs to the same patient, systematic research on possible interactions of drugs widely used in clinical practice seems indispensable.

Among the reasonably adequate types of model arrhythmias, those elicited by occlusion of a major coronary artery deserve mention. In these model arrhythmias, the underlying pathologic changes and their consequences are very similar to those occurring after acute myocardial infarction in man, although the slowly developing atherosclerotic changes of the vascular intima in the patient and the sudden constriction by a ligature around the vessel in the experimental animal are by no means equal phenomena.

Heart rhythm disturbance is rarely due to one factor only. Usually, simultaneous changes in several, mainly electrophysiologic parameters are needed to produce a lasting arrhythmia. In addition, analysis of the different types of arrhythmias has shown (SZEKERES and PAPP, 1971) that sometimes the factors eliciting arrhythmia can be clearly distinguished from those responsible for the perpetuation of the disorder. We showed recently (SZEKERES, 1973) that, although arrhythmias appearing soon after coronary ligation are usually elicited by the ectopic firing originating from the ischemic area, the appearance of the heart rhythm disturbance is also greatly dependent on the actual metabolic state of the working myocardium not directly affected by coronary ligation. BURN et al. (1955) showed that in auricular fibrillation produced in a heart-lung preparation by acetylcholine infusion and simultaneous high frequency electrical stimulation, the electrical stimulation is the eliciting factor, since arrhythmia persists even after cessation of stimulation as long as the acetylcholine infusion, the factor responsible for perpetuation of the arrhythmia, is continued. In the experiments of SWAIN and CURTIS (1966), auricular fibrillation in the dog heart-lung preparation elicited by electrical stimulation for 2 seconds, and not lasting longer than a few seconds, could be prolonged for more than an hour using hypertonic NaCl or mannitol for perpetuation of the arrhythmia. HOLLAND et al. (1957) showed that in isolated atria, electrical stimulation may elicit fibrillation; however, the presence of acetylcholine and of reduced potassium concentration in the medium is necessary to maintain it.

In other cases, however, the factors eliciting arrhythmia cannot be clearly distinguished from those responsible for its preservation. Often one and the same substance may evoke and maintain arrhythmia, such as aconitine, which must be removed to stop the heart rhythm disturbance.

In most cases, only a synergism of two or more factors facilitating the appearance of arrhythmia can be established with certainty. For instance epinephrine in doses not sufficient to evoke ventricular fibrillation alone, may produce fibrillation in animals treated with chloroform (LEVY, 1914), cyclopropane (MEEK et al., 1937) or benzene (NAHUM and HOFF, 1934). This synergism is based upon changes in the cardiac muscle itself, increasing its responsiveness to arrhythmogenic impulses originating partly in the myocardium, as ectopic firing from ischemic areas, or to extrinsic (electrical, mechanical, thermal, chemical, osmotic) stimuli.

Since the coordinated rhythmic contractions of the heart are based mainly on the dominance of the sino-atrial pacemaker, which controls the entire cardiac function, additionally, on the predetermined pathways and conduction velocity of the impulses, and finally on the relatively long refractory period of the heart muscle, changes in these parameters may facilitate the appearance of arrhythmia. Accordingly, these changes may be present in the form of a depressed sino-atrial automaticity and/or increased ectopic activity, further, as depressed conduction, reduced refractory period, increased excitability, uneven propagation of impulses and non-uniform recovery of excitability. Changes of the predetermined pathway due to a local and/or unidirectional block may also be present. The main factors responsible for these changes are: general and local hypoxia or ischemia (the latter due mainly to disturbances in the local myocardial circulation), increased neurovegetative tone, accumulation of catecholamines etc. Interventions facilitating the appearance of these alterations may play an important role in the pathomechanism of experimental arrhythmias, and as far as possible, will be carefully analyzed when describing the different methods.

Choice of the right type of experimental preparation, as well as that of the species, is of crucial importance in the production of adequate experimental arrhythmias. As shown by HALLE and WOLLENBERGER (1962) and WOLLENBERGER (1964), even in single myocardial cells of chick embryos cultured *in vitro*, digitoxin may alter the spontaneous rhythmic contractile activity to fibrillation-like undulations. Aconitine arrhythmia has been produced not only in the heart *in situ* and in heart-lung preparations, but also in isolated atria (WEST, 1964) and on Purkinje fibers (HEISTRACHER and PILLAT, 1962). Similarly, acetylcholine, as mentioned previously, produced auricular fibrillation in isolated atria if reduced potassium concentration was present and electrical shocks were applied to elicit the heart rhythm disturbance.

The advantage of isolated preparations lies in the fact that they are free from extracardiac (neural or hormonal) influences; in fact, in many preparations of this type, instability of the O_2 supply due to changes in the local circulation can also be eliminated, and so the pathomechanism of the arrhythmia in question may be analyzed in a much simplified system. However, this simplification is also a disadvantage if immediate conclusions as to the mechanism of the pathological processes occurring in man have to be drawn. On the other hand, in the whole animal, as in the patient, the extra- and intracardiac factors are always present, and their influence on the heart rhythm disturbance as well as any modification of their action by antiarrhythmic drugs can be studied.

As regards species, arrhythmias induced in cold-blooded animals are so different from those produced in warm-blooded ones, especially mammals, that nowadays they are rarely used as subjects for arrhythmic models. Occasionally the toad heart was used to investigate certain theoretical problems (BROOKS et al., 1955). Among the mammals, for practical reasons, we can distinguish animals with relatively small hearts—the rat, the guinea pig, the rabbit and the cat—and those with comparatively larger hearts—the dog, the pig and the monkey. Members of the first group are capable of spontaneous recovery from cardiac fibrillation because of the shorter pathway of the impulses enabling the latter to be extinguished at areas still refractory—and so prolonged circus movement of the abnormal excitation wave is less probable (GARREY, 1944). The rat lends itself especially well to serial experiments, when a large number of animals are required for statistical evaluation. Guinea pig and rabbit hearts are very suitable for isolated preparations. In addition, the latter species, being quiet by nature and with easily accessible ear veins for injection, is very useful for studying experimental arrhythmias in the unanesthetized animal. The cat represents the largest species still capable of spontaneous defibrillation. At the same time it can be regarded as a very tough species, lending itself well to surgical interventions such as thoracotomy and fixation of electrodes on the heart. On the other hand, the cat is sufficiently sensitive to cardioactive drugs. Animals belonging to the second group, i.e. possessing a relatively large heart, seldom show spontaneous defibrillation, though it is still more likely to occur in younger animals than in older ones. However, owing to its large-sized heart, at the level of the heart *in situ*, the most important investigations of the basic electrophysiologic phenomena involved in the genesis of arrhythmias have been carried out in the dog. In addition, the dog is very sensitive to arrhythmogenic stimuli; its tendency to develop arrhythmias or even fibrillation is higher than that of man. As a representative of a higher stage of development than the dog, the monkey would be an even better subject for experimental arrhythmias, but its use is restricted because of the high cost of maintenance. Today, the miniature pig, whose coronary vascular system is very similar to that of man, is becoming more and more popular, especially for the study of arrhythmias produced by coronary ligation.

For practical reasons, it seems useful to classify the experimental arrhythmias according to the techniques used for their production. These are:

a) electrical stimulation of the heart;

b) mechanically or thermally produced local blocks and ectopic foci in the heart;

c) drugs or other chemical agents administered intravenously or applied topically to the heart;

d) direct excitation of the central nervous system.

B. Production of Cardiac Arrhythmias by Electrical Stimulation of the Heart

Electrical stimulation represents one of the oldest methods still in use for producing arrhythmia in experimental animals. This is mainly due to its marked advantages over all other types of arrhythmia-producing interventions: its effect —except for extremely intensive stimuli—is fully reversible, causing no harm to the myocardium; the analogy with the natural impulse is closer than with all other methods and finally, the parameters characterizing the stimulus, e.g. its strength and duration, can be accurately determined and controlled. Moreover, a deeper analysis of the influence of electrical current on the heart is necessary for practical, i.e. clinical considerations, especially in view of the steadily increasing use of various artificial pacemakers, defibrillators and instruments used for cardioversion, which operate on the principle of external electrical shock, not to speak of the unfortunately, markedly increasing number of electrical shock accidents.

Arrhythmia or fibrillation in the heart can be produced by electrical stimulation either by applying 1. one single electrical shock, or 2. serial shocks, with progressively increasing intensity, or 3. progressively increasing rate, using suprathreshold stimuli; finally 4. by prolonged application of galvanic current.

To understand the mechanism by which electrical stimulation evokes the heart rhythm disturbance, it is advisable to start from the analysis of the action of a single shock, since all other types of electrical stimulation can be explained on the basis of this model.

I. Single Electrical Shock

If the myocardium is stimulated by a monopolar electrode corresponding to the cathode, the electrical stimulus, if strong enough, will depolarize the cardiac membrane in a manner similar to that of the natural impulse originating from the pacemaker cells. When using suprathreshold stimuli, the response of the heart will be determined mainly by two factors—the duration of the stimulus and its position within the cardiac cycle.

If the stimulus is made after the repolarization phase at identical times in diastole, but with current of variable intensity and duration, a strength duration curve can be constructed, showing that the intensity of current required for generation of impulses is fairly constant for stimuli of 1 msec duration or longer.

If the duration of the cathodal stimulus is constant, but its intensity and position within the cardiac cycle are changed, an intensity interval curve can be constructed, depicting the changes of excitability. These curves rendered possible the accurate determination of the absolute and relative refractory periods as well as that of the so-called vulnerable period, i.e. when the heart is most susceptible to the fibrillation-eliciting effect of a single DC or AC stimulus (WIGGERS and WEGRIA, 1940). The vulnerable period occurs at the end of systole and coincides with the dip in the excitability curve, as shown by BROOKS et al. (1951).

If the monopolar electrode corresponds to the anode, the stimulation will hyperpolarize the membrane, but if the stimulus is not too long in duration, the hyperpolarization will discharge upon its interruption, i.e. depolarization will occur. For clinical as well as for theoretical purposes, mainly bipolar electrodes are used. One drawback is that it is not possible to determine which electrode gives the stimulus at a given moment; another is, that the two regions of the heart to which the electrodes are applied recover their excitability at different times. However, in the case of closely located bipolar electrodes, the stimulus will originate from the electrode which is more effective at the time of stimulation (cathodal stimulus is more effective during diastole and anodal stimulus just before completion of repolarization).

If the stimulus is not strong enough, it may only temporarily reduce the transmembrane potential which may soon return to its initial value after interruption of the stimulus. In terms of the ionic theory, depolarizing action of the sodium entry into the cell is counterbalanced by the potassium efflux. If the stimulus is strong enough to reduce the membrane potential to a critical value (the so-called threshold potential), then the sodium entry will follow an explosion-like spontaneous course, prevailing over the repolarizing action of potassium efflux, and the membrane will become fully depolarized, giving rise to a propagating wave of depolarization. The minimal current intensity applied in diastole and required for the induction of a propagating wave of excitation, i.e. the stimulus just depolarizing the membrane to the threshold potential, is the "diastolic threshold", a measure of the excitability of the heart. WIGGERS and WÉGRIA (1940) showed that weak electrical shocks applied to the vulnerable period elicited only extrasystoles, but that increasing the intensity resulted in the appearance of fibrillation above a certain limit (the so-called "fibrillation threshold"). However, even with shocks of high intensity, fibrillation could never be elicited; only extra beats appeared, if the stimulus was applied after complete recovery of excitability, i.e. diastole.

In order to explain these phenomena, it is advisable to discuss the propagation of the depolarization wave starting from the electrically stimulated site. It is known that cardiac fibers are not uniform and that there are clearly measurable differences between adjacent fibers with respect to excitability, conductivity and refractoriness. Especially the latter, indicating the development of recovery of excitability, is of great importance, since it is not uniform even in the normal myocardium. Therefore, the demarcation line between the refractory area left behind by the advancing excitation wave and the areas already recovering their excitability is of an irregular shape, which means that at points situated at the same distance from the site of stimulation, some of the fibers may be excitable again, whereas adjacent fibers may still be refractory to excitation. If, at the earliest possible time after the natural or artificially induced excitation wave, i.e. in the vulnerable period, a second stimulus just strong enough to produce a propagating depolarization wave is applied, then the latter will spread over the myocardium in the wake of, but outside of, the retreating border of the absolute refractory zone of the preceding excitation wave and will appear in the form of an extrasystole. If, however, the intensity of the electrical shock reaches the fibrillation threshold, the depolarization will extend to a larger area and, at places, it may reach the irregular boundary of the preceding wave of excitation. At these sites the second wave of depolarization will be extinguished whereas at other places its propagation is undisturbed. Accordingly, a difference in phase in the spreading of excitation will arise between certain nearby sections of the myocardium, and since there is no continuous refractory zone behind the wave of excitation, circus movement of the latter becomes possible. All this may lead to gradually increasing disorganization of the contractions, ending in fibrillation.

II. Serial Electrical Shocks of Progressively Increasing Intensity

The mechanism of the arrhythmogenic effect of serial electrical shocks can be explained on the basis of the foregoing considerations. If serial shocks of gradually increasing intensity and of high frequency (10 to 20 c/s) are applied to the myocardium, first extrasystoles, later tachycardia, flutter and finally fibrillation will appear irrespective of the form of stimuli used, e.g. rectangular pulses, faradic current or simple alternating current (Fig. 1). Accordingly, the most important clinical forms of arrhythmia can be reproduced with the help of electrical stimulation. A possible explanation of these findings is the following: Electrical stimulus of low intensity but higher than the diastolic threshold may elicit an extra beat. However, the next shock is not strong enough to break through the refractory phase of the preceding excitation wave. If the current intensity is sufficiently high, then the second or one of the following shocks may elicit a propagating response also in the relative refractory phase of the first stimulus. The cycle length and with this the absolute refractory period will become shorter, so that in the next cycle, the extra beat can be elicited earlier. The number of contractions per minute will progressively increase, the developing tachycardia will smoothly change into flutter. With progressively shorter refractory periods, the stimuli are given more opportunities to hit the myocardium in the vulnerable period and if the stimuli are strong enough, they may evoke fibrillation.

III. Electrical Stimulation of Continuously Increasing Frequency Rate

LEWIS et al. (1920) chose another way to produce fibrillation by serial shocks. They used suprathreshold stimuli of fixed intensity, but the stimulation rate was progressively increased until fibrillation appeared. The mechanism by which arrhythmia is produced using this type of stimulation is very similar to that of the preceding method, i.e. with progressively shorter cycle length the refractory period also becomes shorter and therefore, the extra beats elicited by stimulation may appear more and more early in the cardiac cycle. The heart rate increases as long as the heart is able to follow the stimulation. Tachycardia developing to flutter will appear. The maximal stimulation rate is determined by the so-called "effective refractory period"—i.e. the shortest interval between two stimuli to which the heart responds with contraction. If the rate of stimulation is increased above the maximal frequency that the heart is able to follow, then soon one or more stimuli will hit the heart in the vulnerable period, and if sufficiently strong, may precipitate fibrillation.

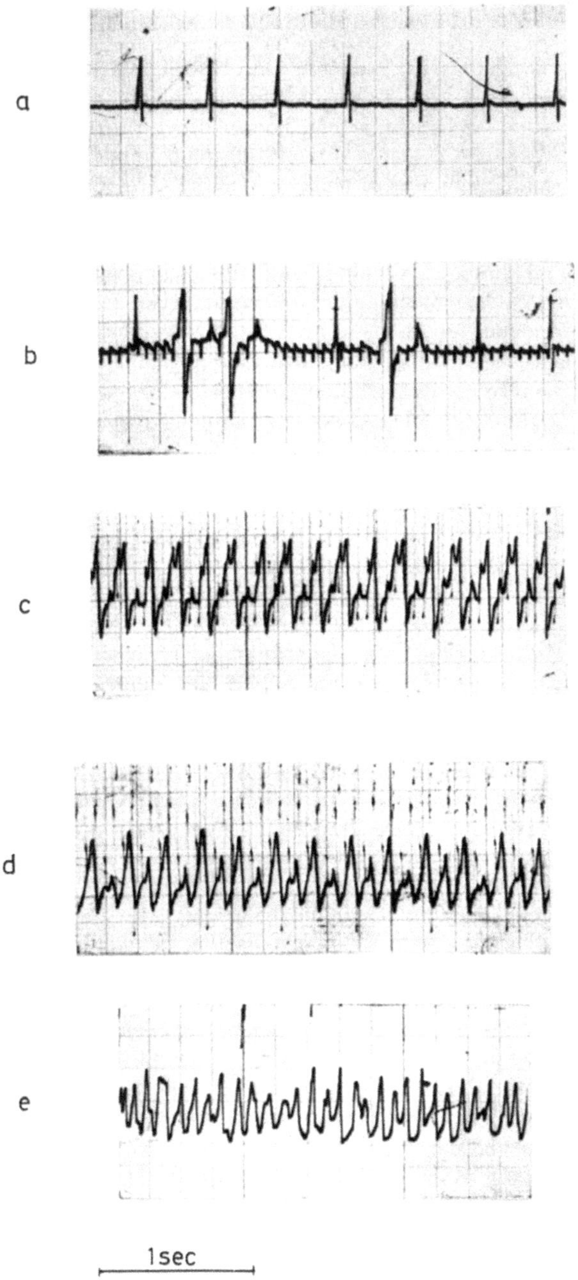

Fig. 1a—e. *Effect of serial electrical shocks of gradually increasing intensity applied to the right ventricle of the cat heart.* Electrocardiogram was recorded in lead II. — Rectangular impulses of 1 msec duration and 20 c/s were used. (a) control; (b) extrasystoles at 0.75 mA; (c) and (d) tachycardia at 1.50 and 1.80 mA, respectively; (e) ventricular fibrillation at 2.50 mA

IV. Prolonged Application of Galvanic Current

Weak but prolonged galvanic current may also depolarize the cardiac membrane sufficiently to elicit arrhythmia or even fibrillation. The mechanism by which this intervention produces arrhythmia can be explained on the basis of the observations of TRAUTWEIN and KASSEBAUM (1961), who found that weak depolarizing current increases the steepness of the slope of the slow diastolic depolarization in Purkinje fibers, thus enhancing their firing rate. It can be assumed, therefore, that the galvanic current may increase the automaticity of the latent heterotopic pacemakers, establishing favorable conditions for irregular cardiac activity. Presumably similar electrotonic injury current arises in myocardial ischemia or infarction, representing one of the main factors responsible for the arrhythmias appearing under these pathological conditions.

Since the ultimate goal of producing experimental arrhythmias in animals is the better understanding of the processes involved in the mechanism of the different types of heart rhythm disturbances, analysis of the factors facilitating or inhibiting the appearance of arrhythmias seems equally important. The great advantage of the electrical stimulation methods lies in the fact that they are not only able to produce one or another form of the heart rhythm disturbances similar to those seen in patients, but they allow the quantitative determination of the effort by which these arrhythmias are produced or on the contrary, abolished; in other words, they may reflect the tendency of the heart to arrhythmia (flutter or fibrillation). In addition, to the possibility of an easier or of a more difficult induction of arrhythmia, this concept covers another phenomenon, namely the tendency of the elicited heart rhythm disturbance to persist or to cease spontaneously. The two events do not necessarily concur. Sometimes electrical stimulation of very high intensity is required to induce fibrillation owing to the reduced excitability of the myocardium as in the case of severe hypoxia or ischemia of the myocardium. However, once induced, it may persist and prove very resistant to all antifibrillatory measures. On the other hand, fibrillation is occasionally easy to produce and yet may end spontaneously, especially in young animals and in those with relatively small hearts. In cardiosurgery, the degree of susceptibility to arrhythmogenic stimuli, such as manipulation of the heart, is of great importance, since ventricular fibrillation once evoked can hardly be expected to cease spontaneously in the large human heart. In the assay of antiarrhythmic agents, it is important to know how easily flutter or fibrillation is elicited by external stimuli, since after pretreatment with antiarrhythmic drugs, electrical stimulation of much higher intensity is required to evoke flutter or fibrillation.

Therefore, a method which follows closely the changes in the tendency of the auricles and ventricles to develop arrhythmia (flutter or fibrillation) on external stimuli is needed. This can be accomplished very accurately with the aid of the electrical fibrillation threshold method based on the determination of the minimal current intensity just able to evoke auricular or ventricular fibrillation. The lower the current intensity needed for this purpose, the higher is the susceptibility or tendency of the respective auricle or ventricle to fibrillation. On the basis of the mechanism of fibrillation induced by electrical stimulation discussed previously, the electrical fibrillation threshold may be defined as the minimal current intensity capable of producing depolarization of the cardiac membrane extending to the boundary of the fibers still refractory to excitation in the wake of the preceding excitation wave. Thus, the fibrillation threshold indicates above all the vulnerability of the myocardium.

There are several ways to determine the electrical fibrillation threshold. WIGGERS and WÉGRIA (1940) used in their classical experiments the single shock method, i.e. they increased gradually the intensity of a single shock applied in the vulnerable period until fibrillation appeared. However, this method has a number of inherent difficulties and has never become popular for the assay of antiarrhythmic drugs. Thus, in order to apply the fibrillation-evoking shock exactly within the vulnerable period, either the sino-atrial pacemaker must be excluded by crushing or by chemical agents and the heart driven by an electrical pacemaker—or if the heart rate is constant and the second, fibrillating shock is sufficiently long to fall within the vulnerable period, this extra stimulus can be controlled by one of the ECG waves, usually the R wave. In both instances exact timing of the fibrillating stimulus is necessary; therefore, specially built stimulators with an adjustable interval between the two stimuli, are needed. In addition, in the case of the ECG-controlled extra stimulus, spontaneous or drug-induced changes in the cycle length may require repeated readjustment of the delay. One of the greatest disadvantages of the single shock method is that it requires a current of rather high intensity which may irreversibly injure the myocardium at the site of stimulation; thus reproduction of initial values is not possible. The danger of myocardial damage is even greater if, in order to enable continuous measurement of the threshold by steadily increasing the intensity, the stimuli are applied to each cycle. — VAN TYN and MCLEAN (1961) showed that in order to avoid myocardial injury, a period corresponding to 10–15 cycles should separate two successive extra stimuli. Consequently, rapidly changing processes may escape the investigator. A further factor retarding estimation of the fibrillation threshold with the single shock method is that animals with larger hearts—such as the dog—rarely defibrillate spontaneously, so electrical defibrillation is required. Since the high intensity current needed for electrical defibrillation alters the electrical properties of the myocardium, a 10–30 min recovery period between two determinations seems necessary if complete recovery is to be expected at all. In most cases the hypoxic injury due to the standstill of circulation as well as to the mechanical damage caused by cardiac massage (often necessary pior to defibrillation) may alter the basic electrophysiologic properties of the myocardium in such a way that complete recovery to the initial state is no longer possible.

In view of these inadequacies of the single shock method, we used in most experiments serial shocks with progressively increasing intensity for the production of the different forms of arrhythmias, as discussed, as well as for the determination of the fibrillation and the flutter thresholds. The latter is a new concept—introduced by us (SZEKERES and PAPP, 1971) and corresponds to the minimal current intensity just able to produce auricular or ventricular flutter. The advantage of the latter is that it requires a lower current intensity than that needed for determination of the fibrillation threshold. Although cats and smaller animals tend to return spontaneously to normal rhythm even from ventricular fibrillation, strong serial shocks may sometimes evoke persistent cardiac fibrillation requiring electrical defibrillation. We showed (SZEKERES and PAPP, 1971) that there is a good correlation between the fibrillation threshold and the flutter threshold measured in the same animal, the intensity of current needed for the latter is only one third to one fourth of the fibrillation threshold. Hemodynamic consequences of both methods are the same, i.e. the cardiac pumping mechanism is heavily impaired; therefore circulation is minimal or stops completely and blood pressure falls abruptly. Like the fibrillation threshold, the flutter threshold has a sharply defined margin—it is highly reproducible and frequently repeated, and it tends to return to the initial value even after different interventions. Since the flutter so produced stops immediately after discontinuance of the stimulation in the relatively small cat heart, it may be used to determine from minute to minute the susceptibility of the myocardium to arrhythmogenic stimuli, which allows one to follow closely the rapidly changing processes.

The techniques employed for determination of the flutter threshold are described in detail elsewhere (SZEKERES and PAPP, 1971) and here will be only briefly summarized. Cats weighing 3 kg on the average are anesthetized with a dial-urethan solution (4% allylbarbiturate + 16% urethan), artificially ventilated and thoracotomized. The bipolar stimulating silver electrodes embedded in plastic holders are stitched to the anterior surface of the right ventricle and clipped to the left auricle, respectively. Stimuli of only 1 msec duration are used, so the risk of polarization can be excluded (KLENSCH, 1954; BROOKS et al., 1955). The intensity of the current passing through the heart can be directly read in mA from one beam of a two channel dual-beam oscilloscope. The diagram of the experimental set-up for determination of the flutter (and fibrillation) threshold, which is, in addition, capable of measuring the refractory periods, conductivity and excitability, is shown in Fig. 2. For precipitation of flutter or fibrillation, serial rectangular impulses of 1 msec duration and 20 c/s frequency may be used. The intensity is progressively increased until flutter appears. The appearance of flutter can be established by direct inspection of the heart or by the abrupt fall of the blood pressure, as well as by an ECG. Appearence of fibrillation can be verified only from the ECG, since fibrillo-flutter of very high frequency is barely separable from fibrillation by direct inspection of the heart and since the abrupt fall in blood pressure appears in both types of arrhythmia.

In animals with relatively large hearts, which have a great tendency to develop persistent fibrillation to external stimuli, even serial shocks may precipitate prolonged ventricular fibrillation. For this reason, a milder, less dangerous intervention was recommended for estimation of the tendency to develop arrhythmia to external stimuli by HOFFMAN et al. (1951). This method is the so-called "multiple response threshold", i.e. the lowest current intensity of a single shock applied in the vulnerable period, which is just able to elicit multiple ventricular response. This multiple response appears usually in form of a few successive extrasystoles, although sometimes fibrillation-like potentials may appear for a short time. Persistent ventricular fibrillation is, however, seldom observed, and since HAN et al. (1964) showed that changes of the multiple response threshold run fairly parallel with those of the "true" fibrillation threshold, this method seems to be a very useful estimation of the susceptibility of the relatively large hearts of dogs, monkeys and pigs to external arrhythmogenic stimuli. It is highly reproducible and its advantage over the single shock method is that, owing to the immediate recovery, the determinations can be repeated within short intervals, and the tendency of the heart to arrhythmia can be followed very closely—as with the serial shock method in cats. Estimation of the multiple response threshold is carried out in anesthetized thoracotomized dogs with artificially driven hearts. The heart is driven through bipolar electrodes applied to the sinoatrial region using a somewhat higher driving frequency than that of the sino-atrial pacemaker, so the heart will follow the artifical pacemaker and chemical or mechanical destruction of the sino-atrial node is not necessary. The second stimulus of 10 msec duration and of an intensity about four times that of the diastolic threshold is applied at the line of demarcation of the absolute and the relative refractory periods, and by slowly proceeding towards the end of the cycle at the site where multiple extrasystoles appear, the vulnerable phase is established. The intensity

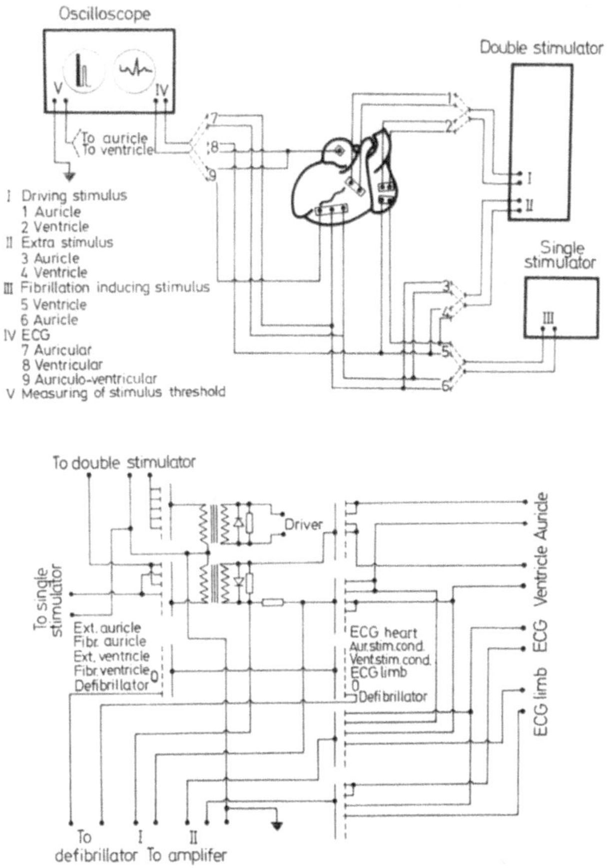

Fig. 2. *Experimental arrangement for determination of electrical fibrillation threshold, conductivity, excitability and refractoriness in the cat heart*

is then regulated to give a stimulus just strong enough to produce multiple ventricular response.

Analysis of the factors facilitating or inhibiting the appearance of arrhythmia also requires determination of other basic cardiac electrophysiologic parameters such as excitability, conductivity and refractoriness. The experimental set-up shown in Fig. 2 allows also estimation of these parameters. In the artificially driven heart the second stimulus will be applied in diastole, and the diastolic threshold, i.e. the lowest stimulus intensity just evoking a single extrasystole, will be determined first. Then by gradually approaching the extra stimulus toward the beginning of the cycle, the duration of the relative and absolute refractory periods can be established. For estimation of the conductivity in the auricle, the distance between the stimulus artifact evoked by the driving electrodes attached to the right auricle, and the elicited action potential recorded from left auricle can be measured. Intraventricular conduction can be estimated either by measuring the width of the QRS complex or by driving the ventricle by means of bipolar electrodes attached to the base of the right ventricle and by determining the distance between the stimulus artifact and the potential recorded from the apex.

Conduction of the atrioventricular impulse can be similarly characterized in two ways. The simpler procedure is to measure the PQ distance in the ECG. A more sensitive method, also yielding more information, is the determination of the A-V functional refractory period according to KRAYER et al. (1951). Briefly: the auricular driving frequency is increased until the ventricles are unable follow the driving and escape as a consequence of the fact that the atrioventricular transmission is just refractory to the successive driving stimuli.

C. Cardiac Arrhythmias Evoked by Local Blocks and Spontaneously Firing Ectopic Foci Produced by Local Myocardial Ischemia and Thermal or Mechanical Injury of the Myocardium

All methods listed in this chapter have in common that they alter the basic electrophysiologic parameters of the heart within a circumscribed area only. Their arrhythmogenic action may be due to local hypoxia or ischemia produced by reduction or complete stoppage of the local blood supply, to local heating or cooling of the myocardium, and finally, to mechanical crushing. The latter two interventions act mainly by inhibition of impulse propagation through the myocardium. However, all of the preceding procedures may give rise to local blocks and spontaneously firing ectopic foci leading to asynchronous recovery of excitability in adjacent fibers and accordingly to asynchronous propagation of impulses. Although each of these factors alone may contribute to the development of arrhythmia, their arrhythmogenic effect is even more expressed if they act simultaneously. Special emphasis should be placed on this fact, because, as was shown by us in local myocardial ischemia due to coronary ligation, the most irregularly firing ectopic focus alone may not be sufficient to evoke arrhythmia unless the surrounding normal heart muscle is rendered susceptible to the irregular impulses (SZEKERES et al., 1972a, b). We demonstrated that transient ischemia developing in the working myocardium not affected directly by coronary occlusion may evoke changes in the electrophysiologic parameters of that area, thus facilitating the appearence of arrhythmia. These electrophysiologic changes include shortening of the repolarization phase as well as asynchronous recovery of excitability in nearby areas. We assume, therefore, that the arrhythmogenic action of local foci depends on at least two factors: a) on the presence of a spontaneously discharging focus outside the pacemaker area—firing independently of the pacemaker; b) on certain metabolic and electrophysiologic changes in the "normal" myocardium surrounding the ectopic focus, which may increase its responsiveness to the irregular impulses originating from the focus.

I. Local Myocardial Ischemia

Heart rhythm disturbance due to local ischemia evoked by ligation of a coronary artery seems to fulfil fairly well the criteria of the adequate model-arrhythmia discussed in the introduction, since the pathomechanism is similar to that of arrhythmia occurring in patients after myocardial infarction. From the point of view of a better understanding of the pathophysiology as well as of the therapy of these arrhythmias, analysis of the changes occurring in the early phase, i.e. immediately after coronary occlusion, is of special importance, since these arrhythmias, which sometimes develop to ventricular fibrillation, may have fatal

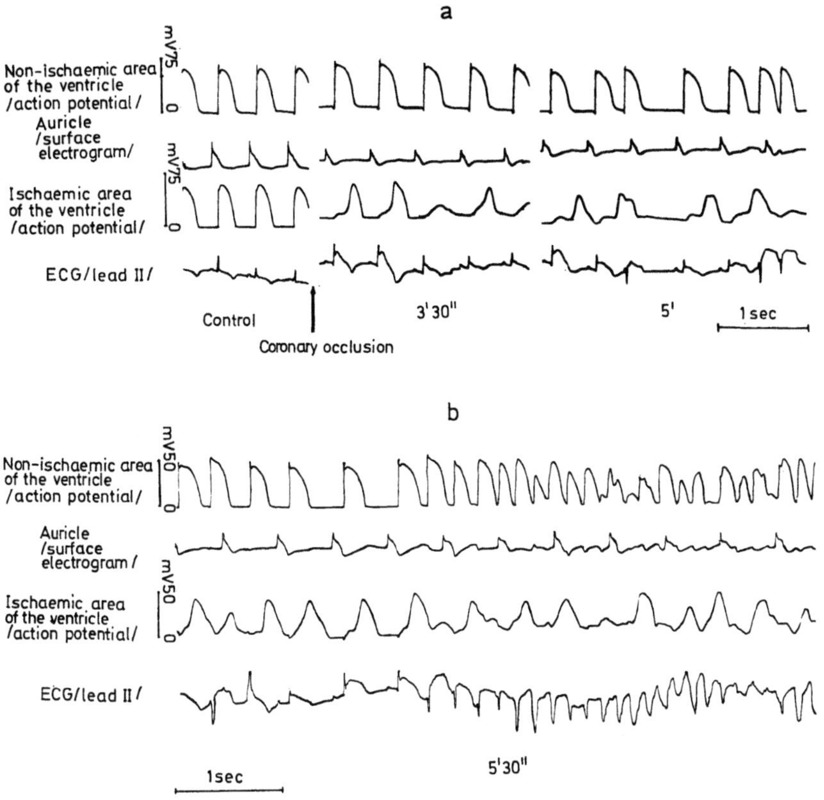

Fig. 3a and b. *Electrical activity of various parts of the heart following sudden occlusion of the left descending coronary artery in a pentobarbital-anesthetized dog.* Monophasic action potentials from the ischemic and nonischemic ventricular areas, surface electrogram from the right atrium, as well as electrocardiogram (lead II) were recorded. Panels (a) and (b) represent two consecutive periods of the same experiment. (See text for details)

consequences. Often there is no time left for the transport of these patients to the coronary care unit—they may die immediately or within one hour after the onset of myocardial infarction.

This increased susceptibility may be due to increased sympathetic and vagal tone, since surgical or chemical denervation of the heart (Szekeres et al., 1972b) prevents the appearance of early arrhythmias after coronary occlusion. The characteristic electrophysiologic changes occurring soon after myocardial infarction are displayed in Fig. 3a. The monophasic action potentials recorded from the ischemic zone as well as from that not directly affected by coronary occlusion show that there is little change in the normal area. On the other hand, in the ischemic zone early decrease of the amplitude, shortening of the repolarization, slowing of the depolarization phase and increasing asynchrony between the potentials of the ischemic and unaffected myocardium are present. This may lead to scattered extrasystoles, and as seen in Fig. 3b, in parallel with a progressively increasing firing rate in the ischemic area, to ventricular fibrillation.

As mentioned previously, however, sometimes even the most expressed asynchrony of the discharges between the ectopic focus and the normal heart rhythm was not able to produce arrhythmia. It may be for this reason that Varma and

MELVILLE (1963) observed only a 30% incidence of ventricular fibrillation after ligation of the left descending coronary artery in dogs. However, when coronary ligation was associated with hypothermia—an intervention increasing susceptibility to fibrillation, as shown by SZEKERES et al. (1961)—the incidence of ventricular fibrillation increased from 30 to 100% (VARMA and MELVILLE, 1963). Hypothermia alone caused a 40% incidence of ventricular fibrillation.

In order to avoid acute ventricular fibrillation, HARRIS (1950) introduced the two-stage ligation technique. For this purpose he first occluded the left descending coronary artery only partially and then performed total occlusion after a minimum interval of 30 min. After having completed the second ligation, the chest was closed under aseptic conditions and spontaneous respiration restored. Five to 7 h after the operation, arrhythmia in the form of ventricular tachycardia may appear, but the maximal ectopic activity develops only on the second day after operation. According to WINBURY and HEMMER (1955) and CLARK and CUMMINGS (1956), this is the most suitable time for the assay of antiarrhythmic agents. The two-stage coronary ligation method was applied by MALING and MORAN (1957) and MORAN et al. (1962) as an intervention increasing the arrhythmogenic action of epinephrine and norepinephrine in dogs. Similar observations were made by WINBURY et al. (1962) in pigs.

In view of the theory discussed previously, the use of these drugs may sensitize the myocardium to the ectopic firing of the infarcted area produced by coronary ligation. In the experiments of MORAN et al. (1962), 10 μg/kg epinephrine or norepinephrine was given on the fourth or fifth day following the ligation, when the arrhythmia evoked by ligation had already ceased and cardiac activity had returned to the normal rhythm. On administration of the catecholamines, the latent pacemaker areas were activated again and extrasystoles, as well as ventricular tachycardia, appeared. This method proved useful also for the evaluation of antiarrhythmic agents.

II. Local Heating or Cooling of the Myocardium

Local heating of the myocardium may give rise to increased ectopic activity. Moreover, the refractory period becomes shorter in the heated area and at the same time conduction velocity increases. But as BROOKS et al. (1955) pointed out, this method is not used to produce arrhythmia, because in order to reach a temperature difference sufficient to disorganize cardiac activity, the circumscribed area should be heated to a temperature which would impair the myocardium.

Local cooling seems to be less harmful and, according to SCHERF and SCHOTT (1935), local temperature differences high enough to evoke arrhythmia may be more easily established. According to HOFF and STANSFIELD (1949), local cooling may produce an injury current between the cooled and the normothermic area which is able to initiate a propagated excitation wave. Also conduction is slowed down in the cooled area, thus providing the possibility for a prolonged circus movement of impulses.

III. Mechanical Injury of the Myocardium

ROSENBLUETH and GARCIA-RAMOS (1947) introduced the method of crushing the inter-vena-caval bridge of the atria and simultaneous application of electrical stimulation in order to produce atrial flutter in anesthetized thoracotomized dogs. This flutter-model was considered for a long time as the main argument in favor of the circus movement theory. SCHERF and BLUMENFELD (1954), however, showed that the flutter so produced did not stop even after ligation of the supposed pathway of the circular movement; thus they concluded that this type of atrial flutter cannot be explained by the circus movement theory but is probably due to spontaneously firing ectopic foci.

D. Induction of Cardiac Arrhythmias by Intravenous Administration or Topical Application of Drugs or Other Chemical Substances

A wide variety of drugs and other chemical substances with different pharmacologic properties are capable of producing arrhythmias. Our present knowledge regarding the precise mode of action of many of these agents, as well as the correlation between their arrhythmogenic activity and chemical structure, is far from complete, so that the use of these compounds remains mainly empirical. In spite of this, drug-induced model-arrhythmias proved to be useful both in studying the nature of changes underlying the appearance of various arrhythmias and in assaying antiarrhythmic action. Accordingly, much information has become available on the direct effect of arrhythmogenic agents on the fundamental electrophysiologic characteristics of the heart which are thought to be essential in the development or maintenance of disorders of cardiac rhythm. In addition, the influence of some of these compounds on extracardiac arrhythmogenic (nervous or humoral) factors has also been studied. On the other hand, analysis of the effects of new, potential antiarrhythmic drugs in model-arrhythmias has become an important part of the normal assay procedure. By using such techniques, useful information can be obtained about the possible mode of action of the antiarrhythmic drug in question.

The most important compounds known to exert arrhythmogenic activity are listed in this section, and the essential data providing evidence for their arrhythmogenic action are summarized. When describing the individual compounds and the experimental techniques used to produce arrhythmias, special attention is given to the mode of action of these agents, chiefly to their characteristic effects on the fundamental parameters of cardiac electrical activity.

From the practical point of view, drug-induced model-arrhythmias are based either on the *intravenous injection* or the *topical application* of various substances.

I. Intravenous Administration of Arrhythmogenic Agents

When an arrhythmogenic substance is administered through the blood stream, i.e. mainly intravenously, arrhythmia is produced either by the direct influence of the compound on the cardiac tissue or by an action exerted at extracardiac sites, such as the autonomic neuro-humoral control of the heart, but both mechanisms can be operative at the same time. In spite of the many variables which play a part in the genesis of arrhythmias under these conditions, the net effects of the arrhythmogenic agents can be interpreted in terms of disorders of cardiac impulse formation, e.g. production of rapidly firing ectopic foci by aconitine, digitalis, etc., disorders of impulse conduction, e.g. slowing of conduction due to veratrine alkaloids, cardiac glycosides, etc., or a combination of both processes. — Arrhythmias can be induced by the administration of *one agent* or combined injection of *several compounds*.

1. Administration of One Arrhythmogenic Agent

a) Cardiac Glycosides

One of the most important manifestations of digitalis intoxication is the appearance of cardiac arrhythmia. Although this fact became known very long ago, until recently relatively little attention has been paid to the possibility of using cardiac glycosides for the production of model-arrhythmias in animal experiments. Even DAWES' detailed review on experimental cardiac arrhythmias, published in 1952, does not contain any information on cardiac glycosides as arrhythmogenic agents. It is now fully recognized that digitalis intoxication is one of the most common causes of serious disorders of cardiac rhythm in various clinical situations (MASON et al., 1973a, b; SINGH and NORRIS, 1973), and cardiac glycosides are being used extensively to produce experimental dysrhythmias.

Several cardiac glycosides (ouabain, acetylstrophanthidin, digitoxin, digoxin, deslanoside, etc.) have been shown to be capable of inducing model-arrhythmias, but the most frequently applied agent is ouabain (G-Strophanthin).

Usually about 50–60% of the lethal dose of a given glycoside has to be administered intravenously to produce severe arrhythmias (FARAH and MARESH, 1948; MOE and MENDEZ, 1951). Although almost every type of cardiac arrhythmia can be produced by these toxic doses, the occurrence of ectopic beats (chiefly of ventricular origin) is the most common phenomenon to be observed in animal experiments. The usual sequence of events is: T-wave flattening or inversion on the electrocardiogram, ventricular or nodal extrasystoles, occasionally bigeminal rhythm, ventricular tachycardia of monofocal or multifocal origin, and finally, ventricular fibrillation (KATZUNG, 1968). In addition to the increase in ectopic impulse formation, in most cases, there is a decrease in A-V conduction after about 20% of the lethal dose, and partial or complete A-V block occurs at approximately 50% of the lethal dose (MOE and MENDEZ, 1951). Detailed description of these arrhythmias has been given by several authors (SCHERF and SCHOTT, 1953; VASSALLE et al., 1963; GREENSPAN and STEINMETZ, 1966).

Sudden intravenous injection of toxic doses of cardiac glycosides may lead to an early ventricular fibrillation followed by cardiac arrest. In order to produce long-lasting arrhythmias it is, therefore, advisable to administer these agents in graded doses. In anesthetized dogs, *ouabain* is usually injected intravenously in an initial dose of about 40 μg/kg, followed by further doses of 10–20 μg/kg 30 min later and every 10 min thereafter until the desired arrhythmia (in the majority of cases persistent nodal or ventricular tachycardia) is established (GARRETT et al., 1964; KATZUNG, 1968; PAPP and SZEKERES, 1972). The sensitivity of dogs to the arrhythmogenic action of ouabain is variable; the dose required to produce severe arrhythmia is about 70 to 80 μg/kg in general, but sometimes more than 100 μg/kg may be necessary (CLARK and CUMMINGS, 1956; WINBURY and PAPIERSKI, 1956). Since the intoxication due to cardiac glycosides is a progressive process, it is hard to standardize the arrhythmia. Nevertheless, in most cases the ouabain-induced arrhythmia persists for more than 60 to 90 min (its duration of action is considerably longer than that of acetylstrophanthidin) (KATZUNG, 1968), so that there is sufficient time available to determine, at least semi-quantitatively, whether a drug or another factor is capable of influencing (reverting to sinus rhythm or aggravating) the dysrhythmia (WINBURY and PAPIERSKI, 1956; LUCCHESI and HARDMANN, 1961; MOE, 1961; MOKLER and VAN ARMAN, 1962; GARRETT et al., 1964; HEISTRACHER et al., 1965; SOMANI and LUM, 1965; SOMANI et al., 1966; LUCCHESI and IWAMI, 1968). In the same way, ouabain-arrhythmia can consistently be produced also in the dog heart-lung preparation. This technique is used

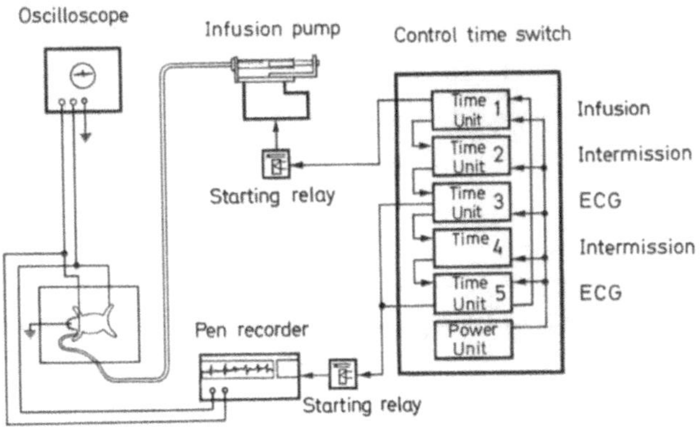

Fig. 4. *Diagram of an automated intermittent-infusion technique used for the determination of the dose of ouabain required to produce arrhythmia in anesthetized guinea pigs*

occasionally to assess direct antiarrhythmic effects of drugs on the heart (SOMANI and LUM, 1966; LADDU and SOMANI, 1969; LADDU, 1970).

Ouabain-induced arrhythmias can also be produced by the so-called intermittent infusion technique, which has been used in anesthetized guinea pigs (SEKIYA and VAUGHAN WILLIAMS, 1963; PAPP and VAUGHAN WILLIAMS, 1969a, b; SINGH and VAUGHAN WILLIAMS, 1970a, b, 1972). In Fig. 4 the arrangement of an automated version of this method is demonstrated. Ouabain is infused intermittently into the right jugular vein from the syringe of a constant rate infusion pump. Every 2 min, 6 μg/kg ouabain are injected during 30 sec. After each infusion period ECG records (lead II) are taken by a pen recorder at times and the ECG is monitored continuously by an oscilloscope. The operation of the infusion pump and the pen recorder is automated by using an electronic time switch attached to starting relays. In each period lasting usually for 2 min, the sequence of events is a follows: infusion of ouabain for 30 sec; intermission for 25 sec; ECG recording for 5 sec; intermission for 55 sec; ECG recording for 5 sec. The duration of the infusion and recording periods, as well that of the intermissions, is adjustable at will. When using this technique, successively increasing doses of ouabain will produce supraventricular arrhythmias with prolonged P-R and unequal R-R intervals on the ECG (at about 80 to 90 μg/kg), followed by occasional ectopic extrasystoles (at approximately 180 to 200 μg/kg), ventricular rhythm (at about 220 to 240 μg/kg), ventricular fibrillo-flutter or clear fibrillation (at about 260 to 280 μg/kg) and cardiac arrest (at about 310 to 330 μg/kg). ECG records taken from an experiment of this kind are shown in Fig. 5. The method is especially suitable for studying the protective action of various compounds against ouabain-induced arrhythmias, when changes in the dosage of ouabain required to produce various dysrhythmias is measured. A similar technique has recently been applied to the induction of ouabain-arrhythmia in the cat (KELLIHER and ROBERTS, 1972).

Continuous intravenous infusion of *acetylstrophanthidin* at a rate of 80 μg/min has also been used to produce model-arrhythmias in dogs (LUCCHESI and SHIVAK, 1964). The onset of action of this glycoside is faster than that of ouabain, so that the dosage necessary to produce arrhythmia can be determined even more rapidly (KATZUNG, 1968). Acetylstrophanthidin has been used to induce dysrhythmias not only *in vivo*, but also in isolated rabbit hearts (LUCCHESI and IWAMI, 1968). In the

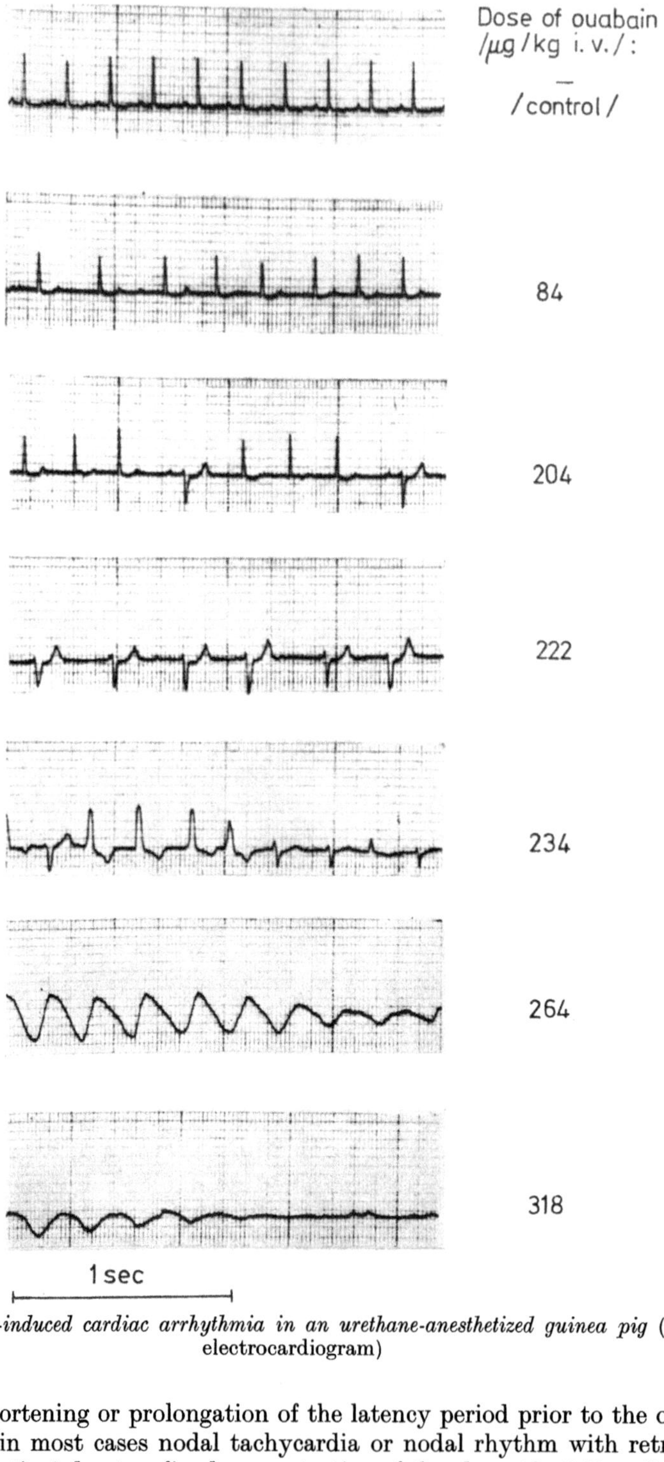

Fig. 5. *Ouabain-induced cardiac arrhythmia in an urethane-anesthetized guinea pig* (Lead II electrocardiogram)

latter case, shortening or prolongation of the latency period prior to the onset of arrhythmias (in most cases nodal tachycardia or nodal rhythm with retrograde P-wave conduction) due to a fixed concentration of the glycoside (640 µg/l) is used as an indicator of action.

In addition to ouabain and acetylstrophanthidin, other cardiac glycosides administered intravenously, have also been used occasionally for the production of model-arrhythmias. These include *digoxin* (SODHI et al., 1966), digitoxin (BAZIKA et al., 1966), *deslanoside* (GILLIS et al., 1971, 1973) and *K-strophanthin* (CHARLIER and VANDERSMISSEN, 1955a, b, c; SCHMITT and SCHMITT, 1960).

In some cases intravenous injection of large doses of cardiac glycosides represents only one of the factors faciliting the appearance of model-arrhythmias, and in order to elicit the disturbance of cardiac rhythm, other arrhythmogenic interventions are applied simultaneously. Accordingly, acetylstrophanthidin (CIOFALO et al., 1966; LEVITT and ROBERTS, 1966) or ouabain (BARRETT and CULLUM, 1968) has been used in combination with vagal stimulation to produce ventricular arrhythmias. The method is based on the fact that in animals whose sino-atrial nodal rate is slowed by vagal stimulation to a critical point giving rise to ventricular escape, relatively small amounts of glycosides are required to raise the automaticity of subatrial pacemaker centers. The intensity of vagal stimulation is adjusted to produce a marked sinus bradycardia and the smallest dose of the glycoside necessary to induce ventricular extrasystole is determined. This dose can be regarded as a quantitative measure of ventricular automaticity. It should be mentioned that in this case the glycoside itself, in the doses used, does not evoke arrhythmia in the absence of vagal stimulation. A variant of this method consists of intravenous administration of acetylstrophanthidin to dogs with atrioventricular block induced by ligating the bundle of His (ROBERTS et al., 1963).

Although typical model-arrhythmias involving the combined use of electrical stimulation of the heart and intravenous administration of a digitalis glycoside have not been developed as yet, it is of interest to note that in digitalized animals the threshold to electrical shock is changed; the discharge energy required to produce ventricular tachycardia is reduced in the digitalized heart (LOWN et al., 1965). Digitalis glycosides also lower the threshold for repetitive extrasystoles in response to pacemaker stimuli (LOWN et al., 1967). Although paired electrical pacing has been shown to be an effective means of preventing or suppressing digitalis-induced arrhythmias in experimental animals, the lethal dose of digitalis is decreased under these conditions, and when using this technique in overdigitalized animals or patients, there is considerable danger of inducing ventricular fibrillation (FROMMER et al., 1965; MASON et al., 1973b).

There is ample evidence to suggest that the arrhythmogenic action of cardiac glycosides is related to both cardiac and extracardiac mechanisms. — Results of many observations, reviewed recently by LEE and KLAUS (1971), make it apparent that the Na^+, K^+-activated (transport) ATPase associated with the myocardial cell membrane, is directly and strongly inhibited by toxic amounts of cardiac glycosides. In addition, a temporal correlation between the toxic cardiac electrophysiologic effects of these glycosides and the glycoside-induced inhibition of transport ATPase activity has also been established (TEN EICK et al., 1973). In view of the known function of transport ATPase, cardiac glycosides will inhibit at the same time the Na^+, K^+ exchange mechanisms resulting in a loss of intracellular K^+ and concomittant increase in the intracellular Na^+ concentration. Most of the theoretically predicted electrophysiologic consequences of an inhibition of the myocardial transport ATPase (decrease in resting membrane potential and depolarization rate, etc.) are, in fact, observable also in the presence of large concentrations of digitalis. Simultaneous measurements of intracellular potassium concentration, potassium flux and membrane potential in Purkinje fibers revealed that severe dysrhythmia caused by toxic concentrations of cardiac glycosides could be due to a decrease in the intracellular potassium concentration. On increasing the intracellular concentration of the potassium ion the glycoside-induced reduction in membrane potential was restored and the arrhythmia was suppressed (MÜLLER, 1963; CARMELIET and VERDONCK, 1967). Considering these observations it seems reasonable to assume that inhibition of the transport ATPase constitutes, at least in part, the basis of the intricate mechanism of the toxic, direct arrhythmogenic action of cardiac glycosides. In view of this, the fundamental mechanism of the toxic and therapeutic (positive inotropic) action of digitalis seems to be different, since the latter effect has been attributed to alterations in the calcium transport across the cardiac membrane or to changes in the intracellular calcium binding (LÜLLMANN and HOLLAND, 1962; NAYLER, 1967; LEE and KLAUS, 1971).

The electrophysiologic actions of cardiac glycosides are manifold and depend on a large number of variables (see reviews by TRAUTWEIN, 1963; SZEKERES and PAPP, 1968, 1971; LEE and KLAUS, 1971; MASON et al., 1973a). From the point of view of the development of arrhythmias, alterations in the electrical activity of the specialized impulse-generating and -conducting tissue of the heart are of crucial importance. In Purkinje fibers a marked reduction in the maximum diastolic potential accompanied by a major increase in automaticity and appearance of rapidly firing ectopic foci with series of spontaneous action potentials ("extrasystoles") is most characteristic of digitalis excess. Following an incomplete repolarization, spontaneous depolarizations begin at low resting membrane potentials, and action potentials of low amplitude and short duration (after-potentials) develop, leading to the generation of multiple discharges and low amplitude oscillations (MÜLLER, 1963; HOFFMAN and SINGER, 1964; CARMELIET and VERDONCK, 1967; DUDEL and TRAUTWEIN, 1958; PASTELIN and MENDEZ, 1972; ROSÉN et al., 1973a, b).

In the whole heart the known direct (also indirect, see below) depressant effect of cardiac glycosides on the sino-atrial pacemaker tissue (JAMES and NADEAU, 1960) leading to partial or complete loss of sinus dominance, also gives rise to the development of rapid ectopic rhythms. In the presence of toxic concentrations of cardiac glycosides the rate of depolarization is decreased (DUDEL and TRAUTWEIN, 1958; KASSEBAUM, 1963) with concomitant depression in impulse conduction, especially in the atrioventricular node (MOE and MENDEZ, 1951; WATANABE and DREIFUS, 1966) and in the Purkinje fibers (SWAIN and WEIDNER, 1957). In addition to the decreased resting membrane potential, a diminution in the membrane responsiveness, i.e. a shift to the right of the rate of depolarization/resting potential curve, also contributes to this effect (DUDEL and TRAUTWEIN, 1958; KASSEBAUM, 1963). The combination of the enhancement of Purkinje fiber automaticity and the depression of its conductivity favors the development of glycoside-induced ventricular fibrillation.

In Purkinje fibers, high concentrations of glycosides produce an acceleration of the repolarization phase (DUDEL and TRAUTWEIN, 1958; KASSEBAUM, 1963; PASTELIN and MENDEZ, 1972) which can serve as a basis for shortening the ventricular refractory period (MÉNDEZ and MÉNDEZ, 1953; HAN and MOE, 1964) and precipitate the development of severe arrhythmia. Cardiac excitability is usually reduced in the presence of toxic digitalis concentrations (MOE and MÉNDEZ, 1951), and simultaneously with a major reduction of the resting membrane potential, excitability is lost completely (PASTELIN and MENDEZ, 1972). A slightly increased excitability has been observed with small doses of cardiac glycosides (MOE and MÉNDEZ, 1951).

Many of the characteristic electrophysiologic alterations due to digitalis excess (decrease in the resting membrane potential, shortening of the action potential duration, etc.) can also be observed in the non-specialized working myocardial tissue. As regards the arrhythmogenic effects, it is of particular interest to note that the working myocardium (mainly the ventricular muscle) is much less sensitive to the toxic concentrations of cardiac glycosides than is the specialized conducting tissue (Purkinje fibers) (VASSALLE et al., 1962; SWAIN and WEIDNER, 1957). Accordingly, arrhythmogenic concentrations of digitalis may have different effects on the neighboring areas of the ventricular myocardium, which is known to precipitate the development of arrhythmia. Indeed, inhomogeneity in recovery of excitability, as measured at various points of the right ventricle, has been shown to be increased in ouabain intoxication (HAN and MOE, 1964).

Cardiac glycosides, in addition to their direct cardiac actions, are known to increase the central vagal influence to the heart (KRAYER, 1944), to enhance the sensitivity of the sinoatrial node to the depressant effect of vagal activity or acetylcholine (GREMELS, 1935; SZEKERES et al., 1951; GAFFNEY et al., 1958) and to activate vagal reflexes (HEYMANS et al., 1932). These effects can facilitate the appearance of arrhythmias, especially in the presence of excess catecholamines (SCHERF et al., 1961; ROBERTS and BAER, 1960; ROBERTS et al., 1956). The significance of a vagal component in the arrhythmogenic action of digitalis is shown by the fact that the glycoside-induced shortening in the atrial refractory period, which is known to precipitate the development of certain arrhythmias (SZEKERES and PAPP, 1971), can be prevented or diminished by section of the vagi or administration of atropine (FARAH and LOOMIS, 1950). Moreover, the pronounced prolongation of the functional refractory period of the atrioventricular transmission system, leading ultimately to atrioventricular block, is, at least in part, also a vagally mediated effect of cardiac glycosides (MÉNDEZ and MÉNDEZ, 1953).

The arrhythmogenic action of cardiac glycosides appears to be dependent also on adrenergic mechanisms. It has been shown that surgical removal of the sympathetic nerves and the adrenals increased the lethal dose of ouabain and decreased the incidence of digitalis-induced ventricular fibrillation (MÉNDEZ et al., 1961; ERLIJ and MÉNDEZ, 1964; BOYAJY and NASH, 1966). Digitalis increases cardiac sympathetic nerve activity just prior to or simultaneously with inducing ventricular arrhythmia (GILLIS, 1969; GILLIS et al., 1971). In favor of these observations sympathetic blockade by pharmacologic means also protected against arrhythmia due to digitalis intoxication. — Accordingly, adrenergic neuron blocking agents, such as bretylium (PAPP and VAUGHAN WILLIAMS, 1969a; GILLIS et al., 1973), guanethidine (RAINES et al., 1968), reserpine (ROBERTS et al., 1963; ERLIJ and MÉNDEZ, 1963, 1964; CIOFALO et al., 1966; LEVITT and ROBERTS, 1966; ROBERTS et al., 1967), when given several hours prior to digitalis intoxication, reduced the occurrence or delayed the development of digitalis arrhythmias. — Although the dual (specific and non-specific) actions of the majority of the adrenergic beta-receptor blocking compounds resulted in considerable difficulties in the interpretation of the mode of action of these drugs in glycoside-induced arrhythmias, it has been clearly demonstrated that relatively small doses of beta-adrenergic antagonists with weak or negligible non-specific actions are capable of preventing or terminating heart rhythm disturbances produced by digitalis (RAPER and WALE, 1968, 1969; PAPP and VAUGHAN WILLIAMS, 1969b, c; KELLIHER and ROBERTS, 1972). In addition, levo-propranolol (which is about 100 times more potent as a beta-receptor blocker than the dextro isomer) proved to be more active in preventing arrhythmias due to an acute digitalis intoxication than the d-isomer (BARRETT and CULLUM, 1968; DOHADWALIA et al., 1969). Quite recently, similar observations were also made with levo- and dextro-practolol (KELLIHER and RO-

BERTS, 1972). Whatever the explanation for the beneficial effect of beta-receptor blockers in digitalis arrhythmias might be, it is beyond any doubt that these compounds provide significant protection against the beta-receptor stimulating action of catecholamines released and circulating even under normal conditions without any increase in the basal sympathetic activity. In view of the foregoing results obtained with sympathectomy, this effect of beta-blockers can be considered as an "antiarrhythmic" measure in digitalis arrhythmia. It is also pertinent that injection of catecholamines or stimulation of adrenergic cardiac nerves has been shown to increase the toxic, arrhythmogenic actions of cardiac glycosides on the heart (SEKILYA and VAUGHAN WILLIAMS, 1963; BECKER et al., 1962; RAPER and WALE, 1969). — On the whole it seems that in digitalis intoxication a sympathetic involvement is not of utmost significance for precipitation of cardiac arrhythmia; nevertheless under certain conditions, especially in the presence of an increased vagal activity, it can contribute to the development of disorders of cardiac rhythm.

b) Barium Chloride

Since the first observation on the arrhythmogenic action of the barium ion, made in the frog heart (BOEHM, 1875), $BaCl_2$ has been shown to produce severe disorders of cardiac rhythm in other species, such as dogs, cats and rabbits (NALEFSKI et al., 1949; ROTHBERGER and WINTERBERG, 1911; LEVY, 1914; SMITH et al., 1940; MCMILLAN and WOLFERTH, 1928; VAN DONGEN, 1936, 1937; BIJLSMA and VAN DONGEN, 1939; BLUMENTHAL and OPPENHEIMER, 1939; BOVET et al., 1939; SCHMITT and SCHMITT, 1960; PAPP et al., 1967; SZEKERES and PAPP, 1971).

In order to produce arrhythmias with $BaCl_2$, administered intravenously, the rabbit has been favored by several investigators (VAN DONGEN, 1936, 1937; SCHMITT and SCHMITT, 1960; PAPP et al., 1967; HADHÁZY et al., 1968; SZEKERES and PAPP, 1971). This species is rather sensitive to the arrhythmogenic effect of $BaCl_2$, and its calmness and readily accessible marginal ear veins make it easy to carry out experiments also in unanesthetized animals. Under appropriate conditions the $BaCl_2$-arrhythmia induced in rabbits is of sufficient severity and duration, it is reversible and reproducible and has been shown to be suitable even for assaying antiarrhythmic action. — The intravenous dose of $BaCl_2$ required to produce arrhythmia varies between 1–5 mg/kg depending on the strain of rabbit and on the experimental conditions. In unanesthetized rabbits, 4 mg/kg $BaCl_2$ will produce scattered extrasystoles of ventricular origin, followed by typical bigeminy or polytopic ventricular extrasystoles leading sometimes to short periods of ventricular tachycardia. If $BaCl_2$ is injected slowly (in about 20 sec) and the concentration of the solution does not exceed 2%, fatal arrhythmia does not occur. The rhythm disorder will last for more than 20 min and will be fully reversible. An example of the lasting and reversible bigeminy produced by intravenous administration of 4 mg/kg $BaCl_2$ to an unanesthetized rabbit is given in Fig. 6. — As jugded from the incidence and kind of arrhythmia, as well as from the duration of action, the same dose administered repeatedly over 24–48 h intervals, has practically the same effect. It is of interest to note, however, that daily $BaCl_2$ treatment for a longer time will cause exhaustion of the animals and even evoke fatal arrhythmias. — The severity of arrhythmia produced by $BaCl_2$ in unanesthetized rabbits greatly depends on the dose. After intravenous administration of 5 mg/kg $BaCl_2$, an initial ventricular fibrillo-flutter or fibrillation often develops, but in the relatively small rabbit heart the fibrillation usually ceases spontaneously and is followed by ventricular arrhythmia until complete recovery occurs (Fig. 7).

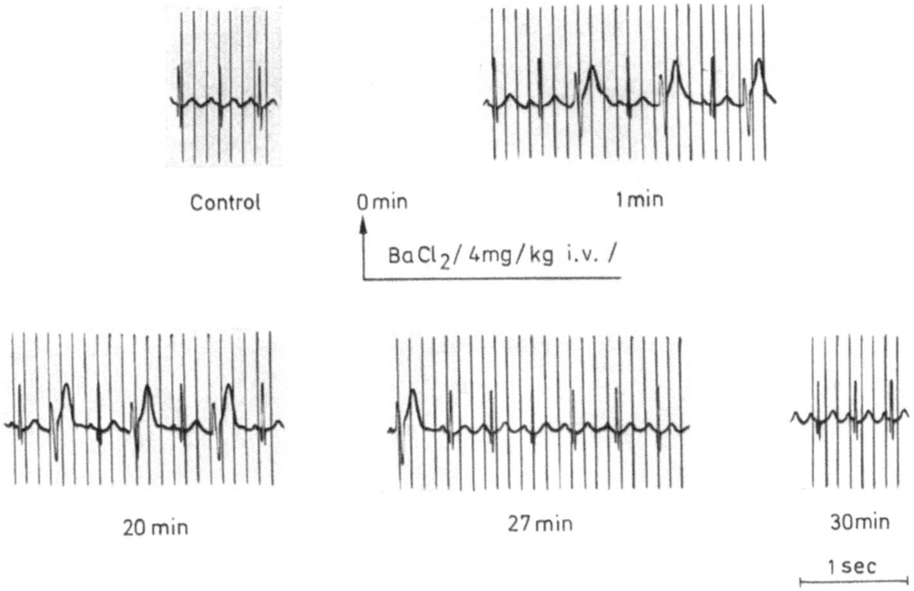

Fig. 6. *Cardiac arrhythmia induced by barium chloride in an unanesthetized rabbit* (Electrocardiogram was recorded in a precordial lead corresponding to position V_4)

The available information regarding the mode of action of $BaCl_2$ in producing cardiac arrhythmias is scanty. Ventricular fibrillation can be induced by $BaCl_2$ not only under *in situ* conditions, but also in the isolated heart (BLUMENTHAL and OPPENHEIMER, 1939), so that the development of arrhythmia could be attributed, at least in part, to a direct cardiac effect. Indeed, a marked increase in the rate of slow diastolic depolarization, i.e. in the automaticity of isolated Purkinje fibers, has been observed under the influence of $BaCl_2$ (ANTONI and OBERDISSE, 1965), and spontaneous pacemaker activity with typical slow diastolic depolarization has been induced by barium ions in the non-specialized working myocardium, including both atrial and ventricular muscle fibers (ANTONI and OBERDISSE, 1965; ANTONI, 1968, 1971). This "automatotropic" (ANTONI, 1971) effect seems to be responsible also for the barium-induced spontaneous activity observed in quiescent left atrial (KRUTA, 1934; ROTHBERGER and SACHS, 1939) or ventricular (GREINER and GARB, 1950; DEUTSCH and LUNDIN, 1946) preparation. In Purkinje fibers of the sheep the changes caused by barium ions are mainly brought about by an increase in sodium inward current (SHIBATA, 1973). The initiation of latent or manifest pacemaker areas in the ordinary ventricular myocardium together with an increase in the automaticity of Purkinje fibers can lead to disorganized electrical activity, when coordinated activation of the ventricle is no longer maintained. As a result, extrasystoles, runs of aberrant ventricular beats and ventricular fibrillation may develop. — It is relevant that the ability of barium ions to initiate rhythmic activity and to facilitate the appearance of occasional repetitive discharges has been proved also in nervous tissue (FENG, 1937; DUN and FENG, 1940); barium ions can cause depolarization and a significant increase in the after-potentials (LORENTE DE NÓ and FENG, 1946).

DAWES (1952) suggested that an extracardiac, adrenergic mechanism might also contribute to the arrhythmogenic action of barium chloride, since the barium-

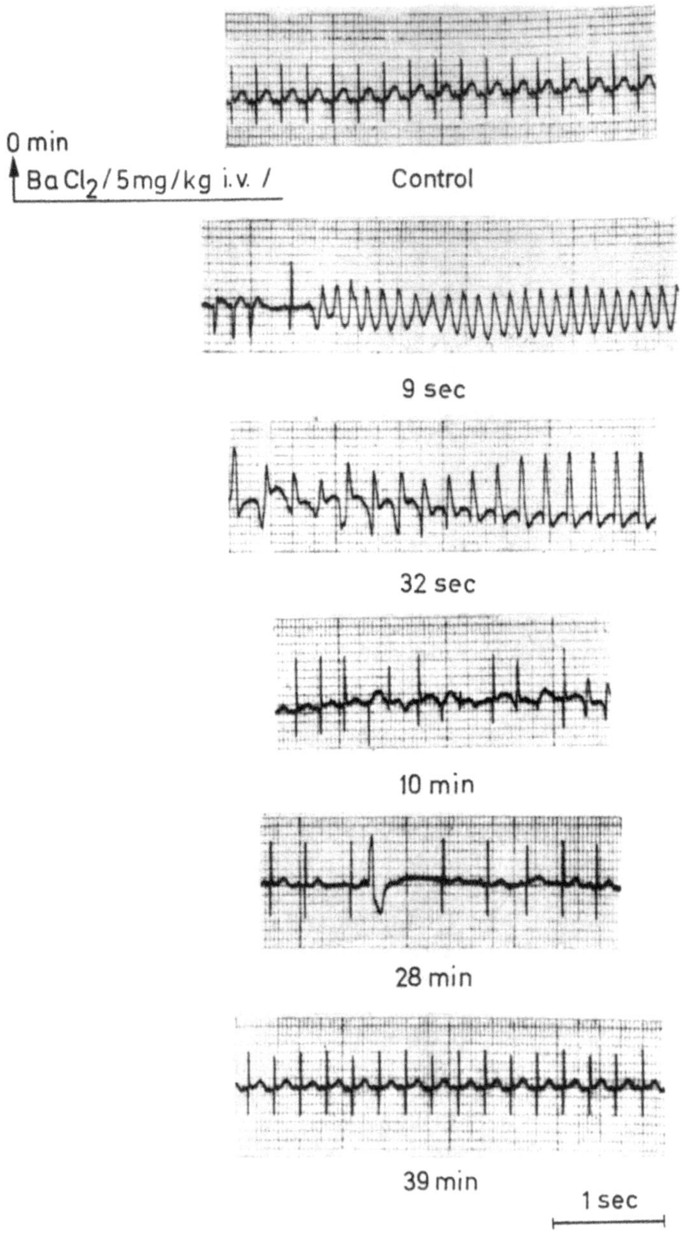

Fig. 7. *Reversible ventricular fibrillo-flutter induced by barium chloride in an unanesthetized rabbit* (Electrocardiogram was recorded in a precordial lead corresponding to position V_4)

induced increase in blood pressure could be abolished by yohimbine, a sympatholytic agent (Hazard and Quinquaud, 1945). In favor of this assumption it has recently been found that beta-adrenergic receptor antagonists are capable of reverting to normal sinus rhythm dysrhythmias produced by intravenous injection of $BaCl_2$ (Papp et al., 1967). However, in view of the known non-specific actions of adrenergic beta-blockers, further studies are required to make sure that an increase in sympathetic activity does play a part in the genesis of barium-induced arrhythmias.

c) Calcium Chloride

Ventricular fibrillation is a frequent occurrence when the serum calcium ion level is three or four times higher than the normal concentration (BROOKS et al., 1955). Intravenous injection of high doses of calcium chloride will invariably precipitate the development of serious dysrhythmias in various experimental animals, such as dogs and mainly rats (ROTHBERGER and WINTERBERG, 1911; HOFF and NAHUM, 1937; HOFF et al., 1939; WINKLER et al., 1939; MALINOW et al., 1953a, b, c, 1954a, b, 1955a, b; NIESCHULZ et al., 1955; WINBURY and HEMMER, 1955; SCHMITT and SCHMITT, 1960; FEKETE and BORSY, 1964; PAPP et al., 1966; SETNIKAR et al., 1966; CUPARENCU et al., 1969). When administered intravenously, the dose of calcium chloride needed to elicit severe cardiac arrhythmias in anesthetized rats varies from 120 mg/kg (FEKETE and BORSY, 1964; SETNIKAR et al., 1966) to 200 mg/kg (MALINOW et al., 1953a, b, c; NIESCHULZ et al., 1955; WINBURY and HEMMER, 1955; SCHMITT and SCHMITT, 1960; TURNER, 1965). The reason for this wide range of doses is that in the different rat strains there is a considerable difference in sensitivity to calcium chloride. Moreover, the concentration of calcium chloride solution and the speed of its injection has not been standardized by the various authors. — In a series of experiments (PAPP et al., 1966) arrhythmia was produced by rapid intravenous injection of 140 mg/kg calcium chloride given as a 2.5% solution. Within a few seconds after injection, two types of response could be observed. In about 80% of the animals, lethal ventricular fibrillation occurred within 60 to 90 sec (Fig. 8a). In the remaining animals ventricular extrasystoles in association with sinus bradycardia and/or atrioventricular block appeared, which passed into short runs of ventricular tachycardia or spontaneously reversible ventricular fibrillation. The latter animals survived, and a practically normal ECG could be recorded after about 30 min (Fig. 8b). In a few animals, calcium chloride produced an immediate and lasting apnea with progressively developing signs of asphyxia leading ultimately to severe bradycardia and cardiac arrest. Upon final evaluation of the results, most authors do not take into account that the latter group of animals responded with immediate apnea and consecutive asphyxia (TURNER, 1965).

The model-arrhythmias produced by calcium chloride are most severe and hard to influence. In spite of this, the ability of new compounds to provide some protection against these arrhythmias has frequently been used for the assay of antiarrhythmic activity (MALINOW et al., 1955a, b; NIESCHULZ et al., 1955; WINBURY, 1956; FEKETE and BORSY, 1964; TURNER, 1965). Usually the decrease in incidence of lethal ventricular fibrillation is the measure of protection, but rather high doses of antiarrhythmics have to be given to produce a significant effect.

The mechanism by which calcium chloride exerts its arrhythmogenic action is complex and not fully understood. It is clear, however, that chiefly cardiac and to some extent also extracardiac factors are involved.

The significance of a direct cardiac action is shown by the fact that on elevation of the calcium concentration severe arrhythmias, including ventricular fibrillation, occur also in the isolated heart (GROSS, 1903; GRUMBACH et al., 1954). Although approximately a fourfold increase in the calcium ion level decreases the excitability of Purkinje fibers by lowering the threshold potential (WEIDMANN, 1955), this change is not uniform in tissues from all parts of the heart. The non-specialized

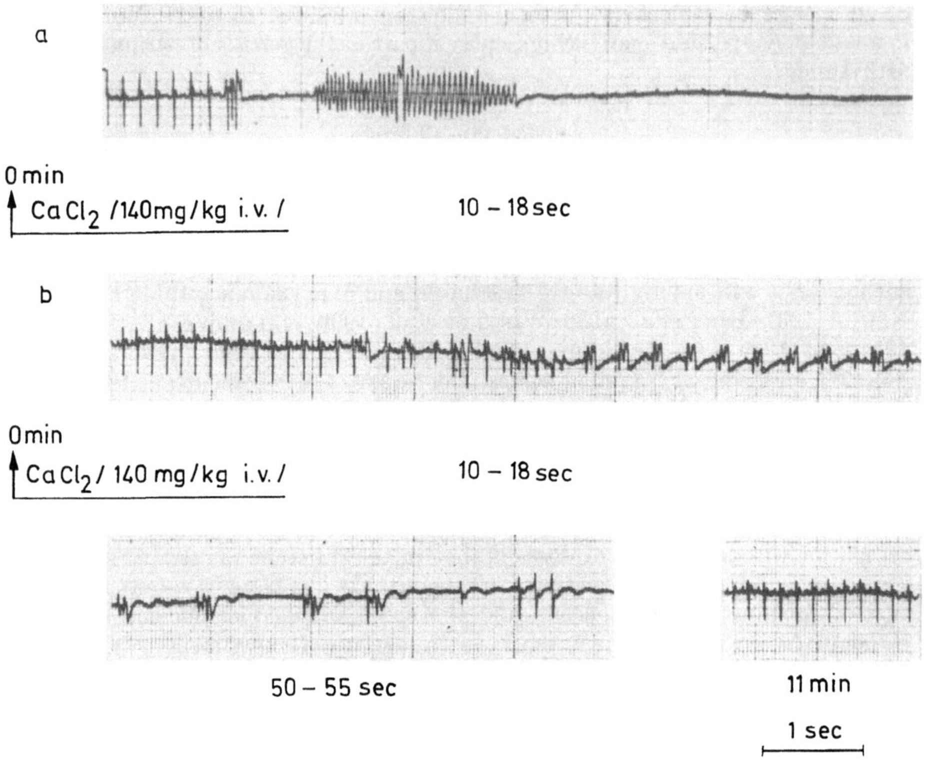

Fig. 8a and b. *Two types of cardiac arrhythmia induced by calcium chloride in urethane-anesthetized rats* (Lead II electrocardiogram)

working myocardium of the ventricle is more resistant to this effect of calcium than the Purkinje fibers (BROOKS et al., 1955; HOFFMAN and SUCKLING, 1956; HOFFMAN and CRANEFIELD, 1960). Accordingly, excitability may even be lost completely in one area of the heart when other regions are still excitable. This may favor the development of local blocks and can increase the asynchrony of impulse propagation, thereby facilitating the appearance of arrhythmias. — On the other hand, an increase in calcium concentration results in a marked acceleration in the repolarization of non-specialized working muscle fibers (HOFFMAN and SUCKLING, 1956; HOFFMAN and CRANEFIELD, 1960). In addition, the same (four times normal) calcium concentration which causes a complete loss of plateau in ventricular muscle, does not appreciably affect the time course of the action potential in Purkinje fibers (BROOKS et al., 1955). This latter difference in sensitivity to high calcium concentrations may lead to an increase in the asynchrony of recovery of excitability of the ventricle, which is known to be one of the most important electrophysiologic alterations underlying the development of arrhythmias. — In the presence of high calcium concentrations the S-shaped curve relating the maximum rate of depolarization (dV_{max}/dt) to the resting membrane potential, is shifted to the left, i.e. the sodium conductance and thus the membrane responsiveness is increased, because of the enhancement of the available sodium carrier (WEIDMANN, 1955). Accordingly, when calcium ions are in excess, the inward sodium current is greater even at low resting membrane potentials (i.g. at an early stage of repolarization) and an early recovery of excitability occurs, giving rise to extrasystoles. — The spontaneous activity of isolated Purkinje fibers is not enhanced under the influence of high calcium concentrations; on the contrary, there is a considerable decrease in automaticity because of the diminished threshold potential (WEIDMANN, 1955). This is also valid for the sinoatrial pacemaker activity (SEIFEN et al., 1964; WEST, 1972).

In addition to the direct cardiac effects, the arrhythmias induced by intravenous injection of calcium chloride appear to be due, at least in part, to an indirect action mediated through the autonomic nervous system. In rats the appearance of these arrhythmias was partially prevented by surgical destruction of certain areas of the central nervous system which are thought to be related to the sympathetic pathways running to the heart, whereas bilateral vagotomy was without effect. Ganglionic blocking agents also afforded some protection (MALINOW et al., 1953a). Although the possible role of a sympathetic involvement in the genesis of calcium chloride-induced arrhythmia cannot be excluded, the direct cardiac action of calcium ions seems to be far more important than the extracardiac adrenergic mechanisms. Adrenergic neuron blocking agents administered several hours prior to the intravenous injection of calcium chloride to rats, exerted only a minor protective action (PAPP et al., 1966), and in dogs the effect of various sympatholytic agents capable of delaying the development of calcium chloride-induced ventricular fibrillation did not seem to be specific either (CUPARENCU et al., 1969). — It must be borne in mind, however, that under the influence of high calcium concentrations catecholamines can be released from the peripheral adrenergic structures even in an isolated heart (LISSÁK, 1938), resulting in an increase of the tendency towards arrhythmia.

d) Aconitine

Intravenous administration of aconitine has long been known to cause severe disorders of cardiac rhythm in various experimental animals (for earlier references see BOEHM, 1920; TRIPOD, 1951). In recent studies, cats (NIESCHULTZ et al., 1955) and mostly rats (FEKETE and BORSY, 1964; SZEKERES and PAPP, 1971) have been used for this purpose. The intravenous dose of aconitine used to produce model-arrhythmias is usually about 30 to 50 μg/kg, under the influence of which ventricular (or nodal) extrasystoles, sometimes typical bigeminal ventricular tachycardia of monofocal or multifocal origin and, frequently, even ventricular fibrillation, develop. Depending on the species and other experimental conditions (anesthesia, etc.), there is about 1 to 5 min latency period prior to the onset of the persistent arrhythmia which lasts for at least 15 to 20 min, but sometimes for more than an hour, and occasionally irreversible ventricular fibrillation leading to the death of the animal ensues. An example of the aconitine-induced arrhythmia with characteristic bigeminal rhythm is presented in Fig. 9. — Various compounds are capable of delaying the onset of these arrhythmias (FEKETE and BORSY, 1964), and aconitine-induced rhythm disorders can also be suppressed by drugs (NIESCHULTZ et al., 1955; SZEKERES and PAPP, 1971), so that this model-arrhythmia is suitable for assaying antiarrhythmic action.

Although the possible role of some extracardiac factors in the arrhythmogenic action of aconitine cannot be entirely neglected (BOEHM, 1920), it is the direct cardiac effect of aconitine which is of decisive importance in the induction of arrhythmia. In the isolated heart of the rabbit or the cat, dysrhythmia of about the same type and severity as observed in the *in situ* heart, can be produced by using a nutrient solution containing low concentrations (10^{-8} to 10^{-7} g/ml) of aconitine (TRIPOD, 1951). Decapitation did not significantly alter the arrhythmo-

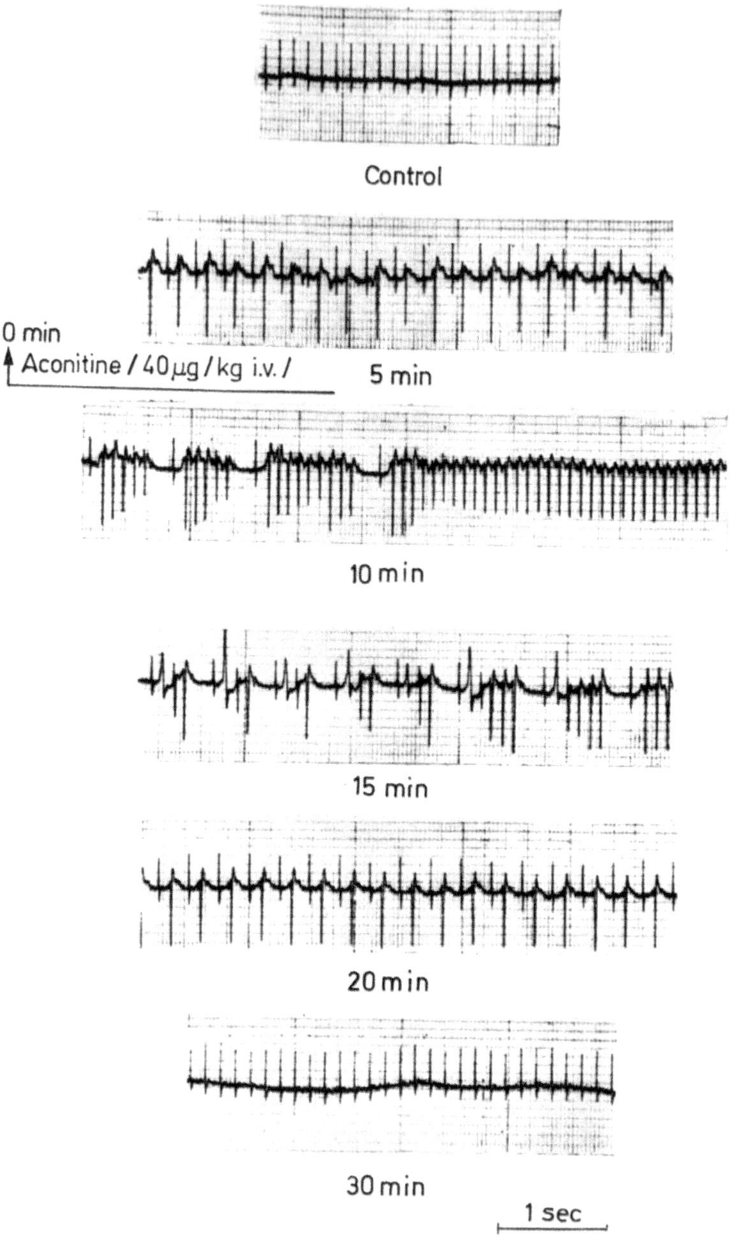

Fig. 9. *Aconitine-induced cardiac arrhythmia in a pentobarbital-anesthetized rat* (Lead II electrocardiogram)

genic effect of aconitine given intravenously in a dose of 30 μg/kg to cats (NIESCHULTZ et al., 1955). In view of this, production of arrhythmia by topical application of aconitine to various parts of the heart has been favored by many investigators and is being used far more frequently for the assay of antiarrhythmic compounds than the intravenous aconitine test. — Details regarding the topical application and the mode of action of aconitine will be treated under Section II.3.

e) Veratrum Alkaloids

Intravenous injections of high doses of veratrine (about 0.5 to 1.5 mg/kg of the crude alkaloidal mixture) and the purified veratrum alkaloids (cevadine, cryptenamine) have been shown to be capable of producing ventricular extrasystoles, ventricular tachycardia and fibrillation in animal experiments (KRAYER and ACHESON, 1946; KRAYER et al., 1953; BENFORADO, 1957). Although there are quantitative and also qualitative differences in the arrhythmogenic action of the individual alkaloids, practically all these agents have in common the property of inducing ventricular fibrillation (MATSUDA et al., 1953; BENFORADO, 1957; SWAIN and MCCARTHY, 1957; SWAIN and WEIDNER, 1957). In view of this it is surprising that these agents are not used extensively for the assay of antiarrhythmic activity.

In spite of the fact that relatively little information is available concerning the mechanism of veratrine-induced arrhythmia in the whole heart, analysis of the effects of veratrum alkaloids on various cardiac tissues resulted in some new data which can provide some explanation for the genesis of these heart rhythm disturbances. The mode of action of various tertiary amine ester alkaloids (veratridine, cevadine, protoveratrin A and B, etc.), has already been studied to some extent. It was found that under the influence of these agents, ventricular automaticity is increased, and rapidly firing ectopic foci and ventricular tachycardia develop (BENFORADO, 1957; SWAIN and MCCARTHY, 1957; SWAIN and WEIDNER, 1957). Similarly to aconitine, veratrine is capable of inducing repetitive discharges in reponse to a single stimulus in Purkinje fibers and also in non-specialized auricular or ventricular myocardium (GOLDENBERG and ROTHBERGER, 1936; MATSUDA et al., 1953; BROOKS et al., 1955). Excitability is decreased in the auricle and also in the ventricle with concomitant slowing of conduction in various parts of the heart (BROOKS et al., 1955). It is of interest to note that conduction is more depressed in Purkinje fibers than in the ventricular myocardium (SWAIN and MCCARTHY, 1957), which may increase the inhomogeneity of the spread of excitation leading to disorganized electrical activity. The action potential duration and the re- fractory period of auricular and ventricular muscle are prolonged in the presence of veratrum alkaloids (MATSUDA et al., 1953; BROOKS et al., 1955; SWAIN and MCCARTHY, 1957). In spite of this, susceptibility to fibrillation induced by single electrical shocks is increased although the vulnerable period falls later in the cycle because of the prolongation of the refractory period (GILSON, 1939; BROOKS et al., 1955).

Under *in situ* conditions intravenous injection of veratrum alkaloids of tertiary amine ester type causes a severe reflex bradycardia which can be prevented by sectioning the vagi (DAWES, 1947). On the contrary, another group of veratrine alkaloids (secondary alkylamines, such as veratramine, veratrosine, etc.) have a *direct* depressant effect on sinoatrial (and also on atrioventricular) nodal pacemaker activity without depressing spontaneous automaticity in the ventricle, i.e. in the Purkinje fibers (KRAYER and ACHESON, 1946; KRAYER, 1949; KRAYER and REITER, 1950; KRAYER et al., 1955; INNES et al., 1956). Depression of the sinoatrial rate by veratramine occurs periodically, for reasons not yet known (KOSTERLITZ et al., 1955). Whatever the intricate mechanism of the marked bradycardia produced by various veratrum alkaloids might be, the resultant decrease in sinus dominance gives rise to the development of ectopic foci leading to ventricular extrasystoles, tachycardia or fibrillation.

f) Large Doses of Antiarrhythmic Agents

When given in large doses, antiarrhythmic agents are capable of exerting a paradoxical effect, i.e. they may elicit severe arrhythmia, including ventricular

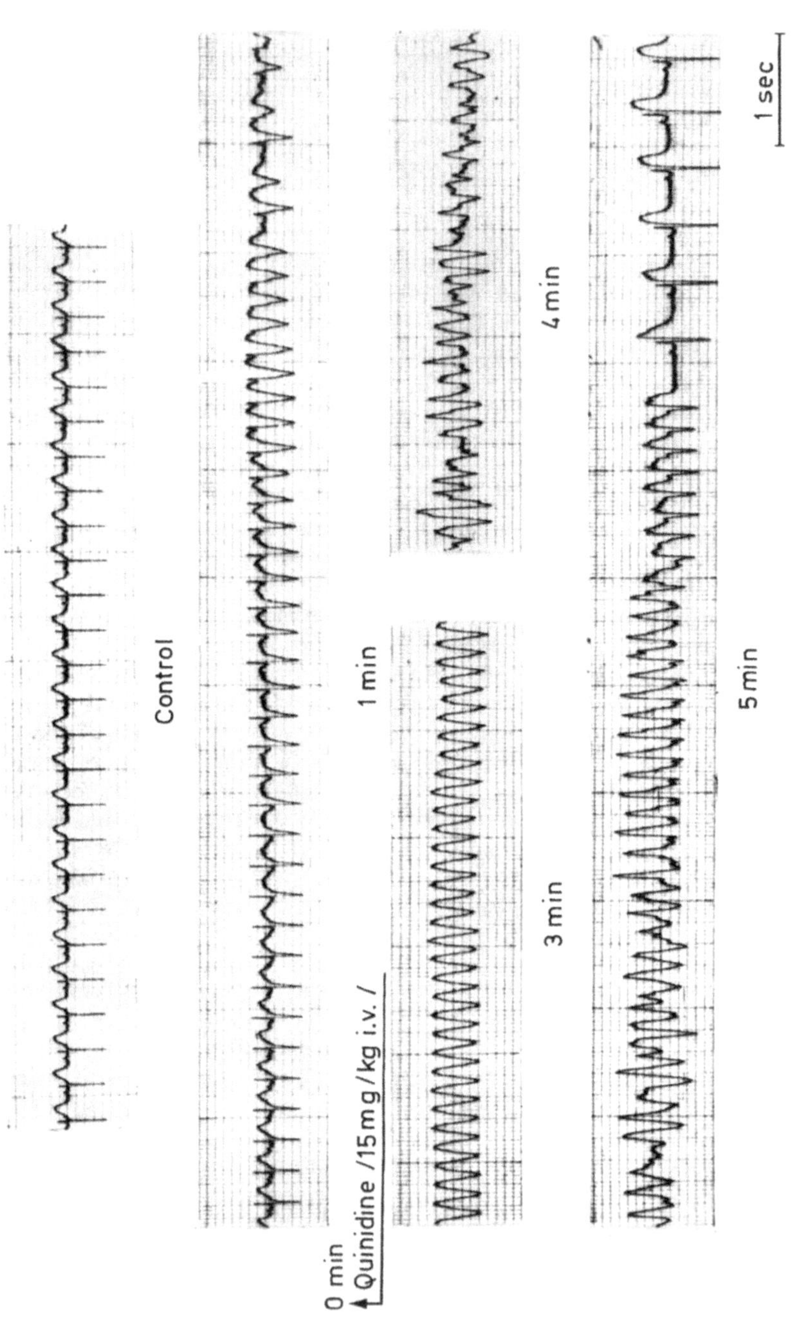

Fig. 10. *Ventricular flutter and reversible fibrillation induced by quinidine in an unanesthetized rabbit* (Electrocardiogram was recorded in a precordial lead corresponding to position V_4)

fibrillation. In addition, arrhythmia may be induced even by smaller doses of antiarrhythmics, when susceptibility to arrhythmia is increased or a manifest disorder of cardiac rhythm is already present. — Such an arrhythmogenic effect has been observed with quinidine (SPANG, 1964; NYE and ROBERTS, 1966), procainamide in hypothermia (COVINO et al., 1955), procaine administered together with adrenalin

(GRUMBACH, 1956), papaverine (WÉGRIA and NICKERSON, 1942), ajmaline (SPANG, 1964), N-propyl-ajmaline (NAKAYAMA et al., 1973), quinidine, propranolol and pronethalol in the presence of $BaCl_2$-induced arrhythmia (PAPP et al., 1967). — The effect of 15 mg/kg quinidine, administered intravenously to an unanesthetized rabbit, is shown in Fig. 10. Under the in- fluence of this large dose of quinidine, ventricular flutter leading to fibrillation occurred which, in the relatively small rabbit heart, ceased spontaneously.

In the foregoing cases, decrease in excitability and slowing of conduction may reach a certain critical value when coordinated activation of the heart is impossible. In this respect it is noteworthy that in quinidine intoxication (20 to 30 mg/kg i.v. to dogs), the pronounced prolongation of the refractory period is not uniform in the various parts of the ventricle, and the temporal dispersion of recovery of excitability (i.e. inhomogeneity) is increased to such an extent that the latter effect alone would be sufficient to serve as a basis for the development of severe dysrhythmia (HAN and MOE, 1964).

g) Miscellaneous Compounds

In addition to the preceding agents, intravenous administration of some other compounds will also produce arrhythmia. These include thiopental, certain propylene glycols, amarin, a propiophenone derivative called "U-0882" and also some of the adrenergic and cholinergic stimulants. In the absence of another arrhythmogenic intervention the arrhythmia induced by these compounds appears only occasionally and is usually short-lived.

When given in an intravenous dose of 20 to 25 mg/kg to dogs, *thiopenthal* causes scattered ventricular extrasystoles which can be prevented by various antiarrhythmic drugs (GRUBER et al., 1953; NIESCHULTZ, 1955). — The monomethylesters of certain mono-, di- and tri*propylene glycols* will cause auricular fibrillation (SHIDEMAN and PROCITA, 1951). — A cyclic amidine derivative *amarin* (2,4,5-triphenyl-dihydro-imidazole) in doses larger than 15 mg/kg i.v. frequently produces marked bradycardia associated with ventricular arrhythmias (FASTIER and SMIRK, 1948; BROOKS et al., 1955). The propiophenon derivative "*U-0882*" when given intravenously in a dose of 10 mg/kg, is capable of producing severe ventricular arrhythmia, including ventricular fibrillation (MOORE and SWAIN, 1960a). Since in the presence of high catecholamine concentrations both amarine and U-0882 exert a more pronounced arrhythmogenic effect, analysis of the arrhythmias so produced as well as their mode of action will be treated in some detail under Section 2.a.

Of the autonomic drugs, *adrenaline*, *noradrenaline* and *mephentermine* have been shown to increase ectopic pacemaker activity in the auricle and the ventricle leading to the appearance of a number of extrasystoles of ventricular origin (GILBERT et al., 1958, 1959). Model-arrhythmias suitable for assaying antiarrhythmic action have been frequently elicited by a large intravenous dose of adrenalin in dogs and cats (SOMANI and LUM, 1965; PAPP, 1966; SOMANI et al., 1966). Rapid intravenous injection of 100 μg/kg adrenalin results in the development of runs of uni- and multifocal ventricular tachycardia with occasional premature beats. The arrhythmia thus produced lasts for about 3 to 6 min. When evaluating the results the total number of beats per minute, as well as the number of sinus and ectopic beats per minute, is considered for each successive 30 sec period in the manner described by MALING and MORAN (1957). The mode of action of catecholamines in producing these arrhythmias is described under Section 2.a. — Intravenous injection of noradrenaline has not been used frequently to produce arrhythmia, but in combination with sub-arrhythmic multiple electrical stimulation of the ventricle, it can cause even ventricular fibrillation (GILBERT, 1959). — Intravenous injection (0.5 to 5 μg/kg) or infusion (10 μg/kg/min) of *acetylcholine* causes short-lived "spontaneous" atrial or ventricular arrhythmia in a few cases only (SZEKERES and PAPP, 1965, 1971). As mentioned in the introduction, however, combined application of acetylcholine infusion and electrical stimulation results in persistent auricular fibrillation (BURN et al., 1955).

2. Combined Administration of Several Arrhythmogenic Agents

a) Adrenergic Stimulants and Sensitizing Agents

The arrhythmogenic effect of adrenergic stimulants described in Section 1.g is greatly enhanced after "sensitization" of the myocardium. All the model-arrhythmias of this type are based on Levy's early observation that under light chloroform anesthesia, intravenous injection of adrenaline caused ventricular fibrillation (LEVY, 1914). Much of our knowledge regarding the fundamental nature of disorders of cardiac rhythm has been derived from experiments carried out with these complex methods, involving also the use of certain inhalant anesthetics of clinical significance (halothane, ether, cyclopropane, etc.). Moreover, these techniques have gained widespread use in the assay of antiarrhythmic compounds.

The experimental technique was first standardized by MEEK et al. (1937) and consisted originally of the induction of a constant anesthesia with chloroform or cyclopropane in dogs or cats for a period of 30 to 40 min. At the end of this time about 10 μg/kg epinephrine was injected intravenously to evoke fibrillation. — In a recent variant of this method (SOMANI and LUM, 1965; SOMANI et al., 1966), the myocardium is "sensitized" to epinephrine by 0.1 ml/kg methylchloroform administered intratracheally to pentobarbital-anesthetized dogs. Fifteen to 30 sec later rapid intravenous injection of 10 μg/kg epinephrine invariably produces ventricular fibrillation. When studying the antiarrhythmic potency of various substances, the decrease in the incidence of ventricular fibrillation following the administration of the compound to be tested is the measure of protection. Animals in which fibrillation does not occur because of the protective effect of the antiarrhythmic agents, can be rechallenged at approximately 30 min intervals, and the duration of the antiarrhythmic action can also be assessed. More quantitative versions of the methylchloroform-epinephrine arrhythmia are represented by some techniques in which the threshold dose of epinephrine required to produce a definite number of extrasystoles per minute is determined, or the occurrence of extrasystoles evoked by a fixed smaller dose of epinephrine is measured (KATZUNG, 1968). — In a more recent study *petroleum ether* (a mixture of lower aliphatic hydrocarbons) was used as a "sensitizing" agent administered intratracheally in a dose of 0.05 ml/kg in vaporized form to pentobarbital-anesthetized dogs, and the dose of epinephrine producing severe ventricular arrhythmias amounted to only 5 μg/kg (VIANA and OSSWALD, 1971). In urethan-anesthetized cats, larger doses of petroleum ether (0.1 ml/kg intratracheally) and epinephrine (30 μg/kg intravenously) were required to produce severe ventricular arrhythmia (NIESCHULTZ et al., 1955).

During the past decades a large number of compounds have been shown to be able to "sensitize" the heart to adrenergic stimulants, and various sympathomimetics have been applied in combination with these agents to produce ventricular arrhythmias. In addition to *chloroform* and *cyclopropane* (MEEK et al.,

1937; ALLEN et al., 1940; DETERLING et al., 1954; DRESEL et al., 1960; KATZ, 1965), *halothane* (RAVENTOS, 1956; ANDERSEN and JOHANSEN, 1963; TAKAORI and LOEHNING, 1965; SOMANI and LUM, 1966), *halopropane* (KATZ, 1964a, b, 1966) and *various hydrocarbons* (CHENOWETH, 1946; GARB and CHENOWETH, 1948; RIKER et al., 1955), *ether* (MEEK et al., 1937; DETERLING et al., 1954), *benzene* (WÉGRIA and NICKERSON, 1943; NAHUM and HOFF, 1934) and also *amarin* (FASTIER and SMIRK, 1948; BROOKS et al., 1955), as well as the propiophenon derivative "*U-0882*" (MOORE and SWAIN, 1960a, b) also possess the ability to increase the sensitivity of the heart to the arrhythmogenic action of epinephrine. On the other hand, severe disorders of cardiac rhythm may be elicited by combined application of a "sensitizing" agent and *norepinephrine* (MEEK, 1941; GARB and CHENOWETH, 1948; ANDERSEN and JOHANSON, 1963), *isoproterenol* (MORAN et al., 1962; KATZ, 1965; KABELA and MENDEZ, 1966), *dopamine* (KATZ et al., 1967; PAPP and SZEKERES, 1972c); *desoxyepinephrine* and *tyramine* (LEVY, 1914), *cobefrin* (corbasil) and *kephrine* (stryphnon) (MEEK, 1941). Although *ephedrine* was found ineffective in precipitating ventricular arrhythmias in the presence of inhalant anesthetics (MEEK, 1941), it was capable of inducing ventricular fibrillation in cats pretreated with large doses of ouabain (VAN DONGEN, 1936).

Of the preceding adrenergic stimulants, epinephrine has by far been used most widely for the production of model-arrhythmias in combination with other agents. While discussing the possible mechanism of these arrhythmias, it seems, therefore, justified to concentrate first on the mode of action of this catecholamine. From the point of view of the arrhythmogenic properties of epinephrine, some of its direct cardiac effects are of fundamental significance. In isolated Purkinje fibers the most striking change due to epinephrine is an increase in rate of the slow diastolic depolarization resulting in a markedly enhanced automaticity. Under the influence of epinephrine, depolarization occurs even in quiescent Purkinje fibers leading to oscillations and development of a pacemaker (OTSUKA, 1958; TRAUTWEIN and SCHMIDT, 1960; TRAUTWEIN, 1963). Further studies are required to elucidate the mechanism of these effects, nevertheless in Purkinje fibers epinephrine shifts the relation between activation of the potassium current and membrane potential in a depolarizing direction; there is a decline in potassium conductance following an action potential which could result in enhanced pacemaker activity (HAUSWIRTH et al., 1968). — Although the *direct* effect of epinephrine on the sinoatrial node is to increase the slope of the slow diastolic depolarization with concomitant increase in the frequency of pacemaker discharge (WEST et al., 1956; HOFFMAN and CRANEFIELD, 1960; WEST, 1972), under *in vivo* conditions reflex bradycardia develops (LENEL et al., 1948; RIKER et al., 1955), leading to a decrease in the sinus dominance and facilitating the appearance of ectopic foci originating mainly from the Purkinje fibers. The direct stimulating effect of epinephrine on the ectopic pacemaker cells in combination with its indirect depressant action on the sinus node account mainly for the arrhythmogenic properties of this agent.

The epinephrine-induced alterations in excitability and refractoriness are much less prenounced than those occurring in pacemaker activity. On infusing epinephrine or norepinephrine into dogs, a slight increase in ventricular excitability followed by a decrease, has been observed (HAN et al., 1964; SZEKERES, 1964; PAPP and SZEKERES, 1968b). In most cases epinephrine and norepinephrine caused a slight shortening, but occasionally also a prolongation, of the auricular or ventricular refractory period (BROOKS et al., 1955; HAN and MOE, 1964; HAN et al., 1964; PAPP and SZEKERES, 1968b). Under the influence of epinephrine some reduction in the action potential duration of the auricle and the ventricle has also been observed (BROOKS et al., 1955; GILBERT et al., 1968; HOFFMAN and CRANEFIELD, 1960), although prolongation in plateau duration (presumably due to an increase of inward calcium current—REUTER, 1966, 1967; VASSORT et al., 1969; CARMELIET and VEREECKE, 1969) was found in Purkinje fibers. From the point of view of the development of arrhythmias of adrenergic origin, it is of crucial importance that the epinephrine-, or norepinephrine-induced shortening in the refractory period, as measured at various points of the ventricle, is non-uniform, and as a result, the temporal dispersion of recovery of excitability, i.e. inhomogeneity, is increased (HAN and MOE, 1964; HAN et al., 1964; PAPP and SZEKERES, 1968b). The appearance and time course of this enhanced inhomogeneity are closely related to epinephrine-, or norepinephrine-induced decrease in electrical fibrillation threshold (SZEKERES, 1964; PAPP and SZEKERES, 1968a, b; SZEKERES and PAPP, 1971). In this respect it is worth noting that epinephrine, administered intravenously, causes arrhythmia in about 30 sec (NICKERSON and NOMAGUCHI, 1949; FAWAZ, 1951), and the marked reduction of the electrical fibrillation threshold is also confined to the very beginning of the action of various catecholamines (SZEKERES, 1964; PAPP and SZEKERES, 1968a, b; SZEKERES and PAPP, 1971). The reason for this phenomenon is not yet completely understood. One possible explanation is that during the first minutes some degree of inhomogeneous distribution of catecholamines is present in the ventricular myocardium with concomitant increase in asynchrony of recovery of excitability (HAN and MOE, 1964). In addition, the epinephrine-, or norepinephrine-induced reflex bradycardia is most marked in the first minute after injection (LENEL et al., 1948; RIKER et al., 1955), and the maximum increase in blood pressure also occurs in this period. The arrhythmogenic effect of sympathomimetics exhibiting a marked increase in blood pressure can partially be attributed to a mechanical overloading and lasting stretch of the ventricular myocardium leading to incipient heart failure, which is known to enhance the liability of the heart to arrhythmia (PAPP and SZEKERES, 1967, 1968a; SZEKERES and PAPP, 1971). As to the intricate mechanism of catecholamine-induced alterations in cardiac electrical activity at the receptor level, electrophysiologic studies with highly specific and selective beta-receptor blockers have recently shown that all the direct arrhythmogenic changes due to catecholamines are mediated via the beta-adrenergic receptors of the heart (PAPP and SZEKERES, 1968a, b; HAUSWIRTH et al., 1968), more precisely via the receptors of $beta_1$ type (PAPP and SZEKERES, 1972a, b).

Some information has become available on the possible mechanism by which the "sensitizing" agents exert their arrhythmogenic influence on the heart. Chloroform has been shown to increase the asynchrony in recovery of excitability in the ventricular myocardium, thereby facilitating the appearance of arrhythmias (HAN and MOE, 1964). In the non-specialized working myocardium low concentrations of chloroform may increase excitability slightly, but the characteristic effect, especially at higher concentrations, is a marked depression (ACIERNO and DIPALMA, 1951; BROOKS et al., 1955) leading to local blocks and presumably to an enhanced asynchrony in spread of excitation. The same applies also to cyclopropane and ether (ACIERNO and DIPALMA, 1951). Under the influence of these agents, the refractory period is shortened in isolated auricle and markedly prolonged in the heart *in situ* (ACIERNO and DIPALMA, 1951; BROOKS et al., 1955). Ventricular dysrhythmias appear occasionally under the influence of chloroform alone, and in this case the increased sensitivity of the heart to catecholamines of endogenous origin may account for the development of arrhythmias (LEVY, 1914; MEEK et al., 1937; HUTCHEON, 1951). It is of interest that chloroform alone has recently been applied to produce tachycardia and ventricular fibrillation in the mouse and that this model-arrhythmia proved to be suitable for rapid screening of antiarrhythmic compounds (LAWSON, 1968).

The effects of halothane on cardiac electrical activity have been analyzed in detail (HAUSWIRTH and SCHAER, 1967; HAUSWIRTH, 1969). From these studies, it might be concluded that the arrhythmogenic effect of halothane is probably due to a marked shortening of the refractory period both in specialized and non-specialized cardiac tissue, an increased inhomogeneity between the refractory periods in Purkinje and ventricular muscle fibers and a marked decrease in conduction velocity of Purkinje fibers (HAUSWIRTH, 1969).

The mode of action of amarin is similar to that of large doses of quinidine (see Section I.f), because it decreases excitability and conduction velocity and prolongs the refractory period (FASTIER and SMIRK, 1948; BROOKS et al., 1955; MOORE and SWAIN, 1960b). All these effects are very marked and lead to the appearance of local blocks and inhomogeneous spread of excitation in the heart. The enhanced automaticity in ectopic pacemaker areas due to certain adrenergic stimulants (e.g. epinephrine) together with depressed excitability and conduction induced by amarin inevitably leads to the development of arrhythmia. — In contrast to amarine, U-0882 has no significant effect on intracardiac conduction in doses which prolong markedly the refractory period of the ventricular myocardium. Under such conditions epinephrine, by increasing the sinoatrial rate, moves the QRS complex of the ECG earlier, while the Q-T interval is prolonged. As soon as the T-wave becomes superimposed on the QRS complex, ventricular fibrillation occurs (MOORE and SWAIN, 1960a, b). The reason for this effect may be that because of the prolongation of the refractory period, the natural impulses spread through the ventricular fibers at a time when they are still relatively refractory (MOORE and SWAIN, 1960a). Thus, the action potentials generated in the ventricle may be different as to their depolarization rate, duration, etc., and the inhomogeneity of impulse conduction (and probably that of the recovery of excitability) is increased, resulting in disorganized activation of the ventricle and in the appearance of arrhythmia.

b) Hormones Combined with Other Agents

Thyrotoxicosis has long been known to cause supra-ventricular arrhythmia, chiefly atrial fibrillation (WILSON, 1924; WISHART, 1929; NAHUM and HOFF, 1935; SCHERF and SCHOTT, 1953). On the basis of clinical observations, LEVÉQUE (1956) tried te evoke atrial fibrillation in hyperthyroid dogs by rapid intravenous injection of large doses of acetylcholine, and in 81% of the animals, atrial fibrillation of very short duration (less than 60 sec) appeared. In euthyroid animals the same arrhythmia was induced by acetylcholine in only 31% of the cases. In more recent studies it has been shown that the arrhythmogenic action of ouabain and of calcium chloride is also increased in animals made hyperthyroid by prolonged treatment with thyroxine or triiodothyronine (PAPP and SZEKERES, 1971). So far no attempt has been made to standardize these arrhythmias and to use them for the assay of antiarrhythmic action. In addition, the mechanism by which thyroid hormones enhance the susceptibility of the heart to arrhythmia, is not fully understood. The recent observation that the repolarization phase of the action potential is shortened in electrically driven hyperthyroid atria, suggests that a shortening in the absolute refractory period might contribute to the development of atrial dysrhythmias (FREEDBERG et al., 1970). Some increase in the diastolic excitability and a shortening of the effective refractory period have also been found in atria of thyroxine-treated animals (ARNSDORF and CHILDERS, 1970).

Under clinical conditions several authors have observed various arrhythmias during insulin-hypoglycemia (STROUSE et al., 1932; JUDSON and HOLLANDER, 1956; EGELI and BERKMEN, 1960; LEAK and STARR, 1962). Measurements of blood sugar, serum potassium and the urinary excretion of catecholamines revealed that the appearance of arrhythmia is accompanied not only by hypoglycemia, but also by hypokalemia, and that an increased catecholamine excretion is also present. It has, therefore, been suggested that these dysrhythmias may be due to the action of catecholamines on the heart, which is abnormally sensitive to arrhythmogenic factors as a result of hypokalemia (LEAK and STARR, 1962).

Similarly, the insulin-induced decrease in blood potassium level seems to be of crucial importance in model-arrhythmias elicited by the combined administration of insulin, glucose and acetylcholine (LEVÉQUE, 1964a, b, 1965, 1966; BOGER and LEVÉQUE, 1968). The procedure consists of the intravenous injection of insulin (2 units/kg) to pentobarbital-anesthetized dogs followed in 3 min by the administration of glucose in a dose of 200 mg/kg i.v. This results in a relatively stable hypokalemic state, which occurs in 30 min and remains stationary for about 90 min. During this period of hypokalemia the sensitivity of the dog heart to the arrhythmogenic action of acetylcholine is enhanced. Large doses (about 0.2 to 0.5 mg/kg) evoke atrial flutter or fibrillation in at least 80% of the animals, depending on the plasma potassium concentration. Prolongation of arrhythmias may be achieved by infusing acetylcholine intravenously at a rate of 1 mg/min. A major advantage of this method is that the pentobarbital-anesthetized dogs are not damaged and may be used repeatedly for such experiments. The technique is suitable for the assay of antiarrhythmic activity and has been used to study the antiarrhythmic effect of various adrenergic neuron-blocking agents (LEVÉQUE, 1964b, 1965, 1966; BOGER and LEVÉQUE, 1968). In this case either the incidence of acetylcholine-induced atrial fibrillation or the amount of acetylcholine necessary to produce atrial fibrillation is the measure of antiarrhythmic potency. — Although in these model-arrhythmias insulin seems to act indirectly, by inducing hypokalemia, no sufficient information is available on its possible direct cardiac action, which may also play a role.

c) Succinyldicholine and Sensitizing Agents

An interesting clinical observation is that disorders of cardiac rhythm occur when succinyldicholine (a muscle-relaxing agent) is administered repeatedly to patients under halothane or cyclopropane anesthesia (WILLIAMS et al., 1961). Hexafluorenium exerts a protective effect against these dysrhythmias, and they do not develop under thiopental anesthesia (SCHOENSTADT and WHITCHER, 1963). The precise mechanism underlying the appearance of these arrhythmias has not yet been studied in detail. It has been suggested that an increased blood level of choline formed during hydrolysis of succinyl-dicholine could facilitate the development of dysrhythmias (SCHOENSTADT and WHITCHER, 1963).

II. Topical Application of Arrhythmogenic Agents to the Heart

1. Cholinergic Stimulants

Development of various arrhythmias of atrial origin can be facilitated not only by intravenous administration, but also by topical application, of acetylcholine and other cholinergic stimulants. In this respect the first observation was that *methacholine* (acetyl-beta-methylcholine, mecholyl), applied to localized regions on the auricular surface of the dog heart, produced atrial fibrillation without any further arrhythmogenic interventions (HOFF and NAHUM, 1940). In these experiments small strips of filter paper (0.2 × 1 cm) soaked in a methacholine solution of rather high concentration (1:500 to 1:2000) were used. Under similar conditions local application of *acetylcholine* to small areas of the auricle has also been shown to produce atrial fibrillation (SCHERF and CHICK, 1951). These techniques have not been standardized and are not used frequently for the assay of antiarrhythmic action. It is rather the foregoing superfusion of acetylcholine combined with potassium deficiency and electrical stimulation in isolated atria, which is recommended and used more extensively (HOLLAND et al., 1957; MACLEOD and REYNOLDS, 1962; TURNER, 1965). Nevertheless, atrial fibrillation induced by topically applied methacholine was prevented by local application of atropine (HOFF and NAHUM, 1940), and it could be suppressed by various antiarrhythmic agents (HIRSCHFELDER and TAMCALES, 1942; GERTLER and KARP, 1947).

The mechanism of these atrial arrhythmias is fairly well understood. The action potential duration and the refractory period are markedly shortened by both acetylcholine (BURGEN and TERROUX, 1953; TRAUTWEIN and DUDEL, 1958a; HOFFMAN and CRANEFIELD, 1960) and methacholine (HOFFMAN and CRANEFIELD, 1960), and the degree of shortening is not the same in different fiber regions (HOFFMAN and CRANEFIELD, 1960). In the presence of acetylcholine, spread of excitation is also non-uniform (TRAUTWEIN and DUDEL, 1958b; MARSHALL and VAUGHAN WILLIAMS, 1959). Both processes facilitate inhomogeneity and apperance of arrhythmias. Under the influence of acetylcholine, re-entry (circus movement) has been directly traced by microelectrodes in isolated atria, and it was found that a critical mass of auricular tissue (30 mg at least) is required in order to induce fibrillation (WEST and LANDA, 1962). Thus, the mechanism of acetylcholine-induced atrial arrhythmias supports the re-entry theory of fibrillation.

2. Aconitine

The decisive role of a direct cardiac effect in the arrhythmogenic action of aconitine has been shown most clearly by SCHERF (1947, 1948), who found that topical application of this alkaloid to the left atrium resulted in the development of atrial tachycardia or fibrillation. This technique and its variants have been used extensively to produce model-arrhythmias and to test antiarrhythmic compounds (WINBURY, 1956; MACLEOD and REYNOLDS, 1962; TURNER, 1965; KATZUNG, 1968; NAKAYAMA et al., 1971).

The usual method utilizes an anesthetized open-chest dog under artificial respiration. Aconitine is injected subepicardially (0.05 ml of a 0.5% solution) in the wall of the left atrium, or a small cotton pledget soaked in a 0.05% solution of aconitine is placed on the left auricular appendage. Atrial tachycardia or fibrillation with atrioventricular block of different grades and irregular ventricular rhythm ensues within about 2 min and persists for approximately an hour. By clamping off the site of application of aconitine from the rest of the atrium or by cooling the artificial "ectopic focus" the arrhythmia can be suppressed. The difficulty with this technique is that the aconitine solution readily disperses from the site of application and the severity of arrhythmia cannot be controlled. On the other hand, it is not easy to remove the applied aconitine solution from the atrial surface. To overcome these difficulties aconitine-arrhythmia has recently been produced by the so-called "cup method" in dogs (NAKAYAMA et al., 1971). The technique is based on the use of a cup-shaped container made of rubber which is glued upside-down with bio-tissue adhesive on the right atrial surface. Two polyethylene tubes are introduced through the bottom of the cup so that the tip of one tube is very close to the atrial wall. The cup is filled through one of the tubes with aconitine solutions of various concentrations (0.001 to 1%), and aconitine can be removed by washing thoroughly the inside of the cup with Ringer's solution. Under these conditions arrhythmia of relatively uniform severity can be produced which will last as long as the aconitine solution is present in the cup, i.e. in a restricted area of about 10 square mm of the atrial surface.

In order to produce fast ectopic rhythm, aconitine has been applied topically also to *isolated* rabbit atria (MACLEOD and REYNOLDS, 1962). A filter paper disk of 2 mm in diameter is soaked in 2.5% aconitine and placed on the tip of the left atrial appendage for a period of 1.5 min only. During the latter procedure the fluid level in the bath is first lowered, and after application and removal of the disk it is raised again to cover the atrium completely. The firing rate of the ectopic pacemaker thus produced is very high, the atrial frequency is usually increased by about 100 to 150%. Various antiarrhythmic substances act by abolishing or delaying the development of the aconitine-induced ectopic pacemaker center or by depressing its firing rate.

The mechanism of the arrhythmogenic action of aconitine is based on the production of an ectopic focus, concerning which significant information has been obtained from microelectrode studies on working muscle (MATSUDA et al., 1959; SCHMIDT, 1960; TAMAI et al., 1961; HEISTRACHER and PILLAT, 1962) and Purkinje fibers (SCHMIDT, 1960; HEISTRACHER and PILLAT, 1962; PEPER and TRAUTWEIN, 1967). The most striking electrophysiologic effect of aconitine is the production of long-lasting "depolarizing" after-potentials with concomitant shorter or longer trains of rhythmic discharges. Thus, following an incomplete repolarization, action potentials of low amplitude and short duration will develop leading to high frequency focal activity. This effect can be observed both in ordinary muscle (MATSUDA et al., 1959; SCHMIDT, 1960) and also in Purkinje fibers (SCHMIDT, 1960; HEISTRACHER and PILLAT, 1962), and it is related to an increase in sodium conductance together with a delayed inactivation of the sodium current, resulting in a highly unstable membrane (PEPER and TRAUTWEIN, 1967).

3. Delphinine

A long-lasting auricular flutter or ventricular tachycardia can be produced by local application of delphinine (an alkaloid akin to aconitine) to the auricular or ventricular surface of the dog heart (SCHERF et al., 1960, 1963). These arrhythmias appear after about a 2 to 4 min latency period, last for approximately 40 min and —in contrast to aconitine-induced dysrhythmias—never change into auricular (or ventricular) fibrillation. Although this technique has not been widely used for the production of model-arrhythmias, it may be significant from the point of view of the assay of antiarrhythmic activity, since diphenylhydantoin has been shown to suppress the high frequency ectopic rhythm produced by delphinine in atria.

4. Cardiac Glycosides

Arrhythmias (chiefly coupled extrasystoles of bigeminal type) have occasionally been produced by cardiac glycosides applied locally to the surface of the heart (KISCH, 1944; SCHERF, 1944). This procedure has not been introduced as a routine technique for the production of model-arrhythmia, but it serves as an important evidence for the ability of cardiac glycosides to induce focal automaticity at ectopic pacemaker areas.

5. Veratrum Alkaloids

Topical application to the heart of high concentrations of veratrine (the impure alkaloidal mixture) and those of other pure alkaloids, such as veratridine and cevadine, has been shown to produce cardiac arrhythmias (SCHERF and CHICK, 1951). Methods based on this observation have not been developed, but the phenomenon itself provides some evidence to suggest that abnormal impulse formation from an ectopic center might contribute to the appearance of veratrine-induced arrhythmias.

E. Production of Cardiac Arrhythmias by Direct Stimulation of the Central Nervous System

Various disorders of cardiac rhythm can also be induced by direct stimulation of the central nervous system. Most of the methods suitable for this purpose are rather elaborate. In addition, they are usually not reproducible and have not been standardized either. In view of this, it is not surprising that these techniques are not used for the assay of antiarrhythmic action. They are, however, most suitable for producing certain pathologic processes which are frequently encountered in the clinic and which lead to the appearance of arrhythmias. For this reason they can provide useful qualitative information about the effectiveness of drugs in cardiac arrhythmias of central origin and also about the possible mode of action of substances antagonizing or facilitating the development of arrhythmias. The techniques in question include electrical stimulation of various parts of the central nervous system, injection of drugs or chemical substances into the cerebral ventricles and also mechanical procedures, such as cerebral compression or other measures increasing intracranial pressure. Little is known about the complex nature of these arrhythmias and in this respect only limited conclusions can be drawn. It is beyond any doubt, however, that destruction or blockade of the various nervous pathways connecting the brain and the heart is capable of preventing or diminishing the arrhythmogenic actions of electrical, chemical or mechanical stimuli applied directly to the central nervous system.

I. Electrical Stimulation of the Central Nervous System

Electrical stimulation of various cortical areas, such as the gyrus orbitalis or gyrus frontalis, has been shown to produce ventricular extrasystoles in curarized unanesthetized cats under artificial respiration (SINITSIN and KISIN, 1964). Thiopental, hexamethonium and to some extent also papaverine provided protection against these arrhythmias. Nodal and ventricular extrasystoles, as well as ventricular techycardia, were elicited by stimulation of the limbic lobe and the amygdala (CAROLL et al., 1961). The appearance of these dysrhythmias was inhibited by chlordiazepoxide. On stimulation of the hypothalamus, cardiac rhythm disorders developed in various species, such as the dog, the cat and the rabbit (BEATTIE et al., 1930; ALLEN, 1931; VAN BOGAERT, 1936; FOSTER and WEINBERG, 1960; WEINBERG and FOSTER, 1960; ATTAR et al., 1963; MELVILLE et al., 1963). The same applies to the electrical stimulation of the mesencephalic (ATTAR et al., 1963) and bulbar (BURIAK, 1963, 1964) reticular formations, as well as to the stimulation of certain nuclei of the brain stem (MAUCK and HOCKMAN, 1967). Arrhythmias evoked by stimulation of the anterior hypothalamic region could partially be antagonized by section of the vagi (MELVILLE et al., 1963). Similarly, vagal section and also methyl-scopolamine were capable of antagonizing dysrhythmias due to electrical stimulation of certain diencephalic areas (MANNING and COTTEN, 1962). In the latter case extirpation of the stellate ganglia also led to a decrease of the incidence of arrhythmia, so that both the sympathetic and the parasympathetic systems seem to play a role in the genesis of these dysrhythmias.

II. Injection of Drugs or Other Chemical Substances into the Cerebral Ventricles

Injection of *picrotoxin* (0.1 mg) into the lateral ventricle of anesthetized rabbits (VARMA et al., 1961, 1962) or cats (MELVILLE and SHARE, 1963) produced paroxysmal auricular or ventricular tachycardia, most frequently ventricular extrasystoles and occasionally also ventricular fibrillation. On injecting the same agent in a dose of 2 μg/kg into the fourth ventricle of the dog, atrioventricular block, extrasystoles (including bigeminy) and ventricular tachycardia were observed in unanesthetized, succinyldicholine-treated dogs (BIRCHER et al., 1963). The occurrence of the latter arrhythmias was reduced by central cholinolytics, such as ethylbenztropine, but a complete protection was only achieved when the sympathetic nerves and the vagi were blocked simultaneously.

Small quantities of other agents, such as *acetylcholine*, *caffeine* or *nicotine*, injected into the lateral cerebral ventricle of the anesthetized and vagotomized cat are also capable of producing dysrhythmias (DIKSHIT, 1934). Similar observations have been made with *pentamethylenetetrazol* (5 mg/kg) or *deslanoside* (4 μg/kg) injected into the fourth ventricle (BIRCHER et al., 1963), and with *potassium chloride* (0.5 ml of 0.25 M solution) administered into the lateral cerebral ventricle (BENDIKOV, 1964). The appearance of dysrhythmia produced by potassium chloride was completely prevented by sympathectomy, but vagotomy and administration of atropine were without effect. *Tryptamine-strophanthidine* (125 to 250 μg) injected into the fourth cerebral ventricle produced ventricular extrasystoles and paroxysmal ventricular tachycardia, and the development of these arrhythmias was inhibited by intravenous administration of chlorpromazine (WEINBERG and HALEY, 1956). Under the same conditions injection of chlorpromazine into the fourth ventricle did not exert any protective action, so that in this case the antiarrhythmic effect of chlorpromazine seems to be due not so much to central as to peripheral mechanisms.

III. Increased Intracranial Pressure or Cerebral Compression

On the basis of clinical observations it has become known that an increase in intracranial pressure results in marked alterations of the electrocardiogram, including the appearance of various cardiac arrhythmias (SCHAPER, 1955; EFFERT et al., 1961; FENTZ and GORMSEN, 1962; HUGENHOLTZ, 1962). Sudden insufflation of air into the lateral cerebral ventricle produced similar effects in unanesthetized rabbits (SHKHVATSABAYA, 1964). Cranial trauma caused by a blow or a hammerstroke at the parieto-occipital region of the guinea pig (EICHBAUM and PEREIRA, 1964; EICHBAUM et al., 1965b) led to the development of ventricular extrasystoles and sometimes, in the guinea pig, to the appearance of ventricular fibrillation. Various measures (epidural insufflation of air, intracerebral injection of blood or paraffin, etc.) resulting ultimately in cerebral compression, produced practically the same effect, though independently of the primary site of intervention. It is, therefore, probable that from the point of view of the appearance of these arrhythmias indirect excitation of certain subcortical (mainly hypothalamic) regions is of decisive importance. The observed disorders of cardiac rhythm were prevented by the administration of reserpine, or simultaneous transection of the spinal cord and the cervical vagi, whereas vagal section alone or intravenous injection of atropine did not provide significant protection. Thus, the predominant role of sympathetic activity in the genesis of these arrhythmias is not in doubt (EICHBAUM et al., 1965a).

References

ACIERNO, L. J., DIPALMA, J. R.: The effects of ether, cyclopropane and chloroform on the isolated auricle of the cat. Anesthesiology **12**, 567 (1951).

ALLEN, C. R., STUTZMAN, J. W., MEEK, W. J.: The production of ventricular tachycardia by adrenalin in cyclopropane anesthesia. Anesthesiology **1**, 159 (1940).

ALLEN, W.: Experimentally produced premature systolic arrhythmia (pulsus bigemus) in rabbits; effective areas in brain. Amer. J. Physiol. **98**, 344 (1931).

ANDERSEN, N., JOHANSEN, S. H.: Incidence of catechol-amine-induced arrhythmias during halothane anesthesia. Anesthesiology **24**, 51 (1963).

ANTONI, H.: Die Entstehung ektopischer Schrittmacher durch Funktionswandel des nicht-automatischen Arbeitsmyokards. In: Herzrhythmusstörungen. — Neue experimentelle klinische und therapeutische Gesichtspunkte. Stuttgart-New York: F. K. Schattauer Verlag 1968.

ANTONI, H.: Electrophysiological mechanisms underlying pharmacological models of cardiac fibrillation. Naunyn-Schmiedeberg's Arch. exp. Path. Pharmak. **269**, 177 (1971).

ANTONI, H., OBERDISSE, E.: Elektrophysiologische Untersuchungen über die Barium-induzierte Schrittmacher-Aktivität im isolierten Säugetiermyokard. Pflügers Arch. ges. Physiol. **284**, 259 (1965).

ARNSDORF, F. M., CHILDERS, R. W.: Atrial electrophysiology in experimental hyperthyroidism in rabbits. Circulat. Res. **26**, 575 (1970).

ATTAR, H. J., GUTIERREZ, M. T., BELLET, S., RAVENS, J. R.: Effect of stimulation of hypothalamus and reticular activating system on production of cardiac arrhythmia. Circulat. Res. **12**, 14 (1963).

BARRETT, A. M., CULLUM, V. A.: The biological properties of the optical isomers of propranolol and their effects on cardiac arrhythmias. Brit. J. Pharmacol. **34**, 43 (1968).

BAZIKA, V., LANG, T. W., PAPPELBAUM, S., CORDAY, E.: Ajmalin, a rauwolfia alkaloid for the treatment of digitoxic arrhythmias. Amer. J. Cardiol. **17**, 227 (1966).

BEATTIE, J., BROW, G. R., LONG, C. N. H.: Physiological and anatomical evidence for existence of nerve tracts connecting hypothalamus with spinal sympathetic centres. Proc. roy. Soc. B **106**, 253 (1930).

BECKER, D. J., NONKIN, P. M., BENNETT, L. D., KIMBALL, S. G., STERNBERG, M. S., WASSERMAN, F.: Effect of isoproterenol in digitalis cardiotoxicity. Amer. J. Cardiol. **10**, 242 (1962).

BENDIKOV, A. E.: Effects produced by amizyl, iprazid and nitroglycerin upon the coronary circulation with experimentally induced spasms of the cardiac vessels. Farmakol. i Toksikol. **27**, 695 (1964).

BENFORADO, J. M.: Studies on veratrum alkaloids. XXVI. Comparison of the cardiac action of various tertiary amine ester alkaloids. J. Pharmacol. exp. Ther. **120**, 412 (1957).

BIJLSMA, U. G., VAN DONGEN, K.: Experimentelle Therapie des Flatterns und Flimmerns des Herzens. Ergebn. Physiol. **41**, 25 (1939).

BIRCHER, R. P., KANAI, T., WAND, S. C.: Mechanism of cardiac arrhythmias and blood pressure changes induced in dogs by pentylenetetrazol, picrotoxin and deslanoside. J. Pharmacol. exp. Ther. **141**, 6 (1963).

BLUMENTHAL, B., OPPENHEIMER, E. T.: Method for the study of ventricular fibrillation. Amer. Heart J. **18**, 363 (1939).

BOEHM, R.: Über die Wirkungen der Barytsalze auf den Tierkörper nebst Bemerkungen über die Wirkung des Wasserschierlings auf Frösche. Naunyn-Schmiedeberg's Arch. exp. Path. Pharmak. **3**, 216 (1875).

BOEHM, R.: Heffter's Handbuch der experimentellen Pharmakologie. II. **1**, 283 (1920).

Boger, D. C., Levêque, P. E.: The anti-arrhythmic effect of (—) N-(l-Phenylethyl) guanidine. Arch. int. Pharmacodyn. **175**, 129 (1968).

Bovet, D., Fourneau, E., Tréfouel, J., Strickler, H.: Le diéthylaminoéthoxy-2-diphényle (1262 F). Propriétés pharmacologiques et activité sur la fibrillation du cœur. Arch. int. Pharmacodyn. **62**, 234 (1939).

Boyajy, L. D., Nash, C. B.: Alteration of ouabain toxicity by cardiac denervation. Toxicol. appl. Pharmacol. **9**, 199 (1966).

Brooks, C. McC., Hoffman, B. F., Suckling, E. E., Orias, O.: Excitability of the heart. New York: Grune and Stratton, Inc. 1955.

Brooks, C. McC., Orias, O., Gilbert, J. L., Siebens, A. A., Hoffman, B. F., Suckling, E. E.: Auricular fibrillation: relationship of "vulnerable period" to "dip" phenomenon of auricular excitability curve. Amer. J. Physiol. **164**, 301 (1951).

Burgen, A. S. V., Terroux, K. G.: On the negative inotropic effect in the cat's auricle. J. Physiol. (Lond.) **120**, 449 (1953).

Buriak, M. A.: The action of neurotropic drugs on experimental arrhythmias produced by local stimulation of bulbar reticular formation. In: Problems of pharmacology of reticular formation and synaptic transmission. Leningrad 1963.

Buriak, M. A.: Chloracizine effects on experimental arrhythmias of central origin. Farmakol. i Toksikol. **27**, 579 (1964).

Burn, J. H., Vaughan Williams, E. M., Walker, J. M.: The effects of acetylcholine in the heart-lung preparation including the production of auricular fibrillation. J. Physiol. (Lond.) **128**, 277 (1955).

Carmeliet, E. E., Verdonck, F.: Interaction between ouabain and butidrine, a beta-adrenergic blocking substance, on the heart. Europ. J. Pharmacol. **1**, 269 (1967).

Carmeliet, E. E., Vereecke, J.: Adrenaline and the plateau phase of the cardiac action potential. Importance of Ca^{++}, Na^{+} and K^{+} conductance. Pflügers Arch. ges. Physiol. **313**, 300 (1969).

Caroll, M. N., Jr., Hoff, E. C., Kell, J. F., Jr., Suter, C. G.: The effects of ethanol and chlordiazepoxide in altering autonomic responses by isocortical and paleocortical stimulation. Biochem. Pharmacol. **8**, 15 (1961).

Charlier, R., Vandersmissen, L.: Propriétés antiarythmiques d'une diphénylbutylamine substituée. Arch. int. Pharmacodyn. **101**, 377 (1955a).

Charlier, R., Vandersmissen, L.: A propos de quelques substances douées de propriétés antiarythmiques. Arch. int. Pharmacodyn. **102**, 419 (1955b).

Charlier, R., Vandersmissen, L.: Propriétés antiarythmiques de la 4-4 (4′ méthoxyphényl) (3″ méthyl 4″ oxyphényl) butylamine 2. Arch. int. Pharmacodyn. **104**, 61 (1955c).

Chenoweth, M. B.: Ventricular fibrillation induced by hydrocarbons and epinephrine. J. industr. Hyg. **28**, 151 (1946).

Ciofalo, F., Levitt, B., Roberts, J.: Some aspects of the anti-arrhythmic activity of reserpine. Brit. J. Pharmacol. **28**, 44 (1966).

Clark, B. B., Cummings, J. R.: Arrhythmias following experimental coronary occlusion and their response to drugs. Ann. N.Y. Acad. Sci. **64**, 543 (1956).

Covino, B. G., Hegnauer, A. H.: Ventricular excitability cycle. Its modification by pH and hypothermia. Amer. J. Physiol. **171**, 553 (1955).

Cuparencu, B., Ticsa, I., Safta, L., Csutak, V., Barzu, T., Mocan, R.: A pharmacological analysis of the fibrillatory effect of calcium chloride in dogs. Abstracts of the lectures of the IVth International Congress on Pharmacology Basel 1969.

Dawes, G. S.: Studies on veratrum alkaloids. VII. Receptor areas in the coronary arteries and elsewhere as revealed by the use of veratridine. J. Pharmacol. exp. Ther. **89**, 325 (1947).

Dawes, G. S.: Experimental cardiac arrhythmias and quinidine-like drugs. Pharmacol. Rev. **4**, 43 (1952).

Deterling, R. A., Ngai, S. H., Laragh, J. H., Papper, E. M.: The cardiovascular effects of continuous intravenous infusion of norepinephrine, epinephrine and neosynephrine during cyclopropane and ether anesthesia in the dog. Anesthesiology **15**, 11 (1954).

Deutsch, A., Lundin, G.: Effects of minute amounts of barium on cardiac muscle. Acta physiol. scand. **11**, 373 (1946).

Dikshit, B. B.: The production of cardiac irregularities by excitation of the hypothalamic centres. J. Physiol. (Lond.) **81**, 382 (1934).

Dohadwalla, A. N., Freedberg, A. S., Vaughan Williams, E. M.: The relevance of β-receptor blockade to digitalis-induced cardiac arrhythmias. Brit. J. Pharmacol. **36**, 257 (1969).

Dresel, P. E., McCannell, K. L., Nickerson, M.: Cardiac arrhythmias induced by minimal doses of epinephrine in cyclopropane-anesthetized dogs. Circulat. Res. **8**, 948 (1960).

DUDEL, J., TRAUTWEIN, W.: Elektrophysiologische Messungen zur Strophanthinwirkung am Herzmuskel. Naunyn-Schmiedeberg's Arch. exp. Path. Pharmak. **232**, 393 (1958).

DUN, F. T., FENG, T. P.: Studies on the neuromuscular junction. XX. The site of origin of the junctional after-discharge in muscles treated with quanidine, barium or eserine. Chin. J. Physiol. **15**, 433 (1940).

EFFERT, S., GROSSE-BROCKHOFF, F., RIPPERT, R.: Elektrokardiographische Befunde bei Subarachnoidalblutungen. Dtsch. med. Wschr. **86**, 1508 (1961).

EGELI, E. S., BERKMEN, R.: Action of hypoglycemia on coronary insufficiency and mechanism of ECG alterations. Amer. Heart J. **59**, 527 (1960).

EICHBAUM, F. W., GAZETTA, B. H., BISSETTI, P. C.: Mechanism of encephalogenic heart injury. Z. ges. exp. Med. **139**, 735 (1965a).

EICHBAUM, F. W., GAZETTA, B. H., BISSETTI, P. C., PEREIRA, C. B.: Electrocardiographic disturbances following acute increase of intracranial pressure. Experiments in dogs. Z. ges. exp. Med. **139**, 721 (1965b).

EICHBAUM, F. W., PEREIRA, C. B.: Effect of cranial trauma on the electrocardiogram experiments in guinea-pigs. Cardiologia (Basel) **44**, 46 (1964).

ERLIJ, D., MÉNDEZ, R.: Modification of digitalis intoxication by exclusion of sympathetic system. Fed. Proc. **22**, 148 (1963).

ERLIJ, D., MÉNDEZ, D.: Adrenergic actions on heart rate, atrioventricular refractory period and intraventricular conduction in dogs. Arch. int. Physiol. **72**, 44 (1964).

FARAH, A., LOOMIS, T. A.: The action of cardiac glycosides on experimental auricular flutter. Circulation **2**, 742 (1950).

FARAH, A., MARESH, G.: Determination of the therapeutic, irregularity and lethal doses of cardiac glycosides in the heart-lung preparation of the dog. J. Pharmacol. exp. Ther. **92**, 32 (1948).

FASTIER, F. N., SMIRK, F. H.: Some properties of amarin, with special reference to its use in conjunction with adrenaline for the production of idio-ventricular rhythms. J. Physiol. (Lond.) **107**, 318 (1948).

FAWAZ, G.: The mechanism by which N:N-dibenzyl-chloroethylamine protects animals against cardiac arrhythmias induced by sympathomimetic amines in presence of cyclopropane or chloroform. Brit. J. Pharmacol. **6**, 492 (1951).

FEKETE, M., BORSY, J.: On the antiarrhythmic effect of some thymoleptics: Amitriptylene, Imipramine, Trimepropimine and Desmethylimipramine. Med. exp. (Basel) **10**, 93 (1964).

FENG, T. P.: Studies on the neuromuscular junction. VII. The eserine-like effects of barium on motor nerve endings. Chin. J. Physiol. **12**, 177 (1937).

FENTZ, V., GORMSEN, J.: Electrocardiographic patterns in patients with cerebrovascular accidents. Circulation **25**, 22 (1962).

FOSTER, J. M., WEINBERG, J.: Bioelectrical changes of the heart cycle induced by stimulation of diencephalic regions. Exp. Neurol. **2**, 26 (1960).

FREEDBERG, A. S., PAPP, J. GY., VAUGHAN WILLIAMS, E. M.: The effect of altered thyroid state on atrial intracellular potentials. J. Physiol. (Lond.) **207**, 357 (1970).

FROMMER, P. L., ROBINSON, B. F., BRAUNWALD, E.: Studies on digitalis-induced arrhythmias. J. Pharmacol. exp. Ther. **151**, 1 (1965).

GAFFNEY, T. E., KAHN, J. B., VAN MAANEN, E. F., ACHESON, G. H.: A mechanism of the vagal effect of cardiac-glycosides. J. Pharmacol. exp. Ther. **122**, 423 (1958).

GARB, S., CHENOVETH, M. B.: Studies on hydrocarbon-epinephrine induced ventricular fibrillation. J. Pharmacol. exp. Ther. **94**, 12 (1948).

GARRETT, J., GONCALVES MOREIRA, M., OSSWALD, W., GUIMARÃES, S.: Antiarrhythmic activity of N,N-diisopropyl-N'-isolamyl-N'-diethylaminoethylurea hydrochloride (P-286). J. Pharmacol. exp. Ther. **143**, 243 (1964).

GARREY, W. E.: Nature of fibrillary contraction of the heart: Its relation to tissue mass and form. Amer. J. Physiol. **33**, 397 (1914).

GERTLER, M. M., KARP, D.: Effect of atebrine on auricular fibrillation in the dog. Proc. Soc. exp. Biol. (N.Y.) **64**, 213 (1947).

GILBERT, J. L., LANGE, G. G., BROOKS, C. McC.: Influence of sympathomimetic pressor drugs on arrhythmias caused by multiple stimuli. Circulat. Res. **7**, 417 (1959).

GILBERT, J. L., LANGE, G., POLEVOY, I., BROOKS, C. McC.: Effects of vasoconstrictor agents on cardiac irritability. J. Pharmacol. exp. Ther. **123**, 9 (1958).

GILLIS, R. A.: Cardiac sympathetic nerve activity: Changes induced by ouabain and propranolol. Science **166**, 508 (1969).

GILLIS, R. A., CLANCY, M. M., ANDERSON, R. J.: Deleterious effects of bretylium in cats with digitalis-induced ventricular tachycardia. Circulation **47**, 974 (1973).

GILLIS, R. A., MCCLELLAN, J. R., SAUER, T. S., STANDAERT, F. G.: Depression of cardiac sympathetic nerve activity by diphenylhydantoin. J. Pharmacol. exp. Ther. **179**, 599 (1971).

GILSON, A. S.: Agents causing cardiac supernormality. Proc. Soc. exp. Biol. (N.Y.) **41**, 1 (1939).
GOLDENBERG, M., ROTHBERGER, C. J.: Über die Wirkung von Veratrin auf den Purkinjefaden. Pflügers Arch. ges. Physiol. **238**, 295 (1936).
GREENSPAN, K., STEINMETZ, E.: Digitalis and potassium: pharmacodynamic relationship. In: Mechanism and therapy of cardiac arrhythmias. New York, London: Grune and Stratton 1966.
GREINER, T. H., GARB, S.: The influence of drugs on the irritability and automaticity of heart muscle. J. Pharmacol. exp. Ther. **98**, 215 (1950).
GREMELS, H.: Über die Wirkung des Vagus auf die Herztätigkeit. Naunyn-Schmiedeberg's Arch. exp. Path. Pharmak. **179**, 360 (1935).
GROSS, E.: Die Bedeutung der Salze der Ringer'schen Lösung für das isolierte Säugetierherz. Pflügers Arch. ges. Physiol. **99**, 264 (1903).
GRUBER, C. M., JR., GRUBER, C. M., KWANG SOO LEE: Papaverine hydrochloride in thiobarbiturate anesthesia in dogs. Arch. int. Pharmacodyn. **93**, 248 (1953).
GRUMBACH, L.: The initiation of ventricular tachycardia and fibrillation in isolated hearts by potassium chloride. Circulat. Res. **4**, 293 (1956).
GRUMBACH, L., HOWARD, J. W., MERRIL, V. I.: Factors related to the initiation of ventricular fibrillation in the isolated heart: Effect of calcium and potassium. Circulat. Res. **2**, 452 (1954).
HADHÁZY, P., KECSKEMÉTI, V., VIZI, E. S., ILLÉS, P.: Antiarrhythmic effect of some naphthylalkylamine derivatives. Acta physiol. Acad. Sci. hung. **33**, 185 (1968).
HALLE, W., WOLLENBERGER, A.: Beiheft zum Forschungsfilm: Rhythmische Kontraktion kultivierter isolierter Herzzellen und ihr Verhalten gegenüber Digitoxin. Berlin: Deutsches Zentralinstitut für Lehrmittel 1962.
HAN, J., JALON, P. G., MOE, G. K.: Adrenergic effects on ventricular vulnerability. Circulat. Res. **14**, 516 (1964).
HAN, J., MOE, G. K.: Nonuniform recovery of excitability in ventricular muscle. Circulat. Res. **14**, 44 (1964).
HARRIS, A. S.: Delayed development of ventricular ectopic rhythms following experimental coronary occlusion. Circulat. Res. **1**, 1318 (1950).
HAUSWIRTH, O.: Effects of halothane on single atrial, ventricular and Purkinje fibers. Circulat. Res. **24**, 745 (1969).
HAUSWIRTH, O., NOBLE, D., TSIEN, R. W.: Adrenaline: mechanism of action on the pacemaker potential in cardiac Purkinje fibres. Science **162**, 916 (1968).
HAUSWIRTH, O., SCHAER, H.: Effects of halothane on the sinoatrial node. J. Pharmacol. exp. Ther. **158**, 36 (1967).
HAZARD, R., QUINQUAUD, A.: L'yohimbine, paralysant de barium vasoconstricteur. C. R. Soc. Biol. (Paris) **139**, 601 (1945).
HEISTRACHER, P., HELL, E., KRAUPP, O.: Untersuchungen über die antifibrillatorische Wirkung von N,N'-dimethyl- bzw. N,N'-Diäthyl-N,N'-bis-[3-(3',4',5'-trimethoxy-benzoxy)-propyl]-äthylendiamin. Arzneimittel-Forsch. **15**, 146 (1965).
HEISTRACHER, P., PILLAT, B.: Elektrophysiologische Untersuchungen über die Wirkung von Chinidin auf die Aconitinvergiftung von Herzmuskelfasern. Naunyn-Schmiedeberg's Arch. exp. Path. Pharmak. **244**, 48 (1962).
HEYMANS, C., BOUCKAERT, J. J., REGNIERS, P.: Sur le mechanisme reflexe de la bradycardie provoquée par les digitaliques. C. R. Soc. Biol. (Paris) **110**, 572 (1932).
HIRSCHFELDER, A. D., TAMCALES, F.: Inhibition of experimental auricular fibrillation by procaine and other substances. Proc. Soc. exp. Biol. (N.Y.) **50**, 272 (1942).
HOFF, H. E., NAHUM, L. H.: An analysis of the cardiac irregularities produced by calcium and their prevention by sodium amytal. J. Pharmacol. exp. Ther. **60**, 425 (1937).
HOFF, H. E., NAHUM, L. H.: Production of auricular fibrillation by application of acetyl-β-methylcholine chloride to localized regions on the auricular surface. Amer. J. Physiol. **129**, 428 (1940).
HOFF, H. E., SMITH, P. K., WINKLER, A. W.: Electrocardiographic changes and concentration of calcium in serum following intravenous injection of calcium chloride. Amer. J. Physiol. **125**, 162 (1939).
HOFF, H. E., STANSFIELD, H.: Ventricular fibrillation induced by cold. Amer. Heart J. **38**, 193 (1949).
HOFFMAN, B. F., CRANEFIELD, P. F.: Electrophysiology of the heart. New York-Toronto-London: McGraw-Hill Book Co. Inc. 1960.
HOFFMAN, B. F., GORIN, E. F., WAX, F. S., SIEBENS, A. A., BROOKS, C. McC.: Vulnerability to fibrillation and the ventricular excitability curve. Amer. J. Physiol. **167**, 88 (1951).
HOFFMAN, B. F., SINGER, D. H.: Effects of digitalis on electrical activity of cardiac fibers. Progr. cardiovasc. Dis. **7**, 226 (1964).

HOFFMAN, B. F., SUCKLING, E. E.: Effect of several cations on transmembrane potentials of cardiac muscle. Amer. J. Physiol. **186**, 317 (1956).

HOLLAND, W. C., BURN, J. H., SCHÜMANN, H. J.: Production of auricular fibrillation by electrical stimulation of isolated rabbit auricles in the presence of acetylcholine. J. Pharmacol. exp. Ther. **119**, 153 (1957).

HUGENHOLTZ, P. G.: Electrocardiographic abnormalities in cerebral disorders. Report of six cases and review of the literature. Amer. Heart J. **63**, 451 (1962).

HUTCHEON, D. E.: Susceptibility to ventricular fibrillation during chloroform and cyclopropane anaesthesia. Brit. J. Pharmacol. **6**, 31 (1951).

INNES, I. R., KOSTERLITZ, H. W., KRAYER, O.: Studies on veratrum alkaloids. XXIV. The inhibition by veratramine and veratrosine of the cardioaccelerator effect of electrical stimulation of the accelerator nerves. J. Pharmacol. exp. Ther. **117**, 317 (1956).

JAMES, T. N., NADEAU, R. A.: The chronotropic effect of digitalis studied by direct perfusion of the sinus node. J. Pharmacol. exp. Ther. **139**, 42 (1960).

JUDSON, W. E., HOLLANDER, W.: The effects of insulin-induced hypoglycemia in patients with angina pectoris. Amer. Heart J. **52**, 198 (1956).

KABELA, E., MENDEZ, R.: Action of propranolol on the atrio-ventricular node and on its response to adrenaline and isoprenaline. Brit. J. Pharmacol. **26**, 473 (1966).

KASSEBAUM, D. G.: Electrophysiological effects of strophanthin in the heart. J. Pharmacol. exp. Ther. **140**, 329 (1963).

KATZ, R. L.: Antiarrhythmic action of N,N-bis (phenylcarbamoylmethyl)-dimethyl ammonium chloride (QX-572). Anesthesiology **25**, 291 (1964a).

KATZ, R. L.: Antiarrhythmic and cardiovascular effects of synthetic oxytocin. Anesthesiology **25**, 653 (1964b).

KATZ, R. L.: Effects of alpha and beta adrenergic blocking agents on cyclopropane-catecholamine cardiac arrhythmias. Anesthesiology **26**, 289 (1965).

KATZ, R. L.: Neural factors affecting cardiac arrhythmias induced by halopropane. J. Pharmacol. exp. Ther. **152**, 88 (1966).

KATZ, R. L., LORD, C. O., EAKINS, K. E.: Anesthetic-dopamine cardiac arrhythmias and their prevention by beta adrenergic blockade. J. Pharmacol. exp. Ther. **158**, 40 (1967).

KATZUNG, B.: Evaluation of drugs affecting the contractility and the electrophysiological properties of the heart. In: Selected pharmacological testing methods. London: Edward Arnold Ltd., New York: Marcel Dekker Inc. 1968.

KELLIHER, G. J., ROBERTS, J.: The effect of d(+)- and l(—)-practolol on ouabain-induced arrhythmia. Europ. J. Pharmacol. **20**, 243 (1972).

KISCH, B.: Strophanthin: Clinical and experimental experiences of the past 25 years. New York: Brooklyn Med. Press 1944.

KLENSCH, H.: Einführung in die biologische Registriertechnik. Stuttgart: Georg Thieme Verlag 1954.

KOSTERLITZ, H. W., KRAYER, O., MATALLANA, A.: Studies on veratrum alkaloids. XXII. Periodic activity of the sinoauricular node of the denervated cat heart caused by veratramine. J. Pharmacol. exp. Ther. **113**, 460 (1955).

KRAYER, O.: A difference in cardioaccelerator action between digitoxin and digitoxigenin. Proc. Soc. exp. Biol. (N.Y.) **57**, 167 (1944).

KRAYER, O.: IX. The inhibition by veratrosine of the cardioaccelerator action of epinephrine and of norepinephrine. J. Pharmacol. exp. Ther. **97**, 256 (1949).

KRAYER, O., ACHESON, G. H.: The pharmacology of the veratrum alcaloids. Physiol. Rev. **26**, 383 (1946).

KRAYER, O., ARORA, R. B., MEILMAN, E.: Studies on veratrum alkaloids. XXI. The action of veratramine upon impulse generation in the dog heart. J. Pharmacol. exp. Ther. **113**, 446 (1955).

KRAYER, O., KUPCHAN, S. M., DELIWALA, C. V., ROGERS, B. H.: Untersuchungen über die Veratrumalkaloide. XVIII. Die chemischen und pharmakologischen Beziehungen zwischen den Zyganeusalkaloiden und den Veratrumalkaloiden. Naunyn-Schmiedeberg's Arch. exp. Path. Pharmak. **219**, 371 (1953).

KRAYER, O., MANDOKI, J. J., MENDEZ, C.: Studies on veratrum alkaloids. XVI. The action of epinephrine and of veratramine on the functional refractory period of the auriculoventricular transmission in the heart-lung preparation of the dog. J. Pharmacol. exp. Ther. **103**, 412 (1951).

KRAYER, O., REITER, M.: Studies on veratrum alkaloids. XI. Jervine and pseudojervine, antagonists to the cardioaccelerator action of epinephrine and of accelerans stimulations. Arch. int. Pharmacodyn. **4**, 409 (1950).

KRUTA, V. L.: Sur l'activité automatique de l'oreilette gauche isolée du cœur du mammifére. Arch. int. Physiol. **40**, 140 (1934).

LADDU, A. R.: Antiarrhythmic activity of 1-(DI-2,6-xylylmethoxy)-3-(isopropylamino) propanol-2-hydrochloride (BS-7977-D) in the dog heart lung preparation. Europ. J. Pharmacol. **9**, 129 (1970).
LADDU, A. R., SOMANI, P.: Antiarrhythmic actions of 4-(2-hydroxy-3-isopropyl-amino-propoxy)-acetanilide (ICI 50,172) in the dog heart-lung preparation. J. Pharmacol. exp. Ther. **170**, 79 (1969).
LAWSON, J. W.: Antiarrhythmic activity of some isoquinoline derivatives determined by a rapid screening procedure in the mouse. J. Pharmacol. exp. Ther. **160**, 22 (1968).
LEAK, D., STARR, P.: The mechanism of arrhythmias during insulin-induced hypoglycemia. Amer. Heart J. **63**, 688 (1962).
LEE, K. S., KLAUS, W.: The subcellular basis for the mechanism of inotropic action of cardiac glycosides. Pharmacol. Rev. **23**, 193 (1971).
LENEL, R., VANLOO, A., RODBARD, S., KATZ, L. N.: Factors involved in the production of paroxysmal ventricular tachycardia induced by epinephrine. Amer. J. Physiol. **153**, 553 (1948).
LEVÉQUE, P. E.: Production of atrial fibrillation in dogs by thyroid administration and acetylcholine injection. Circulat. Res. **4**, 108 (1956).
LEVÉQUE, P. E.: Guanethidine as an antifibrillatory agent. Nature (Lond.) **203**, 1389 (1964a).
LEVÉQUE, P. E.: A simple repeatable standardized procedure for the production of auricular fibrillation in the intact dog. Arch. int. Pharmacodyn. **149**, 297 (1964b).
LEVÉQUE, P. E.: Anti-arrhythmic action of bretylium. Nature (Lond.) **207**, 203 (1965).
LEVÉQUE, P. E.: Bethanidine: a new antifibrillatory agent. Arch. int. Pharmacodyn. **163**, 422 (1966).
LEVITT, B., ROBERTS, J.: Effect of quinidine and pronethalol on acetylstrophanthidin-induced ventricular arrhythmia in cats treated with reserpine. Circulat. Res. **19**, 662 (1966).
LEVY, A. G.: The genesis of ventricular extrasystoles under chloroform with special reference to consecutive ventricular fibrillation. Heart **5**, 299 (1914).
LEWIS, R., FIL, H. S., STROUD, W. D.: Observations upon flutter and fibrillation. Part II. The nature of auricular flutter. Heart **7**, 191 (1920).
LISSÁK, K.: The effect of calcium on the output of sympathin in the frog's heart. Amer. J. Physiol. **123**, 256 (1938).
LORENTE DE NÓ, R., FENG, T. P.: Analysis of the effect of barium upon nerve with particular reference to rhythmic activity. J. cell. comp. Physiol. **28**, 397 (1946).
LOWN, B., CANNON, R. L., III, ROSSI, M. A.: Electrical stimulation and digitalis drugs: Repetitive response in diastole. Proc. Soc. exp. Biol. (N.Y.) **126**, 698 (1967).
LOWN, B., KLEIGER, R., WILLIAMS, J.: Cardioversion and digitalis drugs: Changed threshold to electric shock in digitalized animals. Circulat. Res. **17**, 519 (1965).
LUCCHESI, B. R., HARDMANN, H. F.: The influence of dichlorisoproterenol (DCI) and related compounds on ouabain and acetylstrophanthidin-induced cardiac arrhythmias. J. Pharmacol. exp. Ther. **132**, 372 (1961).
LUCCHESI, B. R., IWAMI, T.: The antiarrhythmic properties of ICI 46037, a quaternary analog of propranolol. J. Pharmacol. exp. Ther. **162**, 49 (1968).
LUCCHESI, B. R., SHIVAK, R.: Effect of quinidine and procaine amide upon acetylstrophanthidin cardiotoxicity. J. Pharmacol. exp. Ther. **143**, 366 (1964).
LÜLLMANN, H., HOLLAND, W. C.: Influence of ouabain on an exchangeable calcium fraction, contractile force, and resting tension of guinea-pig atria. J. Pharmacol. exp. Ther. **137**, 186 (1962).
MACLEOD, D. P., REYNOLDS, A. K.: Studies on some rauwolfia preparations with special reference to their effect on cardiac arrhythmias. Arch. int. Pharmacodyn. **138**, 437 (1962).
MALING, H., MORAN, N. C.: Ventricular arrhythmias induced by sympathomimetic amines in unanesthetized dogs following coronary artery occlusion. Circulat. Res. **5**, 409 (1957).
MALINOW, M. R., BATTLE, F. F., MALAMUD, B.: Nervous mechanisms in ventricular arrhythmias induced by calcium chloride in rats. Circulat. Res. **1**, 554 (1953a).
MALINOW, M. R., BATTLE, F. F., MALAMUD, B.: Prevention of neurogenic ventricular arrhythmias in the rat by autonomic blocking drugs. Amer. J. Physiol. **175**, 8 (1953b).
MALINOW, M. R., BATTLE, F. F., MALAMUD, B.: A standardized method for the neurogenic and cardiogenic production of ventricular arrhythmias in the rat. Acta physiol. lat.-amer. **3**, 216 (1953c).
MALINOW, M. R., BATTLE, F. F., MALAMUD, B.: Neurogenic and cardiogenic production of ventricular arrhythmias in the rat. Acta Cardiol. (Brux.) **9**, 201 (1954a).
MALINOW, M. R., BATTLE, F. F., MALAMUD, B.: Prevention of experimental ventricular arrhythmias in the rat by atropine. Arch. int. Pharmacodyn. **99**, 458 (1954b).
MALINOW, M. R., BATTLE, F. F., MALAMUD, B.: The pharmacology of experimental ventricular arrhythmias in the rat. 1. Antihistaminic drugs. Arch. int. Pharmacodyn. **102**, 55 (1955a).

MALINOW, M. R., BATTLE, F. F., MALAMUD, B.: The pharmacology of experimental ventricular arrhythmias in the rat. 2. Mechanism of action of nupercaine hydrochloride. Arch. int. Pharmacodyn. **102**, 266 (1955b).

MANNING, J. W., COTTEN, M. V.: Mechanism of cardiac arrhythmias induced by diencephalic stimulation. Amer. J. Physiol. **203**, 1120 (1962).

MARSHALL, J. M., VAUGHAN WILLIAMS, E. M.: Pacemaker potentials. The excitation of isolated rabbit auricles by acetylcholine at low temperatures. J. Physiol. (Lond.) **131**, 186 (1959).

MASON, D. T., DEMARIA, A. N., AMSTERDAM, E. A., ZELIS, R., MASSUMI, R. A.: Antiarrhythmic agents. II. Therapeutic considerations. Drugs **5**, 292 (1973b).

MASON, D. T., ZELIS, R., AMSTERDAM, E. A., MASSUMI, R. A.: Mechanism of digitalis arrhythmias: Electrophysiologic and myocardial subcellular considerations. In: Cardiac arrhythmias. New York: Grune and Stratton 1973a.

MATSUDA, K., HOFFMAN, B. F., ELLNER, C. N., KATZ, M., BROOKS, C. MCC.: Veratrine induced prolongation of repolarisation in the mammalian heart. Abstr. 19th int. Physiol. Congr. 1953.

MATSUDA, K., HOSHI, T., KAMEYAMA, S.: Effects of aconitine on the cardiac membrane potential of the dog. Jap. J. Physiol. **9**, 419 (1959).

MCMILLAN, T. M., WOLFERTH, C. C.: An untoward effect of barium chloride in producing short runs of aberrant ventricular beats. J. Lab. clin. Med. **14**, 839 (1928).

MEEK, W. J.: Some cardiac effects of the inhalant anesthetics and the sympathomimetic amines. Harvey Lect. **36**, 188 (1941).

MEEK, W. J., HATHAWAY, H. R., ORTH, O. S.: The effects of ether, chloroform and cyclopropane on cardiac automaticity. J. Pharmacol. exp. Ther. **61**, 240 (1937).

MELVILLE, K. I., BLUM, B., SHISTER, H. E., SILVER, M. D.: Cardiac ischemic changes and arrhythmias induced by hypothalamic stimulation. Amer. J. Cardiol. **12**, 781 (1963).

MELVILLE, K. I., SHARE, N. N.: Cardiovascular response following injection of picrotoxin into the lateral cerebral ventricle. Rev. canad. Biol. **22**, 265 (1963).

MÉNDEZ, C., ACEVES, J., MÉNDEZ, R.: The anti-adrenergic action of digitalis on the A-V transmission system. J. Pharmacol. exp. Ther. **131**, 199 (1961).

MÉNDEZ, R., MÉNDEZ, C.: The action of glycosides on the refractory period of heart tissues. J. Pharmacol. exp. Ther. **107**, 24 (1953).

MOE, G. K., MÉNDEZ, R.: The action of several cardiac glycosides on conduction velocity and ventricular excitability in the dog heart. Circulation **4**, 729 (1951).

MOE, R. A.: Some pharmacological properties of RO 2-5803, an anti-arrhythmic compound. Arch. int. Pharmacodyn. **132**, 295 (1961).

MOKLER, C. H., VAN ARMAN, C. G.: Pharmacology of a new antiarrhythmic agent, γ-diisopropyl-amino-α-phenyl-α-(2-pyridyl)-butyramide (SC-7031). J. Pharmacol. exp. Ther. **136**, 114 (1962).

MOORE, J. O., SWAIN, H. H.: Sensitization to ventricular fibrillation. I. Sensitization by a substituted propiophenon, U-0882. J. Pharmacol. exp. Ther. **128**, 243 (1960a).

MOORE, J. I., SWAIN, H. H.: Sensitization to ventricular fibrillation. II. Sensitization by amarine and congeners of U-0882. J. Pharmacol. exp. Ther. **128**, 253 (1960b).

MORAN, N. C., MOORE, J. I., HOLCOMB, H. K., MUSHET, G.: Antagonism of adrenergically induced cardiac arrhythmias by dichloroisoproterenol. J. Pharmacol. exp. Ther. **136**, 327 (1962).

MÜLLER, P.: Kalium und Digitalistoxizität. Cardiologia (Basel) **42**, 1 (1963).

NAHUM, L. H., HOFF, H. E.: The mechanism of sudden death in experimental acute benzol poisoning. J. Pharmacol. exp. Ther. **50**, 336 (1934).

NAHUM, L. H., HOFF, H. E.: Auricular fibrillation in hyperthyroid patients. J. Amer. med. Ass. **105**, 254 (1935).

NAKAYAMA, K., KOIKE, H., OSHIMA, T., HASHIMOTO, K.: Antiarrhythmic potency of N-propyl ajmaline with untoward response of ventricular fibrillation in excess dose. Jap. J. Pharmacol. **23**, 9 (1973).

NAKAYAMA, K., OSHIMA, T., KUMAKURA, S., HASHIMOTO, K.: Comparison of the effects of various β-adrenergic blocking agents with known antiarrhythmic drugs on aconitine-arrhythmia produced by the cup method. Europ. J. Pharmacol. **14**, 9 (1971).

NALEFSKI, L. A., GILBERT, N. C., FENN, G. K.: Cardiovascular changes observed following the experimental administration of barium chloride. J. Lab. clin. Med. **34**, 1733 (1949).

NAYLER, W. G.: Calcium exchange in cardiac muscle: a basic mechanism of drug action. Amer. Heart J. **73**, 379 (1967).

NICKERSON, M., NOMAGUCHI, G.: Mechanism of dibenamine protection against cyclopropane-epinephrine cardiac arrhythmias. J. Pharmacol. exp. Ther. **95**, 1 (1949).

NIESCHULZ, O., POPENDIKER, K., HOFFMAN, I.: Weitere pharmakologische Untersuchungen über N-Methyl-piperidyl-(3)-methyl-phenylthiazin. Arzneimittel-Forsch. **5**, 680 (1955).

NYE, C. E., ROBERTS, J.: The reactivity of atrial and ventricular pacemakers to quinidine. J. Pharmacol. exp. Ther. **152**, 67 (1966).
OTSUKA, M.: Die Wirkung von Adrenalin auf Purkinje-Fasern von Säugetierherzen. Pflügers Arch. ges. Physiol. **266**, 512 (1958).
PAPP, J. GY.: Importance of the neurovegetative blocking action of antiarrhythmic drugs in cardiac arrhythmias of various origin. Proc. IVth Hung. Conf. Ther. Pharmacol. Res. Budapest: Publishing House of the Hungarian Academy of Sciences 1966.
PAPP, J. GY., FÖRSTER, W., SZEKERES, L., RÖSSLER, V.: Action of β-receptor blocking sympatholytics on $CaCl_2$-induced arrhythmias in rats. Experientia (Basel) **22**, 524 (1966).
PAPP, J. GY., SZEKERES, L.: Influence of stretch and dynamic functional state of the myocardium on tendency of the heart to arrhythmia. Acta physiol. Acad. Sci. hung. **32**, 163 (1967).
PAPP, J. GY., SZEKERES, L.: The arrhythmogenic action of sympathomimetic amines. Europ. J. Pharmacol. **3**, 4 (1968a).
PAPP, J. GY.,SZEKERES, L.: Analysis of the mechanism of adrenergic actions on ventricular vulnerability. Europ. J. Pharmacol. **3**, 15 (1968b).
PAPP, J. GY., SZEKERES, L.: Cardiac electrophysiological changes due to oxyfedrine. In: Action of oxyfedrine. Stuttgart-New York: Schattauer Verlag 1972.
PAPP, J. GY., SZEKERES, L.: On the nature of adrenergic receptors involved in catecholamine-induced changes in the electrical activity of the heart. Diss. pharm. pharmacol. **23**, 622 (1972a).
PAPP, J. GY., SZEKERES, L.: Receptors mediating alterations in cardiac electrical activity due to adrenergic stimulants. Abstracts of Papers of the Fifth International Congress on Pharmacology. San Francisco 1972b.
PAPP, J. GY., SZEKERES, L.: The electrophysiological mechanism of dopamine and l-dopa-induced cardiac arrhythmias and the protective effect of β-adrenoceptor blocking agents. Rev. esp. Cardiol. Symposia, Mesas Redondes y Communicaciones, Madrid, Communic. A/3. 1972c.
PAPP, J. GY., SZEKERES, L., SZMOLENSZKY, T.: The effects of quinidine, ajmaline, papaverine and adrenergic β-receptor inhibitors in experimental $BaCl_2$-arrhythmia developed for the quantitative assay of antiarrhythmic drugs. Acta physiol. Acad. Sci. hung. **32**, 365 (1967).
PAPP, J. GY., VAUGHAN WILLIAMS, E. M.: The effect of bretylium on intracellular cardiac action potentials in relation to its antiarrhythmic and local anaesthetic activity. Brit. J. Pharmacol. **37**, 380 (1969a).
PAPP, J. GY., VAUGHAN WILLIAMS, E. M.: A comparison of the antiarrhythmic actions of I.C.I. 50172 and (−)-propranolol and their effects on intracellular cardiac action potentials and other features of cardiac function. Brit. J. Pharmacol. **37**, 391 (1969b).
PAPP, J. GY., VAUGHAN WILLIAMS, E. M.: The effect of some catecholamine β-receptor blocking compounds on the toxicity to the heart of ouabain. Brit. J. Pharmacol. **36**, 178P (1969c).
PASTELIN, G., MÉNDEZ, R.: Singular effects of a new short acting cardiac glycoside in Purkinje cells. Europ. J. Pharmacol. **19**, 291 (1972).
PEPER, K., TRAUTWEIN, W.: The effect of aconitine on the membrane current in cardiac muscle. Pflügers Arch. ges. Physiol. **296**, 328 (1967).
RAINES, A., MOROS, D., LEVITT, B.: The effect of guanethidine on ouabain-induced ventricular arrhythmias in the cat. Arch. int. Pharmacodyn. **174**, 373 (1968).
RAPER, C., WALE, J.: Propranolol, MJ 1999 and Ciba 39089 Ba in ouabain and adrenaline-induced cardiac arrhythmias. Europ. J. Pharmacol. **4**, 1 (1968).
RAPER, C., WALE, J.: Cardiac arrhythmias produced by interaction of ouabain and β-receptor stimulation. Europ. J. Pharmacol. **6**, 223 (1969).
RAVENTOS, J.: The action of fluothane—a new volatile anaesthetic. Brit. J. Pharmacol. **11**, 394 (1956).
REUTER, H.: Strom-Spannungsbeziehungen von Purkinje-Fasern bei verschiedenen extracellularen Calcium-Konzentrationen und unter Adrenalin-Einwirkung. Pflügers Arch. ges. Physiol. **287**, 357 (1966).
REUTER, H.: The dependence of slow inward current in Purkinje fibres on the extracellular calcium-concentration. J. Physiol. (Lond.) **192**, 479 (1967).
RIKER, W. F., DEPIERRE, F., ROBERTS, J., ROY, B. B., REILLY, J.: The epinephrine and hydrocarbon-epinephrine disturbance in the cat. J. Pharmacol. exp. Ther. **114**, 1 (1955).
ROBERTS, J., BAER, R.: A method for the evaluation of depressants of subatrial rhythmic function in the heart of intact animal. J. Pharmacol. exp. Ther. **129**, 36 (1960).
ROBERTS, J., ITO, R., REILLY, J., CAIROLI, V. J.: The influence of reserpine and βTM10 on digitalis-induced ventricular arrhythmia. Circulat. Res. **13**, 149 (1963).
ROBERTS, J., LEVITT, B., STANDAERT, F. G.: Autonomic nervous system and control of cardiac rhythm. Nature (Lond.) **214**, 912 (1967).

ROBERTS, J., STANDAERT, F., KIM, Y. I., RIKER, W. F., JR.: The initiation and pharmacologic reactivity of a ventricular pacemaker in the intact animal. J. Pharmacol. exp. Ther. **117**, 374 (1956).

ROSÉN, M., GELBAND, H., HOFFMAN, B. F.: Correlation between effects of ouabain on canine electrocardiogram and on transmembrane potentials of isolated Purkinje fibers. Circulation **47**, 65 (1973a).

ROSÉN, M. R., GELBAND, H., MERKER, C., HOFFMAN, B. F.: Mechanism of digitalis toxicity. Effects of ouabain on phase four of canine Purkinje fiber transmembrane potentials. Circulation **47**, 681 (1973b).

ROSENBLUETH, A., GARCIA-RAMOS, J.: Studies on flutter and fibrillation. II. The influence of artificial obstacles on experimental auricular flutter. Amer. Heart J. **33**, 677 (1947).

ROTHBERGER, C. J., SACHS, A.: Rhythmicity and automatism in the mammalian left auricle. Quart. J. exp. Physiol. **29**, 69 (1939).

ROTHBERGER, C. J., WINTERBERG, H.: Über die experimentelle Erzeugung extrasystolischer ventriculärer Tachykardie durch Acceleransreizung. (Ein Beitrag zur Herzwirkung von Barium und Calcium.) Pflügers Arch. ges. Physiol. **142**, 461 (1911).

SCHAPER, G.: Elektrokardiographische Untersuchungen während der Pneumencephalographie. Mschr. Kinderheilk. **103**, 14 (1955).

SCHERF, D.: Experimental digitalis and strophanthin extrasystoles. Exp. Med. Surg. **21**, 70 (1944).

SCHERF, D.: Studies on auricular tachycardia caused by aconitine administration. Proc. Soc. exp. Biol. (N.Y.) **64**, 233 (1947).

SCHERF, D.: Effect of fagarine on auricular fibrillation. Proc. Soc. exp. Biol. (N.Y.) **67**, 59 (1948).

SCHERF, D., BLUMENFELD, S.: Mechanism of auricular flutter caused by crushing and electric stimulation. Cardiologia (Basel) **24**, 193 (1954).

SCHERF, D., BLUMENFELD, S., TANER, D., YILDIZ, M.: Cardiac arrhythmias provoked by focal application of delphinine. Arch. Kreisl.-Forsch. **33**, 4 (1960).

SCHERF, D., BLUMENFELD, S., YILDIZ, M.: Experimental study on ventricular extrasystoles provoked by vagal stimulation. Amer. Heart J. **62**, 670 (1961).

SCHERF, D., BLUMENTHAL, S., YILDIZ, M.: Experimental study of ectopic impulse formation in the left atrium. Cardiologia (Basel) **43**, 133 (1963).

SCHERF, D., CHICK, F. B.: Experimental parasystole. Amer. Heart J. **42**, 212 (1951).

SCHERF, D., SCHOTT, A.: Extrasystoles and allied arrhythmias. London: William Heineman, Ltd. 1953.

SCHMIDT, R. F.: Versuche mit Aconitin zum Problem der spontanen Erregungsbildung im Herzen. Pflügers Arch. ges. Physiol. **271**, 526 (1960).

SCHMITT, H., Mme SCHMITT, H.: Sur la pharmacologie de l'ajmaline. Arch. int. Pharmacodyn. **127**, 163 (1960).

SCHOENSTADT, D. A., WHITCHER, C. E.: Observations on the mechanism of succinyl dicholine-induced cardiac arrhythmias. Anesthesiology **24**, 358 (1963).

SEIFEN, E., SCHAER, H., MARSHALL, J. M.: Effect of calcium on the membrane potentials of single pacemaker fibers and atrial fibers in isolated rabbit atria. Nature (Lond.) **202**, 1223 (1964).

SEKIYA, A., VAUGHAN WILLIAMS, E. M.: The effects of pronethalol, dichloroisoprenaline and disopyramide on the toxicity of the heart to ouabain and anaesthetics. Brit. J. Pharmacol. **21**, 462 (1963).

SETNIKAR, I., MAGISTRETTI, M. J., TIRONE, P.: Cardiovascular and other pharmacological activities of three β-phenoxy-ethylamines with local anesthetic activity. Arzneimittel-Forsch. **16**, 1275 (1966).

SHIBATA, J.: The effects of barium on the action potential and the membrane current of sheep heart Purkinje fibers. J. Pharmacol. exp. Ther. **185**, 418 (1973).

SHIDEMAN, F. E., PROCITA, L.: The pharmacology of the monomethyl ethers of mono-, di-, and tripropylene glycol in the dog with observations on the auricular fibrillation produced by these compounds. J. Pharmacol. exp. Ther. **102**, 79 (1951).

SHKHVATSABAYA, I. K.: Experimental reproduction of arrhythmias by stimulation of central nervous system. Fed. Proc. **23** (Trans. Suppl.), 1211 (1964).

SINGH, B. N., NORRIS, R. M.: The clinician's approach to antiarrhythmic therapy. Drugs **5**, 257 (1973).

SINGH, B. N., VAUGHAN WILLIAMS, E. M.: Local anaesthetic and antiarrhythmic actions of alprenolol relative to its effect on intracellular potentials and other properties of isolated cardiac muscle. Brit. J. Pharmacol. **38**, 749 (1970a).

SINGH, B. N., VAUGHAN WILLIAMS, E. M.: A third class of anti-arrhythmic action. Effects on atrial and ventricular intracellular potentials, and other pharmacological actions on cardiac muscle, of MJ 1999 and AH 3474. Brit. J. Pharmacol. **39**, 675 (1970b).

SINGH, B. N., VAUGHAN WILLIAMS, E. M.: A fourth class of anti-dysrhythmic action, effect of verapamil on ouabain toxicity, on atrial and ventricular intracellular potentials, and on other features of cardiac function. Cardiovasc. Res. **6**, 109 (1972).

SINITSIN, L. N., KISIN, I. E.: The effect of thiopental, hexamethonium and papaverine on cardiac disturbances in stimulation of the brain cortex. Farmakol. i Toksikol. **27**. 138 (1964).

SMITH, P. K., WINKLER, A. W., HOFF, H. E.: Cardiovascular changes following intravenous administration of barium chloride. J. Pharmacol. exp. Ther. **68**, 113 (1940).

SODHI, H. K., BOOKER, W. M., BHAGAT, B.: The effects of mephentermine on digitalis-induced arrhythmias. Arch. int. Pharmacodyn. **161**, 132 (1966).

SOMANI, P., FLEMING, J. G., CHAN, G. K., LUM, B. K. B.: Antagonism of epinephrine-induced cardiac arrhythmias by 4-(2-isopropylamino-1-hydroxyethyl)-methanesulfon-anilide (MJ 1999). J. Pharmacol. exp. Ther. **151**, 32 (1966).

SOMANI, P., LUM, B. K. B.: The antiarrhythmic actions of beta adrenergic blocking agents. J. Pharmacol. exp. Ther. **147**, 194 (1965).

SOMANI, P., LUM, B. K. B.: Blockade of epinephrine- and ouabain-induced cardiac arrhythmias in the dog heart-lung preparation. J. Pharmacol. exp. Ther. **152**, 235 (1966).

SPANG, K.: Formen, Ursachen und klinische Auswirkungen des akuten Herzstillstandes. Verh. dtsch. Ges. Kreisl.-Forsch. **30**, 56 (1964).

STROUSE, S., SOSKIN, S., KATZ, L. N., RUBINFELD, S. H.: Treatment of older diabetic patients with cardiovascular disease. J. Amer. med. Ass. **98**, 1703 (1932).

SWAIN, H. H., CURTIS, G. P.: The use of hypertonic solutions to produce atrial fibrillation in the dog heart-lung preparation. J. Pharmacol. exp. Ther. **151**, 438 (1966).

SWAIN, H. H., MCCARTHY, D. A.: Veratrine, protoveratrine and andromedotoxin arrhythmias in the isolated dog heart. J. Pharmacol. exp. Ther. **121**, 379 (1957).

SWAIN, H. H., WEIDNER, C. L.: A study of substances which alter intraventricular conduction in the isolated dog heart. J. Pharmacol. exp. Ther. **120**, 137 (1957).

SZEKERES, L.: Discussion of Dr. West's paper. In: Pharmacology of cardiac function. Proc. 2nd Int. Pharmacol. Mtg., Prague. Oxford: Pergamon Press 1964.

SZEKERES, L.: Pharmacological interventions against arrhythmias appearing after coronary occlusion. Abstracts of papers presented to the IVth Congress of the Polish Pharmacological Society. Łódz 1973.

SZEKERES, L., ARATÓ, M., KOVACSICS, J.: Über die Vagus-Wirkung der Herzglykoside. Acta physiol. Acad. Sci. hung. **1**, 22 (1951).

SZEKERES, L., MÉHES, J., PAPP, J. GY.: Mechanism of increased susceptibility to fibrillation of the hypothermic mammalian heart in situ. Brit. J. Pharmacol. **17**, 167 (1961).

SZEKERES, L., PAPP, J. GY.: The effect of vagal stimulation and acetylcholine on susceptibility to fibrillation of the mammalian heart at different body temperatures. Acta physiol. Acad. Sci. hung. **26**, 277 (1965).

SZEKERES, L., PAPP, J. GY.: Antiarrhythmic compounds. Fortschr. Arzneimittelforsch. **12**, 292 (1968).

SZEKERES, L., PAPP, J. GY.: Experimental cardiac arrhythmias and antiarrhythmic drugs. (A monograph.) Budapest: Publishing House of the Hungarian Academy of Sciences (Akadémia Kiadó) 1971.

SZEKERES, L., PAPP, J. GY., UDVARY, É.: Early electrophysiological and biochemical changes in the non-infarcted myocardium and their relation to arrhythmias appearing soon after coronary occlusion. Rev. esp. Cardiol. VI. Congreso Europeo de Cardiologia. Symposia, Mesas Redondas y Communicaciones, Madrid. Communic. A/3. 1972a.

SZEKERES, L., PAPP, J. GY., UDVARY, É.: Pharmacological interventions against arrhythmias appearing after coronary occlusion. Abstract of Papers of the Fifth International Congress on Pharmacology. San Francisco 1972b.

TAKAORI, M., LOEHNIG, R. W.: Ventricular arrhythmias during halothane anesthesia: Effect of isoproterenol, aminophylline and ephedrine. Canad. Anaesth. Soc. J. **12**, 275 (1965).

TAMAI, T., YANAGA, T., GOTO, M.: On the transmission of excitation in the atrial muscle during aconitine-induced fibrillation. Jap. J. Physiol. **11**, 656 (1961).

TEN EICK, R. E., BASSETT, A. L., OKITA, G. T.: Dissociation of electrophysiological and inotropic actions of strophanthidin-3-bromoacetate: Possible role of adenosine triphosphatase in the maintenance of the myocardial transmembrane Na^+ and K^+ gradients. J. Pharmacol. exp. Ther. **185**, 12 (1973).

TRAUTWEIN, W.: Generation and conduction of impulses in the heart as affected by drugs. Pharmacol. Rev. **15**, 277 (1963).

TRAUTWEIN, W., DUDEL, J.: Zum Mechanismus der Membranwirkung des Acetylcholin an der Herzmuskelfaser. Pflügers Arch. ges. Physiol. **266**, 324 (1958a).

TRAUTWEIN, W., DUDEL, J.: Hemmende und erregende Wirkungen des Acetylcholins am Warmblüterherzen. Zur Frage der spontanen Erregungsbildung. Pflügers Arch. ges. Physiol. **266**, 653 (1958b).
TRAUTWEIN, W., KASSEBAUM, D. G.: On the mechanism of spontaneous impulse generation in the pacemaker of the heart. J. gen. Physiol. **45**, 317 (1961).
TRAUTWEIN, W., SCHMIDT, R. F.: Zur Membranwirkung des Adrenalin an der Herzmuskelfaser. Pflügers Arch. ges. Physiol. **271**, 715 (1960).
TRIPOD, J.: Fibrillation cardiaque et activité antifibrillante sur le cœur isolé de mammifére. Arch. int. Pharmacodyn. **85**, 121 (1951).
TURNER, R. A.: Screening methods in pharmacology. New York: Academic Press 1965.
VAN BOGAERT, A.: Hypothalamus et réactions cardio-vasculaire d'origine centrale. Arch. int. Pharmacodyn. **53**, 137 (1936).
VAN DONGEN, K.: The action of some drugs on fibrillation of the heart. Arch. int. Pharmacodyn. **53**, 80 (1936).
VAN DONGEN, K.: The action of hydrocupreine and hydrocupreidine on fibrillation of the heart. Arch. int. Pharmacodyn. **56**, 193 (1937).
VAN TYN, R. A., MCLEAN, L. D.: Ventricular fibrillation threshold. Amer. J. Physiol. **201**, 457 (1961).
VARMA, D. R., MELVILLE, K. I.: Ventricular fibrillation induced by coronary occlusion during hypothermia in dogs and the effects of quinidine, quinacrine and oxytocin. Canad. J. Biochem. **41**, 511 (1963).
VARMA, D. R., SHARE, N. N., MELVILLE, K. I.: Cardiovascular responses following injection of picrotoxin into the lateral cerebral ventricle of rabbits. Biochem. Pharmacol. 8, 135 (1961).
VARMA, D. R., SHARE, N. N., MELVILLE, K. I.: Cardiovascular responses following injection of picrotoxin into the lateral cerebral ventricle of rabbits. Int. J. Neuropharmacol. **1**, 203 (1962).
VASSALLE, M., GREENSPAN, K., HOFFMAN, B. F.: An analysis of arrhythmias induced by ouabain in intact dogs. Circulat. Res. **13**, 132 (1963).
VASSALLE, M., KARIS, J., HOFFMAN, B. F.: Toxic effects of ouabain on Purkinje fibers and ventricular muscle fibers. Amer. J. Physiol. **203**, 433 (1962).
VASSORT, G., ROUGIER, O., GARNIER, D., SAUVIAT, M. P., CORABOEUF, E., GARGOUÏL, Y. M.: Effects of adrenaline on membrane inward currents during the cardiac action potential. Pflügers Arch. ges. Physiol. **309**, 70 (1969).
VIANA, A. P., OSSWALD, W.: Antiarrhythmic action of atropine. Arch. int. Pharmacodyn. **192**, 238 (1971).
WATANABE, Y., DREIFUS, L. S.: Electrophysiological effects of digitalis on A-V transmission. Amer. J. Physiol. **211**, 1461 (1966).
WÉGRIA, R., NICKERSON, N. D.: The effect of papaverine, epinephrine and quinidine on the fibrillation threshold of the mammalian ventricles. J. Pharmacol. exp. Ther. **75**, 50 (1942).
WÉGRIA, R., NICKERSON, N. D.: The benzol-adrenalin test as a reliable method of estimating changes in the sensitivity of the dog's ventricles to fibrillation. Application of the method to the study of quinidine sulfate. Amer. Heart J. **25**, 58 (1943).
WEIDMANN, S.: The effects of calcium ions and local anaesthetics on electrical properties of Purkinje fibers. J. Physiol. (Lond.) **129**, 568 (1955).
WEINBERG, S. J., FOSTER, J. M.: Electrocardiographic changes produced by localized hypothalamic stimulations. Ann. intern. Med. **53**, 332 (1960).
WEINBERG, S. J., HALEY, T. J.: Effect of chlorpromazine on cardiac arrhythmias induced by intracerebral injection of tryptamine-strophanthidin. Arch. int. Pharmacodyn. **105**, 209 (1956).
WEST, T. C.: Fibrillatory and antifibrillatory drugs. In: Pharmacology of cardiac function. Proc. 2nd Int. Pharmacol. Mtg. Oxford: Pergamon Press **5**, 133 (1964).
WEST, T. C.: Electrophysiology of the sinoatrial node. In: Electrical phenomena in the heart. New York-London: Academic Press 1972.
WEST, T. C., FALK, F., CERVONI, P.: Drug alteration of transmembrane potentials in atrial pacemaker cells. J. Pharmacol. exp. Ther. **117**, 245 (1956).
WEST, T. C., LANDA, J. F.: Minimal mass required for induction of sustained arrhythmia in isolated atrial segments. Amer. J. Physiol. **202**, 232 (1962).
WIGGERS, C. J., WÉGRIA, R.: Quantitative measurement of the fibrillation thresholds of the mammalian ventricles with observation on the effect of procaine. Amer. J. Physiol. **131**, 296 (1940).
WILLIAMS, C. N., DEUTSCH, S., LINDE, H. W., BULLOUGH, J. W., DRIPPS, R. D.: Effects of intravenously administered succinyldicholine on cardiac rate rhythm and arterial pressure in anesthetized man. Anesthesiology **22**, 947 (1961).

WILSON, F. N.: The cardiac disturbances associated with diseases of the thyroid gland. J. Amer. med. Ass. **82**, 1754 (1924).

WINBURY, M.: Relation between atrial and ventricular antiarrhythmic assay methods, rationale for a screening program. Ann. N.Y. Acad. Sci. **64**, 564 (1956).

WINBURY, M. M., HAUSLER, L. M., PRIOLI, N. A., ZITOWITZ, L.: Effect of epinephrine on cardiac rhythm in the miniature pig before and after coronary occlusion. J. Pharmacol. exp. Ther. **138**, 287 (1962).

WINBURY, M. M., HEMMER, M. L.: Action of quinidine, procaine amide and other compounds on experimental atrial and ventricular arrhythmias in the dog. J. Pharmacol. exp. Ther. **113**, 402 (1955).

WINBURY, M. M., PAPIERSKY, D. H.: Suppression of experimental ventricular arrhythmias in the unanesthetized dog with N-(γ-isopropylaminopropyl)-α, α-diphenylacetamide hydrochloride. Arch. int. Pharmacodyn. **108**, 215 (1956).

WINKLER, A. W., HOFF, H. E., SMITH, P. K.: Electrocardiographic changes and concentration of calcium in serum following intravenous injection of calcium chloride. J. Physiol. (Lond.) **125**, 162 (1939).

WISHART, S. W.: Cardiac irregularities associated with diseases of the thyroid gland. Amer. J. Surg. **7**, 329 (1929).

WOLLENBERGER, A.: Rhythmic and arrhythmic contractile activity of single myocardial cells cultured in vitro. Circulat. Res. Suppl. to Vols. **14–15**: II–184 (1964).

Experimental Production of Cerebral Vascular Disorders

E. Betz

With 12 Figures

A. Introduction

Diseases of the coronary and cerebral vascular systems are the two most frequent causes of death in man. It is therefore not surprising that experimental pathophysiological and therapeutic models have met with wide interest in cerebral circulatory research. Disturbances of the cerebral circulation are mostly caused by total or partial occlusion of a brain vessel. Moreover, there exist a number of other factors causing disturbance of blood flow which do not have a suitable equivalent in this respect in other organs. Variation of pressure within the inflexible skull can influence cerebral blood flow (CBF). The walls of the brain vessels themselves have much less muscle than comparable vessels in other parts of the body, and the edema of the tissue is of much greater significance for tissue perfusion than in other organs.

The regulation of CBF can be principally influenced by two systems, as the rough graph in Fig. 1 shows. The factors represented in the upper part of the diagram in Fig. 1 affect the effective blood pressure, and their influence can be recorded with the nitrous oxide technique for measuring blood flow through the total brain (Kety and Schmidt, 1948a). The components listed in the lower part of Fig. 1 affect local cerebral vascular resistance. These components

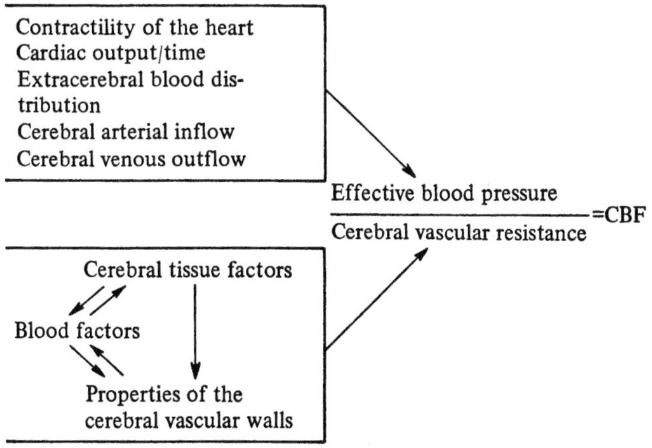

Fig. 1. CBF as a quotient of blood pressure and cerebral vascular resistance (CVR). The components which influence CBF are classified according to factors which mainly affect systemic blood pressure and those which influence CVR

consist of blood- and tissue factors. As in the other organs, local vascular resistance is not equal in each cerebral region but is regulated according to the local conditions. Therefore it is understandable that local variations of blood flow cannot be recorded with techniques for measuring the over-all cerebral blood flow. Local blood flow measurements of the brain were introduced by GIBBS (1933b), who measured flow by means of heated thermocouples. The techniques have been extended by the introduction of blood flow measurements which allowed the local blood flow in living animals and in man to be quantified (LEWIS et al., 1960; LASSEN and INGVAR, 1961; MÜLLER-SCHAUENBURG and BETZ, 1969; MÜLLER-SCHAUENBURG, 1972).

Table 1. Regional cerebral blood flow in conscious cats (1st and 2nd column) and in cats anesthetized with thiopental (3rd column). The values of column 1 are obtained with the ^{131}J-trifluoroiodomethane and those in column 2 with ^{14}C antipyrine technique. The same technique was used for the local blood flow studies in light thiopental anesthesia. The reduction of blood flow can be seen mainly in the cortex and in the basilar ganglia, whereas insignificant decreases occur in the white matter

	1 LANDAU et al. (1955) 10 consc. cats	2 REIVICH et al. (1969) 6 consc. cats	3 SOKOLOFF et al. (1961) 11 cats anesthetized with thiopental
	Superficial cerebral structures		
Cortex			
Sensory motor	1.38 × 0.12	1.09 × 0.04	0.65 × 0.07
Auditory	1.30 × 0.05	1.22 × 0.11	0.72 × 0.07
Visual	1.25 × 0.06	1.17 × 0.04	0.77 × 0.09
Miscellaneous association	0.88 × 0.04	0.81 × 0.05	0.67 × 0.06
Olfactory	0.77 × 0.06	0.74 × 0.05	0.62 × 0.07
White matter	0.23 × 0.02	0.21 × 0.01	0.26 × 0.04
	Deep cerebral structures		
Medical geniculate body	1.22 × 0.04	1.43 × 0.11	0.81 × 0.09
Lateral geniculate body	1.21 × 0.08	1.64 × 0.14	0.79 × 0.07
Caudate nucleus	1.10 × 0.08	1.02 × 0.07	0.91 × 0.11
Thalamus	1.03 × 0.05	1.06 × 0.06	0.71 × 0.09
Hypothalamus	0.84 × 0.05	0.68 × 0.06	0.55 × 0.06
Basal ganglia and amygdala	0.75 × 0.03		0.58 × 0.05
Amygdala		0.54 × 0.03	
Hippocampus	0.61 × 0.03	0.62 × 0.04	0.59 × 0.04
Optic tract	0.27 × 0.02	0.20 × 0.01	0.22 × 0.08
	Midbrain and pons		
Inferior colliculus	1.80 × 0.11	1.74 × 0.08	1.41 × 0.14
Superior olive	1.17 × 0.13	1.08 × 0.07	1.56 × 0.27
Superior colliculus	1.15 × 0.07	1.10 × 0.16	0.82 × 0.10
Inferior olive		0.75 × 0.03	
Reticular formation	0.59 × 0.05	0.65 × 0.03	0.49 × 0.06
	Cerebellum and medulla		
Cerebellum			
Nuclei	0.79 × 0.05	0.84 × 0.03	0.56 × 0.08
Cortex	0.69 × 0.04	0.83 × 0.03	0.57 × 0.05
White matter	0.24 × 0.01	0.24 × 0.01	0.29 × 0.06
Medulla			
Vestibular nuclei	0.91 × 0.04	0.92 × 0.03	0.84 × 0.10
Cochlear nuclei	0.87 × 0.07	0.95 × 0.11	0.99 × 0.14
Pyramid	0.26 × 0.02	0.22 × 0.02	0.28 × 0.03

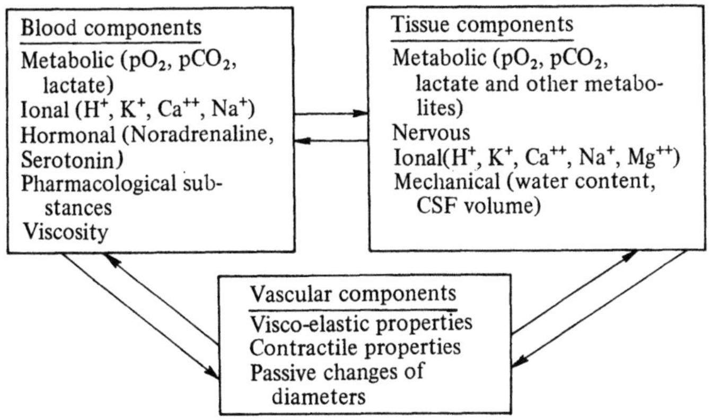

Fig. 2. The graph shows interactions of various blood-, tissue- and vascular components which take part in the regulation of cerebral vascular resistance

Measurements made by LANDAU et al. (1955), SOKOLOFF (1961), FIESCHI et al. (1965, 1966a, 1968c), REIVICH et al. (1969a) revealed considerable differences in the rate of blood flow in different cerebral regions. Such differences exist not only between the gray and the white matter but also within the various parts of the gray matter (see Table 1 and also: FIESCHI, 1967, 1968c; FIESCHI et al., 1968a; HEISS et al., 1969, 1971; SVEINSDOTTIR et al., 1969, 1971/72; WILKINSON et al., 1969; IWABUCHI et al., 1971; OLESEN, 1971; MCHENRY et al., 1971; BARKER, 1971/72; SOKOLOFF et al., 1971/72; BROWN and DONALDSON, 1971/72; RISBERG and INGVAR, 1971/72; INGVAR and FRANZEN, 1973; SVEINSDOTTIR and LASSEN, 1973).

The knowledge of local changes is especially meaningful for the most commonly occurring form of human cerebral vascular diseases, vascular occlusion. An analysis of metabolites in the arterial and cerebral venous blood yields an unsatisfactory picture of what is happening in single tissue sections. The blood appearing in the jugular venous bulb or in large cerebral veins is mixed blood from various tissue regions. If one part of the tissue is undersupplied, the metabolites of this area will appear more slowly and in smaller quantities in the venous blood, thus increasing the discrepancy between the true tissue conditions and the measured values in the blood. There are indeed reciprocal effects between blood and tissue components, as represented in Fig. 2, but the delay in obtaining equilibria prevents conclusions being made from blood analysis about tissue conditions, at least in local blood flow disturbances.

Experiments in animals therefore consist mainly of such pathophysiological analyses, which for obvious reasons cannot be carried out in humans. In man it is not possible to excise tissue samples of the brain tissue for experimental, diagnostic or therapeutic purposes without a hazardous operation, possibly causing considerable damage. This is different if one needs e.g. a muscle tissue sample. Because of all these difficulties, one is more dependent on animal experiments in the elucidation of pathogenetic, pathophysiological and therapeutic mechanisms in disorders of the cerebral circulation than in the case of other organs. It must, however, be stated that there are differences between the conditions in an animal brain and those in a human brain; so all models can be applied to clinical questions only with reservation. Thus no one has yet managed to produce analogous models of cerebral vascular sclerosis in sufficient quantities in small experimental animals. Only in aging pigs does one find sclerosis of cerebral vessels which is similar to that in humans (LUGINBÜHL, 1966; RAFCLIFFE et al., 1970; INFANGER and LUGINBÜHL, 1972). However, for pathophysiological experiments blood flow measurements offer considerable difficulties in these old and mostly fat animals. When using animals one also has to consider the fact that the potentials between blood and cerebral spinal fluid (CSF)-space may be vary from species to species and that the concentrations of substances (e.g. ions) in human CSF are not directly comparable to those from all animals. It should be added that there are differences between the blood supplies in animals and in the human brain and that a large number of animals have an anatomically different vascular network.

B. Acute Experimental Occlusion

The effect of an occlusion of a single brain vessel in humans is extraordinarily variable. In a number of cases an intracerebral occlusion of a vessel causes no disturbance of the total brain function whatsoever, whereas in other cases severe damage of functions and structures result. After occlusion of one carotid artery the disturbance in some animals is transient and of no significance for cerebral function whereas in other cases the occlusion causes an infarction which affects the whole hemisphere. This fact was recognized very early by WILLIS (1664), and thus the function of the arterial anastomotic connections at the basis of the brain could be deduced. Blood flow measurements showing the functions of the cerebral vascular anastomoses have been conducted for more than 20 years (SHENKIN et al., 1951; RICHTER, 1953; DENNY-BROWN and MEYER, 1957; MEYER and DENNY-BROWN, 1957; SYMON, 1960; FIELDS et al., 1965; BETZ, 1969a; SYMON and ROSS-RUSSELL, 1971). All these experiments show evidence of the great variability of the collateral supply to single brain regions.

It has been demonstrated that, during continuous registration of local blood flow of cortical regions of both hemispheres in cats and dogs, a sudden occlusion of a carotid artery leads to a rapid and steep reduction of blood flow in both hemispheres. The initially strong decrease in local cortical blood flow, however, does not remain low but flow increases again towards the initial value. This second rise in local CBF shows considerable individual variation. The cortical flow in the contralateral hemisphere rises in sometimes above the level prior to the occlusion, whereas CBF in the ipsilateral hemisphere sometimes returns to the initial level (in about 30% of cats with one carotid artery occluded) and in other cases remains more or less below the value before ligation of the artery (BETZ and SCHMAHL, 1966). After occlusion of a cerebral vessel there are two factors which mainly determine the fate of the tissue:

1. Number and volumes of preformed collateral network;
2. a time factor which is efficient for the development of collateral channels after the occlusion or narrowing of vessels and which causes a gradual re-establishment of a sufficient blood supply.

This gradual vascular dilatation could be one of the reasons for the smaller number of severe apoplectic insults when the vascular occlusion develops slowly as compared with the severe damage after sudden occlusions or narrowing in normal vessels.

In 1960 BUNCE ligated one or two common carotid arteries and/or one or both vertebral arteries in dogs and found that all animals survived longer than

3 months. In the animals in which he interrupted the carotid and vertebral circulation, the intelligence and alertness was somewhat impaired; the physical condition was poor, with marked emaciation, loss of hair and edema of the extremities. The groups of animals in which either the common carotids were occluded or the vertebral arteries were interrupted or in which two carotid arteries and one vertebral artery were occluded appeared normal 4 months after the operation. This led to the conclusion that in dogs permanent interruption of the vertebral and the carotid arteries is not incompatible with life and that collateral circulation was sufficient to sustain life for the observation period of 4 months. Corresponding results were obtained by ANTHONY et al. (1963). SYMON and ROSS-RUSSELL (1971) conducted similar experiments in baboons. In subsequent operations with several weeks' intervals between each operation they dissected the vessels and repeatedly recorded the ophthalmic artery-pressure. Immediately after the operation the ophthalmic artery-pressure was significantly lower than some weeks later, indicating a developing collateral supply of the vascular bed of the brain tissue. Some months after ligation of all neck vessels pressure in the ophthalmic artery had increased to 50% of the normal pressure. Measurements of the middle cerebral arterial blood pressure gave values between 24 and 42% of the mean systemic arterial blood pressure.

In rabbits LOWE (1962) observed the development of the collateral circulation by means of serial retinal artery pressure readings and by means of resin casts of cerebral vessels. As in dogs or baboons neither carotid nor vertebral ligations produced any permanent ischemia in their area of supply. In 25 animals in which combined vertebral and carotid occlusions were performed in the course of 24 weeks, a marked lowering of the arterial pressure in the head was obtained. Seven of 25 animals survived. In the experiments of LOWE (1962) no animal developed hypertension until the carotid sinuses were subsequently denervated.

The important role of systemic arterial blood pressure was also pointed out by NOELL (1944), THOMPSON and SMITH (1951) and KONG et al. (1967); see also section E.

With measurements of the local oxygen pressure made by means of tiny platinum wire electrodes, the oxygen pressure on the surface of the brain hemispheres during occlusion of one middle cerebral artery decreased rapidly to low values in the region supplied by the occluded vessel. The local oxygen pressure values were not uniformly low but showed relatively high O_2 pressure spots in an O_2 pressure field in which the distribution of the oxygen pressures even shifted towards lower oxygen pressure values (Fig. 3). This indicates that from the surrounding collateral vessels some channels with high oxygen-containing blood entered the low-perfused area and supplied some districts with oxygen (NEUMANN et al., 1970).

In numerous experiments it has been demonstrated (FIESCHI, 1966; FIESCHI et al., 1968a, b) that not only are the oxygen pressures heterogenous in an infarcted region but also that the local blood flow is very inhomogeneous in such areas;—at least within the first few minutes after the occlusion. In monkeys as a rule a persisting infarction was seen after an occlusion time of more than 15 min duration if the animals were not pretreated with high doses of heparin (SMITH et al., 1969). In heparinized animals with ischemia the chances of improvement of circulation are good.

The development and sufficient functioning of collateral vessels are not only seen after occlusion of the carotid or vertebral arteries. Immediately after occlusion of the middle cerebral artery in cats (SUNDT and WALTZ, 1966), a strong decrease of blood flow in the area which is supplied by this vessel can be seen.

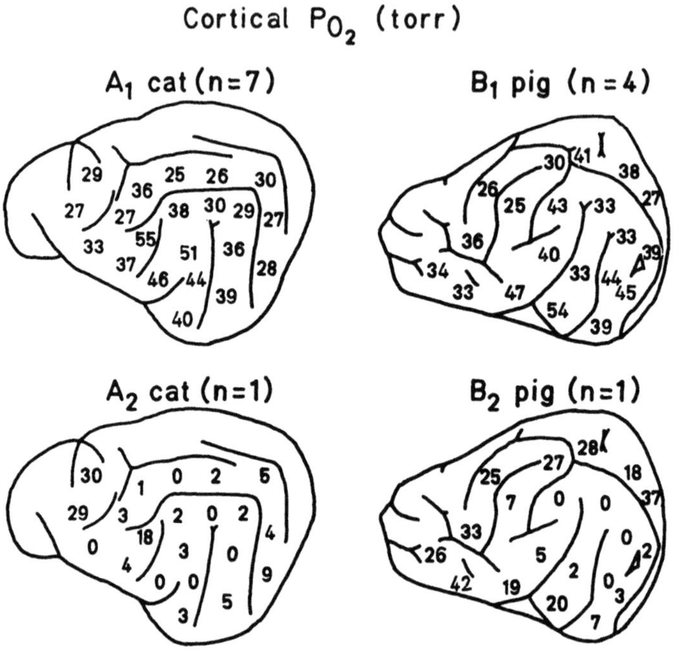

Fig. 3. Cartographical distribution of oxygen pressure on the cortical surface. A_1: mean values in 7 cats before ligating the middle cerebral artery (m.c.a.). A_2: typical P_{O_2} distribution in a single cat after ligature of the m.c.a. B_1: mean values in 4 pigs before occlusion of the m.c.a. B_2:P_{O_2} distribution in a single pig brain after occlusion. The animals were anesthetized with 25 mg/kg pentobarbital. Note the spots with high P_{O_2} values within the surrounding low oxygen pressure values (From Neumann et al., 1970)

Just as with the effects in carotid occlusion, local blood flow tends to reincrease to a certain extent. However, the initial value is very seldom obtained. The collateral vessels are developed here to a lesser degree than in the circle of Willis.

If the ligation of a cerebral vessel is released after a brief occlusion a reactive hyperemia occurs. Besides a strong increase in blood flow a significant increase above normal values in the oxygen pressure of the venous blood drained from the disturbed tissue appears in the phase of reactive hyperemia (Feindel, 1968; Feindel et al., 1966, 1967, 1968; Høedt-Rasmussen et al., 1967; Yamamoto et al., 1970; Blair et al., 1970).

After a brief occlusion, the reactive hyperemia in the affected tissue returns to normal blood flow values within some minutes. The effects of long-lasting occlusions are similar to the reactions in man after removal of intravascular thrombi or in the vicinity of areas receiving low supplies. In such cases reactive hyperemic regions have been observed for some days after the apoplexia (Paulson, 1968, 1969, 1970; Paulson et al., 1970; Lassen, 1973). The focal abnormalities consisted of hyperemic foci, ischemic foci and focal vasoparalysis. The autoregulation of the vessels (see p. 192) ceases for a considerable time within the affected region (Lassen and Paulson, 1969; Symon et al., 1972) or is at least severely disturbed (Rees et al., 1970; Fein, 1973; Sengupta et al., 1973). Because of the development of techniques which enable recording of the regional circulation in man (e.g. the epicerebral angiography by fluorescin,

FEINDEL et al., 1967, 1968), the animal experiment has lost its significance with regard to the relation between cerebral vascular occlusion and regional flow pattern. The experiment, however, is still of great importance for the problems of local metabolism, intracerebral flow distribution or problems of investigating new substances for the therapy of blood flow disturbances. Measurements of regional blood flow during occlusive diseases already exist in man in such a huge quantity that here only recently published symposia, reviews and textbooks will be mentioned (McDOWALL, 1969; BROCK et al., 1969; ROSS-RUSSELL, 1971; FIESCHI, 1972; GÄNSHIRT, 1972; PURVES, 1972).

Long-term observations of animals in which cerebral vessels were occluded showed that under certain circumstances the animals survived despite occlusion of both carotid and both vertebral arteries, as described previously.

C. Dysregulation of the Intracerebral Blood Distribution

The pattern of the flow distribution after an occlusion of a brain vessel does not remain constant with time. The change in blood flow distribution during the course of the time after the occlusion is dependent on a number of factors which in turn are not only dependent on the reactions in the disturbed region. In the preceding chapter the effects of systemic blood pressure on the low residual flow through the disturbed region were mentioned. A decrease in the perfusion pressure causes a further fall in blood flow through the affected region so that flow may reach a critical low value here whereas the normal regions compensate for the fall in blood pressure by dilating their arteries. Thus a disturbance of blood flow distribution aggravates the effect of vascular occlusion. In 1961 a reversed flow through the vertebral arteries was observed during increased activity of the arm muscles in cases in which the brain vessels were narrowed. This reversed flow appeared when the vascular resistance of the arm vessels decreased to an extreme degree whereas the cerebral vessels did not (REIVICH et al., 1961). This phenomenon was designated "subclavian steal syndrome" (FISCHER, 1962), and has been found in the carotid arteries also. Since then it has often been described (JANEWAY et al., 1964; SAMMARTINO and TOOLE, 1964; HANDA et al., 1965; TOOLE, 1965; RAMIREZ-BOETTNER, 1966; HARPER et al., 1967; KATO et al., 1969; BARNETT et al., 1970). Ligature of the brachiocephalic trunk in dogs and monkeys regularly causes a reversal of the blood flow in the right vertebral artery whereas it is maintained in the carotid in its normal direction. Blood flow in the contralateral arteries is always increased (DORNDORF and GÄNSHIRT, 1972). These experiments indicate that dilatation of one vascular region causes in such experimental conditions deterioration of the already low-supplied brain tissue.

In principle similar changes in the blood flow distribution can also be seen within the brain during an intracerebral vascular occlusion. Such changes have been demonstrated when flow was measured within the low-supplied region and in its vicinity. These dysregulations of blood flow distribution are of essential significance during the application of vascular dilators which reduce the cerebral vascular resistance. In 1966 it was shown (BETZ and SCHMAHL, 1966) that during the occlusion of one carotid artery in cats the injection of papaverine caused variations in the flow pattern through the affected and unaffected hemispheres. In some of the experiments the dilatory stimulus caused a decrease of the cortical flow in the affected side whereas CBF in the normal hemisphere increased. In other cases no reaction at all could be seen in the low-supplied hemisphere when

Before ligature of R_2	After ligature of R_2			
		Reactions of the vascular regions after injection of a dilator		
Initial value ($I=\frac{P}{R}$)	I (total) remains constant	1st possibility	2nd possibility	3rd possibility
Total flow $10=\frac{100}{10}$	$10=\frac{100}{10}$	$12=\frac{96}{8}$	$12=\frac{96}{8}$	$12=\frac{96}{8}$
Partial flow R_1 $5=\frac{100}{20}$	$5=\frac{100}{20}$	$7.4=\frac{96}{13}$	$6.9=\frac{96}{14.1}$	$6.9=\frac{96}{14.1}$
Partial flow R_2 $5=\frac{100}{20}$	$5=\frac{50}{10}$	$4.6=\frac{46}{10}$	$5.1=\frac{46}{9}$	$5.1=\frac{51}{10}$
		P is lowered by 4%; maximal decrease of resistance in R_2; collateral vessel maximally dilated	P is lowered by 4%; the resistance in R_2 is lowered by additional dilatation	P is lowered by 4%; maximal decrease of resistance in R_2; the resistance of the collateral vessel was lowered by dilatation

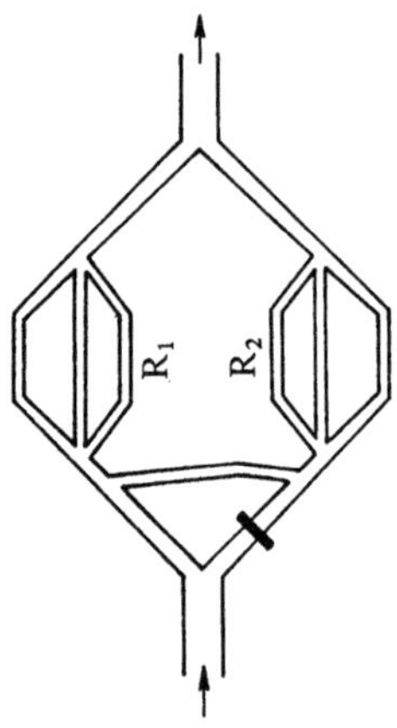

Fig. 4. Schematic diagram of two equal vascular regions, connected by a collateral vessel. In the first column the situation before ligature is demonstrated. The total flow is defined by the ratio: blood pressure (P) and resistance (R). Total flow is the sum of the flow through the resistances R_1 and R_2 [5 (ml)/unit of time]. 2nd column: After ligature. It is assumed that total flow remains as high as before ligature in both resistances (R_1 and R_2). This is possible if the vascular resistance decreases proportionally to the lowered blood pressure. In columns 3, 4 and 5 examples of the reactions of blood pressure and vascular resistance after intravenous application of a vascular dilator are given. The examples show in column 3 a "steal phenomenon" in which flow in the normal resistance (R_1) increases while in R_2, flow is lowered In columns 4 and 5 it is shown by which mechanisms flow may increase within the low supplied R_2

flow increased in the normal hemisphere, and in about 1/3 of the experiments flow increased in the affected side as well as in the unaffected side. On analyzing these various types of flow pattern, it became obvious that KIRCHHOFF's rules of current distribution in a network of resistances are the basis of this mechanism. Fig. 4 contains a model of the effects of a dilatory stimulus in two equivalent vascular beds (or current circuits) connected by a collateral connection. The experimentally obtained evidence of the existence of blood flow distributions which disfavor the low-supplied area has been confirmed not only in the brain but also in other organs (within the myocardium by measurements of the local blood flow in various myocardial regions during the occlusion of a coronary vessel) (BETZ et al., 1961, 1964). Meanwhile it has also been demonstrated that dysregulations which disfavor poorly supplied cerebral regions exist also in patients with local cerebral vascular diseases. By analogy with the subclavian steal phenomenon they have been designated as local steal phenomenon (LASSEN and PALVÖLGYI, 1968; SYMON, 1968, 1969; PAULSON, 1968; NEUMANN et al., 1970).

As mentioned previously, the low blood flow in certain regions of the brain immediately after occlusion can be transiently increased in some of the experiments by the application of dilating agents (HØEDT-RASMUSSEN, 1969). This increase can be seen despite the fact that there is no increase in systemic arterial blood pressure. In a few cases blood flow has been observed to increase for a short time even somewhat above the initial value (BETZ and SCHMAHL, 1966). This indicates that the vascular reactions of the animal organism in which all cerebral vessels except the ligated vessel and those in the region supplied by the ligated vessel are normal, do not involve all reserves for maintaining blood flow as high as possible in the disturbed region. On the other hand it has been demonstrated that in some of the animals the same dosage of dilating drugs decreased local flow in the low-supplied area and increased flow in the normal tissue. These differences in responsiveness of local blood flow or local oxygen pressure (HALSEY, 1970) after the injection of cerebral vasodilators are dependent on:

1. The change in the ratio: blood pressure/CVR in the badly supplied area (if the vessels within this region are already maximally dilated, a dilating agent cannot cause additional dilation).

2. The responses of the vessels in the vicinity of the low-perfused area.

It is assumed that the responses of the vessels in the border zone of the low-supplied area are mediated by chemical stimuli e.g. metabolites (FIESCHI, 1967, 1968; LASSEN, 1968; LASSEN and INGVAR, 1968; PAULSON, 1970; NEUMANN et al., 1970 and others). Because of the irritation of the perifocal area the vessels in this zone are often dilated (FIESCHI et al., 1968a, b). In the vicinity of this perifocal area many vessels are still able to dilate after the application of vasoactive dilating agents. These vessels react in the normal manner because dilating vasoactive agents released from the tissue of the low-supplied area do not reach the vascular smooth muscle cells by diffusion. Consequently those arteries or arterioles in the vicinity of the perifocal area remain in a normal metabolic state, and dilating agents are able to increase blood flow even if the arterial blood pressure decreases. The extent to which this "reserve" is used in favor of the low-supplied region is dependent on the effective blood pressure gradient from the border zone into the low-supplied region, on the ability of additional dilation of the vessels within the perifocal and within the low-supplied area, on the number and diameters of the collateral vessels and on the extravascular fluid content. An increase in the latter causes edema which in turn causes a rise in local vascular resistance (see section J).

The interindividual variations of the responses of local blood flow and local oxygen pressure correspond to those which were observed during angiography in man after occlusion (Lit. see HERRMANN, 1964). The individual variations render more difficult the decision of whether the application of vasodilating agents in the therapy of local disturbances of blood flow is useful or not. There exist controversial opinions about the application of vasodilating agents for the therapy of local blood flow disturbances caused by partial or total vascular occlusion. This controversy has developed in view of the danger of the appearance of a steal phenomenon, which must be prevented at all costs (Gottstein, 1969, 1973; Betz, 1972a; Carpi, 1972).

Comparing the results of animal experiments with the measurements in patients, it must be pointed out that the conditions in patients with arteriosclerotic vessels are different from those in animals with nearly normal vessels. From the available measurements in patients it can be seen that a disfavoring of the already undersupplied area occurs more frequently in patients than in experimental animals (Fieschi, 1967; Lassen and Palvölgyi, 1968; Symon, 1968; Wüllenweber, 1968). Additionally one has to consider that dilatation of the vessels in the vicinity of an infarcted area causes an increase of the effective filtration pressure in those vessels in which the effective blood pressure increases. If osmotically active substances have already accumulated in the extravascular space, the possibility of an increase of fluid content in the extravascular space can not be excluded when the blood flow is not able to wash out the osmotically active agents. The energetics and the fluid content of the brain will be considered in Chapters D and J.

D. Effect of Decreased CBF on Cerebral Tissue Energetics

The most dramatic effects of a decrease in CBF are seen when the effective arterial blood pressure suddenly falls to zero. This conditions is obtained in animal experiments either by blocking all vessels perfusing the brain (Gänshirt et al., 1952a, b; Schneider, 1958; Wolin et al., 1971) or by cardiac arrest. Within a few seconds after such an event, the energetic potential of the brain tissue diminishes steeply (Schmahl et al., 1965; Müller et al., 1970; Siesjö and Nilsson, 1971). Fig. 5 demonstrates an experiment from which it can be seen that the creatine phosphate (Cr$\sim$P) of the cortical tissue sinks within 2 min to nearly zero. There is also an initial, steep decrease of adenosine triphosphate (ATP). After about 1 min, however, the decrease slows down when about 30% of its initial value is reached. Within the following 2–3 min the decrease is distinctly delayed. During the observed time in Fig. 5 considerable amounts of ATP remain unconsumed despite the metabolic activity of the tissue. The latter can be determined from the continuing production of lactate. The amount of lactate production in this phase in the anesthetized animals is about 4 μmol/min·g brain tissue (Thorn and Heitman, 1954; Schmahl et al., 1965; Döring and Olbrisch, 1970). The delayed decrease of ATP has already been reported by Pfleiderer et al. (1955), Scholl et al. (1957) and Minard and Davis (1962). Lowry and co-workers (1964), Lowry and Passoneau, (1964) explain the delay in the decrease of ATP by a shift of the creatine kinase equilibrium $Cr\sim P + ADP = Cr + ATP$ in favor of ATP as a consequence of the pH decrease during ischemia. The assumption of an equilibrium between Cr$\sim$P-, Cr-, ATP- and ADP-contents, which is based on the pH hypothesis, is obviously not conclusive in the experiments of Schmahl et al. (1965). The disappearance of the Cr$\sim$P after 2 min of ischemia during continuing glycolysis and turnover of energy-rich phosphate in the phase of the delayed ATP decrease at a level of about 30% of the initial level, contradicts the pH hypothesis. It is not yet clear why the ATP contents are not diminished at a greater rate.

The effects of longer-lasting complete ischemia on the energy-rich substrates of the brain tissue have been studied also by Hossmann and Lechtape-Grüter

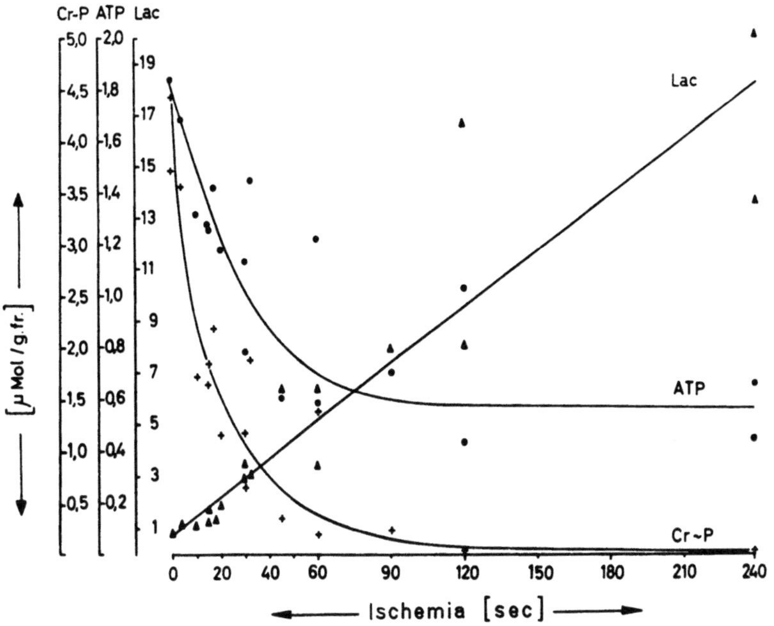

Fig. 5. Effect of complete ischemia on cerebral cortical tissue Cr∼P, ATP and lactate. The values are given in μmol/g tissue (fresh weight). Values were obtained from 28 cats anesthetized with 25 mg/kg pentobarbital (From Schmahl et al., 1965)

(1971/72) and Kobayashi et al. (1973). They noted that ATP finally disappeared after long-term ischemia of more than 5 min (see also Ljunggreen and Siesjö, 1973). After occlusion of a single cerebral vessel the disturbances of cerebral energetics in the area supplied by this vessel are as variable as the collateral supply. Occlusion of a carotid artery in cats caused a significant increase of the lactate content and of the Red/Ox-ratio (lactate/pyruvate) in the ipsilateral hemisphere as compared with the undisturbed contralateral hemisphere (Schmahl et al., 1971/72). The accumulation of lactate is accompanied by a decrease in the local pH. As described in section I, the dilatory stimulus of the resistance vessels is often seen as a consequence of the resulting local acidosis. Fig. 6 demonstrates the effect of an occlusion of the right carotid artery on the local cortical blood flow, which was continuously recorded on the cortical surface of both hemispheres (measuring site: suprasylvian gyrus), on the local cortical oxygen-pressure, on the pH on the cortical surface of the suprasylvian gyrus and on the arterial blood pressure. The decrease in blood flow and in oxygen pressure is initially more pronounced. After initial decrease they return to a value slightly lower than that before ligation. Cortical pH in this region remains low. The injection of papaverine causes a local "steal phenomenon" (see section C). Neither the cytoplasma $NADH/NAD^+$-ratio nor the energy-charge potential of the adenine nucleotide pool (ATP) + 0.5 (ADP) / (ATP) + (ADP) + (AMP) was significantly changed as compared to the controls in these experiments. It was, however, demonstrated (Eklof and Siesjö, 1971) that the effective blood pressure was essential for the changes of Cr∼P, ATP, ADP, AMP and the NADH/NAD^+-ratio of the tissue. If, during carotid artery ligation, the arterial blood pressure was diminished below a mean arterial blood pressure of 100 mmHg,

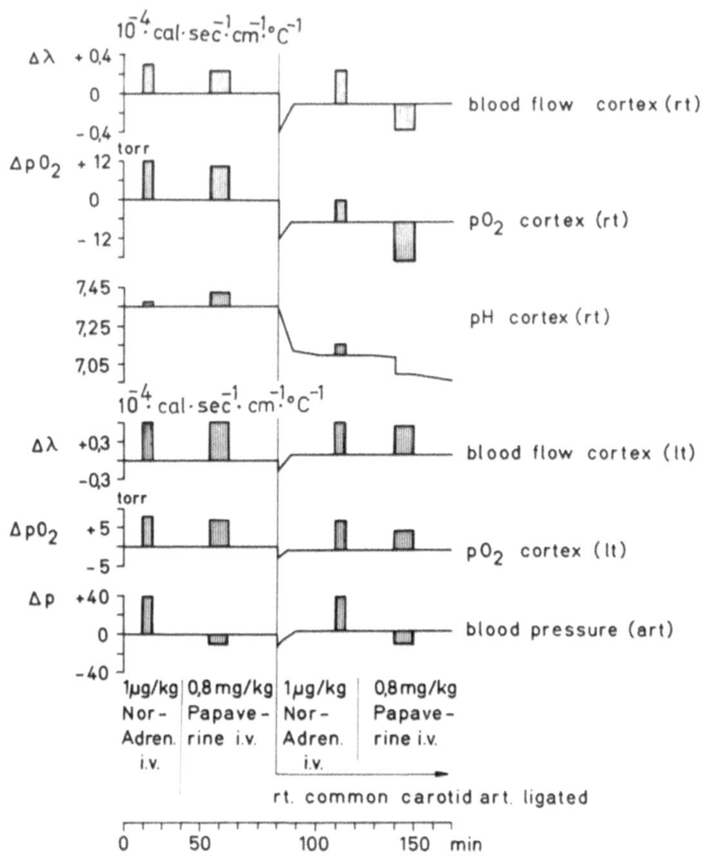

Fig. 6. Occlusion of the right (rt.) common carotid artery in a cat. Cortical blood flow was recorded on both hemispheres by means of heat clearance discs. Cortical oxygen pressure was continuously measured with multiwire platinum electrodes on both hemispheres. The surface-pH on the rt. hemisphere was recorded by a glass electrode the reference of which was placed a very short distance from the sensitive membrane. The measuring site was the suprasylvian gyrus of both hemispheres. Immediately after occlusion local CBF decreased on both hemispheres. It remained lower on the rt. side. Injections of noradrenaline and papaverine caused increases of flow and P_{O_2} prior to the occlusion. During occlusion papaverine led to a decrease of flow and P_{O_2} on the rt. cortex whereas in the lt. cortex flow and P_{O_2} increased. The values are all given as relative changes. The initial values are defined as zero

the substrates showed deviations from normal values in these experiments. Fujishima (1971), however, found a constant oxygen uptake and a constant blood supply in dogs if the arterial blood pressure was not lowered below 50 mmHg. Below this value the lactate concentration and the ratio lactate/pyruvate increased and the CSF-pH decreased. The results clearly indicate not only that the consequences of vascular occlusion for the oxygen- and energy supply of the tissue are dependent on the resulting variation of the blood flow distribution, but also that the arterial blood pressure and the ability for collateral dilatation determine the fate of the tissue.

In dogs with occlusion of a single cerebral vessel, Held et al. (1973) still found in the infarcted area 24 h after the occlusion considerable amounts of

Cr$\sim$P and ATP. Within the perifocal zone a reduction of energy-rich substrate was measured. The glucose metabolism was disturbed not only in the infarcted area but also in tissue samples taken from the non-infarcted tissue of the same hemisphere and the gray and white matter of the contralateral hemisphere. The reduction of glucose was accompanied by an accumulation of lactate. The water content of the tissue rose in the infarcted and in the non-infarcted areas. MICHENFELDER and SUNDT (1971) measured the cerebral ATP and lactate concentrations in monkeys after occlusion of the middle cerebral artery. Within 3 hours after the ligature ATP concentration fell to about 30% of that of the controls, and lactate reached a steady state at a concentration about 8-fold greater than that of normal tissue after an initial steep increase. The effects were found to be potentially reversible, and the authors concluded from their experiments that the anoxic damage of the brain tissue is reversible if the ATP concentration remains above 25% of the normal value. Since the ATP concentration decreases slowly in the ischemic region, there exists a time-span after the occlusion of a great cerebral vessel which can be used for therapy in order to restitute normal flow conditions. This assumption is supported by HOSSMANN and LECHTAPE-GRÜTER (1971/72), who found a partial restitution of EEG functions after 1 h of complete ischemia of the brain. These findings do not agree with those of BRIERLEY et al. (1973). In their experiments they found that moderate hypoxemia with an additional slight decrease in blood supply of no more than 30 min duration leads to irreversible neuronal alterations, and they concluded that the brain cannot tolerate prolonged and total ischemia for more than a few minutes without sustaining irreversible injury (see also GÄNSHIRT et al., 1952b; SCHNEIDER, 1953, 1958, 1957; HIRSCH, 1970; HIRSCH et al., 1955, 1957a, b, 1961, 1970, 1973/74; OBERDÖRSTER et al., 1969). GEHA et al. (1971) studied the cerebral energy metabolism by measuring the lactate and pyruvate concentrations, the pH in the CSF and the arterial blood during occlusion of the carotid and vertebral arteries. They found no significant changes in the clinical behavior of the animals after occlusion of the cervical or the vertebral arteries. Simultaneous occlusion of the cephalic and brachial arteries, however, caused hypoxic changes in the brain, increases in lactate and an irreversible loss of the cerebral functions. LJUNGGREEN and SIESJÖ (1973) induced complete cerebral ischemia in rats by infusing artificial CSF into the cisterna magna. The CSF-pressure was momentarily raised to such a degree that the intracerebral pressure exceeded the arterial blood pressure. The CBF then was zero. The authors found complete energy depletion after 5 min and extended the ischemic period to 15 min. After this long period the energy state of the tissue was completely restituted after re-perfusion, as evaluated from the energy-charge potential of the adenine nucleotide pool. The glutamate concentration, however, remained low in the postischemic phase even when the brains were re-perfused for three hours. The prolonged decrease of glutamate during complete ischemia of 30 to 60 min duration has also been seen by SCHINDLER et al. (unpubl.). There is evidence that the reappearance of tissue glutamate is related to the reappearance of the EEG after the reperfusion of the cerebral vascular system.

GREGERSEN (1962) mentioned in a discussion that the blood within the brain vessels could be one of the reasons causing irreversibility of the resulting brain damage. He reported findings in which it was shown that it was possible to obtain spontaneous respiration and reflexes after 30–40 min of cardiac arrest when, prior to the stopping of blood circulation, the blood was rinsed out of the brain by perfusion of the brain vessels with saline solution.

E. Blood Pressure and Disturbance of the Cerebral Vascular Autoregulation

As described in section B, a sudden fall in the arterial blood pressure causes a decrease in CBF. The decreased flow, however, does not remain at this low level, but is compensated for by the so-called autoregulatory dilatation of the vessels. FOG (1937, 1938, 1939) noticed that pial vessels dilated when the blood pressure was momentarily decreased and that the dilatation of the pial vessels appeared 1–2 min after the decrease of arterial blood pressure. In continuously performed recording of CBF, BETZ (1968a) and KANZOW (1969), and in intermittent recordings RAPELA and GREEN (1964) and ECKSTRÖM-JODAL et al. (1970) found time constants for the appearance of autoregulatory responses of between 30 sec and 2 min. HIRSCH and KÖRNER (1964) observed somewhat longer times. The reincrease of cerebral venous oxygen saturation after blood pressure decrease has similar time constants. The cerebral autoregulation is usually represented as a diagram in which arterial blood pressure and blood flow are related to each other. Its significance has been extensively discussed by LASSEN (1959). In normal man or animals relatively constant blood flow is seen between a mean arterial blood pressure of 70 mmHg and an upper range of 140–170 mmHg. Decreasing systemic arterial pressure to below 70 mmHg usually causes a pressure-passive decrease in CBF. Rapid increase above a critical value leads to an increase of flow. This value is not constant but is dependent on local metabolic conditions. In both cases (strong decrease or increase of pressure) the autoregulatory response is not able to maintain CBF in a normal range. The transitional pressure value at which autoregulation becomes ineffective is the "critical value of autoregulation". The critical threshold is dependent on various parameters:

In individuals with long-lasting increases of arterial blood pressure, the lower threshold for effective autoregulation is elevated to mean arterial blood pressures which can reach 100 mmHg. The upper threshold, on the other hand, can be lowered by the application of dilating agents, e.g. by CO_2-inhalation. It is possible in animal experiments to abolish autoregulation completely. During and shortly after severe hypoxia the CBF is blood pressure-passive over the whole range of pressure values (RAPELA and GREEN, 1964; INGVAR, 1967, 1968, 1969; FREEMAN and INGVAR, 1968a, b; HÄGGENDAL, 1968; LASSEN and PAULSON, 1969). In dogs RAPELA and GREEN (1964) saw after the operation trauma a blood pressure-passive increase of CBF. Loss of autoregulation after cerebral trauma was reported by REIVICH et al. (1969b). Intensive nervous stimuli can also shift the threshold for autoregulation. Fig. 7 shows typical examples of the pressure/flow relations in different cerebral regions in cats. LÜBBERS (1972) has reviewed the mechanisms which contribute to the appearance of cerebral vascular autoregulation. There are three hypotheses on which autoregulation is based:

1. The myogenic hypothesis. Despite elimination of nervous connections the tonus of the walls of the cerebral arteries rises during increasing blood pressure.

2. The metabolic hypothesis. The short-lasting initial increase of blood flow directly after the rise of blood pressure washes out a vasodilating effector-substance so that a constriction results (e.g. a metabolite which normally acts as a dilator); decrease in pressure, on the other hand, would then produce or accumulate the dilator.

3. The tissue-pressure hypothesis. According to this hypothesis, the perivascular pressure increases when blood flow rises. Therefore, in organs with a rigid capsule the vascular resistance increases.

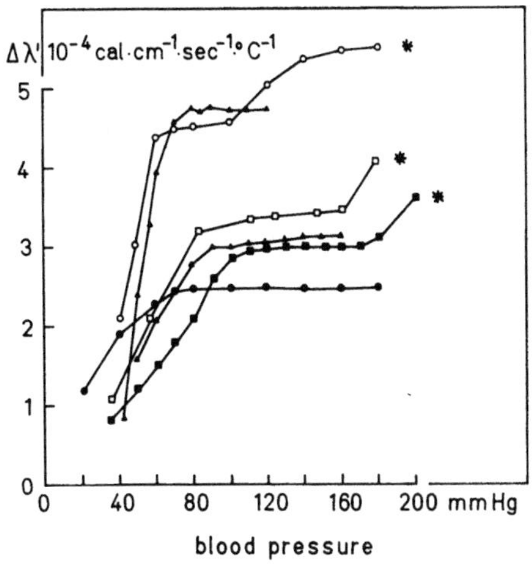

Fig. 7. Local cerebral blood flow ($\Delta \lambda'$) recorded by means of heated thermocouples in the thalamus or hypothalamus of the brain in 6 cats during gradual increase or decrease of blood pressure. Increases were produced by clamping the aorta and in some cases additional infusion of angiotensin. Decreases of flow were produced by bleeding. *indicate experiments in which the upper limit of autoregulation was exceeded. Flow values are given in terms of relative changes of heat clearance (apparent heat conductivity) λ'[cal · cm^{-1} · °C^{-1} · sec^{-1}]. The heat conductivity of the dead brain was defined as initial value (zero)

Autoregulation by myogenic control has the following mechanism (LÜBBERS, 1972): Increase in the intravascular pressure distends the smooth muscle cells of the vascular walls. Some of these cells depolarize and conduct the stimulus along the smooth muscle cells of the vessel. Such pacemaker cells, which cause changes in the membrane potentials of the mooth muscle cells, also reach the upstream structures of the arterial walls. According to HELD et al. (1969) the pulsatory distension of the vascular wall plays an essential role in this type of autoregulation. During pulsating perfusion the autoregulation is more pronounced than during non-pulsating perfusion. The transformation of the mechanical stimulus into the variation of the membrane potential of the cerebral smooth muscle cells has not yet been investigated. The myogenic theory, which was established by BAYLISS (1902), was again taken up by FOLKOW (1949). He showed that after diminution of neural factors the caliber of small vessels varied inversely to the intravascular pressure (GASKELL and BURTON, 1953; JOHANSSON and BOHR, 1966). This finding, however, would mean that in an intact vascular system, the resulting constriction after an increase of blood pressure would cause a further increase in the resistance of the vessels and thus in systemic blood pressure in the form of a positive feedback mechanism.

FOLKOW (1964) tried to solve the problem of explanation by introducing the concept of the pulsating tension variations of the vascular walls. Phasic contractions of vascular smooth muscles are seen as analogous to those which accompany the spontaneously generated depolarizations of the intestinal smooth muscles, the frequency of which is proportional to their tension (BÜLBRING, 1962). Whether the properties of intestinal smooth muscles can be transferred to the cerebral vascular smooth muscle and whether the blood pressure/flow relationships assumed by FOLKOW's model are valid remains to be determined. SIEGEL et al. (1971) found in their investigations on K^{42}_{19} and Na^{24}_{11} efflux curves in smooth muscle cells of isolated carotid arteries, that the Na and K exchange occurs rhythmically. They concluded that the ionic basis of slow waves of the membrane potential lies in electrogenic, rhythmically active ion pumps. The frequency of these waves is the same as the frequency of the spontaneously occurring cerebral blood flow oscillations (Betz, 1967). Weiss and Thiemann (1973) developed a model of single vascular units in which they could demonstrate the possibility of synchronization of oscillations in the diameters, thus explaining that myogenic, oscillatory behavior of vessels leads to autoregulatory responses after a stepwise increase of pressure. These mechanisms, however, have not yet been validated for the appearance of disturbances of cerebral vascular autoregulation. The theory of Folkow and the measurements of Held et al. (1969) concerning the relation between autoregulation and pulsating blood flow lead to objections to the myogenic hypothesis. Indeed, the results of investigations made by Rapela and Green (1964) show that the myogenic hypothesis of autoregulation is one of several possible mechanisms. Only considerable variations of the transmural pressure in the arteriolar vascular bed caused corresponding reactions of blood flow.

Continuous measurements of local tissue pH or PCO_2 demonstrate the high speed of variations of metabolites which influence smooth muscle contraction (see section I. 1.). During a sudden increase in blood pressure, blood flow is increased for a short period. Since the PCO_2 of the arterial blood is lower than the tissue PCO_2, the CO_2 is washed out of the walls of the vessels when arterial inflow increases, and thus a more pronounced alkalosis of the vascular walls occurs.

The alkalotic shift of the vascular pH caused by perfusion with blood of a low PCO_2 is a constrictive stimulus similar to a hypocapnia produced by other means. The organism tends to keep the CSF-pH constant and the constancy of the H^+-concentration during increased blood flow can be obtained by the reduction of flow. Therefore this mechanism for adjusting flow also seems to be plausible for cerebral vascular autoregulation. For extensive reviews on this subject see Purves (1972), Betz (1972a, b), Ingvar et al. (1969).

It can be clearly demonstrated that a metabolic feedback control of blood flow occurs during the spontaneous oscillation of local CBF in which the local pH and the local PCO_2 oscillate with the same frequency as flow and in which the PCO_2 acts as the portioning element for the adjustment of the tissue pH (Betz, 1972b).

A disturbance of the autoregulation acts upon the effective filtration pressure in the tissue. This could be demonstrated in animals exposed to repeated periods of inhalation of high CO_2-concentrations which caused pronounced vascular dilatation and an increase in the fluid content in the brain. After a CO_2-inhalation period of 10–15 min, local cortical blood flow decreased below the initial level. The secondary decrease of flow cannot be explained by a secondary increase of CSF pH or decrease of PCO_2, because CO_2 was brought back to the initial level. In some cases, such repeated increases of CO_2 produced brain edema (Betz and Kozak, 1967) with a concomitant decrease of CBF despite normal systemic arterial blood pressure. Reactions in which the upper, critical value of autoregulation is exceeded have also been found in electrical shock experiments. During electrical stimulation of the brain with AC-current applied through the ears of cats for 2–5 sec, arterial blood pressure increased momentarily together with a strong and steep increase of CBF. Blood flow sometimes declined below the initial value 2–3 min after stimulation and CVR increased despite normalization of pH and PCO_2 (experiments have been reported by Brodersen et al., 1973; they have not yet been published). Since such secondary decreases of the CBF can only be recorded if the electrical shock caused a strong increase of arterial blood pressure, it can be assumed that the upper autoregulatory point has been exceeded. Breakthroughs of the upper threshold of the autoregulatory ability of cerebral vessels have recently been described by ECKSTRÖM-JODAL et al. (1970, 1971/72). Measurements of this breakthrough have so far been relatively rare because the extensive increases of blood flow usually last only a very short time and cannot be seen with measuring techniques, which need several minutes for their performance (e.g. the nitrous oxide technique). Secondary to the break-through, a reactive decrease of blood flow below the initial value can be seen, which is caused by the increased tissue pressure (edema).

F. Changes in Cerebral Activity and Cerebral Blood Flow

Desynchronization of the electroencephalogram by physiological stimuli (optical, acoustical or tactile) usually causes moderate increases in cerebral blood flow (INGVAR, 1958, 1969; KANZOW et al., 1961; KANZOW and KRAUSE, 1962; MOLNAR, 1967).

In experiments in cats it was observed that noise caused rapid, strong increases in CBF. Animals which were exposed to daily repeated periods of noise partially adapted to the stimulus if noise was always applied in the same frequency-spectra. CBF increased only minimally when the animals had been exposed for about 4 weeks daily to 1 h of noise (BETZ, 1965b). If, however, in the experiment the stimulus was applied at night, flow increased again for a very long period, even if the cat was already fully acclimatized to the noise during daytime. In man undesirable sound (noise) caused increases in CBF in all subjects after the onset of noise (random noise 100 phon). Headaches and discomfort were observed in all the subjects (MIYAZAKI, 1972). It is therefore concluded that severe and repeated noise may induce abnormalities of cerebral circulation. If the tympanic nervous plexus but not the receptors of one cerebral hemisphere is stimulated in dogs, an obvious increase of blood flow in the internal carotid artery on the stimulated side was observed. On the stimulated side the tonus of the vertebral artery increased, and on the opposite side it decreased. Systemic arterial blood pressure during noise usually decreased (ROMANOV and GAEVYI, 1971). Experiments of BONDY and MORELOS (1971) showed that unilateral visual deprivation in chicks caused a decrease in velocity of circulation within the corresponding optical lobes of the hemispheres. All these experiments demonstrate that there are close connections between CBF and sensory stimuli and that the responses of CBF partially show adaptive behavior. Direct stimulation of the reticular formation in the brain stem also causes an increase in CBF (MOLNAR and SZANTO, 1964; SHALIT et al., 1969; VYSHATINA, 1970; CZOPF and MOLNAR, 1970). MEYER et al. (1969a, b) demonstrated that parallel to the increased CBF the cerebral oxygen uptake rises if the EEG shows a desynchronization. An increase in blood flow of 10% was accompanied by an increase in oxygen consumption of 7.7%. A similar effect could be observed in man if an arousal reaction was elicited by a stimulus causing pain (MEYER et al., 1966; KRUPP, 1966).

Whether the stimuli act via nervous pathways on the vascular smooth muscles or via local changes in tissue metabolism has been the subject of numerous conferences in the last few years (BROCK et al., 1969; ROSS-RUSSELL, 1971; FIESCHI, 1972; LANGFITT et al., 1973). This problem will be more intensively discussed in the following chapter.

Seizures caused by convulsion lead to great variations in CBF. It was originally thought that epileptic seizures were caused by cerebral ischemia (Hill, 1896; Gibbs, 1933a). However, it could be demonstrated that CBF increased during both spontaneous and experimental convulsions (Florey, 1925; Grant et al., 1947), and a local cerebral acidosis appeared combined with a decrease of potassium and a retention of Na^+ in the brain tissue (Jasper and Erickson, 1941; Bovet et al., 1960; Meyer and Gotoh, 1961; Meyer et al., 1961, 1966). Gibbs (1933b) and Gibbs et al. (1934) found in some of their experiments that an increase in CBF preceded the experimental convulsion.

The experimental approach to studying the relation between seizures and CBF was obtained by the use of electrical current and by convulsion-inducing drugs. In electrically induced seizures in cats the increase in CBF was often accompanied by an increase in systemic blood pressure (Brodersen et al., 1973). If the increase in CBF is not sufficient to overcome the oxygen deficit, the arterio-venous difference in oxygen increases, indicating an increased demand for oxygen (Gänshirt et al., 1959).

The increasing oxygen demand could also be seen from measurements of the cortical oxygen pressure by polarographic techniques (Davies and Remond, 1946; Davies et al., 1948). During convulsions elicited by electrical stimulation local oxygen consumption doubled during and shortly after the stimulation and then fell below the initial level. Therefore initially the arterio-venous cerebral O_2 difference increased and then diminished. The venous blood was then seen to redden. Ruf (1951, 1952) used hyperbaric oxygen for respiration and caused prolonged seizures. He assumes that with normal air the seizures are terminated by tissue hypoxia. Since the oxygen demand is very high in seizures hypoxia cannot be overcome by an increased CBF when normal air is respired. As a consequence of hypoxia the tissue "oxygen pressure field" (Lübbers, 1968) is shifted towards lower PO_2 values during seizures (Ingvar et al., 1962). The variations in local tissue PO_2 occur during the electrical shock and normalize rapidly after the end of the convulsions. Wilson et al. (1952) could not observe a sustained change in CBF or in oxygen consumption in 21 patients after an average of 10 electric shock treatments.

In order to elucidate the role of the reticular formation during convulsions Molnar and Szanto (1964), Meyer et al. (1969b), Czopf and Molnar (1970) and Molnar et al. (1970) stimulated parts of the cerebral trunk and found changes in CBF. Meyer et al. (1969b) observed increases in CBF and in cerebral O_2 consumption; Molnar et al. (1970), however, observed a decrease in cortical blood flow. The problem of discrepancies between findings is still to be solved.

During electrically induced seizures the energy-rich phosphates show a rapid decrease in cortical phospho-creatine and in ATP (King et al., 1967, 1970). The lactate concentration rises considerably, which partly explains the effects on CBF. In experiments of Jasper and Erickson (1941) and in our own experiments (unpublished), it could be demonstrated that the cortical extravascular pH decreased, which is in turn a dilatory stimulus for brain arteries and arterioles. The rapid administration of a convulsant inhalant "flurothyl" (hexafluoro-diethyl ether, Indokolon) to mice had corresponding effects on the energy-rich substrates of the brain so that in principle the energy-rich substrates, and the red/ox systems seem to react in the same way as during electrically induced convulsions. Whether barbiturates, which reduce the CBF and the demand of the cerebral cortex for oxygen (Schmidt et al., 1945; Homburger et al., 1946; Himwich et al., 1947a, b; Kety et al., 1948b; Taylor and McCall, 1951; McCall and Taylor, 1952; McIlvain, 1952; Bernsmeier, 1959; Daweke et al.,

1959; SOKOLOFF, 1959; GOTTSTEIN et al., 1961; PIERCE et al., 1962; NOVACK et al., 1963; LÜBBERS et al., 1964; ROSOMOFF, 1965; SCHMAHL et al., 1965; FIESCHI, 1967; DÖRING and OLBRISCH, 1970) have convulsion-inhibitory effects because of their action on the oxygen consumption of the tissue is still hypothetical but it would explain the phenomenon that barbiturates can suppress the appearance of convulsions.

Electrical stimulation of circumscribed regions of arteries and arterioles causes local constrictions of the vessels (NAGAI and PROSSER, 1963; BETZ et al., 1973) and leads to spasms of the small vessels which have been observed to last more than 10–20 min. The local application of 0.5% strychnine (MCHEDLISHVILI et al., 1967), however, caused dilatation of the pial vessels but narrowed the cortical vessels (MCHEDLISHVILI and BARAMIDZE, 1967). The latter authors concluded from these results that the pial, rather than the cortical, vessels regulate the volume of blood which flows per time unit through the cortical tissue and that it is mainly cortical blood flow that is deficient during convulsions. The actions of various other analeptic drugs on CBF have been discussed in detail by CARPI and CARTONI (1972).

G. Nervous Influences on Cerebral Vessels

During the last few decades there has been repeated discussion about the degree to which neural components participate in the regulation and in disturbances of the CBF. In order to elucidate this problem numerous experiments in animals and investigations in patients have been conducted. NOTHNAGEL (1867) had already found that painful stimuli of peripheral nerves caused changes in the diameters of pial vessels, and in the preceding chapter some experiments were mentioned which clearly show that stimulation of peripheral nervous receptors causes a rise in CBF. From these examples it can also be seen that is difficult to discriminate between local metabolic tissues processes in the vicinity of the resistance vessels which influence CBF and the actions of transmitters at the nerve endings near the smooth muscle cells of the same vessels. The vascular walls of brain arteries and arterioles are well provided with nervous structures (OBERSTEINER, 1898; HUBER, 1899; HUNTER, 1900/01; STOEHR, 1922; HASSIN, 1929; MIKHAILOV, 1956; LAZORTHES, 1961; CARRATO-IBANEZ and FENOLL, 1966; NIELSEN and OWMAN, 1967). For experimental purposes the origin of those nerves which end at the accessible pial vessels are of great interest. The nerve endings do not degenerate immediately after removal of the cervical sympathetic ganglia. From this it was concluded that the perivascular fibers had their origins in ganglia along the great cerebral vessels (CHOROBSKI and PENFIELD, 1932; PENFIELD, 1932). Later investigations, however, showed that 18–20 days after cervical sympathectomy degenerated nervous fibers appeared within the walls of pial arteries and in the choiroid plexus (TSUKER, 1947; ERKHOV, 1965).

Meanwhile, by means of electron microscopy, it became possible to prove that part of the nerve endings at the smooth muscle cells contain dense cored vesicles and that others contain vesicles which are optically empty. The granula-containing endings are identified as noradrenergic nerve endings and the agranular vesicles probably contain acetylcholine (DAHL and NELSON, 1964; NELSON and RENNELS, 1968). Histochemical studies revealed catecholamines within the walls of pial arteries of rabbits (FALCK et al., 1965; OWMAN et al., 1965). In the rat brain (IWOYAMA et al., 1970) and in the cat brain (NIELSEN and OWMAN, 1967) the same types of nerve endings have been found. LEVER et al. (1968) measured the distances between the smooth muscle cells and the nerve endings. They are relatively wide—about 4000 Å. Later investigations by NELSON et al. (1971) showed medullary and nonmedullary fibers in relatively narrow contact with the smooth muscle cells.

Despite the numerous anatomical data, a precise analysis of the nervous influences on CBF is not yet possible, although extensive literature on this problem exists (WOLFF, 1936; KETY and McDOWALL, 1956; HOLMQUIST et al., 1957; LASSEN, 1959; KETY, 1961; MOLNAR, 1967; HIRSCH and SCHNEIDER, 1968; MCHEDLISHVILI, 1968a, b, 1972; LÜBBERS, 1972). The reasons why these obscurities still exist may be partially explained by the fact that the experiments are usually performed with animals under anesthesia. Anesthesia modifies the responses to nervous stimulation. The difficulties may partially result from the measuring methods used, which have not yet reached the necessary degree of refinement.

Stimulation and Blockade of the Cervical Autonomic Nerves

Many efforts have been made to improve the cerebral circulation by changing the sympathetic or vagal activity. It is, therefore, reasonable to induce pathological conditions by stimulation or blockade of the vegetative system. FORBES and WOLFF (1928) had already found that stimulation of the cervical sympathetic chain caused a moderate constriction of pial arteries, and LUBSEN (1940), using the technique of heated thermocouples, found a decrease in cerebral blood flow. Reviews on the action of the sympathetic system on the cerebral vessels were made by INGVAR (1958), KRUPP (1966) and MCHEDLISHVILI (1968b, 1972). SUGIURA (1970), who also found a diminished flow, did not notice any significant influence of the variation of chemical factors in the blood (e.g. by the changes of the CO_2 tension) on the reactions after stimulation or blockade of the sympathicus. This finding conflicts with the results of LUDWIGS and SCHNEIDER (1954) and of HARPER et al. (1970), who found local differences in flow responses after sympathetic stimulation and a dependency on the PCO_2. The vascular effects were found to be maximal at normal arterial PCO_2. In the medullary regions the responses were more pronounced than in the cortex. Sympathectomy caused an increase, and stimulation, a reduction of flow in the experiments of JAMES et al. (1969). Dissection of the sympathetic nerves enhanced the vascular reactions to increased CO_2. Bilateral cervical sympathectomy in monkeys did not disturb cerebral vascular autoregulation (EKLOF et al., 1971). If the vagus was cut in its cervical part the responses of CBF to hypoxia and hypercapnia were reduced. Stimulation of the central part of the vagus caused an increase in CBF which was independent of the arterial PCO_2. Vagotomy did not effect the pial vascular diameters if blood pressure was constant (FORBES et al., 1937), nor the arterial-cerebral venous oxygen difference (USINGER et al., 1966). Vagal stimulation, however, caused pial vascular dilatation. From all these findings it was concluded that the cerebral vascular system is under autonomous reflex control (GOLLWITZER-MEIER and ECKHARDT, 1935; ROSENBLUM, 1971). The action of nervous transmitters of the sympathetic system on the muscular structures corresponds to the results of WAHL et al. (1972a, b), who found a clear constrictive effect during perivascular application of noradrenaline. During intravenous injection of noradrenaline or adrenaline the results, however, do not correspond. The inflow to the brain or the venous outflow was found to increase transiently (INGVAR and SÖDERBERG, 1956; GOTTSTEIN, 1962; IKEDA et al., 1963), or to decrease (DITTMAR et al., 1954; BOVET et al., 1960). The different findings are caused mainly by the resulting increase in blood pressure. As mentioned previously, the relation of arterial blood pressure to cerebral vascular resistance determines the flow rate. The degree of constrictive response in turn is dependent on the degree of variation of blood pressure. Discrepancies in the results are seen not only after injection of noradrenaline but also after the intravenous application of adrenaline (review see SOKOLOFF, 1959; BETZ, 1972a; CARPI, 1972). As yet it is impossible to distinguish how far the metabolic changes in the tissue or the blood interact with direct actions elicited by the nerve endings in the vascular wall.

H. Experimental Investigation of the Smooth Muscles of Brain Vessels

As discussed briefly in the section on autoregulation of cerebral vessels, the basic mechanisms of smooth muscle contraction play an essential role in autoregulatory responses and in reactions to pharmacologic agents. With regard to the reaction of single smooth muscle cells the question of to what degree mechanical or chemical stimuli determine the response of the vascular resistance has to be formulated in another way. Each stimulus which acts on the smooth muscle cell—regardless if it is mechanical, metabolic, nervous or electric—can produce changes in the contractile structures or in the visco-elastic elements and induces a chain of events which finally leads to contraction or relaxation of the smooth muscle fibers. For the understanding of pathologic and physiologic regulation, knowledge of the basic mechanisms in these structures is essential. The investigations in this field, however, are of great methodical difficulty and they have concentrated on the vessels which can be easily exposed: the pial vessels, the great cerebral arteries or the carotid arteries. MCHEDLISHVILI et al. (1967b) tried to discriminate between the reactions of cortical and pial vessels and observed differences in their participation in autoregulation (see also MCHEDLISHVILI, 1972).

For some years many findings have supported the hypothesis that CO_2 does not act in molecular form on the vascular resistance but that the pH of the fluid in which CO_2 is dissolved is the adequate stimulus for cerebral vascular smooth muscle fibers (SEVERINGHAUS, 1966; SEVERINGHAUS et al., 1966; SKINHØJ, 1966; BETZ and KOZAK, 1967; BETZ and HEUSER, 1967; FIESCHI, 1967; LASSEN and INGVAR, 1968; SIESJÖ et al., 1968; AGNOLI, 1968; SKINHOJ, 1969; AGNOLI et al., 1969a, et al.). Any variation of the CO_2 concentration in the blood or in the tissue causes a variation of the pH at the surface and within the smooth muscle cells. In many situations the change in vascular resistance is combined with pH variations (HEUSER, unpublished). A clear dependency of the pial vascular diameters on the pH of mock CSF which was brought into the immediate vicinity of the smooth muscles of the pial vessels by means of microperfusion has been found (WAHL et al., 1970; KUSCHINSKI et al., 1971/72; KNABE and BETZ, 1972). Perivascular acidosis dilatated and perivascular alkalosis constricted local sections of pial arteries and arterioles. These results indicate that cerebral cortical tissue acidosis causes an increase of flow by means of a relaxation of smooth muscle fibers and confirm the results which are discussed in the section on CO_2 action and hypoxia. It has, however, been shown that the smooth muscle tension of cerebral vessels is not exclusively regulated by changes in the extravascular or intramural H^+ concentration (BETZ and HEUSER, 1967; MCDOWALL

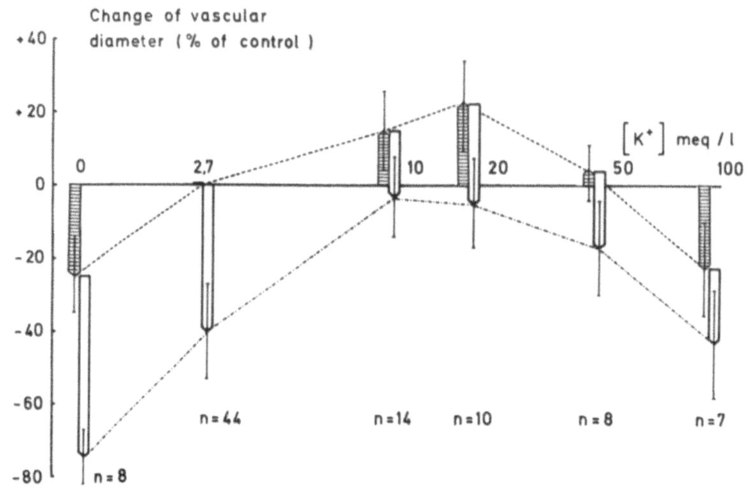

Fig. 8. The effect of varying potassium concentrations in the perivascular space of small pial arteries (80–200 μm diameter) and of electrical stimulation with DC-impulses on the diameters of the stimulated vessels. Mock CSF's of constant pH and different K^+ concentrations were applied by means of microperfusion into the immediate vicinity of pial arteries. The normal CSF potassium concentration in the cats was 2.7 mEq/L. The dark columns indicate the changes of the vascular diameters after application of different K^+ in the CSF. The white columns represent the constrictive reaction after stimulation with tiny AgCl electrodes attached at both sides of the exposed vessel (diameter of current electrode: 0.1 mm, size of the reference electrode: 0.7 · 0.2 · 0.1 mm). Stimulation with square wave impulses (5 mA, 15 Hz, 1 ms/imp., duration of stimulation 10 sec). Blood potassium was normal and constant

and HARPER, 1968a, b). It was shown that an increase in the concentration of Ca^{++} during a decrease in perivascular pH inhibited the dilatation (BETZ et al., 1973; VLAHOV and ENZENROSS, 1973). The application of EGTA or EDTA prevented the constrictive action of alkalosis on pial vessels. The electrical stimulation of single arterial sections of pial arteries with short-lasting DC impulses also caused localized constrictions of the pial arteries which could be blocked by perivascular application of 10 mmol/L EGTA or EDTA. This indicated the central role of Ca^{++} in the constrictive process.

Not only Ca^{++} but also potassium has to be regarded as an essential ion in the regulation of smooth muscle tension. KNABE and BETZ (1972), HEUSER et al. (1971/72), KUSCHINSKI et al. (1971/72) and BALDY-MOULINIER (1971/72, 1973) agree from their experiments that increasing concentrations of potassium above normal up to 20 mEq/l in the extravascular fluid lead to dilatation of the pial vessels, and a decrease below 3 mEq/l causes constriction. Very high potassium concentrations (above 60 mEq/l) also cause constrictions (see Fig. 8). BALDY-MOULINIER (1971, 1972, 1973) mentioned experiments in which it was shown that blocking the ion pump of the cell membranes by intraventricular administration of ouabaine, an inhibitor of the membrane Na-K-ATP-ase, caused a release of intracellular potassium into the extracellular space which was associated with cerebral hyperemia. From the experiments of BÖNING (1972) and KUSCHINSKI et al. (1972) it can be seen that there exists an interaction between the pH-dependent vascular reactions and the potassium concentration in the extravascular space of pial vessels. According to KUSCHINSKY et al. (1972), at a CSF-bicarbonate concentration of over 5 mEq/l, the potassium-induced reaction dominates the pH-dependent response, whereas with bicarbonate concentrations below 5 mEq/l the pH-dependent reactions became apparent.

Since in hyperventilation or severe hypercapnia (HEUSER et al., 1971/72; SCHINDLER et al., 1971/72, 1974) the potassium concentration in the extravascular space changes, this combined action probably explains better than earlier assumptions the complexity of the regulation of CVR. K^+ and Ca^{++} variations in CSF as a cause of vascular disturbances have not yet been regarded as a cause of pathological flow in humans.

The described type of reaction to K^+ variations in pial arteries has not been seen in strips of great cerebral arteries. TODA and FUJITA (1973) found increasing tensions in isolated cerebral arteries of dogs and humans when they increased the K^+ concentration in the bathing solutions. The increase was maximal between K^+ concentrations of 20–30 mM. A strong increase in the tension of strips of basilar, posterior cerebral and middle cerebral arteries was observed during the addition of 10^{-6} M serotonin and 10^{-5} M noradrenaline. Transmural electrical stimulation elicited contractions of the common carotid artery strips.

KUSCHINSKY and WAHL (1973) reported investigations in which they perfused the immediate vicinity of pial vessels with mock CSF containing noradrenaline. No evidence was found that α-receptors participate in the regulation of the tone of pial arteries. This was concluded from the fact that $2.5 \cdot 10^{-6}$ M pentolamine, which reduced the norepinephrine-induced constriction, had no effect when given alone.

I. Disturbances of CBF by Variation of Blood Gases

From the components affecting cerebral circulation the disturbances elicited by changes in the cerebral vascular walls have been discussed in the preceding chapters. It has also been pointed out that changes in systemic arterial or venous pressure are an essential cause of cerebral diseases because of insufficient blood supply through the cerebral vessels. The already mentioned types of disturbance have been considered from the experimental point of view.

Three important causes of the disturbances which affect the cerebrovascular system, however, have not yet been regarded in detail: arterial hypoxia, arterial hypercapnia and hypocapnia during fully maintained circulation. O_2-deficiency and hypercapnia are sometimes combined in human diseases (e.g. during reduced gas diffusion in the lung, in a-v shunts in the lung, during reduced contractility of the heart, etc.).

In animals the three main types of disturbance are analyzed separately in order to discriminate between the reactions of the cerebrovascular system caused by hypoxia or by changes in the PCO_2.

I. Increase in CO_2 and CBF

A large number of books, review articles and single articles exist on the relation between changes in CO_2 and cerebral circulation. Therefore the following references can be only a limited selection of the great number which agree with the finding that hypercapnia causes increases in CBF. Decreases in the cerebral PCO_2 caused by hyperventilation result in a decrease in CBF because of a rise in cerebral vascular resistance (WOLFF and LENNOX, 1930; BENZINGER et al., 1938; NOELL and SCHNEIDER, 1944; KETY and SCHMIDT, 1946, 1948b; SCHIEVE and WILSON, 1953; SCHNEIDER, 1953; NOVACK et al., 1953; PATTERSON et al.,

1955; LASSEN, 1959; BÜHLMANN et al., 1960; MEYER and GOTOH, 1960; HARPER and BELL, 1963; MCHENRY et al., 1964; ALEXANDER et al., 1965; HARPER, 1965, 1966, 1969; HARPER and GLASS, 1965; HÄGGENDAL and JOHANSSON, 1966; SHACKELFORD and HEGEDUS, 1966; SKINHØJ, 1966; FIESCHI, 1967; AGNOLI, 1968; AGNOLI et al., 1969a, b; FENCL et al., 1969; POSNER et al., 1969; RYZHOVA, 1970; HAINING et al., 1970; CRANSTON and ROSENDORFF, 1971; RAICHLE et al., 1971; GÄNSHIRT, 1972; BETZ, 1973).

It cannot be assumed that blood vessels in individual regions of the brain respond to variations of arterial CO_2-pressure ($PaCO_2$) in the same way. HANSEN et al. (1957) found that the responses of blood flow in gray matter and in white matter were different. Between $PaCO_2$ of 35–65 mmHg gray matter flow increased at a rate of approximately 1.4 ml blood/100 g·min·mmHg $PaCO_2$ whereas flow through the white matter increased only at a rate of 0.46 ml/100 g·min·mmHg $PaCO_2$ (JAMES et al., 1969). Since from Table 1 it is evident that within the gray matter and the white matter there are considerable differences in blood flow, the mentioned discrimination of reactions between white and gray matter surely is an oversimplification of the differences in the reactions. Besides these local differences which obscure the pathophysiological aspects of local blood flow disturbances, the normal cerebrovascular response to CO_2 is dependent on the systemic blood pressure. At approximately 50 mmHg mean arterial blood pressure the vascular response to carbon dioxide is abolished, as demonstrated by HARPER and GLASS (1965) in dog experiments. At about 70–90 mmHg $PaCO_2$ in dogs (HARPER and GLASS) or 8–10% CO_2 in the inspired air in cats (BETZ, 1965a), the reactions of CBF to a further increase are diminished or abolished. PATTERSON et al. (1955) tried to find a threshold for the CBF response to increasing CO_2 in the air. They found no effect when they increased the CO_2 concentration by less than 2.5%. They made their measurements, however, in anesthetized individuals. In conscious cats at 1% CO_2 in the air, slight increases in CBF can already be observed (BETZ, 1965a).

Continuous recording of local cerebral blood flow by means of heat clearance techniques indicates a high speed of response of the vascular resistance to CO_2 (BETZ, 1965a, 1972b).

In the preceding section it was discussed whether carbon dioxide could act upon vascular smooth muscle in molecular form or only as a result of its effect in altering the pH of the intra- or extracellular fluid of the vascular smooth muscle. Since CO_2 diffuses freely and rapidly between blood and CSF, changes in $PaCO_2$ are always causing variations in the CSF-pH, and in the pH of the smooth muscle cells. An extensive discussion of this problem is given by PURVES (1972) and BETZ (1972b) and in a symposium (INGVAR, 1969), and will not be dealt with here in detail. One aspect of this problem, however, seems to be important in connection with the production of cerebrovascular disturbances in animals, i.e., chronic exposure to high CO_2 concentration.

If animals are exposed to an increased CO_2 concentration in the inspired air, CBF increases. However, after some hours of exposure the blood flow tends to decrease again despite high CO_2 in the environmental air, and finally reaches the initial value (BETZ, 1965a).

It was shown by AGNOLI (1968) and AGNOLI et al. (1969b) that it is only initially that the CO_2 increase causes a decrease in the CSF-pH. In the course of adaptation to high CO_2, the CSF-pH moves towards normal values. The reason for this secondary increase in pH is an increasing bicarbonate concentration in the CSF. It could be demonstrated by AGNOLI et al. (1969a) that CBF does not return to normal values if the CSF-pH is kept low. This reaction is in accordance with the hypothesis that the extravascular pH plays an essential role in the regulation of CBF (see section on basic mechanisms of flow regulation). ECKSTRÖM-JODAL and HÄGGENDAL (1969) confirmed this behavior of CBF in patients with chronic respiratory insufficiency. In one case in which CBF remained high, the CFS-pH was lower than normal despite a complete return to normal of the blood-pH. This experiment has been taken as partial evidence for the theory that cerebral vascular resistance is regulated mainly by the pH in the extravascular space.

Exposure of cats to 5–6% CO_2 for 6–8 h daily caused a slow decrease in the hypothalamic blood flow during each period of exposure. However, after 12 days of repeated daily exposure the initial rise in CBF was much lower or was absent completely in single cases despite the fact that the cats were kept in normal air in the intervals between the periods of exposure to high CO_2. CSF-pH was not recorded in these animals. It must be assumed, however, that the pH decreased during each single period of exposure of the cats to high CO_2 even after some days. Therefore the variations in pH cannot be the only reason for the adjustment of CVR. According to ADOLPH (1964) adaptive responses to specific stimuli appear when the exposures are only performed for a limited period per day. It cannot be said which other adaptive mechanisms are involved in the exposure to high CO_2. The mentioned experiments, however, explain why, in respiratory acidosis of patients, the CBF need not be found to have increased.

If CO_2 is increased above 10% the EEG amplitudes are reduced and the frequency spectrum is shifted towards slower components. A further increase in the CO_2 concentration of over 10% leads to a blood pressure passive reaction of CBF. At 40–60% CO_2 in O_2 KNEBEL Diss. (1974) Tuebingen and SCHINDLER et al. (1971/72) found blood pressure values of 60–90 mmHg, and CBF was slightly elevated or slightly decreased or unchanged when compared with normal conditions. The changes of Cr $\sim$ P (slight reduction) and lactate (reduction) were caused by the effects of the H^+ increase. If blood flow was reduced during high CO_2 exposure, signs of hypoxia appeared (decrease in ATP, increasing lactate in the tissue). Since EEG is isoelectric in solely severe hypercapnia as well as in hypercapnia plus hypoxia, the EEG cannot be used as a criterion of whether the blood flow is sufficient for the energy supply of the brain or not.

II. Hypoxia and CBF

There are a great number of books, reviews and single articles on the effects of hypoxia on human or animal brain (e.g. CHORNYAK, 1938; KETY and SCHMIDT, 1948b; SCHMIDT, 1950; SCHNEIDER, 1953, 1961; LASSEN, 1959; WOLF, 1959; GLEICHMANN et al., 1962; COHEN, 1965; MCLEDINGHAM, 1966; SHIMOJYO et al., 1966; BETZ, 1968b; KOGURE et al., 1970a, b; MANN, 1970; BARTKO, 1971; BAKAY and KOBAYASHI, 1971; GÄNSHIRT, 1972) which agree with the theory that arterial hypoxia causes an increase in CBF mainly because cerebrovascular resistance decreases.

There are many ways in which the brain tissue can become hypoxic despite maintained circulation. Arterial hypoxia caused by ventilatory or circulatory failure is the most common reason. Venous hypoxia because of diminished O_2 capacity of the blood is another reason for cerebral hypoxia.

It can be seen that in normal conscious animals the first slight increases appear when the O_2 concentration in the inspired air reaches 17–16% (BETZ, 1965a). Fig. 9 shows the relation between O_2 concentration in the inspired air

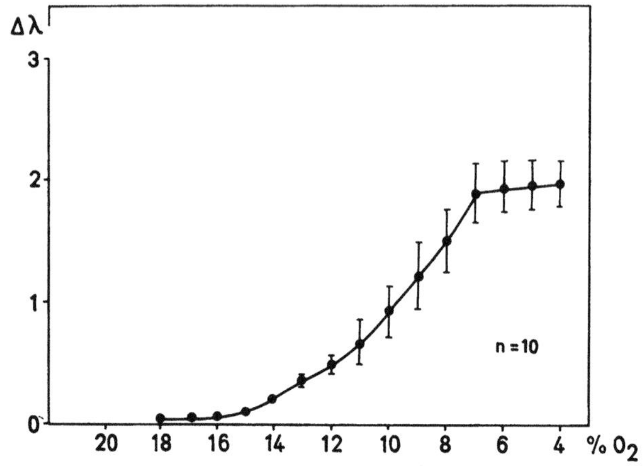

Fig. 9. Increase of local blood flow in the thalamus or hypothalamus in 10 conscious cats during gradual diminution of the oxygen concentration in the inspired air. The rate of decrease was $^1/_2$% O_2/min. Blood flow was continuously recorded in terms of regional heat clearance $\Delta\lambda'$ (see Fig. 7) (From BETZ, 1965a)

and local blood flow in the thalamus and hypothalamus of 10 cats. The correlation of CBF with cerebral venous PO_2 in normocapnia of anesthetized animals shows that increases in CBF start when the PvO_2 decreases to 25–28 mmHg and reaches a maximum at about 20 mmHg PO_2 (NOELL and SCHNEIDER, 1942; SCHAERTLIN, 1961; GROTE et al., 1971). In hypercapnia and in metabolic acidosis the reactions to hypoxia appear at higher venous PO_2 values than in normocapnia (MCDOWALL and HARPER, 1968b; GROTE et al., 1971). The increase in blood flow caused by hypoxia is augmented by additional respiratory acidosis.

The effect of acute hypoxia on cerebral energetics is similar to that during ischemia (THORN et al., 1958; SCHMAHL et al., 1966). Fig. 10a shows the effect of respiring a gas mixture with low O_2 concentration during maintained cerebral circulation on EEG, cortical oxygen pressure, lactate, pyruvate and the energy-rich phosphates. The EEG ceases when Cr∼P has reached 1.5 mmol/L in the brain tissue. At this stage CBF has not yet stopped. After inhalation of a high concentration of O_2 the energy-rich substrates return rapidly to normal values if the hypoxia did not disturb the cardiac functions and if it was of short duration.

In Fig. 10b a gas mixture with low PO_2 was inspired. The PO_2, however, was not as low as in the experiment in Fig. 10a. It can be seen clearly that there is no isoelectric EEG. Cr∼P, however, is already somewhat decreased and the tissue lactate content and the lactate/pyruvate ratio is high. The oxygen pressure is low when measured on different sites of the cortex. If the oxygen pressure is only moderately decreased no significant reaction of the Cr∼P or ATP can be observed. The lactate, however, has already started to increase. This increase is accompanied by a decrease in CVR if normocapnia is maintained. The differences in the contents of energy-rich phosphates and lactate between the reactions with maintained circulation during hypoxia and those results obtained in tissue with reduced blood flow are minimal.

In the experiments of FUJISHIMA et al. (1971) the local effects of hypoxia induced by inhalation of 6% O_2 and 94% N_2 on cortical and hypothalamic blood flow of dogs yielded different results. Local cortical blood flow decreased in $^1/_3$ of the animals during hypoxia, but in all animals local cortical blood flow

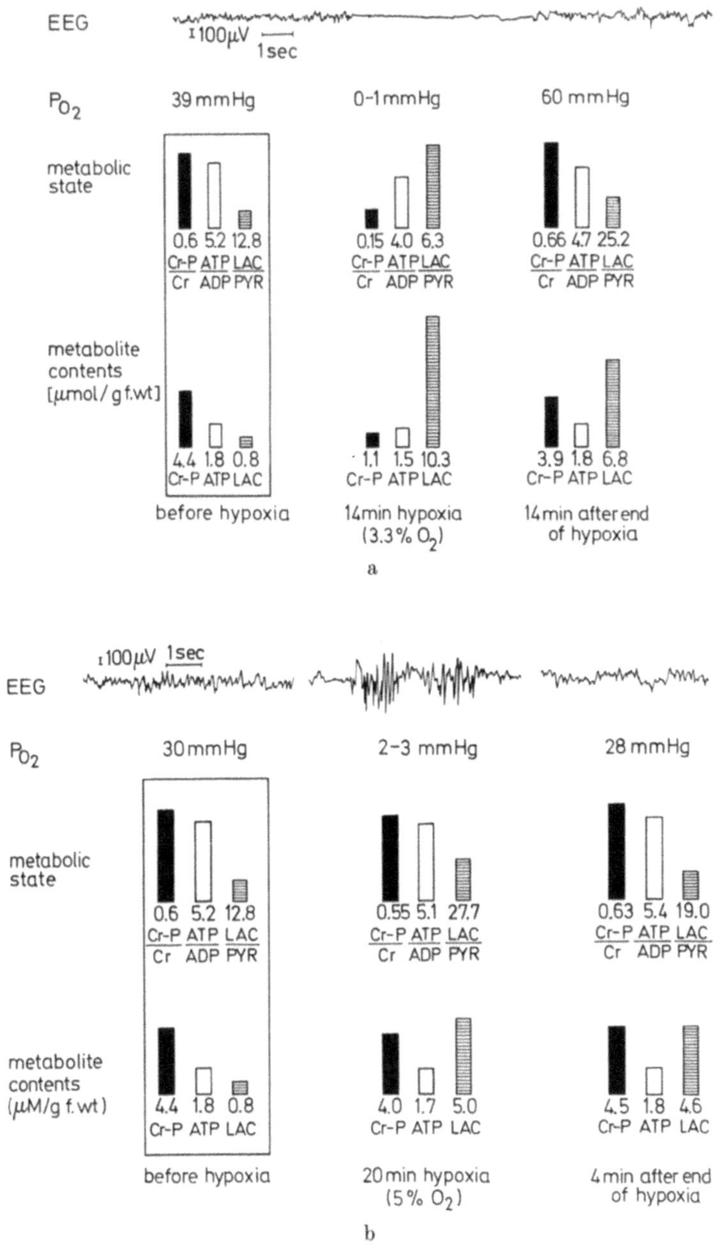

Fig. 10. (a) EEG, cortical P_{O_2} and metabolic state of energy-rich substrates of the cerebral cortex in cats during severe hypoxia (3% O_2, 3.5% CO_2 and 93.5% N_2). Upper line: Sections of the continuous EEG-recording. 2nd line: O_2-pressure recorded with a multiwire platinum electrode on the cortical surface. 3rd line: Contents of metabolites in μmol/g fresh weight. Left column (prior to hypoxia) controls which give the mean values of 10 cats during spontaneous respiration of normal air. The tissue samples were obtained by means of a steal punch which was cooled in liquid air. The amount of each sample was about 100 mg cortical tissue (From Schmahl et al., 1966). (b) EEG, cortical P_{O_2} and metabolic state of the cerebral cortex during hypoxia (5% O_2, 3.5% CO_2, 91.5% N_2). Arrangement as in Fig. 10a. The hypoxia was not so severe that the EEG ceased (From Schmahl et al., 1966)

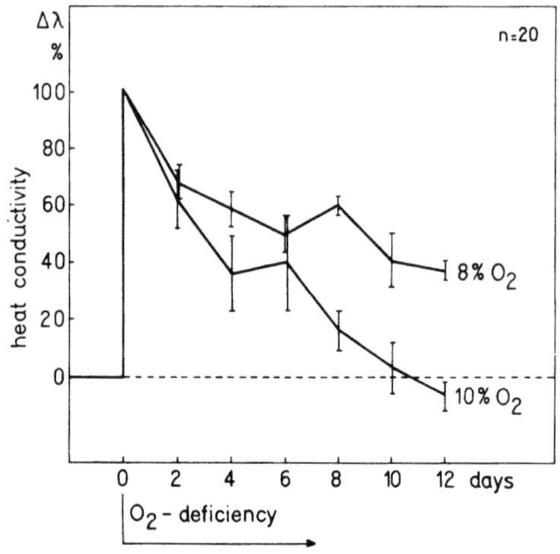

Fig. 11. Mean values of regional cerebral blood flow in 20 conscious cats during daily repeated hypoxia. Duration of exposure to low P_{O_2} daily at least four hours. The animals lived in normal air during the intervals between the exposures. 10 cats were exposed to 10% O_2 and 10 cats to 8% O_2. Blood flow was continuously recorded by heat clearance probes. The initial values in normal atmosphere were defined as $\Delta\ \lambda = 0\%$. The mean increase in cerebral blood flow during the first exposure to 8% O_2 or 10% O_2 as $\Delta\ \lambda = 100\%$. In the course of adaptation the mean values of CBF in the 10 cats which were exposed to 10% O_2 decreased to normal values within 12 days, whereas CBF in those cats which were exposed to 8% O_2 remained elevated (From BETZ et al., 1965)

increased during hypercapnia in all regions studied. These differences are difficult to understand.

Autoregulation is eliminated by hypoxia (FREEMAN and INGVAR, 1968a, b; BALDY and MOULINIER, 1971). Whether this lack of autoregulation is caused by variations in the extravascular H^+ or K^+ concentration or by the action of other vasoactive substances is not yet sufficiently clear (see sections E and H).

Chronic hypoxia can be easily established in animals which are placed in chambers with low oxygen content. Exposure of cats to 10% CO_2 initially causes an increase of CBF. Within 12 hrs of continuous exposure the blood flow decreases again towards its normal value (BETZ, 1965a). During exposure of 10 conscious cats to 10% O_2 or 8% O_2 for several days, each day for at least 6 hrs, an adaptation of CBF to the hypoxic conditions could be observed (Fig. 11). Fig. 11 shows that after 12 days of intermittent exposure (to 10% O_2) CBF remained normal despite decreasing PO_2 in the inspired air. The relatively short time of exposure to hypoxia makes it improbable that adaptation is entirely due to an increase in hemoglobin (WÜNNENBERG, 1964). SEVERINGHAUS (1964) and SEVERINGHAUS et al. (1966) mentioned that during the adaptation of man to a high altitude (3200 m above sea level) an increase in CBF of 24% initially appeared. After 3–5 days, flow fell to 13% above normal.

The mechanisms of adaptation of CBF in this phase seem to be related to the CSF-pH. Cortical blood flow and the H^+ concentration in the CSF increased simultaneously, suggesting the dependency of cerebral cortical blood flow on cortical pH. KOGURE et al. (1970a) assumed that circulating hypoxic products do not affect cerebral blood flow, indicating that the effects of hypoxia on CBF are secondary to local parenchymatous changes in the brain.

Tissue metabolism changes during the adaptation period. DAHL and BALFOUR (1964) saw an increase of anaerobic glycolysis in adapted animals. DETAR and BOHR (1968), who repeatedly exposed helical strips of rabbit aorta to low PO_2, found modified responses in the development of the tension of the helical strips during repeated exposures to low PO_2, which they think are manifestations of adaptation to hypoxic conditions. Strips of adapted smooth muscles developed a much higher tension after the application of epinephrine than non-adapted strips. DETAR and BOHR (1968) explained the mechanism also by their findings of an increased anaerobic glycolysis. In completely acclimatized rats (to 11000 or 18000 feet altitude), no significant changes were observed in the energy-rich phosphates (ALBAUM and CHINN, 1953). The animals, however, were exposed for such a long time that additional adaptations could come into action (e.g. an increase in hemoglobin), which of course would increase the tendency toward CBF normalization. In high altitude in young rats, the CBF adaptation was found to be more pronounced than in old ones and the cerebellar blood flow of rats did not show any adaptation (HAINING et al., 1970).

In repeated anoxic exposures of guinea pigs and cats by immersing the animals in atmospheres of nitrogen for various periods of time, vascular changes (subpial and intracerebral perivascular hemorrhages and coagulation; fibrosis and incrustation of the vascular walls) were found in addition to the cellular degeneration of the brain tissue (THORNER and LEWEY, 1940). During long-term hypoxia the number of capillaries in the brain cortex was higher than in normal animals (DIEMER and HENN, 1965) and the mean arterial diameters increased (MERKER and SCHNEIDER, 1949). However, a relatively high degree of hypoxia was necessary to cause an increased number of capillaries (DIEMER, 1965).

III. Hyperventilation and CBF

In normal animals or men every increase in ventilation causing a decrease of cerebral PCO_2 leads to cerebral vasoconstriction (GIBBS, 1933a; GIBBS et al., 1935, 1942; NOELL and SCHNEIDER, 1944; KETY and SCHMIDT, 1948b; TURNER et al., 1957; LASSEN, 1959; GOTOH et al., 1961, 1965) and to an increase in blood lactate and cerebral tissue lactate (ALEXANDER et al., 1965; ELDRIDGE and SALZER, 1967; GRANHOLM and SIESJÖ, 1967; PLUM and POSNER, 1967; COHEN et al., 1968; GRANHOLM et al., 1969) thus indicating that the cerebral metabolism is not in its normal state.

GIBBS et al. (1942) and NOELL and SCHNEIDER (1944) stated that the total CBF is not further reduced by hyperventilation when the PO_2 in the jugular vein is diminished below 19 mmHg. In voluntarily hyperventilating men, CBF begins to diminish as soon as the arterial PCO_2 has fallen by about 2 mmHg (PATTERSON, 1960). The maximal reduction of CBF during continued or forced hyperventilation was found to be about 40% of normal global CBF (KETY and SCHMIDT, 1946, 1948b). In animals (cats and rats) the ratios of Cr$\sim$P/Cr and ATP/ADP remain normal despite a fivefold increase in the cortical lactate (WEIDNER, 1969). This indicates that the decrease in blood flow need not necessarily cause a decrease in the available energy during hyperventilation. With combined measurements of cortical oxygen pressure, cortical pH, cortical blood flow and PO_2 in the sagittal sinus and in the arterial blood PICKERODT (1971) found together with a decrease in cortical blood flow a decrease in PO_2 in the sagittal sinus. The decrease of PO_2 in the sagittal sinus was not so pronounced as the O_2 pressure fall in numerous spots of the cortical tissue. The PO_2 on the brain surface was recorded with PO_2 microelectrodes. During hyperventilation the distribution of the cortical PO_2 values shifted towards lower values. At many spots the cortical PO_2 was zero during severe hyperventilation. These measurements explain the increased anaerobic metabolism of glucose resulting in an increased lactate concentration in the brain tissue. During sustained hyperventilation the arterial blood pH remains higher than during normal ventilation. The CSF-pH increases initially but then moves towards the values before hyperventilation. In sustained severe hyperventilation it is possible to reach the initial pH again. CBF, however, remains low despite the decreasing pH (McDOWALL and HARPER, 1968a; BETZ, 1969b). The lactate concentration in the brain tissue increases independently of the pH variation in the extravascular cortical space. This indicates that the lactate concentration is not always correlated to the vascular diameter. The dissociation of pH and CVR during severe hyperventilation has not yet been conclusively explained.

One hypothetical explanation is the following: hyperventilation causes a slight increase in arterial PO_2 so that the arterial blood within those vessels which regulate vascular resistance is high enough to provide a sufficient oxygen supply for the vascular walls of the resistance vessels. Since the smooth muscles of these vessels are not hypoxic and the pH of the smooth muscle cells remains high there is no adequate stimulus for a dilatation. The O_2 capacity of the intravascular contents is low because of the strong vasoconstriction. Therefore cells distant to the arteries do not receive sufficient oxygen in order to maintain complete aerobic conditions. From the remaining anaerobic glycolysis some ATP is produced. It compensates partially for the O_2 deficit and prevents a significant fall of the ATP. The glycolysis due to the O_2 deficit causes at least part of the lactate increase; part of the lactate is produced because of the initial alkalosis. The phosphofructokinase activity, in fact, is increased during alkalosis (optimum at pH 7.5 UI, 1966; ADLER et al., 1971) and causes an increased glycolysis (GEVERS and DOWDLE, 1963; KOGURE et al., 1973).

J. Variations of Intracranial Volume and Cerebral Blood Flow

Perfusion pressure of the brain is altered not only by the variations in arterial blood pressure. An alteration in venous blood pressure, which occurs quite often in diseases of the cardiovascular system, has also to be regarded as a factor which triggers variations in CBF. In dogs JACOBSON et al. (1963) altered the sagittal sinus pressure by compression of the superior vena cava. They found that no significant changes in CBF occurred when the perfusion pressure was not reduced to less than 60 mmHg. Similar results were reported by MOYER et al. (1954), who raised the jugular venous pressure by inflating a cuff around the neck. At 60 mmHg there were no significant variations in CBF. Since a sudden rise in venous pressure results in an increase in intracranial blood volume it must be expected that the intracranial pressure rises if venous pressure is increased. This correlation between CSF pressure and intracranial blood volume can also be clearly shown during inhalation of increased CO_2 in the inspired air (Fig. 12). This gas is known to be a strong vasodilator and causes an increase in CBF under physiological conditions. The findings shown in Fig. 12 agree with the experiments of BAUST et al. (1963), who reported that pulsatory variations in arterial blood pressure or sudden increases in the intravascular blood volume without a rise in blood pressure run parallel to variations in CSF pressure (this was confirmed by RISBERG et al., 1969b). A correlation between CBF and cerebral blood volume was measured by NYLIN (1956, 1960, 1961a, b). RISBERG et al. (1969a) also found a high correlation between local blood volume and local blood flow at the same site of the cerebral tissue. From these results the conclusion may be drawn that there is also a close correlation between CBF,

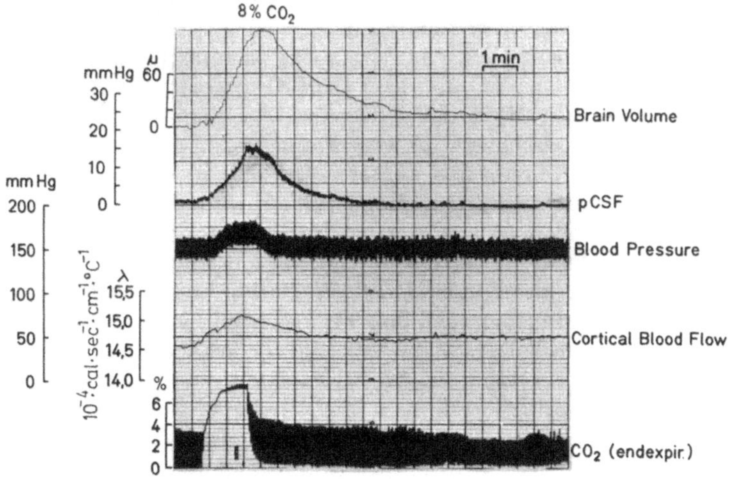

Fig. 12. Combined measurements of the relative changes of brain volume (by means of an implanted displacement transducer), CSF-pressure (p CSF) arterial blood pressure, local cortical blood flow (by means of an implanted heat clearance disc) and end-expiratory CO_2 concentration during short-lasting inhalation of 8% CO_2

cerebral blood volume and CSF pressure. The latter conclusion, however, can be drawn only if the CBF varies rapidly and the flow amplitudes vary moderately. There is a close correlation between the cerebral metabolic rate for O_2 and CSF production (BERING, 1959) but no clear correlation between CSF production and CBF.

During the infusion of acetylcholine into the carotid artery (BAUST et al., 1963) or after the application of papaverine (BETZ and ROOS, 1972), changes in CBF, brain volume and CSF pressure are not parallel. This does not correspond to the results of GOLDENSON et al. (1951), RYDER et al. (1952a, b), RICH et al. (1953), who stated that CBF is always concomitant with CSF pressure.

COURTICE (1940) and FERRIS (1941) reported that they had found decreases in cerebral blood flow as intracranial pressure increased. Direct measurements of CBF and intracranial pressure confirmed that cerebral blood flow was unaffected only if the CSF pressure was not higher than 33 mmHg (KETY et al., 1948a). This behavior of the relation CSF pressure/CBF with somewhat varying critical values for the threshold at which CBF started to decrease during rising intracranial pressure was also observed by several other authors (ZWETNOW et al., 1968; MILLER et al., 1971/72; FITCH et al., 1969; ZWETNOW, 1970; LEWIS and MCLAURIN, 1972; NAGAI et al., 1972a, b). In baboons CBF was maintained in some cases at normal levels despite falling perfusion pressure until the latter decreases below 35–40 mmHg (JENETT et al., 1971). Even at perfusion pressures of less than 10 mmHg some flow through the brain was measured. In other experiments a marked interindividual variation of the relationship between CBF and cerebral perfusion pressure was seen (ROWAN et al., 1972). JOHNSTON et al. (1972) found the critical level at 50 mmHg of intracranial pressure (ICP) when they infused artificial CSF into the cisterna magna. In a group of experiments in baboons they inflated a supratentorial subdural balloon. CBF remained near control level up to ICP's of approximately 60 mmHg. The inflation of a balloon placed within the infratentorial, subdural space caused a variable relationship between

CBF and ICP. These variations were caused by marked changes in arterial blood pressure after inflation of the balloon.

Such experiments have their clinical analogy in intracranial hematoma after head trauma in which CBF is affected if the CSF pressure rises above a certain threshold. HEKMATPANAH (1970, 1972) demonstrated that with rising intracranial pressure the cerebral circulation and perfusion usually decreased and finally ceased. The ceasing of circulation appeared initially in capillaries and later in the larger vessels. After deflation of the balloon, flow returned only in some of the experiments and not in all vascular beds. The failure of the blood flow to return was considered to be due to capillary obstruction. Because of these interrelations between intracranial blood circulation and intracranial pressure, continuous recording of intracranial pressure has been found to be a good gauge of whether a patient will live or die after severe head trauma. It was shown by KUURNE et al. (1972) that in 17 patients with intraventricular pressure above 60 mmHg 14 died, whereas most of the patients survived when ICP was lower than 30 mmHg. The effect of diffuse intracranial hypertension on CBF is not only dependent on the height of the intracranial pressure but also on the rapidity of its development (HEMMER, 1960; LANGFITT et al., 1965a). When an intracranial balloon is inflated rapidly CBF declines immediately. However, with a gradual increase in intracranial pressure the reduction in blood flow may be minimal, when pressure reaches 35–40 mmHg. It is known from patients with brain tumors that despite a high increase in CSF pressure the CBF in the normal brain tissue distant from the tumor remains normal. Because of the difficulties of investigating the compensatory mechanisms which keep the blood flow high in man, this problem is a field of experimental research in animals.

CUSHING (1901, 1902) had already observed an increase in systemic blood pressure during elevated intracranial pressure. The range of the blood pressure increase was sometimes only a few mmHg (GÄNSHIRT, 1957; LANGFITT et al., 1965a; SCHWARTZ and ZAREA, 1969). The rise in arterial blood pressure occurs usually at high CSF pressures not much below 100 mmHg (NAUNYN and SCHREIBER, 1881; CUSHING, 1901; NOELL and SCHNEIDER, 1948; DICKINSON and MCCUBBIN, 1963; RICHARDSON et al., 1965; SAGAWA, 1967; HÄGGENDAL et al., 1970), indicating that this mechanism is of significance for extreme increases in CSF pressure.

This is not the only mechanism for the maintenance of blood flow through the brain during increased CSF pressure. Another compensatory mechanism which tends to keep blood flow high is presumably of the same kind as the cerebral blood flow autoregulation (see section E and MILLER et al., 1973; COOPER and HULME, 1972). Strong evidence for a common basic mechanism for autoregulation of CBF during decreasing arterial blood pressure or increasing CSF pressure is provided by the experiments of KJÄLLQUIST et al. (1969). He observed that even relatively small reductions in the cerebral perfusion pressure brought about by increases of ICP were accompanied by an increased CSF lactate, an increased lactate/pyruvate ratio and by a decreased HCO_3^- concentration, suggesting the appearance of hypoxic CSF lactacidosis in the cerebral tissue (ZWETNOW et al., 1968; ZWETNOW, 1970; NAGAI et al., 1972) which in turn is known as a vasodilator. ZUPPING (1972) also observed CSF acodisis in patients with increased intracranial pressure. In arterial blood the pH was found to be elevated for the patients who were hyperventilated. Their CSF-K^+ was slightly lower than normal. Even at this early stage, venous oxygen tension decreased (TROUPP et al., 1967; NAGAI, 1972), and cerebral venous pH decreased slightly, indicating the occurrence of a tissue acidosis (KJÄLLQUIST et al., 1969). Direct evidence of pial vascular dilatation was given by pial vascular observation through a scull window (WOLFF and FORBES, 1928). If the increase in the intracranial pressure leads to such a reduction in CBF that ischemia occurs for some minutes, a functional recovery of the brain tissue cannot be obtained despite the restitution of normal tissue contents of energy-rich phosphates after decompression (LJUNGGREN et al., 1972; HEKMATPANAH, 1972). During prolonged intracranial hypertension the development of cerebral vasomotor paralysis can be observed (LANGFITT et al., 1965b). The phase after decompression sometimes is described as luxury perfusion (MEYER et al., 1969a; HALSEY and CAPRA, 1971/72), or as prolonged reactive hyperemia (HÄGGENDAL et al., 1967). Long-lasting hyperemic periods after the normalization of the raised cerebrospinal pressure were not only seen if CBF decreased during the increase of intracranial pressure but also if the CBF remained within normal limits during diminuation of the perfusion pressure (HÄGGENDAL et al., 1969). If the CSF-pH is normalized in the period after the decompression, an increase in CBF must be explained by mechanisms other than the pH-dependent vascular reactions. If during impaired autoregulation or vasoparalysis the arterial blood pressure is increased, the water content of the brain tissue rises. The same effect occurs in hypercapnic hypertension (MEINIG et al., 1972). The formation of edema was time-dependent: The longer the arterial hypertension (about 200 mmHg), the higher the water content. A vascular component of hypoxic brain swelling caused by disturbed autoregulation is also assumed by LANGFITT et al. (1970). In the case of local cold injuries of the cortex, local accumulation of edema fluid in the extravascular space appears, enlarges the volume of the affected tissue and increases the local tissue pressure. Regional cerebral blood flow in such regions is closely related to its water content, as documented by MEINIG et al. (1971/72), BRUCE et al. (1972) and MILLER et al. (1973). Moderate hypocapnia increased the local circulation through the edematous area, whereas pronounced hypocapnia had an unfavorable effect on CBF in these regions (WALLENFANG et al., 1973).

Edema augments the cerebral vascular resistance in such a way that autoregulatory dilatation becomes ineffective. Dilating substances (e.g. increasing CO_2 in the inspired air) increase the filtration of fluid into the edema and into the border zone of the edematous focus (BETZ and KOZAK, 1967). An attempt has been made to influence the development of edema by the infusion of osmotically active drugs (sorbitol or mannitol) (BETZ and ROOS, 1971; BETZ et al., 1972; SHALIT, 1972). The effect of these substances depends on the degree of the edema. REED and WOODBURY (1962a) demonstrated that hypertonic urea solution decreased the water content for about 5–6 h. CSF pressure is reduced for only 1–2 h because with the increase of urea concentration in the brain tissue the CSF content reaches its initial level again. The reason for the discrepancy in time is the relatively slow accumulation of urea in the brain tissue. If relatively high doses of hypertonic urea are applied, the initial steep osmotic gradient between blood and brain tissue causes a transport of H_2O from the brain into the blood. From the mode of H_2O variation REED and WOODBURY (1962b) concluded that the diffusion of H_2O in the brain tissue is not uniform. They concluded that there are compartments which lose their water relatively rapidly (e.g. the CSF space) and others from which the water is drained at a low rate. A result of this is a rapid initial decrease in the intracranial water content. The rapid diffusion of urea from the plasma into some compartments of the brain (extracellular space, CSF and some nerve cells) leads rapidly to an osmotic equilibrium between these brain compartments and the plasma, thus reducing the drainage of H_2O from these parts again to zero. On the other hand urea slowly penetrates other brain structures (e.g. glia cells) so that a concentration gradient from the extracellular space into the cells is maintained for some hours. The time and amplitude of the effective concentration gradient of urea determines the duration and the degree of reduction of the water content in the brain tissue. After some hours urea diffuses into the cells and when an equilibrium of the concentrations has been achieved the water content increases again.

K. Conclusion

In this article I have been guided by what seemed to me important lines of investigation in the pathophysiology of cerebral vascular disorders and in the problems which need animal experiments for understanding the mechanisms of dysregulation. Particular interest was shed upon such fields of investigation which seem to propose new points of view for a rational therapy of cerebral vascular disturbaces. When reviewing the very extensive literature, it became apparent that relatively little work has been done on conscious animals. There are numerous differences in the reactions of anesthetized and unanesthetized subjects. The recent and rapid development of methods for measuring CBF in conscious patients with a wide variety of cerebral vascular or metabolic disorders allows not only the recording of total CBF but also of local cerebral circulation. The use of animal experiments should therefore concentrate on those processes which can help to increase our understanding of the development and of the course of vascular diseases. Here the investigations on local tissue metabolism, on basic processes of the smooth muscle cells or on the problems of adaptation of vessels and tissue to abnormal conditions are taken as examples. In order to keep this article within a manageable size, a considerable selection both of topics and references was necessary.

References

ADLER, S., ANDERSON, B., ZEMOTEL, L.: Metabolic acid-base effects on tissue citrate content and metabolism in the rat. Amer. J. Physiol. **220**, 985–992 (1971).

ADOLPH, E. F.: Perspectives of adaptation: some general properties. In: Handbook of physiology, Sect. 4: Adaptation to the environment. Washington: Amer. Physiological Society 1964.

AGNOLI, A.: Adaptation of CBF during induced chronic normooxic respiratory acidosis. Scand. J. clin. Lab. Invest., Suppl. **102**, VII D (1968).

AGNOLI, A., BATTISTINI, N., NARDINI, M., PASSERO, S., FIESCHI, C.: Lack of adaptation of CBF and CSF pH in hypoxic hypercapnia. In: Cerebral blood flow. Berlin-Heidelberg-New York: Springer 1969a.

AGNOLI, A., BOZZAO, L., NARDINI, M., BATTISTINI, N., FIESCHI, C.: Adaptation of cerebral blood flow during induced chronic normooxic respiratory acidosis. In: Pharmakologie der lokalen Gehirndurchblutung. München-Gräfelfing: Werk-Verlag Dr. E. Banaschewski 1969b.

ALBAUM, H. G., CHINN, H. J.: Brain metabolism during acclimatization to high altitude. Amer. J. Physiol. **174**, 141–145 (1953).

ALEXANDER, S. C., COHEN, P. J., WOLLMAN, H., SMITH, T. C., REIVICH, M., MOLEN, R. A. VAN DER: Cerebral carbohydrate metabolism during hypocarbia in man. Anesthesiology **26**, 624–632 (1965).

ANTHONY, L. U., GOLDRING, S., O'LEARY, J., SCHWARTZ, H. G.: Experimental cerebrovascular occlusion in dog. Arch. Neurol. (Chic.) **8**, 515–526 (1963).

BAKAY, L., KOBAYASHI, T.: Cerebral isotope uptake in acute experimental hypercapnic hypoxia. Exp. Neurol. **32**, 303–312 (1971).

BALDY-MOULINIER, M.: Cerebral reflow after anoxia. In: Brain and blood flow. London: Pitman Medical and Scientific Publ. Co. Ltd. 1971.

BALDY-MOULINIER, M.: Cerebral blood flow and membrane ionic pump. Europ. Neurol. **6**, 107–113 (1971/72).

BALDY-MOULINIER, M.: Transport actif ionique et debit sanguin cérébral. Ann. Anesth. franç. Spécial **2**, 37–40 (1972).

BALDY-MOULINIER, M.: Comparative effects of various metabolic inhibitors on cerebral hemodynamics, electrical activity and cation transport. Stroke **4**, 375 (1973).

BARKER, J. N.: Local blood flow and local metabolic activity in aged rat brain. In: Cerebral blood flow and intracranial pressure, part I. Basel-München-Paris-London-New York-Sydney: S. Karger 1971/72.

BARNETT, H. J. M., WORTZMAN, G., GLADSTONE, R. M., LONGHEED, W. M.: Diversion and reversal of cerebral blood flow. Neurology (Minneap.) **20**, 1–14 (1970).

BARTKO, D.: Experimental brain hypoxia. Baltimore-London-Tokyo: University Park Press 1971.

BAUST, W., NIEMCZYK, H., SCHAEFER, H.: Die Beeinflussung des Liquordruckes durch akute hämodynamische Veränderungen. Z. ges. exp. Med. **136**, 619–629 (1963).

BAYLISS, W. M.: On the local reaction of the arterial wall to changes of internal pressure. J. Physiol. (Lond.) **28**, 220–231 (1902).

BENZINGER, TH., OPITZ, E., SCHOEDEL, W.: Durchblutung der Arteria carotis interna bei Sauerstoffmangel und Kohlensäureatmung. Luftfahrtmed. **3** (I), 46–54 (1938).

BERING, E. A.: Cerebrospinal fluid production and its relationship to cerebral metabolism and cerebral blood flow. Amer. J. Physiol. **197**, 825–828 (1959).

BERNSMEIER, A.: Probleme der Gehirndurchblutung. Z. Kreisl.-Forsch. **48**, 278–323 (1959).

BETZ, E.: Adaption of regional cerebral blood flow in animals exposed to chronic alterations of pO_2 and pCO_2. Acta neurol. scand., Suppl. **14**, 120–128 (1965a).

BETZ, E.: Umstellungsreaktionen der Gehirndurchblutung bei chronischem Lärm. Arch phys. Ther. (Lpz.) **17**, 61–65 (1965b).

BETZ, E.: Spontane Schwankungen der Gehirndurchblutung in Narkose und im Wachzustand. Ärztl. Forsch. **21**, 88–93 (1967).

BETZ, E.: Autoregulation of cerebral blood flow studied in the brain of the cat. In: Blood flow through organs and tissues. Edinburgh: Livingstone 1968a.

BETZ, E.: Zur Pathophysiologie der Sauerstoffversorgung. Z. prakt. Anästh. Wiederbeleb. **3**, 261–272 (1968b).

BETZ, E.: Die Hämodynamik des Gehirnkreislaufs bei lokalen Gehirndurchblutungsstörungen. Med. Welt (Stuttg.) **2**, 69–74 (1969a).

BETZ, E.: Influence of cerebrospinal fluid pH on the regulation of cerebral circulation. Int. Anaesthesiol. Clin. **7**, 525–537 (1969b).

BETZ, E.: Pharmakologie des Gehirnkreislaufs. In: Der Hirnkreislauf. Stuttgart: Thieme 1972a.

BETZ, E.: Pathophysiologische Aspekte zur metabolischen Beeinflussung der lokalen Gehirndurchblutung. Ideggyóg. Szle **25**, 493–502 (1972b).

BETZ, E.: Influence of O_2 and CO_2 variations on the coordination of EEG, CBF and energy-rich phosphates in brain tissue. In: Handbook of EEG and Clin. Neurophysiol., vol. 7, Part B, 7B28–7B45 (1973).

BETZ, E., BRAASCH, D., HENSEL, H.: Messung der Myocarddurchblutung mit der Wärmeleitsonde bei Einwirkung von 2,6-Bis(diaethylamino)-4,8-dipiperidino-pyrimido(5,4-d)pyrimidin (Persantin). Verh. dtsch. Ges. Kreisl.-Forsch. **27**, 321–326 (1961).

BETZ, E., ENZENROSS, H. G., VLAHOV, V.: Interaction of H^+ and Ca^{++} in the regulation of local pial vascular resistance. Pflügers Arch. **343**, 79–88 (1973).

BETZ, E., HEUSER, D.: Cerebral cortical blood flow during changes of acid-base equilibrium of the brain. J. appl. Physiol. **23**, 726–733 (1967).

BETZ, E., KOZAK, R.: Der Einfluß der Wasserstoffionenkonzentration der Gehirnrinde auf die Regulation der corticalen Durchblutung. Pflügers Arch. ges. Physiol. **293**, 56–67 (1967).

BETZ, E., KRUG, A., SCHMAHL, F. W.: Die lokale Myocarddurchblutung bei Ligatur von Koronargefäßen. Verh. dtsch. Ges. Kreisl.-Forsch. **30**, 273–279 (1964).

BETZ, E., ROOS, W.: CBF, brain tissue volume and CSF pressure. In: Brain and blood flow. London: Pitman Medical and Scientific Publish. Co. Ltd. 1971.

BETZ, E., ROOS, W., VAMOSI, B., WEIDLER, R.: Subarachnoid pressure dependent drug effect on CSF transport and brain volume. In: Intracranial pressure. Berlin-Heidelberg-New York: Springer 1972.

BETZ, E., SCHMAHL, F. W.: Durchblutung und Sauerstoffdruck in der Gehirnrinde bei Carotisdrosselung und ihre Beeinflussung durch Pharmaka. Pflügers Arch. ges. Physiol. **287**, 368–384 (1966).

BLAIR, R. D. G., WALTZ, A. G.: Regional cerebral blood flow during acute ischemia. Correlation of autoradiographic measurements with observations of cortical microcirculation. Neurology (Minneap.) **20**, 802–808 (1970).

Böning, U.: Der Einfluß von extrazellulären Kalium-, Calcium- und Magnesiumionen auf den Durchmesser pialer Arteriolen. Tübingen: Dissertation 1972.
Bondy, St. C., Morelos, B. S.: Stimulus deprivation and cerebral blood flow. Exp. Neurol. **31**, 200–206 (1971).
Bovet, D., Carpi, A., Virno, M.: Pharmacodynamic de la circulation cérébrale. Experientia (Basel) **16**, 1–20 (1960).
Brierley, J. B., Salford, L. G., Siesjö, B. K., Plum, F.: Moderate hypoxic ischemia irreversibly damages rat brain in 30 min. Stroke **4**, 339 (1973).
Brock, M., Fieschi, C., Ingvar, D. H., Lassen, N. A., Schürmann, K.: Cerebral blood flow. Berlin-Heidelberg-New York: Springer 1969.
Brodersen, P., Paulson, O. B., Bolwig, T. G., Rogon, Z. E., Rafaelsen, O. J., Lassen, N. A.: On the mechanism of cerebral hyperemia in electrically induced epileptic seizures in man. Stroke **4**, 359–360 (1973).
Brown, A. S., Donaldson, A. A.: Clinical vertebral artery cerebral blood flow measurement. In: Cerebral blood flow and intracranial pressure, part I. Basel-München-Paris-London-New York-Sydney: S. Karger 1971/72.
Bruce, D. A., Vapalahti, M., Schütz, H., Langfitt, T. W.: rCBF, $CMRO_2$ and intracranial pressure following a local cold injury of the cortex. In: Intracranial pressure. Berlin-Heidelberg-New York: Springer 1972.
Bühlmann, A., Hossli, G., Hunziker, A.: Respiratorische Acidose und Kreislauf mit besonderer Berücksichtigung des Gehirnkreislaufes. Schweiz. med. Wschr. **90**, 7–21 (1960)-
Bülbring, E.: Electrical activity in intestinal smooth muscle. Physiol. Rev. **42**, Suppl. 5, 160–178 (1962).
Bunce, D. F. M.: Survival of dogs following section of carotid and vertebral arteries. Proc. Soc. Exp. Biol. (N.Y.) **103**, 581–585 (1960).
Carpi, A.: Pharmacology of the cerebral circulation. In: Int. Encyclopedia of pharmacology and therapeutics, sect. 33, vol. I. Oxford-New York-Toronto-Sydney-Braunschweig: Pergamon Press 1972.
Carpi, A., Cartoni, C.: Central nervous system stimulants. In: Int. Encyclopedia of pharmacology and therapeutics, sect. 33, vol. I. Oxford-New York-Toronto-Sydney-Braunschweig: Pergamon Press 1972.
Carrato-Ibanez, A., Abadia-Fenoll, F.: Morphology and origin of the perivascular fibers in the brain substance. Angiology **17**, 771–784 (1966).
Chornyak, J.: The structural changes produced in the human brain by oxygen deprivation (anoxemia) and their pathogenesis. Thesis, University of Pennsylvania School of Medicine. Ann Arbor, Michigan: Edwards Brothers, Inc. 1938.
Chorobski, J., Penfield, W.: Cerebral vasodilator nerves and their pathway from the medulla oblongata. Arch. Neurol. Psychiat. (Chic.) **28**, 1257 (1932).
Cohen, P. H.: The effects of decreased oxygen tension on cerebral circulation, metabolism and function. In: Proc. of the Int. Symposium on the cardiovascular and respiratory effects of hypoxia. Basel-New York: S. Karger 1965.
Cohen, P. J., Alexander, S. C., Wollman, H.: Effect of hypocarbia and of hypoxia with normocarbia on cerebral blood flow and metabolism. Scand. J. Lab. clin. Invest., Suppl. **102**, IV A (1968).
Cooper, R., Hulme, A.: The interdependence of cerebrovascular autoregulation and intracranial pressure. In: Intracranial pressure. Berlin-Heidelberg-New York: Springer 1972.
Courtice, F. C.: The effect of raised intracranial pressure on the cerebral blood flow. J. Neurol. Psychiat. **3**, 293–305 (1940).
Cranston, W. J., Rosendorff, C.: Local blood flow, cerebrovascular autoregulation and CO_2 responsiveness in the rabbit hypothalamus. J. Physiol. (Lond.) **215**, 577–590 (1971).
Cushing, H.: Concerning a definite regulating mechanism of the vasomotor centre which controls blood pressure during cerebral compression. Johns Hopk. Hosp. Bull. **12**, 290–292 (1901).
Cushing, H.: Some experimental and clinical observations concerning states of increased intracranial tension. Amer. J. med. Sci. **124**, 375–400 (1902).
Czopf, J., Molnar, L.: Studies of problems in regulating the cerebral blood flow. II: Effect of cerebral trunk excitation on the blood flow of the stimulated area. Acta physiol. Acad. Sci. hung. **37**, 99–111 (1970).
Dahl, E., Nelson, E.: Electron microscopic observations on human intercranial arteries: II. Innervation. Arch. Neurol. (Chic.) **10**, 158–164 (1964).
Dahl, N. A., Balfour, W. M.: Prolonged anoxia survival due to anoxia pre-exposure: brain adenosine triphosphate, lactate, and pyruvate. Amer. J. Physiol. **207**, 452–456 (1964).
Davies, P. W., Grenell, R. G., Bronk, D. W.: The time course of *in vivo* oxygen consumption of cerebral cortex following electrical stimulation. Fed. Proc. **7**, 25 (1948).

DAVIES, P. W., REMOND, A.: Oxygen consumption of the cerebral cortex of the cat during metrazole convulsions. Res. Publ. Ass. nerv. ment. Dis. **26**, 205–217 (1946).

DAWEKE, H., HAHN, F., OBERDORF, A.: Einfluß von barbituratantagonistischen Analepticis auf EEG, Sauerstoffaufnahme und Durchblutung des Gehirns bei schwerer Veronalvergiftung des Hundes. Naunyn-Schmiedebergs Arch. exp. Path. Pharmak. **235**, 247–260 (1959).

DENNY-BROWN, D., MEYER, J. S.: The cerebral collateral circulation. 2. Production of cerebral infarction by ischemic anoxia and its reversibility in early stages. Neurology (Minneap.) **7**, 567–579 (1957).

DETAR, R., BOHR, D. F.: Adaptation to hypoxia in vascular smooth muscle. Fed. Proc. **27**, 1416–1419 (1968).

DICKINSON, C. J., MCCUBBIN, J. W.: Pressor effect of increased cerebrospinal fluid pressure and vertebral artery occlusion with and without anesthesia. Circulat. Res. **12**, 190 202 (1963).

DIEMER, K.: Über die Sauerstoffdiffusion im Gehirn. II. Mitt. Die Sauerstoffdiffusion bei O_2-Mangelzuständen. Pflügers Arch. ges. Physiol. **285**, 109–118 (1965).

DIEMER, K., HENN, R.: Kapillarvermehrung in der Hirnrinde der Ratte unter chronischem Sauerstoffmangel. Naturwissenschaften **52**, 135–136 (1965).

DITTMAR, H. A., MECHELKE, K., NUSSER, E.: Über die Blutdruck- und Flußänderungen in der Art. carotis communis und Aorta ascendens nach Arterenol und Adrenalin sowie deren Beeinflussung durch Regitin. Naunyn-Schmiedebergs Arch. exp. Path. Pharmak. **223**, 75–88 (1954).

DÖRING, H. J., OLBRISCH, R. R. (unter der Mitarb. v. J. SCHRADER und H. LANG): Elektrocardiogramm, Bestandpotential des Gehirns und energiereiche Phosphatfraktionen der Hirnrinde bei Narkotikum-Überdosierung, Ischämie und Cyanidvergiftung. Pflügers Arch. **319**, 12–35 (1970).

DORNDORF, W., GÄNSHIRT, H.: Die Klinik der arteriellen zerebralen Gefäßverschlüsse. In: Der Hirnkreislauf. Stuttgart: Thieme 1972.

EKLOF, B., INGVAR, D. H., KAGSTROM, E., OLIN, T.: Persistence of cerebral blood flow autoregulation following chronic bilateral cervical sympathectomy in the monkey. Acta physiol. scand. **82**, 172–176 (1971).

EKLOF, B., SIESJØ, B. K.: Cerebral blood flow and cerebral energy states. Acta physiol. scand. **82**, 409–411 (1971).

EKSTRÖM-JODAL, B., HÄGGENDAL, E.: Cerebral blood flow in patients with chronic respiratory insufficiency, with special regard to induced acute changes of the blood gas situation. In: Cerebral blood flow. Berlin-Heidelberg-New York: Springer 1969.

EKSTRÖM-JODAL, B., HÄGGENDAL, E., LINDER, L. E., NILSSON, N. J.: Cerebral blood flow autoregulation and high arterial pressures and different levels of carbon dioxide tension in dogs. In: Cerebral blood flow and intracranial pressure. Europ. Neurol. **6**, 6–10 (1971/72).

EKSTRÖM-JODAL, B., HÄGGENDAL, E., NILSSON, N. J.: Cerebral venous oxygen saturation during rapid changes in the arterial blood pressure: An oximetric study in dogs. Acta physiol. scand. **80**, Suppl. 350, 43–50 (1970).

ELDRIDGE, F., SALZER, J.: Effect of respiratory alkalosis on blood lactate and pyruvate in humans. J. appl. Physiol. **22**, 461–468 (1967).

ERKHOV, I. S.: Material on innervation of the intracerebral vessels. In: Vascular diseases of the brain, No 2, Proc. of the 4th All-Union-Congress of Neuropathologists and Psychiatrists, vol. 2, Moscow, p. 333–336 (1965).

FALCK, B., MCHEDLISHVILI, G. I., OWMAN, C.: Histochemical demonstration of adrenergic nerves in cortex-pia of rabbit. Acta pharmacol. (Kbh.) **23**, 133–142 (1965).

FEIN, J. M.: Focal autoregulatory disturbances in middle cerebral artery vasospasm. Stroke **4**, 333–334 (1973).

FEINDEL, W.: Discussion on cerebral ischemia. In: Cerebral vascular diseases. New York-London: Grune & Stratton 1968.

FEINDEL, W., HODGE, C. P., YAMAMOTO, Y. L.: Epicerebral angiography by fluorescein during craniotomy. Progr. Brain Res. **30**, 471–477 (1968).

FEINDEL, W., YAMAMOTO, Y. L., HODGE, C. P.: The human cerebral microcirculation studied by intra-arterial radio-active tracers, coomassie blue and fluorescein dyes. 4th Europ. Conference on Microcirculation. Cambridge 1966.

FEINDEL, W., YAMAMOTO, Y. L., HODGE, C. P.: Intracarotid fluorescein angiography: A new method for examination of the epicerebral circulation in man. Canad. med. Ass. J. **96**, 1–7 (1967).

FENCL, V., VALE, J. R., BROCH, J. A.: Respiration and cerebral blood flow in metabolic acidosis and alkalosis in humans. J. appl. Physiol. **27**, 67–76 (1969).

FERRIS, E. B., JR.: Objective measurement of relative intracranial blood flow in man with observations concerning the hydrodynamics of the craniovertebral system. Arch. Neurol. Psychiat. (Chic.) **46**, 377–401 (1941).

FIELDS, W. S., BRUETMAN, M. E., WEIBEL, J.: Collateral circulation of the brain. In: Monographs in the surgical sciences, vol. 2. Baltimore: Williams & Wilkins 1965.
FIESCHI, C.: Iperemia reattiva cerebrale focale nelle lesioni ischemiche. Sist. nerv. **18**, 215–220 (1966).
FIESCHI, C.: Fisiologia della circolazione cerebrale. Soc. Ital. Di Cardiol. **1**, 63–94 (1967).
FIESCHI, C.: Regional cerebral blood flow in acute apoplexy, including pharmacodynamic studies. Scand. J. clin. Lab. Invest., Suppl. **102**, XVI: E (1968).
FIESCHI, C.: Cerebral blood flow and intracranial pressure. Basel-München-Paris-London-New York-Sydney: S. Karger I, II 1972.
FIESCHI, C., AGNOLI, A., BATTISTINI, N., BOZZAO, L.: Regional cerebral blood flow in patients with brain infarcts. Arch. Neurol. (Chic.) **15**, 653–663 (1966).
FIESCHI, C., AGNOLI, A., BATTISTINI, N., BOZZAO, L., PRENCIPE, M.: Derangement of regional cerebral blood flow and of its regulatory mechanisms in acute cerebrovascular lesions. Neurology (Minneap.) **18**, 1166–1179 (1968a).
FIESCHI, C., BATTISTINI, N., NARDINI, M.: Experimental cerebral infarction: Focal or perifocal reactive hyperemia and its relationship with the red softening. 4th Int. Symposium of the research group on cerebral circulation. Salzburg 1968b.
FIESCHI, C., BOZZAO, L., AGNOLI, A.: Regional clearance of hydrogen as a measure of cerebral blood flow. Acta neurol. scand., Suppl. **14**, 46–52 (1965).
FIESCHI, C., BOZZAO, L., AGNOLI, A., NARDINI, M., BARTOLINI, A.: The hydrogen method to measure local blood flow in subcortical structures of the brain with a comparative study with the ^{14}C-antipyrine method. Exp. Brain Res. **7**, 111–119 (1969).
FIESCHI, C., ISAACS, G., KETY, S. S.: On the question of heterogeneity of the local blood flow in gray matter of the brain. In: Blood flow through organs and tissues. Edinburgh: Livingstone 1968c.
FISCHER, C. M.: Concerning recurrent transient cerebral ischemia attacks. Canad. med. Ass. J. **86**, 1091–1099 (1962).
FITCH, W., BARKER, J., McDOWALL, D. G., JENNETT, W. B.: The effect of methoxyflurane on cerebrospinal fluid pressure in patients with and without intracranial space-occupying lesions. Brit. J. Anaesth. **41**, 564–573 (1969).
FLOREY, H.: Microscopical observation on the circulation of the blood in the cerebral cortex. Brain **48**, 43–64 (1925).
FOG, M.: Cerebral circulation. The reaction of the pial arteries to a fall in blood pressure. Arch. Neurol. Psychiat. (Chic.) **37**, 351–364 (1937).
FOG, M.: The relationship between the blood pressure and the tonic regulation of the pial arteries. J. Neurol. Psychiat. **1**, 187–197 (1938).
FOG, M.: Cerebral circulation. II. Reaction of pial arteries to increase in blood pressure. Arch. Neurol. Psychiat. (Chic.) **41**, 260–268 (1939).
FOLKOW, B.: Intravascular pressure as a factor regulating the tone of the small vessels. Acta physiol. scand. **17**, 289–310 (1949).
FOLKOW, B.: Description of the myogenic hypothesis. Circulat. Res. **15**, Suppl. 279–287 (1964).
FORBES, H. S., NASON, G. I., WORTMAN, R. C.: Cerebral circulation XLIV. Vasodilation in the pia following stimulation of the vagus, aortic and carotid sinus nerves. Arch. Neurol. Psychiat. (Chic.) **37**, 334–350 (1937).
FORBES, H. S., WOLFF, H. G.: Cerebral circulation III. The vasomotor control of cerebral vessels. Arch. Neurol. psychiat. (Chic.) **19**, 1057–1085 (1928).
FREEMAN, J., INGVAR, D. H.: Elimination of the cerebral blood flow—EEG relationship and autoregulation by hypoxia. In: Blood flow through organs and tissues. Edinburgh-London: Livingstone 1968a.
FREEMAN, J., INGVAR, D. H.: Elimination by hypoxia of cerebral autoregulation and EEG relationship. Exp. Brain Res. **5**, 61–71 (1968b).
FUJISHIMA, M.: Effect of constrictory carotid arteries on cerebral blood flow and on cerebrospinal fluid pH, lactate and pyruvate in dogs. Jap. Heart J. **12**, 467–473 (1971).
FUJISHIMA, M., SCHEINBERG, P., BUSTO, R.: Cerebral cortical blood flow: Variable effects of hypoxia in the dog. Arch. Neurol. (Chic.) **25**, 160–168 (1971).
GÄNSHIRT, H.: Die Sauerstoffversorgung des Gehirns und ihre Störung bei der Liquordrucksteigerung und beim Hirnoedem. Berlin-Göttingen-Heidelberg: Springer 1957.
GÄNSHIRT, H.: Der Hirnkreislauf. Stuttgart: Thieme 1972.
GÄNSHIRT, H., DRANSFELD, L., ZYLKA, W.: Das Hirnpotentialbild und der Erholungsrückstand am Warmblütergehirn nach kompletter Ischämie. Arch. Psychiat. u. Z. Neurol. **189**, 109–125 (1952a).
GÄNSHIRT, H., POECK, K., SCHLIEP, H., VETTER, K., GÄNSHIRT, L.: Durchblutung und Sauerstoffversorgung des Gehirns im Elektrokrampf bei Katze und Hund. Arch. Psychiat. Nervenkr. **198**, 601–621 (1959).

GÄNSHIRT, H., SEVERIN, G., ZYLKA, W.: Die Erholungslatenz des Warmblütergehirns nach kompletter Ischämie. Pflügers Arch. ges. Physiol. **256**, 219–233 (1952b).
GASKELL, P., BURTON, A. C.: Local postural vasomotor reflexes arising from the limb veins. Circulat. Res. **1**, 27–39 (1953).
GEHA, A. S., SALAYMEH, M. T., ABE, T., BAUE, A. E.: Effects of occlusion of the brachiocephalic vessels on cerebral metabolism in the dog. J. surg. Res. **11**, 471–476 (1971).
GEVERS, W., DOWDLE, E.: The effect of pH on glycolysis in vitro. Clin. Sci. **25**, 343–349 (1963).
GIBBS, F. A.: Cerebral blood flow preceding and accompanying experimental convulsions. Arch. Neurol. Psychiat. (Chic.) **30**, 1003–1010 (1933a).
GIBBS, F. A.: A thermoelectric blood flow recorder in the form of a needle. Proc. Soc. exp. Biol. (N.Y.) **31**, 141–146 (1933b).
GIBBS, F. A., GIBBS, E. L., LENNOX, W. G.: Changes in human cerebral blood flow consequent on alterations in blood gases. Amer. J. Physiol. **111**, 557–563 (1935).
GIBBS, F. A., LENNOX, W. G., GIBBS, E. L.: Cerebral blood flow preceding and accompanying epileptic seizures in man. Arch. Neurol. Psychiat. (Chic.) **32**, 257–272 (1934).
GIBBS, F. A., NIMS, L. F., GIBBS, E. L.: Differentiation of the effects of low carbon dioxide on the electrical activity of the cortex. Fed. Proc. **1**, 29–30 (1942).
GLEICHMANN, U., INGVAR, D. H., LÜBBERS, D. W., SIESJÖ, K. B., THEWS, G.: Tissue pO_2 and pCO_2 of the cerebral cortex related to blood gas tensions. Acta physiol. scand. **55**, 127–138 1962).
GOLDENSON, E. S., WHITEHEAD, R. W., PARRY, T. M., SPENCER, J. H., GROVER, R. F., DRAPER, W. B.: Effect of diffusion respiration and high concentrations of CO_2 on cerebrospinal fluid pressure of anaesthetized dogs. Amer. J. Physiol. **165**, 334–340 (1951).
GOLLWITZER-MEIER, K., ECKHARDT, P.: Weitere Untersuchungen über den Nerveneinfluß auf die Hirndurchblutung. Naunyn-Schmiedebergs Arch. exp. Path. Pharmak. **177**, 501–518 (1935).
GOTOH, F., MEYER, J. S., TAKAGI, J.: Cerebral effects of hyperventilation in man. Arch. Neurol. (Chic.) **12**, 410–423 (1965).
GOTOH, F., TAZAKI, Y., MEYER, J. S.: Transport of gases through brain and their extravascular vasomotor action. Exp. Neurol. **4**, 48–58 (1961).
GOTTSTEIN, U.: Der Hirnkreislauf unter dem Einfluß vasoaktiver Substanzen. Einzeldarstellungen aus der theoret. u. klin. Medizin, Bd. 15. Heidelberg: Hüthig-Verlag 1962.
GOTTSTEIN, U.: The effect of drugs on cerebral blood flow especially in patients of older age. Pharmakopsychiat., Neuropsychopharmakol. **2**, 100–109 (1969).
GOTTSTEIN, U.: Was ist gesichert in der medikamentösen Behandlung zerebraler Zirkulationsstörungen? Med. Klin. **68**, 947–951 (1973).
GOTTSTEIN, U., BERNSMEIER, A., LEHN, H., NIEDERMAYER, W.: Hämodynamik und Stoffwechsel des Gehirns bei Schlafmittelvergiftung. Dtsch. med. Wschr. **86**, 2170–2176 (1961).
GRANHOLM, L., LUKJANOVA, L., SIESJÖ, B. K.: The effect of marked hyperventilation upon tissue levels of NADH, lactate, pyruvate, phosphocreatine and adenosine phosphates of rat brain. Acta physiol. scand. **75**, 1–12 (1969).
GRANHOLM, L., SIESJÖ, B. K.: Signs of cerebral hypoxia in hyperventilation. Experientia (Basel) **24**, 337–338 (1968).
GRANT, F. C., SPITZ, E. B., SHENKIN, H. A., SCHMIDT, C. F., KETY, S. S.: The cerebral blood flow and metabolism in idiopathic epilepsy. Trans. Amer. neurol. Ass. **72**, 82–86 (1947).
GREGERSEN, M. I.: Discussion remark. In: Schock, Pathogenese und Therapie. Berlin-Göttingen-Heidelberg: Springer 1962.
GROTE, J., KREUSCHER, H., SCHUBERT, R., RUSS, H. J.: Investigations on the influence of PaO_2 and $PaCO_2$ on the regulation of cerebral blood flow in dogs. In: Brain and blood flow. London: Pitman 1971.
HÄGGENDAL, E.: Elimination of autoregulation during arterial and cerebral hypoxia. Scand. J. clin. Lab. Invest., Suppl. **102**, v:D (1968).
HÄGGENDAL, E., JOHANSSON, B.: Effects of arterial carbon dioxide tension and oxygen saturation on cerebral blood flow autoregulation in dogs. Acta physiol. scand. **66**, Suppl. 258, 27–53 (1966).
HÄGGENDAL, E., LÖFGREN, J., NILSSON, N. J., ZWETNOW, N.: Prolonged reactive hyperemia after periods of increased cerebrospinal fluid pressure. Acta neurol. scand. **43**, 239–256 (1967).
HÄGGENDAL, E., LÖFGREN, J., NILSSON, N. J., ZWETNOW, N.: Influence of induced changès in the cerebrospinal fluid pressure on the cerebral blood flow of dogs. In: Research on the cerebral circulation. Springfield, Ill.: Thomas 1969.
HÄGGENDAL, E., LÖFGREN, J., NILSSON, N. J., ZWETNOW, N.: Effects of varied cerebrospinal fluid pressure on cerebral blood flow in dogs. Acta physiol. scand. **79**, 262–271 (1970).
HAINING, J. L., TURNER, M. D., PANTALL, R. M.: Local cerebral blood flow in young and old rats during hypoxia and hypercapnia. Amer. J. Physiol. **218**, 1020–1024 (1970).

Halsey, J. H., Jr.: Some regional circulatory abnormalities following experimental cerebral infarction. Neurology (Minneap.) **20**, 238–246 (1970).
Halsey, J. H., Capra, N. F.: Intracranial pressure, luxury perfusion, and progression of experimental cerebral infarction. In: Cerebral blood flow and intracranial pressure. Europ. Neurol. **6**, 296–300 (1971/72).
Handa, I., Ishikawa, S., Huber, P., Meyer, J. S.: Experimental production of the "subclavian steal": electromagnetic flow measurements in the monkey. Surgery **58**, 703–712 (1965).
Hansen, D. B., Sultzer, M. R., Freygang, W. H., Sokoloff, L.: Effects of low O_2 and high CO_2 concentrations in inspired air on local cerebral circulation. Fed. Proc. **16**, 54 (1959).
Harper, A. M.: Physiology of cerebral blood flow. Brit. J. Anaesth. **37**, 225–235 (1965).
Harper, A. M.: Autoregulation of cerebral blood flow: influence of the arterial blood pressure on the blood flow through the cerebral cortex. J. Neurol. Neurosurg. Psychiat. **29**, 398–403 (1966).
Harper, A. M.: Regulation of cerebral circulation. In: The scientific basis of medicine. Annual reviews. London: Athlone Press 1969.
Harper, A. M., Bell, R. A.: The effect of metabolic acidosis and alkalosis on the blood flow through the cerebral cortex. J. Neurol. Neurosurg. Psychiat. **26**, 341–344 (1963).
Harper, A. M., Glass, H. I.: Effect of alterations in the arterial carbon dioxide tension on the blood flow through the cerebral cortex at normal and low arterial blood pressures. J. Neurol. Neurosurg. Psychiat. **28**, 449–452 (1965).
Harper, A. M., Rowan, J. O., Deshmukh, V. D., Jennett, W. B.: Studies on possible neurogenic influences on the cerebral circulation. In: Brain and blood flow. London: Pitman 1971.
Harper, J. A., Colding, A. L., Mazzei, E. A.: An experimental hemodynamic study of the subclavian steal syndrome. Surg. Gynec. Obstet. **124**, 1212–1218 (1967).
Hassin, G. B.: The nerve supply of the cerebral blood vessels: a histologic study. Arch. Neurol. Psychiat. (Chic.) **22**, 375–391 (1929).
Heiss, W.-D., Kvicala, V., Prosenz, P., Tschabitscher, H.: Gamma-camera and multichannel analyser for multilocular rCBF measurement. In: Cerebral blood flow. Berlin-Heidelberg-New York: Springer 1969.
Heiss, W.-D., Prosenz, P., Gloning, K., Tschabitscher, H.: Regional and total cerebral blood flow under vasodilating drugs. In: Brain and blood flow. London: Pitman 1971.
Hekmatpanah, J.: Cerebral circulation and perfusion in experimental increased intracranial pressure. J. Neurosurg. **32**, 21–29 (1970).
Hekmatpanah, J.: Irreversible damage and cerebral death in increased intracranial pressure. In: Intracranial pressure. Berlin-Heidelberg-New York: Springer 1972.
Held, K., Gottstein, U., Niedermayer, W.: CBF in non-pulsatile perfusion. In: Cerebral blood flow. Berlin-Heidelberg-New York: Springer 1969.
Held, K., Jacobsen, O., Kraft, K., Berghoff, W.: Regional cerebral metabolism in experimental brain infarction. Stroke **4**, 331 (1973).
Hemmer, R.: Der Liquordruck. Untersuchungen zur Physiologie, Pathophysiologie und medikamentösen Beeinflussung der Liquordynamik. Stuttgart: Thieme 1960.
Herrmann, E.: Die allgemeinen und die herdförmigen, nicht blutungsbedingten Hirnzirkulationsstörungen. Habil.-Schr. Marburg 1964.
Heuser, D., Knabe, U., Gebert, G., Betz, E.: Reactions of pial vessels during variation of local perivascular ionic composition of the CSF. Europ. Neurol. **6**, 96–99 (1971/72).
Hill, L.: The physiology and pathology of the cerebral circulation. An experimental research. London: Churchill 1896.
Himwich, H., Himwich, H. E., Himwich, W. A., Etsten, B.: The functional organization of the central nervous system as observed in pentothal anesthesia. Report of the Int. Physiol. Congr. Jan. 15, 1947a.
Himwich, W. A., Homburger, E., Maresa, R., Himwich, H. E.: Brain metabolism in man: unanesthetized and in pentothal narcosis. Amer. J. Psychiat. **103**, 689–696 (1947b).
Hirsch, H.: Über die Abhängigkeit der Gehirndurchblutung von Blutdruck und die Wiederbelebungszeit des Gehirns. In: Diagnostik und Therapie der zerebralen Gefäßverschlüsse. Stuttgart: Thieme 1970.
Hirsch, H., Euler, K. H., Schneider, M.: Über die Erholung und Wiederbelebung des Gehirns nach Ischämie bei Normothermie. Pflügers Arch. ges. Physiol. **265**, 281–313 (1957a).
Hirsch, H., Euler, K. H., Schneider, M.: Über die Erholung des Gehirns nach kompletter Ischämie bei Hypothermie. Pflügers Arch. ges. Physiol. **265**, 314–327 (1957b).
Hirsch, H., Gleichmann, U., Kristen, H., Magazinovic, V.: Über die Beziehung zwischen O_2-Aufnahme des Gehirns und O_2-Druck im Sinusblut des Gehirns bei uneingeschränkter und eingeschränkter Durchblutung. Pflügers Arch. ges. Physiol. **273**, 213–222 (1961).

HIRSCH, H., KOCH, D., KRENKEL, W., SCHNEIDER, W.: Die Erholungslatenz des Warmblütergehirns bei Ischämie und die Bedeutung eines Restkreislaufs. Pflügers Arch. ges. Physiol. **261**, 392–401 (1955).

HIRSCH, H., KÖRNER, K.: Über die Druck-Durchblutungs-Relation der Gehirngefäße. Pflügers Arch. ges. Physiol. **280**, 316–325 (1964).

HIRSCH, H., OBERDÖRSTER, G., ZIMMER, R., BENNER, K. V., LANG, R.: The recovery of the electrocorticogram of normothermic canine brains after complete cerebral ischaemia. Exp. Brain Res. 1973/74 (in press).

HIRSCH, H., SCHNEIDER, M.: Durchblutung und Sauerstoffaufnahme des Gehirns. In: Handbuch der Neurochirurgie I/2. Berlin-Heidelberg-New York: Springer 1968.

HØEDT-RASMUSSEN, K.: Regional variations in cerebral blood flow in cerebrovascular disease studied under variations of blood pressure and arterial pCO_2. In: Research on the cerebral circulation. Springfield, Ill.: Thomas 1969.

HØEDT-RASMUSSEN, K., SKINHØJ, E., PAULSON, O., EWALD, J., BJERRUM, J. K., FAHRENKRUG, A., LASSEN, N. A.: Regional cerebral blood flow in acute apoplexy. The "luxury perfusion syndrome" of brain tissue. Arch. Neurol. (Chic.) **17**, 271–281 (1967).

HOLMQUIST, B., INGVAR, D. H., SIESJÖ, B.: Cerebral sympathetic vasoconstriction and EEG. Acta physiol. scand. **40**, 146–160 (1957).

HOMBURGER, W., HIMWICH, W. A., ETSTEN, B., YORK, G., MARESA, R., HIMWICH, H. E.: Effect of pentothal anesthesia on canine cerebral cortex. Amer. J. Physiol. **147**, 343–345 (1946).

HOSSMANN, K.-A., LECHTAPE-GRÜTER, H.: Blood flow and recovery of the cat brain after complete ischemia for 1 hour. In: Cerebral blood flow and intracranial pressure. Europ. Neurol. **6**, 318–322 (1971/72).

HUBER, G. C.: Observations on the innervation of the intracranial vessels. J. comp. Neurol. **9**, 1–25 (1899).

HUNTER, W.: On the presence of nerve fibres in the cerebral vessels. J. Physiol. (Lond.) **26**, 465–469 (1900/01).

IKEDA, M., FUJII, J., MURATA, K., TERASAWA, F., OZAWA, T., HOSODA, S., KURIHARA, H. KIMATA, S., OKINAKA, S.: Effect of angiotensin on cerebral circulation in unanesthetized rabbit. Jap. Circulat. J. (En.) **27**, 277–281 (1963).

INFANGER, P., LUGINBÜHL, H.: Arteriosclerosis and ischemic changes in the brains of swine of different age groups. In: Research on the cerebral circulation. 5th Int. Salzburg Conf. Springfield, Ill.: Thomas 1972.

INGVAR, D. H.: Cortical state of excitability and cortical circulation. In:Reticular formation of the brain. Boston, Mass.: Little & Brown 1958.

INGVAR, D. H.: The pathophysiology of the stroke related to findings in EEG and to measurements of regional cerebral blood flow. Stroke (1967) 105–122.

INGVAR, D. H.: Regional cerebral blood flow in cerebrovascular disorders. In: Cerebral circulation. Progr. in brain research, vol. 30. Amsterdam-London-New York: Elsevier 1968.

INGVAR, D. H.: Correlation between cerebral function and cerebral blood flow and its disappearance following anoxia. In: Pharmakologie der lokalen Gehirndurchblutung. München: Banaschewski 1969.

INGVAR, D. H., FRANZEN, G.: Abnormalities in chronic schizophrenia with mental deterioration. Stroke **4**, 553 (1973).

INGVAR, D. H., LASSEN, N. A., SIESJÖ, B. K., SKINHØJ, E.: CBF and CSF. 3rd int. Sympos. on cerebral blood flow and cerebrospinal fluid. Scand. J. clin. Lab. Invest., Suppl. **110** (1969).

INGVAR, D. H., LÜBBERS, D. W., SIESJÖ, B. K.: Normal and epileptic EEG patterns related to cortical oxygen tension in the cat. Acta physiol. scand. **55**, 210–224 (1962).

INGVAR, D. H., SÖDERBERG, K.: A direct method for the measurement of cerebral blood flow. Nature (Lond.) **177**, 339–340 (1956).

IWABUCHI, T., KAWAKAMI, H., UEMURA, K., KUTSUZAWA, T.: Regional cerebral blood flow in apoplexy measured by ^{133}Xe clearance method. Tohoku J. exp. Med. **104**, 1–11 (1971).

IWOYAMA, T., FURNESS, J. B., BURNSTOCK, G.: Dual adrenergic and cholinergic innervation of the arteries cerebral of the rat. An ultrastructural study. Circulat. Res. **26**, 635–646 (1970).

JACOBSON, I., HARPER, A. M., MCDOWALL, D. G.: Relationship between venous pressure and cortical blood flow. Nature (Lond.) **200**, 173–175 (1963).

JAMES, J. M., MILLAR, R. A., PURVES, M. J.: Observations on the extrinsic neural control of cerebral blood flow in the baboon. Circulat. Res. **25**, 77–93 (1969).

JANEWAY, R., CONRAD, M. C., TOOLE, J. F.: Chronic reversal of vertebral artery flow in the dog and its response to reactive hyperemia and change in body position. Neurology (Minneap.) **14**, 258 (1964).

JASPER, H. H., ERICKSON, T. C.: Cerebral blood flow and pH in excessive cortical discharge induced by metrazol and electrical stimulation. J. Neurophysiol. **4**, 333–347 (1941).
JENNETT, W. B., ROWAN, J. O., HARPER, A. M., JOHNSTON, I. H., MILLER, J. D., DESHMUKH, V. D.: Perfusion pressure and cerebral blood flow. In: Brain and blood flow. London: Pitman 1971.
JOHANSSON, B., BOHR, D. F.: Rhythmic activity in smooth muscle from small subcutaneous arteries. Amer. J. Physiol. **210**, 801–806 (1966).
JOHNSTON, I. H., ROWAN, J. O., HARPER, A. M., JENNETT, W. B.: Cerebral blood flow in experimental intracranial hypertension. In: Cerebral blood flow and intracranial pressure. Europ. Neurol. 8, 57–61 (1972).
KANZOW, E.: Diskussion. In: Pharmakologie der lokalen Gehirndurchblutung. München: Banaschweski 1969.
KANZOW, E., GREGL, I. M., HELD, U. P., RICHTERING, I.: Vasomotorische Reaktionen in der Großhirnrinde bei der EEG-Arousal. Pflügers Arch. ges. Physiol. **273**, 288–301 (1961).
KANZOW, E., KRAUSE, D.: Vasomotorik der Hirnrinde und EEG-Aktivität wacher, frei beweglicher Katzen. Pflügers ges. Arch. Physiol. **274**, 447–458 (1962).
KATO, M., TOOLE, J. F., ANAZAWA, W., JANEWAY, R.: Reversed vertebral effects of muscle contraction and hypercapnia. Arch. Neurol. (Chic.) **20**, 172–181 (1969).
KETY, S. S.: Cerebral circulation. In: Handbook of physiology. Washington: Amer. Physiol. Soc. 1961.
KETY, S. S., McDOWALL, R. J. S.: The control of the circulation of the blood. London: Dawson 1956.
KETY, S. S., SCHMIDT, C. F.: The effects of active and passive hyperventilation on cerebral blood flow, cerebral oxygen consumption, cardiac output and blood pressure of normal young men. J. clin. Invest. **25**, 107–119 (1946).
KETY, S. S., SCHMIDT, C. F.: The nitrous oxide method for the quantitative determination of cerebral blood flow in man: Theory, procedure and normal values. J. clin. Invest. **27**, 476–483 (1948a).
KETY, S. S., SCHMIDT, C. F.: The effects of altered arterial tensions of carbon dioxide and oxygen on cerebral flow and cerebral oxygen consumption of normal young men. J. clin. Invest. **27**, 484–492 (1948b).
KETY, S. S., SHENKIN, H. A., SCHMIDT, C. F.: The effects of increased intracranial pressure on cerebral circulatory effects in man. J. clin. Invest. **27**, 493–499 (1948a).
KETY, S. S., WOODFORD, R. B., HARMEL, M. H., FREYHAN, F. A., APPEL, K. E., SCHMIDT, C. F.: Cerebral blood flow and metabolism in schizophrenia: The effects of barbiturate seminarcosis, insulin coma and electro-shock. Amer. J. Psychiat. **104**, 765–770 (1948b).
KING, L. J., SCHOEPFLE, G. M., LOWRY, O. H., PASSONEAU, V., WILSON, S.: Effects of electrical stimulation on metabolites in brain of decapitated mice. J. Neurochem. **14**, 613–618 (1967).
KING, L. J., WEBB, O. L., CARL, J.: Effects of duration of convulsions on energy reserves of the brain. J. Neurochem. **17**, 13–18 (1970).
KJÄLLQUIST, A., SIESJÖ, B. K., ZWETNOW, N.: Effects of increased intracranial pressure on cerebral blood flow and on cerebrospinal fluid HCO_3, pH, lactate and pyruvate in dogs. Acta physiol. scand. **75**, 345–352 (1969).
KNABE, U., BETZ, E.: The effect of varying extracellular K^+-, Mg^{++}- and Ca^{++} on the diameter of pial arterioles. In: Vascular smooth muscle. Berlin-Heidelberg-New York: Springer 1972.
KOBAYASHI, K., KLEIHUES, P., HOSSMANN, K.-A., HOSSMANN, V.: Postischemic recovery of nucleotide metabolism in the cat brain. Stroke **4**, 340 (1973).
KOGURE, K., BUSTO, R., REINMUTH, O., SCHEINBERG, P.: Energy metabolites, water content and catecholamine changes in a model of cerebral embolic infarction. Stroke **4**, 331 (1973).
KOGURE, K., SCHEINBERG, P., FUJISHIMA, M., BUSTO, R., REINMUTH, O. M.: Effects of hypoxia on cerebral autoregulation. Amer. J. Physiol. **219**, 1393–1396 (1970b).
KOGURE, K., SCHEINBERG, P., REINMUTH, O. M., FUJISHIMA, M., BUSTO, R.: Mechanisms of cerebral vasodilatation in hypoxia. J. appl. Physiol. **29**, 223–229 (1970a).
KONG, Y., MOLINARI, G., WHALEN, R. E., HEYMAN, A.: Acute hemodynamic changes during experimental cerebral embolism. Arch. Neurol. (Chic.) **16**, 433–439 (1967).
KRUPP, P.: Cerebrale Durchblutung und elektrische Hirnaktivität. Basel: Schwabe 1966.
KUSCHINSKY, W., WAHL, M.: Alpha-receptors at pial arteries in cats. Pflügers Arch. **343**, Suppl. R 24 (1973).
KUSCHINSKY, W., WAHL, M., BOSSE, O., THURAU, K.: The dependency of the pial arterial and arteriolar resistance on the perivascular H^+ and K^+ concentrations. In: Cerebral blood flow and intracranial pressure. Europ. Neurol. **6**, 92–95 (1971/72).
KUURNE, T., TROUPP, H., KASTE, M., VAPALAHTI, M.: Clinical and experimental intracranial pressure. In: Cerebral blood flow and intracranial pressure. Europ. Neurol. 8, 188–191 (1972).

LANDAU, W. M., FREYGANG, W. H., JR., ROWLAND, L. P., SOKOLOFF, L., KETY, S. S.: The local circulation of the living brain; values in the unanaesthetized and anaesthetized cat. Trans. Amer. neurol. Ass. **80**, 125–129 (1955).

LANGFITT, T. W., KASSELL, N. F., WEINSTEIN, J. D.: Cerebral blood flow with intracranial hypertension. Neurology (Minneap.) **15**, 761–773 (1965a).

LANGFITT, T. W., KUMAR, V., MILLER, J. D.: Cerebral oedema caused by anoxia and changes in intracranial vascular pressures. In: Brain and blood flow. London: Pitman Med. and Sci. Publ. Co. Ltd. 1971.

LANGFITT, T. W., MCHENRY, L. C., JR., REIVICH, M., WOLLMANN, H.: Cerebral circulation and metabolism. 6. Int. CBF Symp. Stroke **4** (1973).

LANGFITT, T. W., WEINSTEIN, J. D., KASSELL, N. F.: Cerebral vasomotor paralysis produced by intracranial hypertension. Neurology (Minneap.) **15**, 622–641 (1965b).

LASSEN, N. A.: Cerebral blood flow and oxygen consumption in man. Physiol. Rev. **39**, 183–238 (1959).

LASSEN, N. A.: On the regulation of cerebral blood flow in diseases of the brain with special regard to the "luxury perfusion syndrome" of brain tissue, i.e. a syndrome characterized by relative hyperemia or absolute hyperemia of the brain tissue. In: Progress in brain research, vol. 30. Amsterdam-London-New York: Elsevier 1968.

LASSEN, N. A., INGVAR, D. H.: Die regionale Durchblutung des Gehirns und ihre Störungen. Verh. dtsch. Ges. Kreisl.-Forsch. **39**, 10–22 (1973).

LASSEN, N. A., INGVAR, D. H.: The blood flow of the cerebral cortex determined by radioactive krypton^{85}. Experientia (Basel) **17**, 42–43 (1961).

LASSEN, N. A., INGVAR, D. H.: Neuere Erkenntnisse über die cerebrale Blutzirkulation (Pathophysiologie). Münch. med. Wschr. **110**, 1491–1493 (1968).

LASSEN, N. A., PALVÖLGYI, R.: Cerebral steal during hypercapnia and the inverse reaction during hypocapnia observed by the ^{133}Xenon technique in man. Scand. J. clin. Lab. Invest., Suppl. **102**, XIII D (1968).

LASSEN, N. A., PAULSON, O. B.: Partial cerebral vasoparalysis in patients with apoplexy: Dissociation between carbon dioxide responsiveness and autoregulation. In: Cerebral blood flow. Berlin-Heidelberg-New York: Springer 1969.

LEVER, J. D., SPRIGGS, T. L., GRAHAM, J. D.: A formol-fluorescence fine-structural and autoradiographic study of the adrenergic innervation of the vascular tree in the intact and sympathectomized pancreas of the cat. J. Anat. (Lond.) **103**, 15–34 (1968).

LEWIS, B. M., SOKOLOFF, S., WECHSLER, R. L., WENTZ, W. B., KETY, S. S.: A method for the continuous measurement of cerebral blood flow in man by means of radioactive krypton (Kr^{79}). J. clin. Invest. **39**, 707–716 (1960).

LEWIS, H. P., MCLAURIN, R. L.: Regional cerebral blood flow in increased intracranial pressure produced by increased cerebrospinal fluid volume, intracranial mass and cerebral edema. In: Intracranial pressure. Berlin-Heidelberg-New York: Springer 1972.

LJUNGGREN, B., GRANHOLM, L., SCHUTZ, H., SIESJÖ, B. K.: Energy state of the brain during and after compression ischemia. In: Intracranial pressure. Berlin-Heidelberg-New York: Springer 1972.

LJUNGGREN, B., SIESJÖ, B. K.: Cerebral metabolic state during postischemic "recovery". Stroke **4**, 343 (1973).

LAZORTHES, G.: Vascularisation et circulation cérébrale. Paris Masson et Cie Ed. 1961.

LOWE, R. D.: Chronic effects on blood pressure of bilateral carotid and vertebral ligation in the rabbit. Circulat. Res. **10**, 73–82 (1962).

LOWRY, O. H., PASSONEAU, J. V.: The relationships between substrates and enzymes of glycolysis in brain. J. biol. Chem. **239**, 32–42 (1964).

LOWRY, O. H., PASSONEAU, J. V., HASSELBERGER, F. X., SCHULZ, D. W.: Effect of ischemia on known substrates and cofactors of the glycolytic pathway in brain. J. biol. Chem. **239**, 18–30 (1964).

LUBSEN, N.: Experimental studies on the cerebral circulation of the unanaesthetized rabbit. I. Stimulation of the cervical sympathetic chain. Arch. néerl. Physiol. **25**, 287–305 (1940).

LUDWIGS, N., SCHNEIDER, M.: Über den Einfluß des Halssympathicus auf die Gehirndurchblutung. Pflügers Arch. ges. Physiol. **259**, 43–55 (1954).

LÜBBERS, D. W.: The oxygen pressure field of the brain and its significance for the normal and critical oxygen supply of the brain. In: Oxygen transport in blood and tissue. Stuttgart: Thieme 1968.

LÜBBERS, D. W.: Physiologie der Gehirndurchblutung. In: Der Hirnkreislauf. Stuttgart: Thieme 1972.

LÜBBERS, D. W., INGVAR, D. H., BETZ, E., FABEL, H., SCHMAHL, F.: Sauerstoffverbrauch der Großhirnrinde in Schlaf- und Wachzustand beim Hund. Pflügers Arch. ges. Physiol. **281**, 58 (1964).

LUGINBÜHL, H.: Comparative aspects of cerebrovascular disease and pathology in different species. In: Cerebral vascular diseases. Transactions of the 5th Princeton Conf. New York: Grune & Stratton 1966.

MANN, L. I.: Effect of hypoxia on fetal cephalic blood flow, cephalic metabolism, and the electroencephalogram. Exp. Neurol. **29**, 336–348 (1970).

MCCALL, M. L., TAYLOR, H. W.: Effects of morphine sulfate on cerebral circulation and metabolism in normal and toxemic pregnant women. Amer. J. Obstet. Gynec. **64**, 1131–1136 (1952).

MCDOWALL, D. G.: Cerebral circulation. Int. Anesthesiology Clinics **7**, No 3 (1969). Boston: Little, Brown 1969.

MCDOWALL, D. G., HARPER, A. M.: CBF and CSF-pH in the monkey during prolonged hypocapnia. Scand. J. clin. Lab. Invest., Suppl. **102**, VIII E (1968a).

MCDOWALL, D. G., HARPER, A. M.: The relationship between blood flow and extracellular pH of the cerebral cortex. In: Blood flow through organs and tissues. Edinburgh: Livingstone 1968b.

MCHEDLISHVILI, G. I.: Functional behaviour of the vascular mechanisms of the brain. Leningrad: Nauka 1968a.

MCHEDLISHVILI, G. I.: Vascular mechanisms of the brain. Library of Congress, Catalog Card 70141241 ISBN/0306–10870–4 1972. Consultants Bureau New York: A Division of Plenum Publ. Corp. New York 10011.

MCHEDLISHVILI, G. I., BARAMIDZE, D. G.: The functional behaviour of cortical blood vessels under conditions of the convulsive activity. Bull. exp. Biol. Med. **11**, 68–71 (1967).

MCHEDLISHVILI, G. I., BARAMIDZE, D. G., NIKOLAISHVILI, L. S.: Functional behaviour of pial and cortical arteries in conditions of increased metabolic demand from the cerebral cortex. Nature (Lond.) **213**, 506–507 (1967).

MCHENRY, L. C., JR., JAFFE, M. E., KENTON, E. J., COOPER, E. S., WEST, J. W., KAWAMURA, J., OSHIRO, T., GOLDBERG, H. I.: Vasodilator responsiveness. — Implications in cerebrovascular disease. In: Brain and blood flow. London: Pitman 1971.

MCHENRY, L. C., JR., SLOCUM, H. C., HAYES, G. J.: The effects of hyperventilation on the cerebral circulation and metabolism. Trans. Amer. neurol. Ass. **89**, 223–225 (1964).

MCILWAIN, H.: Depression by barbiturates of the metabolism of electronically stimulated cerebral tissues. Chem. Abstr. **46**, 8963 (1952).

MCLEDINGHAM, A., MCDOWALL, D. G., HARPER, A. M.: Cerebral cortical blood flow under hyperbaric conditions. III. Int. Conf. on hyperbaric Medicin. Washington: National Academy of Sciences 1966.

MEINIG, G., REULEN, H. J., HADJIDIMOS, A., SIEMON, C., BARTKO, D., SCHÜRMANN, K.: Induction of filtration edema by extreme reduction of cerebrovascular resistance associated with hypertension. In: Cerebral blood flow and intracranial pressure, part II. Basel-München-Paris-London-New York-Sydney: Karger 1971/72.

MEINIG, G., REULEN, H. J., MAGAVLY, C., HASE, U., HEY, O.: Changes of cerebral hemodynamics and energy metabolism during increased CSF pressure and brain edema. In: Intracranial pressure. Berlin-Heidelberg-New York: Springer 1972.

MERCKER, H., SCHNEIDER, M.: Über Capillarveränderungen des Gehirns bei Höhenanpassung. Pflügers Arch. ges. Physiol. **251**, 49–55 (1949).

MEYER, J. S., DENNY-BROWN, D.: The cerebral collateral circulation. 1. Factors influencing collateral blood flow. Neurology (Minneap.) **7**, 447–458 (1957).

MEYER, J. S., GOTOH, F.: Metabolic and electroencephalographic effects of hyperventilation. Experimental study of brain oxygen and carbon-dioxide tension, pH, EEG and blood flow during hyperventilation. Arch. Neurol. (Chic.) **3**, 539–552 (1960).

MEYER, J. S., GOTOH, F.: Interaction of cerebral hemodynamics and metabolism. Neurology (Minneap.) **11**, Suppl. 46–65 (1961).

MEYER, J. S., GOTOH, F., FAVALE, E.: Cerebral metabolism during epileptic seizures in man. Electroenceph. clin. Neurophysiol. **21**, 10–22 (1966).

MEYER, J. S., GOTOH, F., TAZAKI, Y.: Inhibitory action of carbon dioxide and acetazolamide in seizure activity. Electroenceph. clin. Neurophysiol. **13**, 762–775 (1961).

MEYER, J. S., KONDO, A., NOMURA, F., SAKAMOTO, K., TERAURA, T.: Cerebral hemodynamics and metabolism following brain trauma. Demonstration of luxury perfusion following brain-stem laceration. In: Cerebral blood flow. Berlin-Heidelberg-New York: Springer 1969a.

MEYER, J. S., NOMURA, F., SAKAMOTO, K., KONDO, A.: Effect of stimulation of the brain-stem reticular formation on cerebral blood flow and oxygen consumption. Electroenceph. clin. Neurophysiol. **26**, 125–132 (1969b).

MICHENFELDER, J. D., SUNDT, T. M., JR.: Cerebral ATP and lactate levels in the squirrel monkey following occlusion of the middle cerebral artery. Stroke **2**, 319–326 (1971).

MIKHAILOV, S. S.: Structural features of the cavernous sinus. In: Disturbances of the circulation in brain lesions. Moscow: 1956.
MILLER, J. D., GARIBI, J., NORTH, J. B., TEASDALE, G. M.: False autoregulation after cold injury to the cerebral cortex. Stroke **4**, 332 (1973).
MILLER, J. D., STANEK, A. E., LANGFITT, T. W.: A comparison of autoregulation to changes in intracranial and arterial pressure in the same preparation. In: Cerebral blood flow and intracranial pressure. Europ. Neurol. **6**, 34–38 (1971/72).
MINARD, F. N., DAVIS, R. V.: The effects of electroshock on the acid-soluble phosphates of rat brain. J. biol. Chem. **237**, 1283–1289 (1962).
MIYAZAKI, M.: Effect of undesirable sound (noise) on cerebral circulation. Jap. Circulat. J. (En.) **35**, 931–936 (1972).
MOLNAR, L.: Sur le contrôle nerveux de la circulation sanguine régionale des centres cerebraux. Budapest: Akadémiai Kiadó 1967.
MOLNAR, L., KOPA, J. K., POOR, G.: Studies of problems in regulating the cerebral blood flow. III. Recent data on the role of the cerebral trunk in the regulation of the brain blood flow. Acta physiol. Acad. Sci. hung. **37**, 113–124 (1970).
MOLNAR, L., SZANTO, J.: The effect of electrical stimulation of the bulbar vasomotor center on the cerebral blood flow. Quart. J. exp. Physiol. **49**, 184–193 (1964).
MOYER, J. H., MILLER, S. I., SNYDER, H.: Effect of increased jugular pressure on cerebral hemodynamics. J. appl. Physiol. **7**, 245–247 (1954).
MÜLLER, U., ISSELHARD, W., HINZEN, D. H., GEPPERT, E.: Regionaler Energiestoffwechsel im Kaninchengehirn während kompletter Ischämie in Normothermie. Pflügers Arch. **320**, 168–180 (1970).
MÜLLER-SCHAUENBURG, W.: Über einen Ansatz zur Trennung von Wärmeleitung und Wärmeabtransport durch das Blut — ein neues Verfahren zur quantitativen Messung der lokalen Gewebsdurchblutung. Dissertation, Tübingen 1972.
MÜLLER-SCHAUENBURG, W., BETZ, E.: Gas and heat clearance comparison and use of heat transport for quantitative local blood flow measurements. In: Cerebral blood flow. Berlin-Heidelberg-New York: Springer 1969.
NAGAI, H., FURUSE, M., BANNO, K., IKEYAMA, A., MAEDA, S., KUCHIWAKI, H.: Some adjustment mechanism of brain metabolism during increased intracranial pressure. In: Intracranial pressure. Berlin-Heidelberg-New York: Springer 1972a.
NAGAI, H., IKEYAMA, A., FURUSE, M., MAEDA, S., BANNO, K., HASUO, M., KUCHIWAKI, H.: Effect of increased intracranial pressure on cerebral hemodynamics. In: Cerebral blood flow and intracranial pressure. Europ. Neurol. **8**, 52–56 (1972b).
NAGAI, T., PROSSER, C. L.: Patterns of conduction in smooth muscle. Amer. J. Physiol. **204**, 910–914 (1963).
NAUNYN, B., SCHREIBER, J.: Über Gehirndruck. Naunyn-Schmiedebergs Arch. exp. Path. Pharmak. **14**, 1–112 (1881).
NELSON, E., RENNELS, M.: Electron microscopic studies on intracranial vascular nerves in the cat. Scand. J. clin. Lab. Invest., Suppl. **102**, VI A (1968).
NELSON, E., RENNELS, M. L., TAKAYANAGI, T.: Ultrastructural observations on the innervation of intracranial arteries. In: Brain and blood flow. London: Pitman 1971.
NEUMANN, L., BETZ, E., BENZING, H.: Wirkung einer Unterbindung der Arteria cerebri media auf Durchblutung, Sauerstoffdruck und Säure-Basen-Haushalt in deren Versorgungsgebiet. Int. Z. angew. Physiol. **29**, 29–43 (1970).
NIELSEN, K. C., OWMAN, C.: Adrenergic innvervation of pial arteries related to the circle of Willis in the cat (Fluorescent microscopy). Brain Res. **6**, 773–776 (1967).
NOELL, W.: Über die Durchblutung und die Sauerstoffversorgung des Gehirns. V. Mitteilung: Einfluß der Blutdrucksenkung. Pflügers Arch. ges. Physiol. **247**, 528–552 (1944).
NOELL, W., SCHNEIDER, M.: Über die Durchblutung und die Sauerstoffversorgung des Gehirns im akuten Sauerstoffmangel. III. Mitteilung: Die arterio-venöse Sauerstoff- und Kohlensäuredifferenz. Pflügers Arch. ges. Physiol. **246**, 207–249 (1942).
NOELL, W., SCHNEIDER, M.: Über die Durchblutung und die Sauerstoffversorgung des Gehirns. IV. Mitteilung: Die Rolle der Kohlensäure. Pflügers Arch. ges. Physiol. **247**, 514–527 (1944).
NOELL, W., SCHNEIDER, M.: Zur Hämodynamik der Gehirndurchblutung bei Liquordrucksteigerung. Arch. Psychiat. Nervenkr. **118**, 713–730 (1948).
NOTHNAGEL, H.: Die vasomotorischen Nerven der Gehirngefäße (Beitrag zur Lehre von der Epilepsie). Virchows Arch. path. Anat. **11**, 203–213 (1867).
NOVACK, P., KANDA, A., MILLS, L. C., KATZ, S., KATZ, R.: Effects of pentobarbital anesthesia upon cerebral blood flow and metabolism. Fed. Proc. **22**, 480 (1963).
NOVACK, P., SHENKIN, H. A., BORTIN, L., GOLUBOFF, B., SOFFE, A. M.: The effects of carbon dioxide inhalation upon the cerebral blood flow and cerebral oxygen consumption in vascular disease. J. clin. Invest. **32**, 696–772 (1953).

Nylin, G., Blömer, H., Jones, H., Hedlund, S., Rylander, C. G.: Further studies on cerebral blood flow estimated with thorium-B-labelled erythrocytes. Brit. Heart J. **18**, 385–392 (1956).

Nylin, G., Hedlund, S., Regnström, O.: Cerebral circulation studied with labelled red cells in healthy males. Acta radiol. (Stockh.) **55**, 281–304 (1961 a).

Nylin, G., Hedlund, S., Regnström, O.: Studies of the cerebral circulation with labelled erythrocytes in healthy man. Circulat. Res. **9**, 664–674 (1961 b).

Nylin, G., Silverskiöld, B. P., Löfstedt, S., Regnström, O., Hedlund, S.: Studies on cerebral blood flow in man, using radioactive-labelled erythrocytes. Brain **83**, 293–335 (1960).

Oberdörster, G., Saum, R., Benner, U., Gebert, E., Sabota, P., Hirsch, H.: Die Erholung des Elektrocorticogramms nach kompletter Ischämie des Hundehirns in Normothermie. Pflügers Arch. **307**, R. 116 (1969).

Obersteiner, H.: Die Innervation der Gehirngefäße. Arb. Inst. Anat. Physiol. ZNS Wien **5**, 215–220 (1898).

Olesen, J.: The influence of adrenaline, noradrenaline and angiotensin on the cerebral blood flow in man. In: Brain and blood flow. London: Pitman 1971.

Owman, C., Falck, B., Mchedlishvili, G.: Adrenergic structures of the pial arteries and their connections with the cerebral cortex. Bjull. éksp. Biol. Med. **59**, 98–100 (1965).

Patterson, J. L., Jr.: Circulation through the brain. In: Medical physiology and biophysics. Philadelphia: Saunders 1960.

Patterson, J. L., Jr., Heyman, A., Battey, L. L., Ferguson, R. W.: Threshold of response of the cerebral vessels of man to increase in blood carbon dioxyde. J. clin. Invest. **34**, 1857–1864 (1955).

Paulson, O. B.: Regional cerebral blood flow in middle cerebral artery occlusion. Scand. J. clin. Lab. Invest., Suppl. **102**, XVI C (1968).

Paulson, O. B.: Regional cerebral blood flow at rest and during functional tests in occlusive and non-occlusive cerebrovascular disease. In: Cerebral blood flow. Berlin-Heidelberg-New York: Springer 1969.

Paulson, O. B.: Regional cerebral blood flow in apoplexy due to occlusion of the middle cerebral artery. Neurology (Minneap.) **20**, 63–77 (1970).

Paulson, O. B., Lassen, N. A., Skinhøj, E.: Regional cerebral blood flow in apoplexy without arterial occlusion. Neurology (Minneap.) **20**, 125–138 (1970).

Penfield, W.: Intracerebral vascular nerves. Arch. Neurol. Psychiat. (Chic.) **27**, 30–44 (1932).

Pfleiderer, G., Frowein, R. A., Ross, J.: Stoffwechselvorgänge im Gehirn bei akuter Anoxie, akuter Ischämie und in der Erholung. Pflügers Arch. ges. Physiol. **261**, 334–360 (1955).

Pickerodt, V.: Die Wirkung von passiver Hyperventilation auf die Sauerstoffversorgung des Gehirns. Ärztl. Forsch. **25**, 57–67 (1971).

Pierce, E. C., Lambertsen, C. J., Deutsch, S., Chase, P. E., Linde, H. W., Dripps, R. D., Price, H. L.: Cerebral circulation and metabolism during thiopental anaesthesia and hyperventilation in man. J. clin. Invest. **41**, 1664–1671 (1962).

Plum, F., Posner, J. B.: Blood and cerebrospinal fluid lactate during hyperventilation Amer. J. Physiol. **212**, 864–870 (1967).

Posner, J. B., Plum, F., Zee, D.: Ventriculocisternal pH and cerebral blood flow. Arch. Neurol. (Chic.) **20**, 664–667 (1969).

Purves, M. J.: The physiology of the cerebral circulation. Cambridge: University Press 1972.

Rafcliffe, H. L., Luginbühl, H., Pivnik, L.: Coronary, aortic and cerebral atherosclerosis in swine of three age groups: Implications. Bull. Wld Hlth Org. **42**, 225–234 (1970).

Raichle, M. E., Posner, J. B., Plum, F.: Cerebral blood flow during and after hyperventilation. Brain and blood flow. London: Pitman 1971.

Ramirez-Boettner, C. M., Sosa, O. D., Balanza, J., Calcena, R. M.: Subclavian steal syndrome with reversal of blood flow in the right carotid artery. Ann. intern. Med. **44**, 142–144 (1966).

Rapela, C. E., Green, H. D.: Autoregulation of canine cerebral blood flow. Circulat. Res. **15**, Suppl. 1, 205–212 (1964).

Reed, D. J., Woodbury, D. M.: Effect of urea and acetazolamide on brain volume and cerebrospinal fluid pressure. J. Physiol. (Lond.) **164**, 265–273 (1962 a).

Reed, D. J., Woodbury, D. M.: Effect of hypertonic urea on cerebrospinal fluid pressure and brain volume. J. Physiol. (Lond.) **164**, 252–264 (1962 b).

Rees, J. E., Boulay, E. P. G. H. du, Bull, J. W. D., Marshall, J., Russel, R. W. R., Symon, L.: Persistence of disturbance of regional cerebral blood flow after transient ischaemic attacks. In: Brain and blood flow. London: Pitman 1971.

Reivich, M., Holling, H., Roberts, B., Toole, J. F.: Reversal of blood flow through the vertebral artery and its effect on cerebral circulation. New Engl. J. Med. **265**, 878–885 (1961).

Reivich, M., Jehle, J., Sokoloff, L., Kety, S. S.: Measurement of regional cerebral blood flow with C^{14}-antipyrine in awake cats. J. appl. Physiol. **27**, 269–300 (1969a).
Reivich, M., Marshall, W. J. S., Kassell, N.: Loss of autoregulation produced by cerebral trauma. In: Cerebral blood flow. Berlin-Heidelberg-New York: Springer 1969b.
Rich, M., Scheinberg, P., Bell, M. S.: Relationship between cerebrospinal fluid pressure changes and cerebral blood flow. Circulat. Res. **1**, 389–395 (1953).
Richardson, T. Q., Fermoso, J. F., Pugh, G. O.: Effect of acutely elevated intracranial pressure on cardiac output and other circulatory factors. J. surg. Res. **5**, 319–322 (1965).
Richter, H.: Collaterals between the external carotid artery and the vertebral artery in cases of thrombosis of the internal carotid artery. Acta radiol. (Stockh.) **40**, 108–112 (1953).
Risberg, J., Ancri, D., Ingvar, D. H.: Correlation between cerebral blood volume and cerebral blood flow in the cat. Exp. Brain Res. **8**, 321–326 (1969a).
Risberg, J., Ingvar, D. H.: Increase of blood flow in cortical association areas during memorization and abstract thinking. In: Cerebral blood flow and intracranial pressure, part I. Basel-München-Paris-London-New York-Sydney: Karger 1971/72.
Risberg, J., Lundberg, N., Ingvar, D. H.: Regional cerebral blood volume during acute transient rises of the intracranial pressure (plateau waves). J. Neurosurg. **31**, 303–310 (1969b).
Romanov, V. A., Gaevyi, M. D.: Effect of stimulation of the tympanic nervous plexus on cerebral blood circulation and general arterial tension. Fiziol. Ž. (Mosk.) **57**, 697–703 (1971).
Rosenblum, W.: Neurogenic control of cerebral circulation. Stroke **2**, 429–439 (1971).
Rosomoff, H. L.: Adjuncts to neurosurgical anaesthesia. Brit. J. Anaesth. **37**, 246–261 (1965).
Ross-Russell, R. W.: Brain and blood flow. London: Pitman 1971.
Rowan, J. O., Johnston, I. H., Harper, A. M., Jennett, W. B.: Perfusion pressure in intracranial hypertension. In: Intracranial pressure. Berlin-Heidelberg-New York: Springer 1972.
Ruf, H.: Experimentelle Untersuchungen über Krampfverlängerung durch Sauerstoff und Adrenalin: Dauerkrämpfe nach einmaliger elektrischer Reizung oder Cardiazolgabe. Arch. Psychiat. Nervenkr. **187**, 97–127 (1951).
Ruf, H.: Experiments on the prolongation of induced epileptiform convulsions in the cat. J. ment. Sci. **98**, 454–456 (1952).
Ryder, H. W., Espey, F. F., Kimbell, F. D., Penka, E. J., Rosenauer, A., Podolsky, B., Evans, J. E.: Modification of effect of cerebral blood flow on cerebrospinal fluid pressure by variations in craniospinal blood volume. Arch. Neurol. Psychiat. (Chic.) **68**, 170–174 (1952a).
Ryder, H. W., Espey, F. F., Kimbell, F. D., Penka, E. J., Rosenauer, A., Podolsky, B., Evans, J. E.: Influence of changes in cerebral blood flow on the cerebrospinal fluid pressure. Arch. Neurol. Psychiat. (Chic.) **68**, 165–169 (1952b).
Ryzhova, N. M.: Control of local brain circulation by carbon dioxide. Fiziol. Ž. (Mosk.) **56**, 1020–1025 (1970).
Sagawa, K.: Analysis of the CNS ischemic feedback regulation of the circulation. In: Physical basis of circulatory transport. Philadelphia: Saunders 1967.
Sammartino, W. F., Toole, J. F.: Reversed vertebral artery flow. Arch. Neurol. (Chic.) **10**, 590–594 (1964).
Schaertlin, C. E.: Polarographische Messung der Sauerstoffspannung im Hirnblut bei Hypoxie. Helv. physiol. pharmacol. Acta **19**, 255–262 (1961).
Schieve, J. F., Wilson, W. P.: The changes in cerebral vascular resistance of man in experimental alkalosis and acidosis. J. clin. Invest. **32**, 33–38 (1953).
Schindler, U.: Stoffwechsel-Untersuchungen am Cortex cerebri der Katze unter Hypercapnie. Dissertation, Tübingen 1974.
Schindler, U., Betz, E., Pfeiffer, H., Strohm, M.: Cortical metabolites during constant high CO_2 concentrations and their changes during pH variation. In: Cerebral blood flow and intracranial pressure. Europ. Neurol. **6**, 83–87 (1971/72).
Schmahl, F. W., Betz, E., Dettinger, E., Hohorst, H. J.: Energiestoffwechsel der Großhirnrinde und Elektroencephalogramm bei Sauerstoffmangel. Pflügers Arch. ges. Physiol. **292**, 46–59 (1966).
Schmahl, F. W., Betz, E., Talke, H.: Effects of transient carotid occlusion on the extramitochondrial redox system in the disturbed hemisphere. In: Cerebral blood flow and intracranial pressure. Europ. Neurol. **6**, 323–328 (1971/72).
Schmahl, F. W., Betz, E., Talke, H., Hohorst, H. J.: Energiereiche Phosphate und Metabolite des Energiestoffwechsels in der Großhirnrinde der Katze. Biochem. Z. **342**, 518–531 (1965).
Schmidt, C. F.: The cerebral circulation in health and disease. Springfield, Ill.: Thomas 1950.
Schmidt, C. F., Kety, S. S., Pennes, H. H.: The gaseous metabolism of the brain of the monkey. Amer. J. Physiol. **143**, 33–52 (1945).

Schneider, M.: Durchblutung und Sauerstoffversorgung des Gehirns. Verh. dtsch. Ges. Kreisl.-Forsch. **19**, 3–25 (1953).
Schneider, M.: The metabolism of the brain in ischaemia and hypothermia. In: Metabolism of the nervous system. London-New York-Paris-Los Angeles: Pergamon Press 1957.
Schneider, M.: Über die Wiederbelebung nach Kreislaufunterbrechung. Thoraxchirurgie **6**, 95–106 (1958).
Schneider, M.: Zur Pathophysiologie des Gehirnkreislaufs. Acta neurochir. (Wien) **7**, Suppl., 34–50 (1961).
Scholl, H., Pfleiderer, G., Mueldener, B.: Stoffwechselvorgänge im Gehirn bei normaler und herabgesetzter Körpertemperatur unter ischämischer und anoxischer Belastung. J. Neurochem. **2**, 150–165 (1957).
Schwartz, B., Zarea, L.: Cerebral circulation in experimentelly-induced cerebrovascular accidents (rabbit). Exp. Neurol. **23**, 474–484 (1969).
Sengupta, D., Harper, A. M., Jenett, W. B.: Cerebral blood flow in baboon following carotid ligation: Effects of hypoxia and hypotension. Stroke **4**, 330 (1973).
Severinghaus, J. W.: Cerebral blood flow in chronic hypoxia. Acta anaesth. scand. **15**, Suppl. 96 (1964).
Severinghaus, J. W.: Site and mode of action of CO_2 on cerebral blood flow. Federation meetings, Atlantic City, April 1966, p. 12–16.
Severinghaus, J. W., Chiodi, H., Eger, E. J., Brandstrater, B., Hornbein, Th. F.: Role of cerebrospinal fluid pH in normalization of flow in chronic hypocapnia. Circulat. Res. **19**, 274–282 (1966).
Shackelford, R. T., Hegedus, S. H.: Factors affecting cerebral blood flow: Experimental review. Sympathectomy, hypothermia, CO_2-inhalation and papaverin. Ann. Surg. **163**, 771–777 (1966).
Shalit, M. N.: The effects of intra-carotid artery administration of mannitol on cerebral blood flow and intracranial pressure in experimental brain edema. In: Intracranial pressure. Berlin-Heidelberg-New York: Springer 1972.
Shalit, M. N., Reinmuth, O., Shimojyo, B., Scheinberg, P.: A mechanism by which carbon dioxide influences cerebral circulation independent of a direct effect on vascular smooth muscle. In: Research on the cerebral circulation. Springfield, Ill.: Thomas 1969.
Shenkin, H. A., Cabieses, F., Noordt, G. van den, Sayers, P., Copperman, R.: The hemodynamic effect of unilateral carotid ligation on the cerebral circulation of man. J. Neurosurg. **8**, 38–45 (1951).
Shimojyo, B., Reinmuth, O., Kogure, K., Scheinberg, P.: Cerebral blood flow and metabolism at different levels of hypoxia. Trans. Amer. Neurol. Ass. (1966) 338–339.
Siegel, G., Roedel, H., Koepchen, H. P.: Membrane permeability and active transport in vascular smooth muscle. In: 1st Europ. Biophysics Congr. 14.–17. 9. 1971 Baden/Wien. Wien: Med. Akad.-Verl. 1971.
Siesjö, B. K., Kjällquist, Å., Ponten, U., Zwetnow, N.: Extracellular pH in the brain and cerebral blood flow. In: Progr. in brain research, vol. 30. Amsterdam-London-New York: Elsevier 1968.
Siesjö, B. K., Nilsson, L.: The influence of arterial hypoxemia upon labile phosphates and upon extracellular and intracellular lactate and pyruvate concentration in the rat brain. Scand. J. clin. Lab. Invest. **27**, 83–96 (1971).
Skinhøj, E.: Regulation of cerebral blood flow as a single function of the interstitial pH in the brain. Acta neurol. scand. **42**, 604–607 (1966).
Skinhøj, E.: Extracellular pH of the brain and its relation to cerebral blood flow and respiration. In: Research on the cerebral circulation. Springfield, Ill.: Thomas 1969.
Smith, D. R., Ducker, Th. B., Kempe, L. G.: Temporary experimental intracranial vascular occlusion. J. Neurosurg. **30**, 537–544 (1969).
Sokoloff, L.: The action of drugs in the cerebral circulation. Pharmacol. Rev. **11**, 1–85 (1959).
Sokoloff, L.: Local cerebral circulation at rest and during altered cerebral activity induced by anesthesia or visual stimulation. In: Regional chemistry physiology and pharmacology of the nervous system. Oxford: Pergamon Press 1961.
Sokoloff, L., Grave, G. D., Jehle, J. W., Kennedy, Ch.: Postnatal development of the local cerebral blood flow in the dog. In: Cerebral blood flow and intracranial pressure, part I. Basel-München-Paris-London-New York-Sydney: Karger 1971/72.
Stoehr, Ph.: Über die Innervation der Pia mater und des Plexus chorioideus des Menschen. Habil.-Schr. Berlin 1922.
Sugiura, K.: Effect of stellate ganglion block upon carotid blood flow and its relation to cerebral circulation. Brain Nerve (Tokyo) **22**, 33–41 (1970).
Sundt, T. M., Waltz, G.: Experimental cerebral infarction: Retro-orbital, extradural approach for occluding the middle cerebral artery. Proc. Mayo Clin. **41**, 159–168 (1966).

SVEINSDOTTIR, E., LASSEN, N. A.: Detector system for measuring regional cerebral blood flow. Stroke **4**, 365 (1973).

SVEINSDOTTIR, E., LASSEN, N. A., RISBERG, J., INGVAR, D. H.: Regional cerebral blood flow measured by multiple probes: An oscilloscope and a digital computer system for rapid data processing. In: Cerebral blood flow. Berlin-Heidelberg-New York: Springer 1969.

SVEINSDOTTIR, E., TORLÖF, P., RISBERG, J., INGVAR, D. H., LASSEN, N. A.: Monitoring regional cerebral blood flow in normal man with a computer-controlled 32-detector system. In: Cerebral blood flow and intracranial pressure, part I. Basel-München-Paris-London-New York-Sydney: Karger 1971/72.

SYMON, L.: Observations on the leptomeningeal collateral circulation in dogs. J. Physiol. (Lond.) **154**, 1–14 (1960).

SYMON, L.: Experimental evidence for "intracerebral steal" following CO_2 inhalation. Scand. J. clin. Lab. Invest. **102**, Suppl. 102–113 (1968).

SYMON, L.: The concept of intracerebral steal. Int. Anaesth. Clin. **7**, 597–615 (1969).

SYMON, L., HELD, K., DORSCH, N. W. C.: On the myogenic nature of the autoregulation mechanism in the cerebral circulation. In: Cerebral blood flow and intracranial pressure. Basel-München-Paris-London-New York-Sydney: Karger 1972.

SYMON, L., ROSS-RUSSELL, R. W.: The development of cerebral collateral circulation following occlusion of vessels in the neck. An experimental study in baboons. J. Neurol. Sci. **13**, 197–208 (1971).

TAYLOR, H. W., MCCALL, M. L.: The cerebral effects of pentothal sodium in toxemias of pregnancy. J. Philad. Gen. Hosp. **2**, 86–89 (1951).

THOMPSON, R. K., SMITH, G. W.: Experimental occlusion of the middle cerebral artery during arterial hypotension. Trans. Amer. neurol. Ass. **76**, 203–207 (1951).

THORN, W., HEITMANN, R.: pH der Gehirnrinde vom Kaninchen in situ während perakuter, totaler Ischämie, reiner Anoxie und in der Erholung. Pflügers Arch. ges. Physiol. **258**, 501–510 (1954).

THORN, W., SCHOLL, H., PFLEIDERER, G., MUELDENER, B.: Stoffwechselvorgänge im Gehirn bei normaler und herabgesetzter Körpertemperatur unter ischämischer und anoxischer Belastung. J. Neurochem. **2**, 150–165 (1958).

THORNER, M. W., LEWEY, F. H.: The effects of repeated anoxia on the brain. A histopathologic study. J. Amer. med. Ass. **115**, 1595–1600 (1940).

TODA, N., FUJITA, Y.: Responsiveness of isolated cerebral and peripheral arteries to serotonin, norepinephrine, and transmural electrical stimulation. Circulat. Res. **33**, 98–104 (1973).

TOOLE, J. F.: Effect of limb exercise and hypertension on reversed vertebral artery flow (subclavian steal syndrome). In: Cerebral vascular diseases. New York: Grune & Stratton 1965.

TROUPP, H., KUUNE, T., KASTE, M., HUTTUNEN, M.: The effects of raised intracranial pressure on cerebral venous oxygen tension. Acta neurol. scand. **43**, Suppl. 31, 196 (1967).

TSUKER, M.: Innervation of the chorioid plexus. Arch. Neurol. Psychiat. (Chic.) **58**, 474–483 (1947).

TURNER, J., LAMBERTSEN, C. J., OWEN, S. G., WENDEL, H., CHIODI, H.: Effects of .08 and .8 atmospheres of inspired pO_2 upon cerebral hemodynamics at a constant alveolar pCO_2 of 43 mm Hg. Fed. Proc. **16**, 130 (1957).

UI, M.: A role of phosphofructokinase in pH dependent regulation of glycolysis. Biochim. biophys. Acta (Amst.) **124**, 310–322 (1966).

USINGER, W., PLESCHKA, K., ALBERS, C.: Der Einfluß der Vagotomie auf die Hirndurchblutung bei künstlich konstant gehaltenem Blutdruck. Pflügers Arch. ges. Physiol. **291**, 236–240 (1966).

VLAHOV, V., ENZENROSS, H. G.: Einfluß der Ca^{++}-Ionen auf die Kontraktilität der glatten Muskulatur von Piagefäßen. Verh. dtsch. Ges. Kreisl.-Forsch. **39**, 129–132 (1973).

VYSHATINA, A. I.: Regional blood flow changes with electric stimulation of the reticular vasomotor formation of the medulla oblongata. Fiziol. Ž. (Mosk.) **56**, 733–741 (1970).

WAHL, M., DEETJEN, P., THURAU, K., INGVAR, D. H., LASSEN, N. A.: Micropuncture evaluation of the importance of perivascular pH for the arteriolar diameter on the brain surface. Pflügers Arch. **316**, 152–163 (1970).

WAHL, M., KUSCHINSKY, W., BOSSE, O., OLESEN, J., LASSEN, N. A., INGVAR, D.H., MICHAELIS, J., THURAU, K.: Effect of L-norepinephrine on the diameter of pial arterioles and arteries in the cat. Circulat. Res. **31**, 248–256 (1972b).

WAHL, M., KUSCHINSKY, W., BOSSE, O., OLESEN, J., LASSEN, N. A., INGVAR, D. H., THURAU, K.: The effect of perivascular microinjection of norepinephrine and epinephrine on the diameter of pia arteries and arterioles. In: Vascular smooth muscle. Berlin-Heidelberg-New York: Springer 1972a.

WALLENFANG, TH., SCHUBERT, R., REULEN, H. J., SCHÜRMANN, K.: rCBF and regional energy metabolism in cold injury edema as affected by moderate and severe hypocapnia and hypercapnia. Stroke **4**, 332 (1973).

WEIDNER, A.: Energiestatus der Großhirnrinde der Katze während passiver Hyperventilation. Dissertation, Marburg 1970.

WEISS, CH., THIEMANN, V.: Oscillatory pressure induced changes of vascular resistance in autoregulation. Pflügers Arch. **343**, R 25 (1973).

WILKINSON, I. M. S., BULL, J. W. D., DU BOULAY, G. H., MARSHALL, J., ROSS-RUSSELL, R. W., SYMON, L.: The heterogeneity of blood flow throughout the normal cerebral hemisphere. In: Cerebral blood flow. Berlin-Heidelberg-New York: Springer 1969.

WILLIS, TH. W.: Cerebri anatomi, cui accessit nervoru description et usus. London 1664. Gesamtwerk Venedig 1720.

WILSON, W. P., SCHIEVE, J. F., DURHAM, N. C., SCHEINBERG, P.: Effect of series of electric shock treatments on cerebral blood flow and metabolism. Arch. Neurol. Psychiat. (Chic.) **68**, 651–654 (1952).

WOLF, G.: Die Durchblutungsstörungen des Gehirns. Fortschr. Neurol. Psychiat. **27**, 487–548 (1959).

WOLFF, H. G.: The cerebral circulation. Physiol. Rev. **16**, 545–596 (1936).

WOLFF, H. G., FORBES, H. S.: The cerebral circulation. V. Observations of the pial circulation during changes in intracranial pressure. Arch. Neurol. Psychiat. (Chic.) **20**, 1035–1047 (1928).

WOLFF, H. G., LENNOX, W. G.: Cerebral circulation. XII. The effect on pial vessels of variations in the O_2 and CO_2 content of the blood. Arch. Neurol. Psychiat. (Chic.) **23**, 1097–1120 (1930).

WOLIN, L. R.: Tolerance of arrest of cerebral circulation in the rhesus monkey. Exp. Neurol. **30**, 103–115 (1971).

WÜLLENWEBER, R.: "Intracerebral steal" in man recorded by a heat clearance technique. Scand. J. clin. Lab. Invest., Suppl. **102**, XIII c (1968).

WÜNNENBERG, W.: Die lokale Gehirndurchblutung bei akutem und chronischem Sauerstoffmangel. Dissertation, Marburg 1964.

YAMAMOTO, Y. L., PHILLIPS, K. M., HODGE, C. P., FEINDEL, W.: Effects of alterations in arterial carbon dioxide on experimental focal cerebral ischemia. In: Brain and blood flow. London: Pitman Med. and Sci. Publ. Co. 1971.

ZUPPING, R.: Cerebral metabolism in patients with intracranial tumors. J. Neurosurg. **36**, 451–462 (1972).

ZWETNOW, N.: Effects of increased cerebrospinal fluid pressure on the blood flow and on the energy metabolism of the brain. Acta physiol. scand. **339**, Suppl. 1–31 (1970).

ZWETNOW, N., KJÄLLQUIST, Å., SIESJÖ, B. K.: Cerebral blood flow during intracranial hypertension related to tissue hypoxia and to acidosis in cerebral extracellular fluids. In: Progress in brain research, vol. 30. Amsterdam-London-New York: Elsevier 1968.

Experimental Production of Pulmonary Hypertension

H. MEISNER and H. G. BORST

With 8 Figures

A. Introduction

Under normal circulatory conditions, the intravascular pressure of the pulmonary artery is about 22/10 mm Hg, corresponding to a mean pressure of 15 mm Hg (COURNAND, 1947; DEXTER et al., 1950). If the systolic pressure in the pulmonary artery reaches 40 mm Hg, mild pulmonary hypertension is present. A diagnosis of moderate hypertension is associated with a pressure of 40 to 70 mm Hg; above 70 mm Hg the pulmonary hypertension is considered severe. The pressure developed is dependent upon the pressure drop across the pulmonary vascular bed and the volume flow through this system. The ratio of these parameters defines pulmonary vascular resistance which, in contrast to the resistance of the systemic circulation, is low, ranging from 100 to 250 dyne-sec cm^{-5} or 1 to 3 units (WOOD, 1956, 1959; FRIEDBERG, 1966). The pulmonary vascular resistance determines the status of the pulmonary vessels more clearly than the pulmonary pressure only. The smaller the size of the vascular bed, the higher the resistance to flow. Pulmonary vascular resistance is proportional to the pressure, if the volume stays constant (HAMILTON, 1951). Likewise, if the resistance remains constant, pulmonary pressure will vary with the minute volume of flow.

Since the pulmonary vascular bed is highly compliant, pulmonary hypertension can only occur if the limits of vascular distensibility are reached (COURNAND, 1950) or the cross section of the system is reduced (HICKHAM and CARGILL, 1948; RILEY et al., 1948; DEXTER et al., 1950). The former may occur if either of the distending pressures, e.g. pulmonary arterial or pulmonary venous pressure, are elevated excessively (HELLEMS et al., 1948; GORLIN et al., 1951a, b; WOOD, 1954; BORST et al., 1957b). The latter can be the result of amputation, obstruction or luminal narrowing of the vascular bed by physiological or pathological reaction of the vascular wall (ADAMS et al., 1953; FLORES et al., 1954; SCHILLING et al., 1956). Mechanical causes for pulmonary hypertension range from high flow states (LOOGEN, 1958; NAKANA and FISHER, 1965) and pulmonary venous obstruction (DEXTER et al., 1950) to hyperinflation and lung resection (BROFMANN et al., 1957; SCHOENMACKERS, 1966). Changes in vascular tone may be a physiological response to certain drugs (LILJESTRAND, 1958; BAUM and KOT, 1972), to hypoxia (VON EULER and LILJESTRAND, 1946; MOTLEY et al., 1947; LOGARAS, 1947; LILJESTRAND, 1948) and to changes in acidbase balance (VOGEL and BLOUNT, 1965; VILES and SHEPHERD, 1968), as well as to elevated distending pressures (BORST et al., 1957b). Finally pathological luminal narrowing of the pulmonary vessels can be induced by chronic elevation of distending pressures (BLOOMFIELD et al., 1946; COURNAND, 1947; BORDEN et al., 1950), by certain toxic drugs (FERRER et al., 1950; SMITH et al., 1970), and, in rare cases, it may occur without evident noxious stimuli as in primary pulmonary hypertension (EAST, 1940; DRESDALE et al., 1951; WHITAKER and HEATH, 1959). If such changes become irreversible, pulmonary hypertension is termed "fixed", denoting an ominous prognosis for the patient (EISENMENGER, 1897; BIRCKS, 1966; SEBENING, 1967; BÜHLMEYER, 1967; WERTHEIMER et al., 1973).

Experimental research of these problems has focused largely upon the effects of abnormal inspiratory gas mixture and of drugs on the one hand, and upon the consequences of hyperfusion, pulmonary venous congestion and embolization on the other. While the former line of research was designed to clarify the physiological regulation of pulmonary blood flow, the latter was concerned mainly with the mechanisms producing pulmonary hypertension in congenital and acquired heart diseases. Because of the frequency and clinical significance of pulmonary hypertension in cardiac lesions, special emphasis will be given to this problem in this review. Our own attempts to produce pulmonary hypertension, simulating high pulmonary flow states, will be discussed in this context.

B. Pathophysiological Background of the Pulmonary Circulation

Because the normal adult pulmonary vessels are highly distensible, any increase in driving pressure (pulmonary arterial pressure) or in terminal pressure (left atrial pressure) ordinarily will result in a precipitous fall of pulmonary vascular resistance (WILLIAMS, 1954; BORST et al., 1956). Figs. 1 and 2 show resistance data obtained from an *in situ* lung perfusion preparation. There is a rapid reduction of resistance as pulmonary arterial pressure is increased to a range of 22 mm Hg. As the transmural pressure increases, some vascular beds open up or the vessel-caliber increases, and resistance to flow falls. At higher pressures, pulmonary vascular resistance tends to become constant. With a further rise in pressure the vessels seem to approach their limit of distensibility. Similarily, an increase in left atrial (LA) pressure produces distension of the pulmonary vascular bed and therefore a fall in resistance, pulmonary arterial pressure remaining constant. When LA pressure was kept in a selected range (Fig. 2), it again became apparent that in the low LA pressure ranges small variations in PA pressure produced large changes in the resistance, while in the higher ranges, variations in pulmonary arterial pressure produced only slight changes of resistance. In man also, tremendous changes in perfusion volume will not cause an increase in pulmonary atrial pressure: during heavy exercise, for instance, the flow capacity of the pulmonary bed may increase from 6 to 40 l/min without a significant rise in pulmonary arterial pressure (HICKHAM and CARGILL, 1948; SCHWEIZER, 1953; BEVEGARD et al., 1963).

The great distensibility of the pulmonary vascular bed normally is acquired during the first natal weeks and months. A high pulmonary vascular resistance is typical for the fetal state. During this period the open foramen ovale permits communication of the large veins with the left heart. Through the patent ductus arterialized blood flows from the pulmonary artery to the aorta with only one fourth of the blood circulating through the lungs. The reason for this is a high pulmonary vascular resistance; as known from the experiments of DAWES et al. (1954), the pulmonary pressure during fetal life even exceeds the aortic pressure. After the first breaths the pulmonary vascular resistance decreases by 80% within

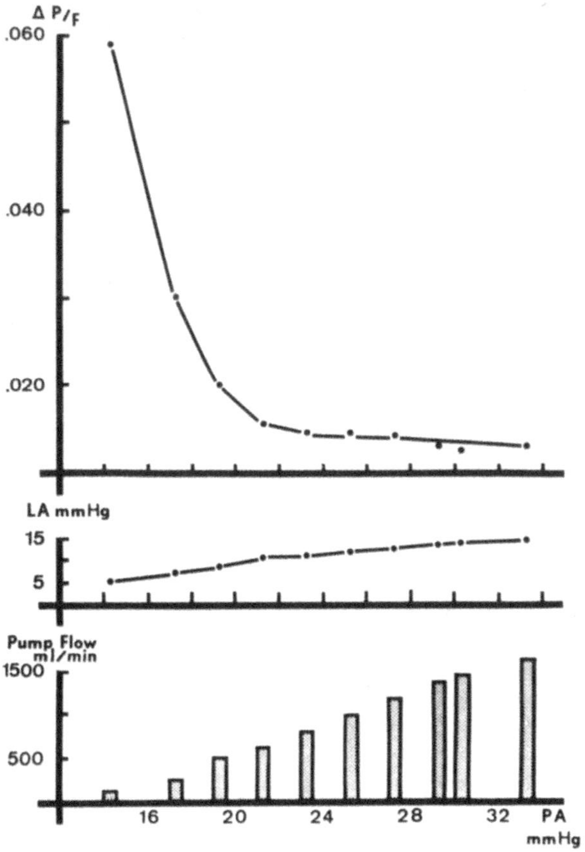

Fig. 1. Experimental results of the relationship between pulmonary resistance to increased perfusion pressure using a pump. Left lung resistance and left atrial mean pressure are plotted against pulmonary arterial mean pressures (abscissa). The columns represent pump output

minutes, the flow increases 3- to 10-fold and pressure in the pulmonary artery drops. Within weeks or months it decreases further to values of 3 to 400 dyne-sec cm^{-5}. The exact mechanisms responsible for these changes are unknown; it is suggested that mechanical stretch of the alveolar capillaries combined with chemosensoric reflexes (Reeves and Leathers, 1964) leads to an increase in lung perfusion (Dawes, 1959). Because the changes from the fetal lung circulation to the normal pulmonary circulation take place slowly in infancy, the pulmonary arterial pressure decreases with age, though gradually. Rudolph et al. (1961) observed 20 infants, aged from 2 to 34 h, with a systolic pressure of 33 to 68 mm Hg and a diastolic pressure of 8 to 42 mm Hg. The youngest baby in his group was 2 h old and had a pressure of 60/42 mm Hg in the pulmonary artery. Deuchar and Knebel (1952) calculated a resistance of 400 dyne-sec cm^{-5} for the age of 5 years, 300 for the age of 10 and 200 dyne-sec cm^{-5} for the adult. These functional results are in good agreement with the vascular architecture of the lung.

Three basic mechanisms leading to pulmonary hypertension in cardiopathies are taken into consideration by the classification of Wood (1958): *Passive*

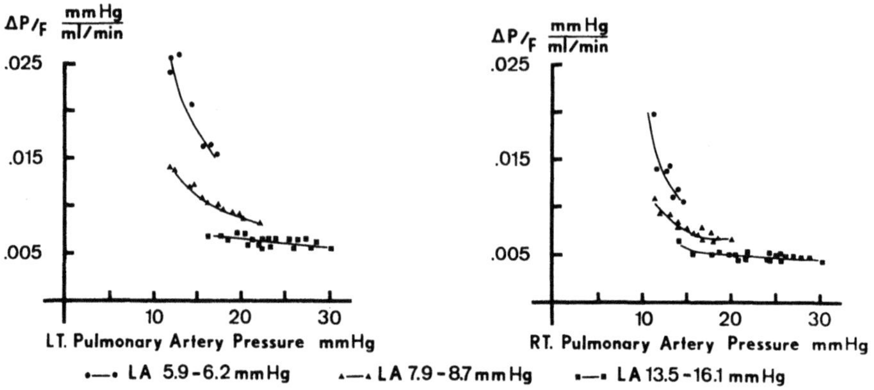

Fig. 2. Lung resistances plotted against pulmonary arterial mean pressures—at various left atrial pressure levels—obtained simultaneously during perfusion of both lungs. It is evident that changes in LA pressure have a greater influence on resistance in the lower ranges than in the high range. Furthermore the resistance was generally lower in the larger right lung

pulmonary hypertension, caused by elevation of pulmonary venous pressure, e.g., by mitral valve disease or pulmonary venous stenosis (JORDAN et al., 1966). In mitral stenosis e.g. pulmonary vascular resistance is increased initially due to vasoconstriction, which can be influenced by the injection of acetylcholine (BURCHELI, 1958; SHEPHERD et al., 1959). Less common causes of obstruction of pulmonary venous flow are pulmonary venous thrombosis, myxoma of left atrium and constrictive pericarditis or endocardial sclerosis (LAWRENCE et al., 1948).

Another form of passive pulmonary hypertension is *hyperkinetic pulmonary hypertension*, caused by increased flow through a patent ductus, ventricular or atrial septal defects or other lesions with a left-right shunt. Any increase of pulmonary blood flow initially produces a fall of resistance and thus prevents a rise of pulmonary arterial pressure. Depending on the lesion present, the pulmonary blood flow may reach values of 20 to 30 l/min. In response to the increased flow the resistance may also rise, thus limiting the quantity of shunt.

In some children with a large left-to-right shunt, the condition of high pulmonary vascular resistance serves as a protection against a large shunt. If the high pulmonary vascular resistance prevents a high pulmonary blood flow, the shunt volume is determined by the relationship between systemic and pulmonary vascular resistances. While some children with such defects maintain a high resistance from birth, others go through a phase of lowered resistance with a subsequent increase often equal to or even surpassing systemic levels. In either case pulmonary resistance may become fixed due to irreversible vascular changes (EDWARDS, 1957). The primary mechanism leading to high resistance in this context gave rise to a number of hypotheses (GILMOUR and EVANS, 1946; CIVIN and EDWARDS, 1951; WOOD, 1959).

Obstructive pulmonary hypertension is caused by massive pulmonary embolism or thrombosis. In such instances thrombotic material may arrive in the lung in the form of showers of emboli or there may be some process which leads to thrombosis *in situ* (SMITH and KROOP, 1957; EDWARDS, 1958). Furthermore pulmonary hypertension may occur if at least two thirds of the total cross section of the pulmonary vascular bed is obstructed (ADAMS et al., 1953).

Obliterative pulmonary hypertension is caused by obliteration of the small vessels, as in emphysema, interstitial lung fibrosis, primary pulmonary hypertension or pulmonary arteriitis (BRAUNSTEIN, 1955).

Vasoconstrictive pulmonary hypertension is induced by acute alveolar hypoxia, acidosis and certain drugs.

Polygenic pulmonary hypertension is the sum of hyperkinetic, obliterative and vasoconstrictive factors, the best example being cor pulmonale in sarcoidosis.

C. Vascular Changes in Pulmonary Hypertension

Microscopic examination of the pulmonary vasculature in fetal life shows thick-walled vessels with muscular hypertrophy of the media, fibrous periadventitial structures and a small lumen. After birth these vessels dilatate; reduction of wall thickness of the media, however, takes 3 to 12 months (CIVIN and EDWARDS, 1951; KÖNN and STORB, 1960; WRIGHT et al., 1964).

The normal pulmonary blood vessels show arterioles consisting of a single elastic lamina (v. HAYEK, 1951). The vast majority of arterioles has no muscular media, even though vessels with a thin muscular media may be found, predominantly in the lingula (HEATH and BEST, 1958). Muscular pulmonary arteries —diameter 100 to 1000 μ—consist of a thin media composed of smooth muscle with occasional collagenous and elastic fibrils bound by internal and external elastic laminae (BRENNER, 1935). Elastic pulmonary arteries—greater than 1000 μ diameter—show a specific pattern of elastic fibrils which predominate in the media (HEATH and EDWARDS, 1958). BRENNER (1935) showed that in adults, intimal fibrosis may occur in all classes of pulmonary blood vessels as a normal age-related change.

Pathological changes of the pulmonary vasculature were described in patients with cardiac anomalies in the last century. The first descriptions of arteriosclerotic depositions in the pulmonary artery were given by ANDRAL (1829), DITTRICH (1850) and BAMBERGER (1857). The first detailed *microscopic* description of pulmonary sclerosis was done by MÖNCKEBERG in 1907. Another summarizing study was written by POSSELT (1909). Many years later pulmonary vascular sclerosis was regarded as the result of pulmonary hypertension rather than its cause (THOMA, 1911; MOSCHCOWITZ, 1927; STEINBERG, 1929; STAEMMLER, 1937). The association with congenital anomalies was studied later in more detail by MULLER and DAMMANN (1952b), HEATH et al. (1956) and HEATH and EDWARDS (1958). The basic microscopic picture of pulmonary hypertension shows media hypertrophy and proliferation of the intima. These vascular lesions can differ as to grade of intimal proliferation (DOWNING et al., 1963; KAPANCI, 1965), increase in elastic tissue (FARRAR et al., 1965) or muscular hypertrophy and hyperplasia (FERGUSON et al., 1953; GOULD, 1968).

In diseases associated *with obstruction to pulmonary venous flow* due to left ventricular failure, the alveoli become thickened with edema fluid, hemosiderin deposition, fibrosis and, primarily, mononuclear cell infiltration. Increased resistance to pulmonary flow exists initially on the basis of vasospasm. In most instances of mitral stenosis, minor forms of medial hypertrophy and ultimately intimal lesions develop in the pulmonary arterioles and muscular arteries (BORDEN et al., 1950; DEXTER et al., 1950; HEATH et al., 1959b), but it is agreed that they are of reversible form (WOOD, 1954). If, however, obstruction of the pulmonary venous return is present prior to birth, the stress on the lungs during fetal life interferes with the normal evolution of the pulmonary vascular bed and produces irreversible, severe vascular changes. FERENCZ and DAMMANN (1957) described 18 patients with medial thickening of the muscular pulmonary arteries, dilatation, tortuosity and intimal proliferation of the arterioles and veins, and increased thickness of the alveolar walls.

HEATH and EDWARDS (1958) distinguished six grades of histologic changes in the pulmonary vessels of patients with congenital heart lesions:

Table 1. Classification of grades of hypertensive pulmonary disease associated with large interventricular shunts showing the type of lesions present in the intima and media of the pulmonary arteries and arterioles. (Modified after HEATH and EDWARDS, 1958)

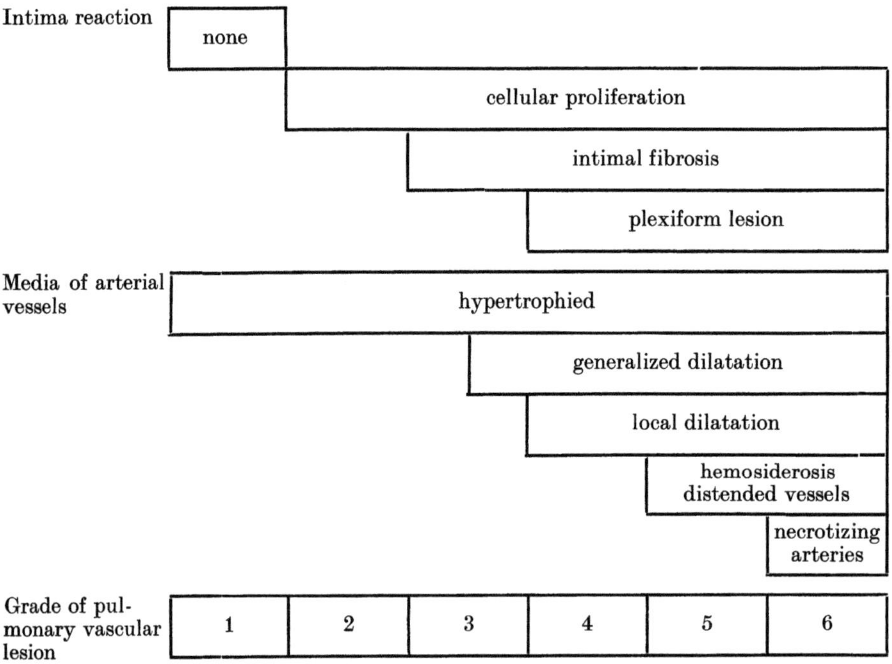

Grade 1 (Table 1) changes are found in patients whose pulmonary arterioles are subjected to systemic blood pressures from birth. The media is thicker, but intimal fibrosis is lacking. There is a close resemblance to the intralobular pulmonary arteries of the fetus. *Grade 2:* in the smaller muscular pulmonary arteries, cellular intimal proliferation is observed. *Grade 3* changes include progressive intimal fibrosis in the muscular arteries and pulmonary arterioles. The most characteristic feature of severe hypertensive pulmonary vascular disease of grade 3, is the occlusion of muscular pulmonary arteries less than 500 μ in diameter by cellular fibrotic tissue and fine elastic fibers. Medial thickening may reach 30% of the external diameter of the vessel. If any dilatation and thinning of the media are found, they are distal to the fibrotic occlusion. In some of the very small muscular pulmonary vessels, distended sacs form, which can be regarded as micro-aneurysms with endothelial proliferation and thrombosis (so-called "dilatation lesions"). These lesions are seen as plexiform, vein-like, angiomatoid and cavernous changes. In the *grade 4* lesions of HEATH and EDWARDS the muscular

pulmonary arteries and the arterioles show dilatation with intimal thickening and onion-skin appearance of the intimal tissue. The microscopic findings in *grade 5* lesions are rigid dilatation and the presence of hyaline intimal fibrosis. Some vessels are widely dilated and surrounded by fibrous acellular tissue. These thin-walled vessels are very fragile and lead to pulmonary hemosiderosis. *Grade 6* changes exhibit necrotizing arteries. Many vessels have acute fibroid necrosis. Some arteries show thrombosis, others gross hypertrophy. The microscopic changes in pulmonary vessels resulting from *destructive disease of the lung parenchyma* differ considerably from this pattern. They will not be regarded in this discussion of the problem of experimental production of pulmonary hypertension.

D. Methods for the Production of Experimental Pulmonary Hypertension

Many experimental conditions have been designed to imitate the clinical situation of cardiopathies leading to pulmonary hypertension in an attempt to study its genesis and reaction to treatment. The particular aim of these studies was to find a distinction between "fixed" pulmonary hypertension—in which operative correction is not advisable—and "reversible" pulmonary hypertension, in which correction carries a lower risk.

First, the production of a temporary increase in pulmonary vascular tone will be discussed, since it may help in understanding the pathogenesis of pulmonary hypertension and the corresponding microscopic changes of the vasculature. Secondly, the most common procedures known from the literature for production of experimental pulmonary hypertension will be reviewed and correlated with the results of our own investigations in that field.

I. The Production of Vasoconstriction in the Pulmonary Vascular Bed

1. Effect of Hypoxia, Hypercapnia and Change in Hydrogen Ion Concentration

v. Euler and Liljestrand in 1946 first demonstrated the production of vasoconstriction of the pulmonary vasculature in the cat by alveolar hypoxia and hypercapnia. This effect later was verified in dogs (Aviado et al., 1952; Stroud and Rahn, 1953; Borst et al., 1957c; Kentera et al., 1964) and in man (Cournand, 1947; McGuire et al., 1951; Fishman et al., 1955; Hertz, 1956a, b; Defares et al., 1960; Rudolph and Yuan, 1966). It was thought to be a protective alveolo-vascular reflex mechanism by Bühlmann et al. (1954), whereby poorly ventilated areas are eliminated from the circulation. Reeves and Leathers (1964) demonstrated the effect of age on pulmonary vasoconstrictor response with hypoxia. In calves breathing 12% oxygen, they found a mean pulmonary arterial pressure of about 100 mm Hg three hours after birth; after five days the pulmonary arterial pressure was only 50 mm Hg and after 4 weeks it remained about 30 mm Hg. This finding suggests that the capacity for marked pulmonary vasoconstriction is extended from life *in utero* to postnatal life. James and Rowe (1957) reported a similar response in a two-day-old infant.

As a mechanism causing vasoconstriction, v. Euler and Liljestrand (1946) suggested local release of lactic acid and carbon dioxide, thereby increasing the hydrogen ion concentration within the muscular smooth muscle. This local reflex is independent of autonomic innervation (LILJESTRAND, 1948; NISELL, 1951a, b; DAGHER et al., 1961). ENSON et al. (1964) showed that variations in the pH of blood may alter the responsiveness of the pulmonary vascular bed to hypoxia in man with chronic lung disease. ENSON et al. (1964) and VOGEL and BLOUNT (1965) described calculations for predicting the pulmonary arterial pressure correlating arterial oxygen tension and pH.

The effect of the hydrogen ion concentration on the pulmonary vasomotor tone is obvious from the experiments of BERGOVSKY et al. (1962) and DOWNING et al. (1965); they found an increase of pulmonary artery resistance in metabolic acidosis which was reversible after the acidosis was equalized. BARER et al. (1967) demonstrated in cats an increase of pulmonary arterial pressure during hypercapnia which was reversible after infusion of alkali. The same group, in another series of experiments using isolated perfusion of one lung lobe, showed that pulmonary arterial pressure rose during inhalation of carbon dioxide and infusion of acids (H_2SO_4, lactic acid, HCl, acetic acid) (BARER et al., 1971). In control and hypoxia states they could demonstrate an increase in pulmonary vascular resistance with decreasing pH: the effect of general hypoxia (PaO_2 23 to 79 mm Hg) on a test lobe was compared at different values of blood pH and at a constant blood flow. In the controls, P_{PA} was raised by acid, while hypoxia caused only a small increment in pressure, probably because the vascular tone was already nearly maximal. Thus acidosis produces pulmonary vasoconstriction and the effect of increased $PaCO_2$ is due to a reduction in pH. An effect of changes in surfactant has also been discussed (AVERY and SAID, 1965). VOGEL and BLOUNT (1965) demonstrated the influence of hydrogen ion concentration in regulating the pulmonary arterial pressure in a patient with alveolar hypoventilation, chronic hypoxia and normal lungs.

2. Effect of Drugs

EDWARDS (1951), HARRIS (1957), BORST et al. (1957a) and AVIADO (1960) studied the effect of pharmacologic agents on the pulmonary circulation in dogs. In a controlled lung perfusion experiment the injection of epinephrine (3.6 μg/kg) or norepinephrine caused vasoconstriction. The same was true after administration of serotonin (5-hydroxytryptamine) using either repeated injections or continuous infusion. The administration of acetylcholine, histamine and aminophylline gave no consistent effects, even though a dilatation would be expected. The authors suggested that the vascular tone is probably very low and no further dilatation of the vessels is possible. In regard to the expected vasoconstrictor effect of serotonin, BLANK et al. (1961) injected newborn albino rats subcutaneously 12 h after birth with 5-hydroxytryptamine 2 to 4 and 10 mg/kg or 5-hydroxytryptophan in a dosis of 5 to 12.5 and 25 mg/kg. They treated the animals for 60 and 90 days, respectively. Pressure recordings gave inconstant right ventricular systolic pressure between 9 and 43 mm Hg. The histologic changes showed medial thickening, but the difference from the control group was not significant, and the method was not regarded as useful for the production of pulmonary hypertension.

II. Effects of Embolization on the Pulmonary Vascular Bed

Both experimental and clinical evidence suggests that in the majority of cases large emboli produce pulmonary hypertension by mechanical obstruction (OWEN et al., 1953; WILLIAMS, 1956; PARASKOS et al., 1972). In contrast small emboli occluding terminal pulmonary arteries are thought to induce pulmonary hypertension by reflex activity (PRICE et al., 1955; WEIDNER and LIGHT, 1958; DEXTER, 1965; SABISTON and WOLFE, 1968). Among the immense numbers of publications on embolization of the pulmonary vascular bed, only those performed with the aim of eliciting pulmonary hypertension will be discussed (compare Table 2).

1. Injection of Autogenous Material

HARRISON (1948) placed clotted human blood into a homogenizer to obtain fragments of not more than 1 mm diameter. Two ml of this clot suspended in saline were injected intravenously into rabbits weekly, and the animals were sacrificed at variable intervals. Initial sections of the lung showed a cellular infiltrate around the vessel wall and edema around the persisting emboli, denoting an inflammatory reaction to the foreign body. After 20 days, shrinkage of the intimal thickening, recanalization and regression of the vascular lesions made this procedure valuable only as a method for producing transient pulmonary hypertension. In 1951 HARRISON used the same experimental set-up, maintaining rabbits up to 22 weeks after the injection. Killing the animals immediately after embolization showed right ventricular hypertrophy due to a suggested rise in pulmonary arterial pressure which was, however, not measured. Twenty weeks after embolization, no ventricular hypertrophy was present, and obstruction of the pulmonary vascular bed was missing. It was suggested that the initial rise in pulmonary blood pressure was due to vasoconstriction.

WARTMANN et al. (1951) and EICHELTER and SCHENK (1969) injected autogenous blood. They observed no significant rise in pulmonary arterial pressure and no progressive lesions in the vascular tree. MUIRHEAD and MONTGOMERY (1951) used human amniotic fluid and blood clots and noted endothelial proliferation, but no rise of pulmonary arterial pressure. BARNARD (1953, 1954a) injected fibrin and red clot emboli in 20 rabbits intravenously twice weekly for up to 368 days. After the 35th injection the symptoms of chronic cor pulmonale developed in some animals and were present in all after 70 injections. In 12 rabbits pressure was measured in the right ventricle, the highest being 36 mm Hg mean, with maximal systolic pressure of 95 and 84 mm Hg. Seven rabbits had pressures below 30 mm Hg. Microscopic sections showed circumferential and eccentric intimal fibrosis, no medial hypertrophy, but medial atrophy. No difference due to the material injected could be demonstrated. Revision of the data reveals that cor pulmonale was diagnosed "by the naked eye" and that 50% of the rabbits died from right ventricular hypertrophy and dilatation. In some, ventricular hypertrophy was present, but pulmonary pressure was normal. An over-all calculation of the volume of material injected revealed that only a part of the clots was retained in the lungs, the rest was re-absorbed, which has also been observed by HEARD (1952). BARNARD (1954b) interpreted the course of events as a combined effect of recurrent vasospasm and impaired intimal nutrition. JAQUES and HYMAN (1957b) injected dogs with autogenous blood clots, ligating in one group the azygos vein. The amount in ml of one half of the body weight (kg) was injected through a 19 gauge needle 2 to 10 times per week for up to 10 weeks. Of 20 injected dogs, 8 died during the experiment. The mean pulmonary pressure, measured at 5 and 10 weeks, respectively, after the injection, was not higher than 35 mm Hg. After one week one dog had a pressure of 55 mm Hg. There was no difference in the dogs with or without azygos vein ligation. On microscopic examination the lungs showed acute congestion, no evidence of medial hypertrophy, but numerous changes in the intima. The clots adhered to the walls and became endothelialized. Eight dogs

Table 2. Summary of most common methods for production of experimental pulmonary hypertension by means of embolization of the pulmonary vascular bed using different material for injection

Authors	Material injected	Animal	Pressure	Histological results
HARRISON, 1948/51	human blood clots	rabbits 22 weeks	transient vent. hypertrophy	transient intimal thickening
WARTMAN et al., 1951	blood emboli	dog 1–5 weeks	normal	small inflammatory reaction
MUIRHEAD, MONTGOMERY, 1951	human amniotic fluid + blood clots		normal	endothelial proliferation
BARNARD, 1953, 1954a, b, 1957	fibrin red clots	rabbits 368 days	RV$\overline{\text{m}}$ 36 mm Hg normal/Pa	intimal fibrosis, medial atrophy
JAQUES, HYMAN, 1957	blood clots azyg. vein lig.	dogs 10 weeks	Pa $\overline{\text{m}}$ 35 mm Hg	congestion, intima changes
HEPINSTALL, 1957	blood clots cholesterol	rabbits	normal	cholesterol deposition
GORE et al., 1962	thromboplastin	rabbits 164 days	Pa $\overline{\text{m}}$ 19.5 mm Hg	thickening of large and medial arteries
GEER et al., 1965	autog. blood clot	dogs 41 weeks	RV transient 35 mmHg	intimal plaque
DALEY et al., 1951	lycopodium spores	dogs	transient Pa 50–90 mm Hg	foreign body reaction
THOMAS et al., 1956	plastic beads	rabbits	right vent. hyp.	—
SINGER et al., 1957	starch	dogs	Pa $\overline{\text{m}}$ 20 mm Hg	edema
WEISBERG et al., 1963/64	starch	dogs, 10–20 months	transient, Pa syst, 35–40 mm Hg	medial thickening, intima proliferation in 5 dogs
KUX, MASSION et al., 1973	glass microspheres	dogs	transient Pa 28 mm Hg	*in vivo* perfused lung lobe
BOEREMA, 1968	air embolism	rabbit	—	medial thickening
BARNARD, 1957	gas embolism	rabbits	right vent. hypertrophy	arteritis, medial hypertr.
GILBERT et al., 1968	air embolism	dogs $7^1/_2$ month	Pa 40–70 mm Hg	intimal fibrosis, medial hypertrophy, necrotizing vasculitis
WALLACE, HAMILTON, 1962	heartworms	dogs	Pa 35 mm Hg	arteritis, medial hypertrophy

showed acute arteritis and infiltration of cells in the media and intima and perivascularly. HEPINSTALL (1957) injected intravenously blood clot from hypercholesterolemic rabbits into animals with and without cholesterol diets. There was a high incidence of cholesterol in the organizing emboli without significant rise in pulmonary arterial pressure. GORE et al. (1962) injected rabbits intravenously with thromboplastin twice a week for up to 164 days. Most of the rabbits, kept up to 30 days, showed thickening of large and medium-sized pulmonary arteries. The mean pressure in the pulmonary artery was 19.5 mm Hg. GEER et al. (1965) injected autogenous clot into dogs; the size of the emboli was estimated to be about $1 \times 3 \times 0.1$ mm. The amount of clot per injection varied in different series from 2 to 42 ml, the number of injections from 1 to 5 per week. It was not possible to produce sustained pulmonary hypertension. In contrast to other authors (HARRISON, 1948; BARNARD, 1954), GEER et al. (1965) noted very little acute inflammation in the walls of the arteries with emboli. The presence of an inflammatory reaction was considered symptomatic of contamination of the embolic material.

2. Injection of Allogenous Material

Because the imitation of clinical pulmonary embolization gave no reliable results in respect to the production of sustained pulmonary hypertension, other investigators injected foreign body material. DALEY et al. (1951), using dogs, injected 20 ml of a 1% suspension of lycopodium spores into the main pulmonary artery or one of its branches. The largest quantity injected was 100 ml. After single injections, the pulmonary arterial pressure rose to 52/40 or 93/47 mm Hg and regained control levels after 2 to 10 min. Repeated injections of lycopodium, failed to elicit a sustained rise in pulmonary arterial pressure. Multiple histological sections showed spores in many large arteries, but not typical lesions.

THOMAS et al. (1956) injected 55 rabbits intravenously with spherical, smooth-surfaced, plastic beads insoluble in body fluids; 20 mg/ml in 5% dextrose were administered. The optimal dose was 200 mg three times a week. The ratio of right ventricle mass to left ventricle mass was measured and seemed significantly increased, i.e., a sign of right ventricular hypertrophy. No pulmonary vascular sclerosis was achieved. SINGER et al. (1957) injected 1 g of starch granules into the pulmonary artery wedge position in dogs. Acute measurements showed a moderate rise in pulmonary arterial pressure (= mean 20 mm Hg). All animals developed pulmonary edema even though the left atrial pressure remained within normal limits. Thus it was suggested that neurohumoral mechanisms influence capillary permeability. WEISBERG et al. (1963) injected a suspension of 2 g of starch in 15 to 20 ml heparinized Ringers solution into the wedge position in dogs. The pulmonary artery pressure rose from 15 to 35 mm Hg or 18 to 40 mm Hg, but only for a short time. In another series of short-term embolization experiments (WEISBERG et al.), the mean pulmonary arterial pressure rose to values between 25 and 32 mm Hg, in one instance to 55 mm Hg. The material was injected, through a wedge catheter into a pulmonary lobe. In the long-term series, the systolic pulmonary arterial pressure reached 30 and 40 mm Hg 10 to 21 months after embolization. Even though starch was administered into one lobe only, the animals developed bilateral pulmonary edema, again invoking an alleged reflex mechanism influencing the permeability of the pulmonary capillary wall (KABINS et al., 1960). No pulmonary edema was found, however, in dogs surviving more than 3 days. Histologically, medial thickening and intimal proliferation were observed in only 5 out of 55 dogs with chronic elevation of pulmonary arterial pressure.

KUX and MASSION (1973) used glass microspheres (50 μm diameter) and an *in vivo* perfusion to demonstrate intrapulmonary reflex vasospasm which seemed to be independent of lung innervation. The mean pulmonary arterial pressures were approximately 25 mm Hg.

3. Effect of Gas Embolization

It has been assumed that the microscopic changes observed after thrombo-embolism are due to organization of blood clots in the intima of the pulmonary vessels. Gas embolization should permit the avoidance of this phenomenon.

BARNARD (1957) reported arterial lesions after intravenous injection of air. In further experiments he injected 6 rabbits with oxygen, nitrogen or argon in steadily increasing doses, starting with 0.1 ml/kg; after three days the dosage was raised by 0.05 to 1.4 ml/kg. Large muscular arteries were affected, exhibiting arteritis, intimal fibrosis and medial hypertrophy. The microscopic alterations seen were independent of the gas used. The changes were thought to be due to occlusion of the vessel by the gas and to vasospasm. BOEREMA (1968) described similar results.

Since the presence of a sphincteric arterial blocking mechanism (WAGENVOORT et al., 1964) in rabbits may influence the result this procedure should preferably be done in dogs. GILBERT et al. (1968) administered 0.5 cc/kg of body weight of air intravenously to dogs. Thereafter this dose was raised to 2.0 cc/kg twice daily for a period of $2^1/_2$ to $7^1/_2$ months. Of 12 dogs, 6 showed chronic elevation of pulmonary arterial pressure (42 to 70 mm Hg). Nine developed lesions of grades 2 to 6, according to the classification of HEATH and EDWARDS (1958), with severe intimal reaction, medial hypertrophy and in one dog necrotizing vasculitis.

4. Effect of Dirofilariasis Immitis

Heartworms (*Dirofilaria immitis*) are nematodes found in dogs from the South and the Atlantic coastal areas of the USA; the intermediate host of the parasite is the mosquito. HENNIGAR and FERGUSON (1957) reported the development of pulmonary hypertension in dogs due to these parasites. WALLACE and HAMILTON (1962) described dogs with an average right ventricular systolic pressure of 42 mm Hg; in one dog in cardiac failure it reached 111 mm Hg and even 158 mm Hg. At autopsy the lung showed severe edema, congestion and hemorrhage. In other dogs treated for nematodes, the right ventricular systolic pressure remained elevated for two years at about 55 mm Hg. At autopsy the lung vessels showed intimal fibrosis. Right ventricular hypertension may be caused only by blockage of the outflow tract of that chamber. It is generally assumed, however, that pulmonary hypertension is produced by some secretion from these worms; furthermore there seems to be an individual susceptibility of some dogs. WALLACE and HAMILTON (1962) reported the use of these parasites for the production of pulmonary hypertension: the worms can be removed from a donor dog by ventriculotomy or pulmonary arteriotomy. If necessary they may be kept briefly in saline and 10% plasma or for several days in modified Earl's solution and 10% plasma (EARL, 1959). In order to transplant the worms, they folded them over the grooved end of a 3 mm diameter plastic rod, about 35 cm long and pushed it down the jugular vein of the recipient. The authors described one dog, 2 months after transplantation of 41 heartworms, in which the right ventricular pressure increased from 30 to 35 mm Hg. In another dog 5 months after transplantation, the pressure increased from 28 to 37 mm Hg. Obviously, a predictable level of hypertension cannot be produced with this procedure.

III. Production of Functional Mitral Stenosis

The pressure in the pulmonary artery may increase as a result of back pressure from the left heart. BARNES et al. (1958) tried to raise the pressure in the pulmonary system: through a thoracotomy the left pulmonary veins were isolated and individually wrapped with cellophane bands. Underneath the cellophane a fibrotic reaction causes pulmonary venous obstruction. Subsequent control catheterizations showed no significant elevation of pulmonary arterial pressure. Two weeks after the first operation in a series of 9 dogs, the pulmonary veins on the right side were treated in the same manner. Two to six weeks after bilateral banding of the pulmonary veins the pulmonary arterial pressure was elevated by 10 to 19 mm Hg. Four to six months after the second operation, in 3 out of 9 dogs the pulmonary arterial pressure was about 30 mm Hg. Only one dog had a pulmonary arterial pressure of 53 mm Hg. Of 9 dogs, 8 showed medial hypertrophy while in some, fibrous thickening of the intima occurred. In 7 of these dogs one or two lobes of the right lung were removed 5 to 8 months later. In only one animal, the pulmonary arterial pressure increased from 30 to 42 mm Hg. In two other dogs with bilateral banding a side-to-side anastomosis between the aorta and the left main pulmonary artery was made. One died of pulmonary edema several hours after the operation, the other showed a rise in pulmonary arterial pressure from 8 mm Hg to 25 mm Hg. The histological changes were as stated previously. The same method was applied by FERGUSON et al. (1959) and yielded a high rate of pulmonary edema (9 out of 13 died) and similar results: slight elevation of pulmonary arterial pressure and medial hypertrophy. Other authors (FERRIN et al., 1951; BOUCEK et al., 1952) confirmed the same results of only a small increase of pulmonary arterial pressure and a high frequency of pulmonary edema.

Graded mitral stenosis is difficult to induce using experimental methods (SHAW et al., 1943). MACCALLUM and MCCLURE (1906) elevated left atrial pressure by placing a distensible balloon in the mitral orifice, with a high incidence of thromboembolism resulting. CONNOLLY (1950) reported reasonable results by placing sutures below the coronary vessels encircling the chordae tendineae in order to produce mitral valve stenosis. ELLISON et al. (1952) used a nylon-covered steel wire to produce stenosis of the base of the mitral ostium: an atraumatic needle was inserted through the wall of the right atrium passing through the interatrial and above the atrio-ventricular groove and emerging anteriorly. The ends of the sutures emanated from the pericardium and were passed through a cannula, permitting tightening from the outside. This was usually done 14 to 21 days after surgery. The authors reported gradual stenosis developing over periods of several weeks. The dogs tolerated a stenosis of 10 mm diameter. Even a mitral narrowing of 5 to 8 mm was possible using delayed tightening of the suture. Pressures in the pulmonary artery of 40/20 mm Hg were measured, and the dogs developed cardiac failure, ascites and edema of the lower extremities. JAQUES and HYMAN (1957a) applied the same technique in dogs. The survival time of these dogs was from 100 to 760 days after the implantation of the purse string suture. To avoid shunts between pulmonary and bronchial venous circulation, the azygos vein was ligated in eight animals. The aperture tolerated was less than 5 mm in diameter. Fifteen dogs developed congestive heart failure. Even though an increase of pulmonary artery and wedge pressure and right ventricular hypertrophy were described, no significant signs of pulmonary hypertension were seen histologically. Medial hypertrophy described by these authors might have been due to heartworm infestation. HADDY et al. (1953) and HANNON et al. (1957) produced a stenotic mitral valve (less than 1 cm diameter) by inversion of the left auricular appendage across the mitral ring above the valve. This procedure caused an elevation of pulmonary venous pressure but only an insignificant rise of pulmonary arterial pressure. Histological examination after three years revealed medial hypertrophy without intimal changes. The average pulmonary arterial pressure in these animals was in normal ranges of 18 to 25 mm Hg, in one animal it was 32 mm Hg.

A similar method was described by VASKO et al. (1967): passing a ligature connected to an Ivalon sponge and Ameroid ellipsoid from the left atrial appendage through the mitral valve and out through the posterolateral wall of the left ventricle, they could invaginate the atrial appendage through the valve ring via the cylinder and thus produce an elevation of left atrial pressure to 15 mm Hg and of the mean pulmonary arterial pressure of 26 mm Hg. HAWE et al. (1970) described a method for producing chronic graded mitral stenosis by suturing a restrictive Teflon-covered metal ring of known orifice into the mitral annulus. The left atrial pressure rose to an average of 14 mm Hg, mean pulmonary arterial pressure ranged from 13 to 30 mm Hg. The size of the orifice varied between 0.63 and 1.04 cm^2.

Generally speaking, therefore, pulmonary venous congestion tends to result in only a small rise in arterial pressure, a probable lowering of resistance and high risk of cardiac failure. The experiment of v. BOGAERT et al. (1957) seem to be an exception: this group described the production of chronic pulmonary hypertension in dogs using anastomosis between the left atrium and the descending aorta. The largest permissible diameter of this shunt was thought to be 6 to 7 mm; otherwise the animals died of lung edema. The pressure in the pulmonary artery rose to 46/20 mm Hg, in the left atrium to 12 to 20 mm Hg, remaining in that range when tested after 60 days. Long-term survivors (up to 7 months) revealed, on microscopic examination, in the arterioles and venoles intimal fibroelastosis and medial hypertrophy of moderate degree.

IV. Production of Hyperkinetic Pulmonary Hypertension

An increase in blood flow to the pulmonary bed can be achieved by three methods: reduction of the total pulmonary vascular bed, creation of septal defects and of communications between systemic and pulmonary circulation.

1. Reduction of the Total Pulmonary Vascular Bed

Normally, pneumonectomy is tolerated well with only insignificant changes of pulmonary arterial pressure (LONGACRE et al., 1937; COURNAND, 1947). In patients without heart disease, occlusion of one pulmonary artery by an intraluminal balloon during exercise results in a rise of pulmonary arterial pressure of only 12 to 50%, while cardiac output may increase as much as threefold (BROFMAN et al., 1957). In cardiac patients a marked elevation in pulmonary arterial pressure occurs, however (SLOAN et al., 1955). The resection of less than one lung in animals induces only minor changes in pulmonary arterial pressure, but if larger amounts of tissue are removed, an elevation in pressure occurs (ADAMS et al., 1953; FLORES et al., 1954; WEIDERANDERS et al., 1964). SCHILLING et al. (1956) imitated the clinical conditions of lung resection by doing a 3-stage operation in dogs, resecting different lobes step by step. When more than 57% of lung tissue was removed, the pulmonary artery systolic pressure was 50 mm Hg, in one dog as high as 84 mm Hg. At autopsy there was right heart hypertrophy and dilatation, the lung parenchyma showing marked arterial medial hypertrophy and fibrosis.

2. Creation of Septal Defects

In man a septal defect at the pretricuspid level sometimes carries a shunt of 15 to 20 l/min for many years without significant elevation of pulmonary arterial pressure (LITTLE et al., 1949; MCGOON et al., 1958; MEISNER, 1966). Large posttricuspid shunts, however, often are associated with pulmonary hypertension (HEATH et al., 1958). HAWLEY et al. (1950) produced an extraventricular shunt between the left and right chamber using an L-shaped cannula of 6 to 7 mm diameter. Although the shunt flow reached almost 50% of the left ventricular stroke volume, the pulmonary arterial pressure increased only 6.3 mm Hg. Experimental interventricular septal defects of 10 mm diameter were produced by HOLMAN and BECK (1925) with a cardiotome and also by GRIFFIN and ESSEX (1951), resulting in a left-to-right shunt of 43 to 84%. All these defects closed spontaneously within 4 months. The only positive results were reported by KAY et al. in 1953. They produced ventricular septal defects of uniform size in dogs by means of a sharpened 12.5 mm cork-borer with suction to remove the plug of septal tissue. From a left thoracotomy an incision was made in the center of a purse-string suture in the outflow tract of the right ventricle and the instrument advanced. Thus a defect slightly larger than the borer was created underneath the semilunar valves, which represents the most frequent anatomical location of congenital defects. Nineteen of 35 animals survived; in three, the defect closed spontaneously. Nine animals were studied 7.5 to 12 months after the operation. In 6 dogs the right ventricular systemic pressure was 55 mm Hg, the pulmonary arterial pressure was 40/10 mm Hg. In one dog the right ventricular pressure increased to 100 mm Hg at a pulmonary arterial pressure of 60/35 mm Hg. The diameter of the remaining ventricular septal defect was 9.3 mm. In 11 dogs lung biopsies were taken 5 to 8 months after the intervention and revealed no histological changes, even though some of the defects were large enough to produce congestive heart failure. Some years later BLANK et al. (1961) attempted to produce interventricular septal defects in fetal puppies *in utero* without success.

3. Production of Vascular Shunts between Systemic and Pulmonary Circulation

Congenital communications between the high and low pressure systems of the circulation, e.g. patent ductus arteriosus, can be associated with pulmonary hypertension, medial hypertrophy and intimal fibrosis of the pulmonary vascular bed. Therefore testing of an equivalent experimental model seemed appropriate (comp. Table 3). In 1939 LEVY and BLALOCK anastomosed the left subclavian artery to the pulmonary artery in 12 dogs, of which 5 survived. After six months none of the dogs showed morphological changes in the pulmonary vasculature. MULLER et al. (1953) designed three groups of similar experiments (see Fig. 3). In the first group 8 mm anastomoses between the left pulmonary artery and the side of the descending aorta were made. Most of the animals (16 out of 21) died of cardiac failure. One animal sacrificed after one year exhibited intimal proliferation and medial hypertrophy in small arteries. Pressures in the pulmonary artery and aorta were almost equal. In another group the left subclavian artery and the superior pulmonary vein were anastomosed. The venous walls were thickened because of medial hypertrophy, but there were no significant changes in the arteries. In the third group the lung circulation was reversed by suturing the proximal end of the left pulmonary artery to the distal end of the superior pulmonary vein or by anastomosing the left arterial appendage with the distal end of the left pulmonary artery. Only slight histologic changes originated in the veins and none in the arteries. FERGUSON et al. (1959) produced a rise in pulmonary arterial pressure from 38 to 60 mm Hg by a subclavian artery-to-left pulmonary artery anastomosis and removal of the left upper lobe in 4 dogs. Constricting the pulmonary veins caused no additional pressure increase. Blood flow on the left side of the lung was reduced by 15% as compared to that in the right lung. Lung biopsies taken 2 to 8 weeks postoperatively demonstrated medial hypertrophy and intimal proliferation. Subsequently FERGUSON and VARCO (1955), using adult dogs, made systemic-pulmonary shunts using two techniques. In one group they anastomosed the left subclavian artery to the left pulmonary artery, the upper or the lower lobe arteries end-to-end (Fig. 3). In the second group they made a side-to-side anastomosis to equivalent areas. Blood flow was calculated by the Fick method. Only the shunt to the left upper lobe resulted in severe pulmonary edema. One dog survived developing medial hypertrophy and intimal proliferation after 16 months. In the shunts to the lower lobe a close relationship between pressure increase and histologic changes was noted. When the mean pulmonary pressure was 61 mm Hg, vascular lesions occurred. At 42 mm Hg, no microscopic changes were discovered. In one animal with a pressure of 100 mm Hg there were grade 3 lesions. In the group with side-to-side anastomosis there was no pulmonary arterial pressure higher than 32 mm Hg mean for up to 64 weeks; the histologic changes were not particularly striking. In six dogs the shunt from the left subclavian artery to the right pulmonary artery was removed and reanastomosed to the previous position. Thereafter pulmonary arterial pressure returned to normal, but the vascular lesions showed no evidence of regression. Best results were obtained by removing the left upper lobe and leaving only the shunt to the lower lobe. The pulsatile thrust of shunt blood flowing through an end-to-end anastomosis was considered important for producing pulmonary hypertension.

More significant results were described by DAMMANN et al. (1955): they produced an end-to-end shunt between the left subclavian artery and the left upper lobe pulmonary artery (Fig. 3). There was a mortality of 30%, while in 25% of the surviving dogs the anastomoses were thrombosed. No animal developed cardiac failure. The pressure was recorded by passing a needle in a retrograde fashion through the anastomosis. The systolic pressure in the pulmonary artery was about 50 mm Hg and reached systemic levels in some dogs. The authors observed a progressive vascular pattern, depending on the time of exposure to an elevated pulmonary arterial pressure. The sequence of events of vascular and parenchymal injury is as follows: the immediate effects of the high pressure are hemorrhage and edema involving the vessels and the adjacent areas. Then fragmentation of the elastica interna and externa and a diffuse inflammatory reaction follow, and overstretched muscle becomes necrotic, leading to vessel destruction. These microscopic changes appear gradually and spread from the site of the shunt toward the periphery of the lung. Eleven weeks after the operation, these changes are—according to DAMMANN et al. (1957)—almost uniform throughout the lobe, showing excessive medial hypertrophy and intimal proliferation with complete obstruction of the lumen. In a few arteries the anatomy was totally destroyed. FERGUSON and BERKAS (1957) in short-term experiments shunted the left subclavian artery to the left pulmonary artery. The mean pressure tolerated without pulmonary edema was about 58 mm Hg. After complete denervation, a pressure in this range produced edema. After the operation, 11 dogs died of pulmonary edema. Three of nine dogs were kept for up to 10 months and developed questionable medial hypertrophy. The same authors (1959), continuing this research, made a shunt from the left subclavian artery to the left lower lobe of the lung. Flow to this lobe was 2 to 3 times normal. If the pressure distal to the anastomosis was above 35 mm Hg, the risk of pulmonary edema was very high. If it was below 30 mm Hg, the chance for development of hypertensive lesions was slim. When a shunt to the main pulmonary artery with bilateral lobe resection was made, pulmonary arterial pressure reached 35 mm Hg and no

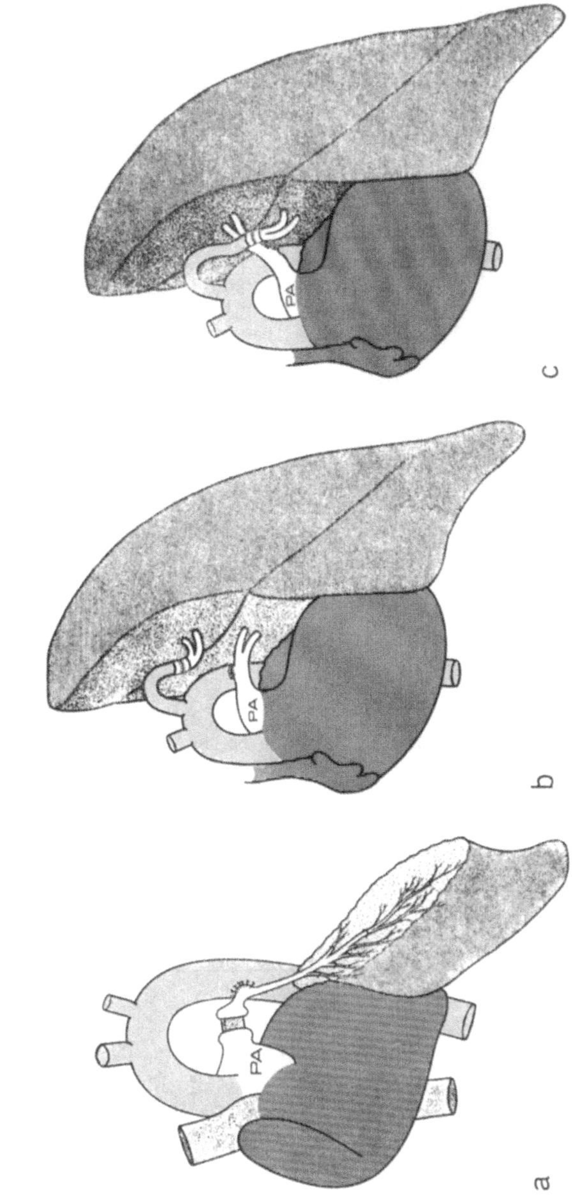

Fig. 3a—c. Summary of experimental procedures associated with the highest probability of hyperkinetic pulmonary hypertension and corresponding vascular lesions. (a) Resection of left upper lobe, anastomosis of pulmonary artery to the descending aorta and banding of the pulmonary branch in order to diminish shunting to the contralateral side. (b) End-to-end anastomosis between the left subclavian artery and the upper lobe. (c) End-to-end anastomosis of the subclavian artery to the pulmonary artery of the lower lobe. Summarized after FERGUSON and VARCO, 1955; BLANK et al., 1961; GLASS et al., 1965; BORST et al., 1966

significant histological changes appeared. HEATH et al. (1959a) described a dog 4 years after an aortopulmonary (Potts) anastomosis of 5 mm diameter, with severe hypertensive pulmonary vascular disease grade 6, according to his classification (1958). The muscular arteries were hypertrophied or occluded by fibrous tissue. Another successful and excellent report on the production of hypertensive lesions in the lung was that by BLANK et al. in 1961. They produced an end-to-end shunt between the subclavian artery and the upper lobe of the left lung in 46 dogs. In 14 animals the left lower lobe pulmonary artery was connected to the aorta or subclavian artery. In 20 dogs the lobar pulmonary artery was re-

Table 3. Summary of the most successful investigations in the production of hyperkinetic pulmonary hypertension. All experimental animals were dogs. The difference in pressure values may be caused by the various techniques applied

Authors	Shunt	Diameter mm	No. of animals	Observation time (months)	Pa pressure mm Hg	Controlled animals	Histology (Grade)
MULLER et al., 1953	aorta, l. pulm. art.	5–8	30	8–12	110/80	5	I–II
FERGUSON, VARCO, 1955	subcl. art.		62	3–8	36 ($\overline{m}$)	3	I–II
	l. pulm. art.				61 ($\overline{m}$)	7	I, II, III
	l. lower lobe	—			—		
	l. upper lobe					1	III
FERGUSON et al., 1955/59	subcl. art.			5	25		
	l. lower lobe	3–8	23	10	40	3	II–III
DAMMANN et al., 1957	subcl. art.				60–90	9	I–III
	l. upper lobe	5–8	41	0.5–2.7			
HEATH et al., 1959a	brachioceph.	1+4		47	31/17	2	—
	pulm. art.		3				
	aorta, pulm. art.	5		46	—	1	VI
BLANK et al., 1961	subcl. art. l. upper lobe		46	9	systemic	4	III
	aorta a. subcl. art., l. lower lobe				—	5	I—II
DOWNING et al., 1963	aorta, l. lower lobe	5	14	3–30	50–80	6	thrombi
						1	plexiform a. angiomat. lesions
GLASS et al., 1963/65	aorta, l. lung lobe	3	66	1–9.5	55–100	11	II–III
						6	IV
BORST et al., 1966	subcl. art.			24	35–50/30	12	II–III
	l. lower lobe	5.7	36				
	l. upper lobe		10	12	80	1	III

anastomosed to the pulmonary artery after 1 h to 9 months. Twenty-four of the animals died in the early postoperative period because of pulmonary edema. The most consistant vascular lesions were seen in animals with shunts to the left upper lobe. In six dogs medial hypertrophy and intimal hyperplasia of the small pulmonary arteries had developed. After reanastomosis the authors described regression of the histological findings.

DOWNING et al. (1963) produced hyperkinetic pulmonary hypertension in dogs by left upper lobectomy and implantation of the lower lobe pulmonary artery end-to-side into the descending thoracic aorta. Four of 14 dogs died of pulmonary congestion and edema. The pressure was measured only once—just after opening the shunt during operation—and it was found to range between 50 to 80 mm Hg. One animal with a large shunt for 16 months had no vascular lesions at all. In another dog, after 30 months, there was great variability of lesions. Thrombi occurred in proximal vessels as well as plexiform and angiomatoid lesions in all stages of development, as described by HEATH and EDWARDS (1958). DOWNING et al. (1963) suggested that mechanical damage at the points of turbulence was

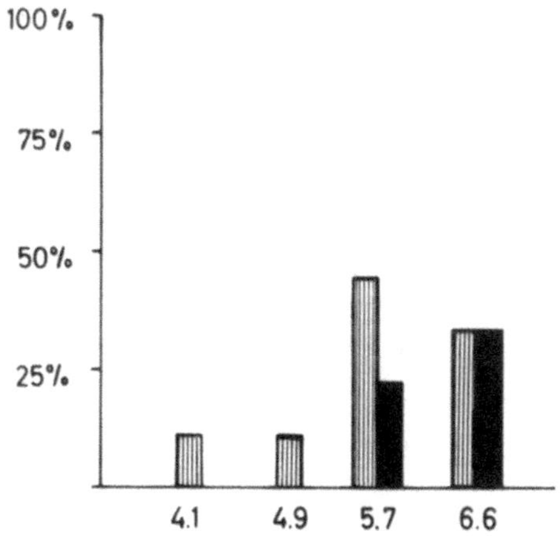

Fig. 4. Operative mortality during production of pulmonary hypertension depending on the diameter of anastomosis between the subclavian artery and the left lower pulmonary lobe. X-axis: diameter of anastomosis in mm. Y-axis: 100% = number of dogs. The black columns signify the dogs lost from pulmonary edema

the cause of these lesions. Such damage at the endothelium may be accompanied by the deposition of a thrombus. The authors found thrombi of various stages and even fibrous mural plaques in such areas. Thrombosis was regarded as a dominant mechanism in the production of irreversible lesions in pulmonary hypertension. In these cases, however, dirofilaria larvae may have played a role. GLASS et al. (1965) succeeded in producing similar pulmonary vascular changes bly employing a modified technique of HEATH and EDWARDS (1958). Using beagoe puppies (2.8 to 8.2 kg), they made a side-to-side aorticopulmonary artery anasthmosis and banded the proximal part of the pulmonary artery to protect the rigt lung and to promote blood flow to the left side. They also varied the procedure by placing the ligatures on the upper and middle lobe arteries or by making an anastomosis between the aorta and lower lobe artery with proximal banding (see Fig. 3). The size of the anastomosis was 3 mm diameter. The mortality was about 50%. Of 66 dogs, 26 developed significant pulmonary arterial pressure elevation of 40%. There was little correlation between the amount of pulmonary arterial pressure and the degree of microscopic vascular lesions. Nine dogs with pulmonary arterial pressures of 55/30 mm Hg up to systemic levels showed no vascular lesions; in contrast grade 2 and 3 lesions were developed at a pressure of 60/30 mm Hg as well as at systemic levels. Grade 3 lesions showing distinct intimal thickening in the muscular arteries and grade 4 with plexiform intimal thickening could be produced in 10 animals. The results were the same with all three methods. Nine dogs were reoperated and the shunt removed, producing normal pulmonary circulatory conditions. Regression of the pulmonary lesions of grades 2 and 3 occurred within 3 to 6 months—no regression was seen in grade 4 changes during an observation period of 14 months.

In 1966/67 our group (BORST et al.) was engaged in such a project and performed two types of experiments. First, the left subclavian artery was anastomosed to the left lower lobe (Fig. 3b); secondly, the subclavian artery was connected with the upper lobe artery (Fig. 3c). In 36 of 46 dogs, the left lower lobe pulmonary artery was anastomosed with the left subclavian artery. Eight of 10 dogs with an anastomosis to the left upper lobe died after the operation of

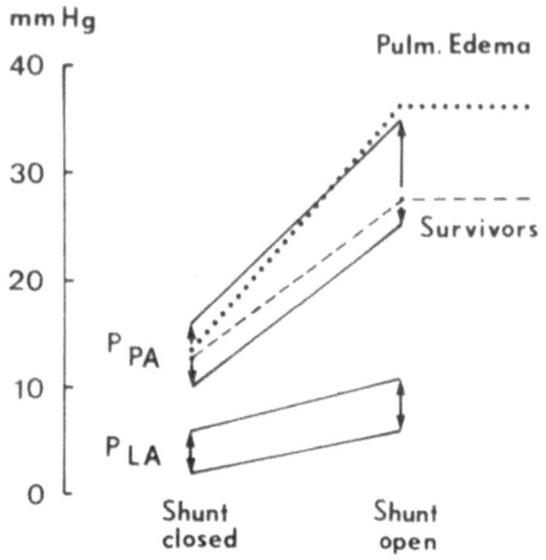

Fig. 5. Results of pressure recordings in the pulmonary artery (PA) and the left atrium (LA) —mean values of 32 animals—after opening and closing of a shunt between the left lower lobe and subclavian artery. The fine dotted line represents the mean PA-pressure of those animals which succumbed to pulmonary edema

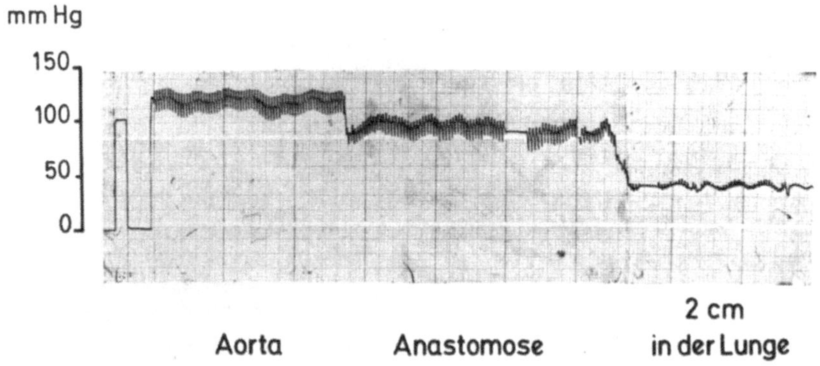

Fig. 6. Systemic-pulmonary fistula to the upper pulmonary lobe in the dog. Pressure was recorded by withdrawl of a catheter from the pulmonary periphery

pulmonary edema or cardiac failure. In order to obtain an anastomosis of defined diameter, we used the suturing apparatus of ANDROSOV (1955). The diameter of the anastomosis varied between 4.1 and 6.7 mm. Of the dogs with the anastomosis to the left lower lobe, 13 survived for periods of up to 2 years. Forty per cent of the deaths were due to lung edema. The correlation is demonstrated in Fig. 4. It is obvious that with the larger shunts, the rate of pulmonary edema increases. In all experiments pressures were recorded in the pulmonary artery, the lobe artery, the left atrium and the ascending aorta. A thin Teflon catheter was advanced through a branch of the subclavian artery through the shunt into the lung periphery (comp. Fig. 6). The pulmonary arterial pressure within the lung was 32 mm Hg. Distal to the anastomosis the catheter passed an area of severe turbulence with varying pressure zones. In the subclavian artery the pressure was systemic. There was no stenosis on the suture line, which indicates that the recording of reliable and undisturbed pressure curves can be problematic. The

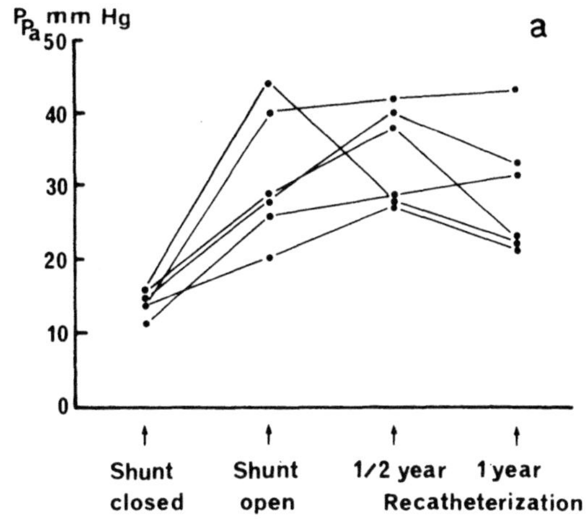

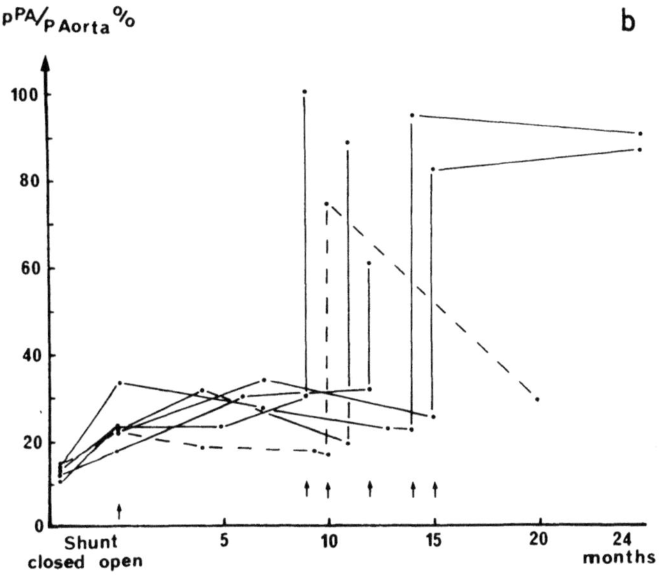

Fig. 7a and b. Summary of the long-term experiments of six dogs with a systemic-pulmonary fistula. (a) After opening of the shunt a significant rise in PA pressure occurs, which shows a small increment during following recatheterization studies (P_{PA} = mean pulm. art. pressure). (b) The same group of dogs after reoperation (↑) where segmental arteries of the lower pulmonary lobe have been ligated, thus decreasing the capacity of the shunted vascular bed. The pressure recordings show an immediate increase of pressure in the pulmonary bed, reaching systemic levels. Y-axis: ratio of pulmonary arterial to aortic pressure

relationship of the systolic and diastolic pressure in the left lower lobe artery and the left atrium before and after opening of the shunt is presented in Fig. 5. These values are calculated from 32 dogs. The pressure in the left lower lobe artery increases to 35/25 mm Hg. The mean pulmonary arterial pressure of dogs, dying of lung edema, is higher. Pressure recordings done in a dog with left subclavian upper lobe anastomosis are seen in Fig. 6. Pulling the catheter back from the lung into the aorta, a pressure of 50 mm Hg was measured 2 cm within the lung

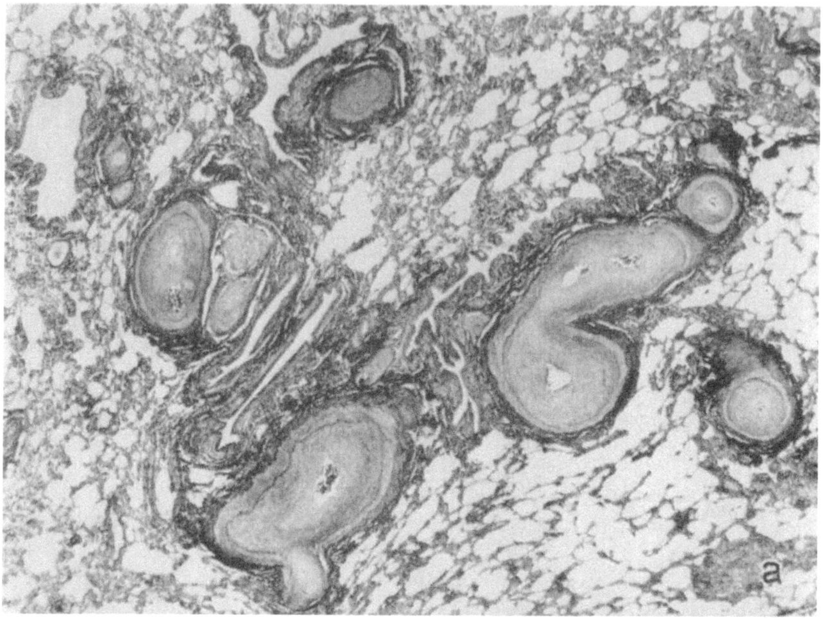

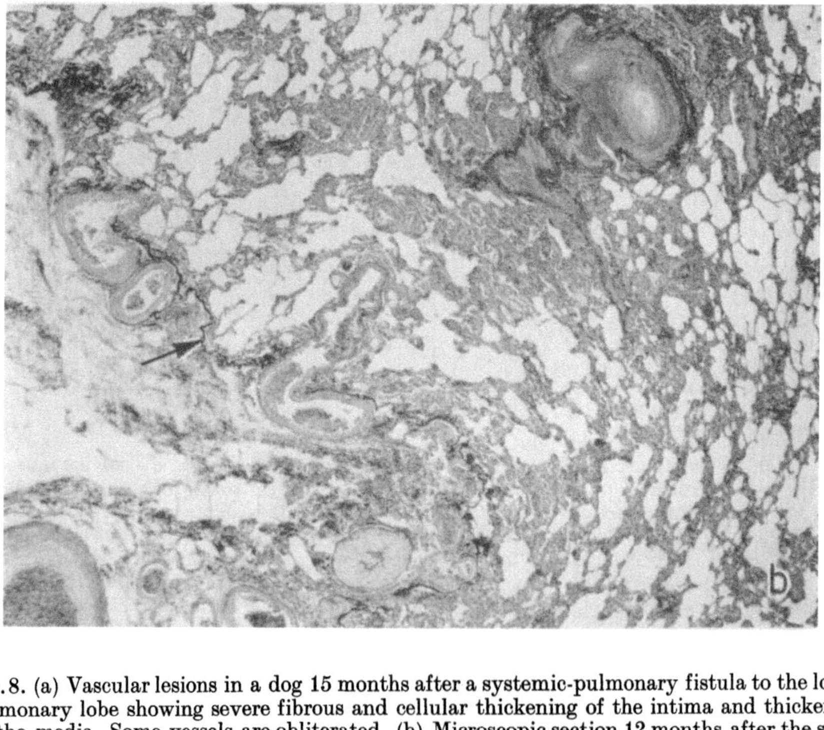

Fig. 8. (a) Vascular lesions in a dog 15 months after a systemic-pulmonary fistula to the lower pulmonary lobe showing severe fibrous and cellular thickening of the intima and thickening of the media. Some vessels are obliterated. (b) Microscopic section 12 months after the same shunt, demonstrating, besides media thickening and intima proliferation in the muscular arteries, perivascular and parenchymatous bleeding. The arrow marks the pleural borderline, showing marked vascularisation of the pleura and communications to bronchial arteries. The microscopic slides are a courtesy of Dr. W. Sebening, Dep. of Pathology, Univ. of Heidelberg (Direktor: Prof. Dr. W. Doerr)

periphery. This agrees in part with the measurements of DAMMANN et al. (1957) who measured almost systemic pressure by needle-puncture distal to the anastomosis. Six of the animals were catheterized by the SELDINGER (1953) technique under light anesthesia at half a year, one and two years. The results are combined in Fig. 7. In all the animals the pulmonary arterial pressure rose immediately after opening of the fistula, levelling off subsequently. After two years recatheterization in two dogs revealed a lobe pressure of 85% respectively 90%, of the aortic pressure. In these dogs we ligated some segmental arteries of the lobe in a second operation in order to decrease the vascular bed in this area. Thereafter in all animals systemic pressure occurred distally to the fistula and no dog died of pulmonary edema.

The pathologic histologic evidence for the presence of vascular lesions due to pulmonary hypertension in these experiments is shown in Fig. 8. Twelve animals were examined 5 to 15 months after a shunt. Five months after an anastomosis to the left lower lobe, perivascular bleeding and hemorrhagic edema were seen. The same fistula after 12 to 15 months in 10 dogs revealed fibrous and cellular proliferation of the intima and in some an occluded lumen; in addition, the media was hypertrophied, resembling changes of grade 3 pulmonary hypertension. In some angiomatoid lesions were observed. The only surviving dog with a shunt to the left upper lobe exhibited intima and media hyperplasia in the muscular arteries and arterioles. A correlation between pulmonary arterial pressure and the type of microscopic lesion present could not be established. Rather, we had the impression that the length of time of an effective fistula was of crucial importance for the creation of pulmonary lesions, which agrees with the report of HEATH et al. (1959a).

These data indicate that the production of experimental pulmonary hypertension in dogs is possible by anastomosing a systemic vessel to one of the lobar pulmonary arteries (Table 3). The effect of such a communication is determined by the diameter of the fistula. When the diameter of the communication is 5 mm or less, the animals show normal or only slightly elevated pulmonary pressure and no changes in the pulmonary vasculature. If the shunt has a diameter of 5 mm or more, fatal pulmonary edema tends to develop rapidly. Thus it would be necessary to produce a fistula of controllable and increasing diameter in order to achieve both survival of the animal and pulmonary hypertension.

V. Production of Pulmonary Hypertension Due to Environmental Influence

1. Effect of High Ambient Gas Pressure

Since the fundamental experiments of v. EULER and LILJESTRAND (1946), it is known that alveolar hypoxia produces vasoconstriction. Chronic alveolar hypoxia is present at an altitude of 3300 to 4000 meters. WILL et al. (1962) produced pulmonary hypertension in cattle living 6 months at an altitude of 3300 meters ($PO_2 \approx 65$ mm Hg) in Colorado. The first increase in pulmonary arterial pressure in these animals was noticed six weeks after arrival, mean pressure reaching values of 27 to 55 mm Hg; two of these animals had a pressure of 100 mm Hg and showed symptoms of right heart failure. These animals showed a significant increase in the weight ratio of the right ventricle to the total ventricular mass as compared to the control. Altitude-induced elevation of pulmonary vascular resistance could be lowered by administration of 100% oxygen. If animals suffering from "high mountain disease" were transported to lower regions, pulmonary arterial pressure regressed to normal within 10 months. Why the pressure reached higher values in some animals than in others is unknown. According to the experiments of REEVES and LEATHERS (1964), the pulmonary vasculature of newborn calves is much more sensitive to hypoxia than that of the adult cattle. BENNETT and SMITH (1934) kept rats in a compressed air (3040 mm Hg) environment ($PO_2 = 635$ mm Hg) for up to 31 days. This is equivalent to an 83.6% mixture of oxygen at normal atmospheric pressure. The highest pulmonary arterial pressure measured was 44 mm Hg. Histologic sections at autopsy showed progressive thickening, narrowing and hyalinization of the pulmonary arteries. VALDIVIA (1957) kept guinea pigs in a chamber simulating a height of 6000 meters for 1 to 5 weeks. The weight of the right heart increased, which was thought to be due to elevated pulmonary arterial pressure; the pressure was, however, not measured. MONGE et al. (1943), ROTTA et al. (1956), HECHT et al. (1959) and SINGH et al. (1965) demonstrated the existence of mountain sickness in native residents of high altitudes associated with the occurrence of right ventricular hypertrophy and marked dilatation of the vascular bed of the lungs. At a hemoglobin (Hb) value of 26 g-%, the arterial HbO_2 was about 74%, blood volume was increased by more than 30%. At an altitude of 4550 meters a pulmonary arterial pressure of 49/27 mm Hg with a mean of 35 mm Hg was measured and pulmonary vascular resistance was markedly elevated. It was suggested, however, that this is a response to polycythemia with an increase of viscosity rather than the effect of vasoconstriction only.

2. Drug-Induced Pulmonary Hypertension

KAY et al. (1967) and CARRILLO and AVIADO (1969) demonstrated a significant increase of pulmonary pressure after administration of pyrrolizidine alkaloids. They described muscular hypertrophy of the pulmonary vasculature, although their findings were not consistent. KAY et al. (1969) deemed it necessary to establish a standard range of normal microscopic values for medial thickness of the pulmonary vessels in rats. They fed ground *Crotalaria spectabilis* seeds to the animals at an initial dose of 0.02% (by weight) for 45 days, and finally increased the dosage to 0.04%. This weed grows in America and Asia, contains the active alkaloids monocrotaline, and belongs to the family of Papilionaceae. Pulmonary vascular changes developed after a period of up to 200 days showing right ventricular hypertrophy, a thick muscular media and, in some animals, acute necrotizing arteritis (cf. SMITH et al., 1970). The pulmonary arteries of some rats showed no intimal fibrosis which might be due to species difference; TURNER and LALICH (1965) found intimal fibroelastosis in pulmonary arteries of the same animals. No dilatation lesions were observed. HEATH (1969) reported systolic pressures in seed-fed rats of 62 to 112 mm Hg (mean 86 mm Hg), the normal range being 27 to 36 mm Hg (mean 29 mm Hg). LÜLLMANN et al. (1972) fed *Crotalaria spectabilis* (250 mg/kg) to rats for 6 weeks which produced an increase of mean PA pressure up to 45 mm Hg, the animals were, however, in poor condition with signs of bleeding probably due to disseminated intravascular coagulopathy. The microscopic sections revealed fresh microthrombi and intimal proliferation of small pulmonary arteries and arterioles. As to the mechanism of production of pulmonary hypertension, it is assumed that the pyrrolizidine alkaloids are metabolized in the liver with some metabolic products acting on the lung vasculature.

Another substance that elevates pulmonary artery pressure is fulvine found in *Crotalaria fulva*. It is used in bush tea in the West Indies. KAY et al. (1971a) fed rats with fulvine. Administration of single doses of 50 mg/kg intraperitoneally or

80 mg/kg by stomach tube resulted in a 55% survival rate for 24 to 37 days, the rats developing pulmonary hypertension and right ventricular hypertrophy. There was thickening of the pulmonary trunk, medial thickening of the muscular pulmonary arteries, and muscularization of the arterioles. Many of the smaller pulmonary arterioles and alveolar capillaries were occluded by thrombi. The pressure was not measured but many animals succumbed to right ventricular failure. Some died earlier of massive hepatic necrosis due to veno-occlusive disease of the liver.

The reports of GURTNER (1969a and b), KAINDL (1969) and LANG et al. (1969) provide clinical evidence for the dietary origin of pulmonary arterial hypertension. These investigators described a high incidence of pulmonary hypertension in patients taking the anorexic drug aminorex fumarate (Menocil) to lose weight. They developed pulmonary vascular lesions typical of pulmonary hypertension, with medial hypertrophy of the muscular pulmonary arteries, intimal fibrosis, plexiform lesions, and occlusion of pulmonary arterioles (BAGHIRZADE and DONATH, 1969). But it was not possible to reproduce such effects in the experimental animal. KRAUPP et al. (1969), BRUNNER and STEPANEK (1970), and KAY et al. (1971b) gave aminorex fumarate (0.05 to 0.3 mg/kg) to dogs and observed only a short-lasting rise of PA pressure (up to 35%), without any morphological changes. HEATH et al. (1970) administered the drug to rats (840 μg/kg for 24 to 302 days) and dogs (6 mg/kg for 20 weeks), but were unable to induce hypertensive pulmonary vascular disease. GROVER and BYRNE-QUINN (1970) gave aminorex to calves but were also unsuccessful in inducing disease. LÜLLMANN et al. (1972) used a series of anorexic agents in rats which increased PA pressure by 30 to 50% microscopic changes however were absent. Similar results have been reported by ENGELHARDT and KALBFLEISCH (1973) who injected (25 to 200 μg/kg) and fed aminorex fumarate to rats for up to 207 days, when the PA pressure increased to 34/22 mm Hg without causing morphological changes of the pulmonary vasculature. It has to be assumed that anorexic drugs act primarily as vasoconstrictors on the pulmonary vessels. It is unknown if this is a direct or indirect action caused by release of vasoactive compounds like serotonin (MIELKE et al., 1972).

According to the investigations of HEATH (1969), HEATH et al. (1970), BURNS (1971), and LÜLLMANN et al. (1972) there are at present three pyrrolizidine alkaloids which are useful in the experimental production of vascular lesions in the lung, i.e. monocrotaline found in *Crotalaria spectabilis*, fulvine found in *Crotalaria fulva*, and senecionine found in *Senecio jacobaea*.

VI. Pulmonary Hypertension in Transplantation

Still a moot point in the literature is the cause of fixed high vascular resistance after lung transplantation (YEH et al., 1962; HARDY et al., 1963; NIGRO et al., 1963; BÜCHERL et al., 1964; KAHN et al., 1965; OTTO and TRENKNER, 1966; TRUMMER and BERG, 1968; WILDEVUUR et al., 1968; ALLGOOD et al., 1968; DAICOFF et al., 1970). MOMMA et al. (1970) describe an increased vascular resistance shortly after transplantation in dogs. NIGRO et al. (1963) in tests made after 2 months and for up to $2^1/_2$ years after unilateral autotransplantation and contralateral pneumonectomy, found an increased mean pulmonary arterial pressure of 38 mm Hg.

While some authors suggested mechanical stenosis on the side of the anastomosis (OTTO and TRENKNER, 1966; VEITH and RICHARDS, 1969; STEVENS et al., 1969), others discussed ischemic damage (MOMMA et al., 1970) or lung denervation as possible causes for pulmonary hypertension (NIGRO et al., 1963; TRUMMER and

BERG, 1968). A detailed study on this subject was made by WILDEVUUR et al. (1968), who describe, several months after unilateral reimplantation and contralateral pneumonectomy, a pressure of 41/15 mm Hg (mean 24 mm Hg) in the pulmonary artery. RHODES et al. (1973) were able to produce mean pulmonary arterial pressures of 38 to 72 mm Hg (average 24 mm Hg) in newborn calves by denervation of the left lung and ligation of the right pulmonary artery. Pulmonary vascular resistance increased fourfold; the experimental procedure, however, was not designed to obtain long-term survivors, so that a description of microscopic changes in the pulmonary vasculature was lacking.

The theory of mechanical stenosis has been refuted by en bloc transplantation of heart and lungs in primates, in which no anastomoses on the pulmonary vessels were required, and in which a pulmonary pressure of 40/17 mm Hg was found (SCHMIDT-HABELMANN et al., 1972). Dogs, however, seem to be more favorable candidates for producing pulmonary hypertension by this technique than baboons (CASTANEDA et al., 1972).

E. Conclusions

The pulmonary vascular tree is a highly distensible segment of the circulatory system. Various acute physiological and pharmacological stimuli by virtue of inducing vasoconstriction, will make this system less distensible and therefore cause an acute increase of pulmonary vascular resistance. By contrast, the experimental production of chronic pulmonary vascular narrowing of a predictable degree appears rather difficult. Among the many methods designed for this purpose, the earliest model was artificial pulmonary embolization. Injection of clot, foreign bodies or air has given variable results.

Experiments imitating the circulatory conditions of clinical pulmonary venous congestion, which is one of the prime causes of pulmonary hypertension in man, have been unsuccessful. On the other hand, the pulmonary hypertension developing in cardiac defects with high pulmonary flow has been reproduced with some success in animals. Also it has been shown that reversal of high pulmonary flow subsequent to its experimental establishment, will reduce some of the vascular lesions produced by hypertension. This finding forms the basis for the so-called "banding operation" for the pulmonary artery as used clinically to protect the lung vessels from the consequences of high flow states (MULLER and DAMMANN, 1952a; DAMMANN et al., 1961). The more severe obstructive pulmonary vascular lesions, by contrast, do not seem to be reversible in either man or animals. For patients with a fixed type of pulmonary vascular hypertension, lung transplantation therefore seems the only useful alternative. Since the yield of experiments imitating high pulmonary flow states is low and the complication rate extremely high, new avenues of producing such pulmonary hypertension should be sought. Promising progress has been reported in connection with lung autotransplantation, a possible cause of pulmonary hypertension being denervation.

Induction of pulmonary hypertension by chronic exposure to low atmospheric pressure, especially in large animals, seems a promising avenue for further research. The effects of high blood viscosity must be eliminated, however, and more histological material presented.

Drug-induced chronic pulmonary hypertension has been of considerable clinical concern recently. Again more experimental data, especially from larger animals, should be accumulated in order to further explore mechanisms, histology and possible modes of treatment.

References

ADAMS, W. E., PERKINS, J. F., CHAO, P., CASTELLANOS, M.: The significance of pulmonary hypertension as a cause of death following pulmonary resection. J. thorac. Surg. **26**, 407–415 (1953).

ALLGOOD, R. J., EBERT, P. A., SABISTON, D. C., JR.: Immediate changes in pulmonary hemodynamics following lung autotransplantation. Ann. Surg. **167**, 352–358 (1968).

ANDRAL, G.: Dictionnaire de Médicine et de Chirurgie Pratiques. Tom 3. Gabon, Méquignan — Marois u. J. B. Baillière. Paris 1829.

ANDROSOV, P. I.: Mechanical suture in surgical treatment of injury to blood vessels and traumatic aneurysms. Vestn. Khir. **3**, 37–44 (1955).

AVERY, M. E., SAID, S.: Surface phenomena in lungs in health and disease. Medicine (Baltimore) **41**, 503–526 (1965).

AVIADO, D. M.: Pharmacology of pulmonary circulation. Pharmacol. Rev. **12**, 159–239 (1960).

AVIADO, D. M., CERLETTI, A., ALANIS, I., BULLE, P. A., SCHMIDT, C. F.: Effects of anoxia on pressure resistance and blood (P^{32}) vol. of pulmonary vessels. Amer. J. Physiol. **169**, 460–470 (1952).

BAGHIRZADE, M. F., DONATH, K.: Menocil-Medikation und pulmonaler Hochdruck (Treatment with Menocil and pulmonary hypertension.) Verh. Dtsch. Ges. Pathologie, 53. Tag., 473–479 (1969).

BAMBERGER, G.: Lehrbuch der Krankheiten des Herzens. Zit. bei KÖHN. Wien: Richter 1857.

BARER, G. R., HOWARD, P., MCCURRIE, J. R.: The effect of carbon dioxide and changes in blood pH on pulmonary vascular resistance in cats. Clin. Sci. **32**, 361–376 (1967).

BARER, G. R., MCCURRIE, J. R., SHAW, J. W.: Effect of changes in blood pH on the vascular resistance of the normal and hypoxic cat lung. Cardiovasc. Res. **5**, 490–497 (1971).

BARNARD, P. J.: Experimental fibrin thromboembolism of the lungs. J. Path. Bact. **65**, 129–139 (1953).

BARNARD, P. J.: Pulmonary arteriosclerosis and cor pulmonale due to recurrent thromboembolism. Circulation **10**, 343–361 (1954a).

BARNARD, P. J.: Thrombo-embolic primary pulmonary arteriosclerosis. Brit. Heart J. **16**, 93–100 (1954b).

BARNARD, P. J.: Pulmonary arteriosclerosis due to oxygen, nitrogen and argon embolism. Arch. Path. **63**, 322–332 (1957).

BARNES, W. H., ELLIS, F. H., GRINDLAY, J. H., EDWARDS, J. E.: Experimental production of pulmonary hypertension. Surgery **44**, 361–371 (1958).

BAUM, M. D., KOT, P. A.: Response of pulmonary vascular segments to angiotensin and norepinephrine. J. thorac. cardiovasc. Surg. **63**, 322–328 (1972).

BENNETT, A. G., SMITH, F. J. C.: Pulmonary hypertension in rats living under compressed air conditions. J. exp. Med. **59**, 181–199 (1934).

BERGOFSKY, E. H., LEHR, D. E., FISHMAN, A. P.: The effect of changes in hydrogen ion concentration on the pulmonary circulation. J. Clin. Invest. **41**, 1942–1502 (1962).

BEVEGARD, S., HOLMGREN, A., JOHNSSON, B.: Circulatory studies in well trained athletes at rest and during heavy exercise. Acta physiol. scand. **57**, 26–32 (1963).

BIRCKS, W.: Chirurgische Gesichtspunkte der pulmonalen Hypertension. Thoraxchirurgie **14**, 521–530 (1966).

BLANK, R. H., MILLER, W. H., JR., DAMMANN, J. F., JR.: Experimental pulmonary arterial hypertension. Amer. J. Surg. **101**, 143–153 (1961).

BLOOMFIELD, R. A., LAUSON, H. D., COURNAND, A., BREED, E. S., RICHARDS, D. W.: Recording at right heart pressures in normal subjects and in patients with chronic pulmonary disease and various types of cardio-circulatory disease. J. Clin. Invest. **25**, 639–664 (1946).

BOEREMA, B.: Appearance and regression of pathological changes in the pulmonary arterial wall after repeated air embolism. J. Cardiovasc. Surg. **6**, 160–162 (1968).

BOGAERT, A. v., FANNES, E., TOSSETTI, R., GENABEEK, S. v., BUYTAERT, L., ARNOLDY, M., VANDAEL, J., HENST, H. v. D.: Hypertension artérielle pulmonaire expérimentale durable chez le chien. Arch. Ma. Coeur **50**, 681–701 (1957).

BORDEN, C. W., EBERT, R. O., WILSON, R. H., WELLS, H. S.: Pulmonary hypertension in heart disease. New Engl. J. Med. **242**, 529–534 (1950).

BORST, H. G., BERGLUND, E., MCGREGOR, M.: The effects of pharmacologic agents on the pulmonary circulation in the dog. J. Clin. Invest. **36**, 669–675 (1957a).

BORST, H. G., BERGLUND, E., WHITTENBERGER, J. L., MEAD, J., MCGREGOR, M., COLLIER, C.: The effect of pulmonary vascular pressures on the mechanical properties of the lungs of anesthetized dogs. J. Clin. Invest. **36**, 1708–1714 (1957b).

BORST, H. G., MEISNER, H., LOIBL, H.: Experimentelle pulmonale Hypertension. Thoraxchirurgie **14**, 481–486 (1966).

BORST, H. G., WHITTENBERGER, J. L., BERGLUND, E.: Influence of pulmonary arterial and left atrial pressures on pulmonary vascular resistance. Circulat. Res. **4**, 393–399 (1956).

BORST, H. G., WHITTENBERGER, J. L., BERGLUND, E., MCGREGOR, M.: Effects of unilateral hypoxia and hypercapnia on pulmonary blood flow distribution in the dog. Amer. J. Physiol. **191**, 446–452 (1957c).

BOUCEK, R. J., GRINDBERG, J. H., BURCHELL, H. B.: Experimental constriction of inflow tracts in heart: analysis of circulatory failure. Amer. J. Physiol. **169**, 442–452 (1952).

BRAUNSTEIN, H.: Periarteritis nodosa limited to the pulmonary circulation. Amer. J. Path. **31**, 837–857 (1955).

BRENNER, O.: Pathology of vessels of pulmonary circulation. Arch. intern. Med. **56**, 211–216 (1935).

BROFMANN, B. L., CHARMS, B. L., KOHN, P. M., ELDER, J., NEWMAN, R., RISIKA, M.: Unilateral pulmonary artery occlusion in man. Control studies. J. thorac. Surg. **34**, 206–227 (1957).

BRUNNER, H., STEPANEK, J.: Drucksteigerungen im kleinen Kreislauf des Hundes durch Aminorex. Naunyn-Schmiedebergs Arch. Pharmakol. **266**, 304–305 (1970).

BÜCHERL, E. S., NASSERI, M. v., PRONDSYNSKI, B.: Lung function studies after homotransplantation, autotransplantation, denervation of the left lung and ligature of the right pulmonary artery. J. thorac. cardiovasc. Surg. **47**, 455–465 (1964).

BÜHLMANN, A., MAIER, C., HEGGLIN, M., KÄLIN, R.: Zur Pathogenese der arteriellen pulmonalen Hypertonie mit besonderer Berücksichtigung des Cor pulmonale beim Emphysem. Cardiologia (Basel) **24**, 96–101 (1954).

BÜHLMEYER, K.: Die pulmonale Hypertension bei angeborenen Herzfehlern im Kindesalter. Bibliotheca Paediatrica Nr. 85. Basel-New York: S. Karger 1967.

BURCHELL, H. B.: Studies in pulmonary hypertension in congenital heart disease. St. Cyres Lecture of the Nat. Heart Hospital. London, Engl., June 4, 1958.

BURNS, J.: The heart and pulmonary arteries of rats fed on Senecio jacobaea. Pathological Society of Great Britain and Ireland. Synopses of papers read at 122nd meeting, Jan. 1971.

CARRILLO, G., AVIADO, D. M.: Monocrotaline-induced Pulmonary Hypertension and p-Chlorophenylalanine (PCPA). Lab. Invest. **20**, 243–248 (1969).

CASTANEDA, A. R., ZAMORA, R., SCHMIDT-HABELMANN, P., HORNUNG, J., MURPHY, W., PONTO, D., MOLLER, J. H.: Cardiopulmonary autotransplantation in primates (baboons): late functional results. Surgery **72**, 1064–1070 (1972).

CIVIN, W. H., EDWARDS, J. E.: Postnatal structural changes in intrapulmonary arteries and arterioles. Arch. Path. **51**, 192–200 (1951).

CONNOLLY, J. E.: Surgical Forum (Amer. College Surgeons). Philadelphia: W. B. Saunders 1950.

COURNAND, A.: Recent observations on the dynamics of pulmonary circulation. Bull. N.Y. Acad. Med. **23**, 27–32 (1947/2).

COURNAND, A.: Some aspects of pulmonary circulation in a normal man and in chronic cardiopulmonary diseases. Circulation **2**, 641–657 (1950).

DAGHER, I. K., MISHALANY, H. G., SIMEONE, F. A., WILSON, J. L.: Mechanisms of pulmonary hypertension in acute hypoxia. J. thorac. cardiovasc. Surg. **42**, 743–754 (1961).

DAICOFF, G. R., ALLEN, P. D., STRECK, C. J.: Pulmonary vascular resistance following lung reimplantation and transplantation. Ann. thorac. Surg. **9**, 569–579 (1970).

DALEY, R., WADE, J. D., MARAIST, F., BING, R. J.: Pulmonary hypertension in dogs induced by injection of lycopodium spores into the pulmonary artery, with special reference to the absence of vasomotor reflexes. Amer. J. Physiol. **164**, 380–390 (1951).

DAMMANN, J. F., BAKER, J. P., MULLER, W. H.: Pulmonary vascular changes induced by experimentally produced arterial hypertension. Surg. Gynec. Obstet. **105**, 16–20 (1957).

DAMMANN, J. F., EACHEN, I. A., THOMPSON, W. M., SMITH, R., MULLER, W. H.: The regression of pulmonary vascular disease after the creation of pulmonary stenosis. J. thorac. cardiovasc. Surg. **42**, 722–734 (1961).

DAMMANN, J. F., JR., SMITH, R. T., MULLER, W. H., JR.: The experimental production of pulmonary vascular disease. Surg. Forum **6**, 155–157 (1955).

DAWES, G. S.: Reflexes originating in the pulmonary circulation. In: Pulmonary Circ. New York-London: Grune & Stratton 1959/2.

DAWES, G. S., MOTT, I. C., WIDDICOMB, J. G.: Fetal circulation in the lamb. J. Physiol. (Lond.) **126**, 563–574 (1954).

DEFARES, J. G., LUNDIN, G., ARBORELIUS, M., JR., STROMBLAD, R., SVANBERG, L.: Effects of "unilateral hypoxia" on pulmonary blood flow distribution in normal subjects. J. appl. Physiol. **15**, 169–174 (1960).

DEUCHAR, C. D., KNEBEL, R.: The pulmonary and systemic circulation in congenital heart disease. Brit. Heart J. **14**, 225–249 (1952/2).

DEXTER, L.: Cardiovascular response to experimental pulmonary embolism. In: Pulmonary Embolic Disease. New York: Grune & Stratton 1965.

DEXTER, L., DOW, J. W., HAYNES, F. W., WHITTENBERGER, J. L., FERRIS, B. G., GOODALE, W. T., HELLEMS, H. K.: Studies of the pulmonary circulation in man at rest. Normal variation and the interrelations between increased pulmonary blood flow, elevated pulmonary arterial pressure and high pulmonary "capillary" pressure. J. Clin. Invest. **29**, 602–613 (1950).

DITTRICH, J.: Über den Laennec'schen Lungeninfarkt und sein Verhältnis zur Erkrankung der Lungenarterien. Zitiert bei KÖHN und RICHTER. Erlangen: Blaesing 1850.

DOWNING, S. E., TALNER, N. S., GARDNER, T. H.: Cardiovascular responses to metabolic acidosis. Amer. J. Physiol. **208**, 237–242 (1965).

DOWNING, S. E., VIDONE, R. A., BRANDT, H. M., LIEBOW, A. A.: The pathogenesis of vascular lesions in experimental hyperkinetic pulmonary hypertension. Amer. J. Path. **43**, 139–765 (1963).

DRESDALE, D. T., SCHULTZ, M., MICHTOM, R. J.: Primary pulmonary hypertension. Amer. J. Med. **11**, 686–705 (1951).

EARL, P. R.: Filariae from the dog in vitro. Ann. N.Y. Acad. Sci. **77**, 163–169 (1959).

EAST, T.: Pulmonary hypertension. Brit. Heart J. **2**, 189–200 (1940).

EDWARDS, J. E.: Functional pathology of the pulmonary vascular tree in congenital cardiac disease. Circulation **15**, 164–196 (1957).

EDWARDS, J. E.: Classification of chronic pulmonary hypertension. Med. Clin. N. Amer. **42**, 1037–1045 (1958).

EDWARDS, W. S.: The effect of lung inflation and epinephrine on pulmonary vascular resistance. Amer. J. Physiol. **167**, 756–762 (1951).

EICHELTER, P., SCHENK, W. G.: Hemodynamic changes following experimental pulmonary embolism. J. thorac. cardiovasc. Surg. **52**, 866–872 (1969).

EISENMENGER, V.: Die angeborenen Defekte der Kammerscheidewand des Herzens. Z. klin. Med. **32**, 1–28 (1897).

ELLISON, R. G., MAJOR, R. C., PICKERING, R. W., HAMILTON, W. F.: Techniques of producing mitral stenosis of controlled degree. J. thorac. Surg. **24**, 154–164 (1952).

ENGELHARDT, R., KALBFLEISCH, H.: Wirkung chronischer Applikation von Aminorexfumarat auf den kleinen Kreislauf der Ratte. Drug. Res. **23**, 1057–1061 (1973).

ENSON, A., GIUNTINI, G., LEWIS, M. L., MARIS, T. Q., FERRER, M. I., HARVEY, R. M.: The influence of hydrogen ion concentration and hypoxia on the pulmonary circulation. J. Clin. Invest. **43**, 1146–1162 (1964).

EULER, U. S. v., LILJESTRAND, G.: Observation on the pulmonary artery blood pressure in the cat. Acta physiol. scand. **12**, 301–320 (1946).

FARRAR, J. F., BLOMFIELD, J., REYE, R. D. K.: The structure and composition of the pulmonary circulation in congenital heart disease. J. Path. Bact. **90**, 97–105 (1965).

FERENCZ, CH., DAMMANN, J. F., JR.: Significance of the pulmonary vascular bed in congenital heart disease. Circulation **16**, 1046–1056 (1957).

FERGUSON, D. J., BERKAS, E. M.: Effect of lung denervation on pulmonary hypertension and edema. Circulat. Res. **5**, 310–314 (1957).

FERGUSON, D. J., BERKAS, E. M., VARCO, R. L.: Circulatory factors contributing to alterations in pulmonary vascular histology. Surg. Forum **4**, 267–269 (1953).

FERGUSON, D. J., BERKAS, E. M., VARCO, R. L.: Experimental methods for the production of pulmonary hypertension. In: Pulmonary Circulation. New York-London: Grune & Stratton 1959.

FERGUSON, D. J., VARCO, R. L.: The relation of blood pressure and flow to the development and regression of experimentally induced pulmonary arteriosclerosis. Circulat. Res. **3**, 152–158 (1955).

FERRER, M. I., HARVEY, R. M., CATHART, R. T., WEBSTER, C. A., RICHARDS, D. W., COURNAND, A.: Some effects of Digoxin upon the heart and circulation in man. Circulation **1**, 161–186 (1950).

FERRIN, A. L., ADAMS, W. L., BARNOFSKY, I. D.: Evolution of experimental methods of producing functional mitral stenosis. Surg. Forum **2**, 206–211 (1951).

FISHMAN, A. P., HIMMELSTEIN, A., FRITTS, H. W., JR., COURNAND, A.: Blood flow through each lung in man during unilateral hypoxia. J. Clin. Invest. **34**, 637–646 (1955).

FLORES, A., ADAMS, W. E., PERKINS, J. F., JR.: Reduction of pulmonary reserve-1. Technique for reducing pulmonary capacity to fifteen percent, with measurements of right heart pressures and arterial blood oxygen saturation in dogs at rest and during exercise. Arch. Surg. **68**, 627–636 (1954).

FRIEDBERG, C. K.: Diseases of the heart. Philadelphia-London: W. B. Saunders Co. 1966.

GEER, J. C., GLASS, B. A., ALBERT, H. M.: Pulmonary vascular lesions in the dog produced by autogenous clot embolism. Exp. molec. Path. **4**, 391–398 (1965).

Gilbert, J. W., Jr., Berglund, E., Dahlgren, S., Ovenfas, C. O., Barnes, R.: Experimental pulmonary hypertension in the dog. J. thorac. cardiovasc. Surg. **55**, 565–571 (1968).

Gilmour, J. R., Evans, W.: Primary Pulmonary Hypertension. J. Path. a. Bact. **58**, 687–697 (1946).

Glass, B. A., Geer, J. C., Albert, H. M.: Experimental studies on the reversibility of pulmonary hypertension. Ann. thorac. Surg. **1**, 159–169 (1965).

Glass, B. A., Geer, J. C., Albert, H. M.: Experimental Studies on the Reversibility of Pulmonary Hypertension. Ann. thorac. Surg. **1**, 159–169 (1965).

Glass, B. A., Harold, A. M., Geer, J. C.: Experimental Studies on Reversibility of Pulmonary Hypertension. Surg. forum **14**, 224–227 (1963).

Gore, I., Tanaka, I., Nakashima, I., Larkey, B. J.: Pulmonary vascular lesions following the repeated intravascular administration of thromboplastin. Amer. J. Path. **41**, 77–93 (1962).

Gorlin, R., Haynes, F. W., Goodale, W. T., Sawyer, C. G., Dow, J. W., Dexter, L.: Studies of the circulation dynamics in mitral stenosis. Amer. Heart J. **41**, 30–45 (1951a).

Gorlin, R., Lewis, B. M., Haynes, F. W., Spiegl, R. J., Dexter, L.: Factors regulating pulmonary "capillary" pressure in mitral stenosis. Amer. Heart J. **41**, 834–854 (1951b).

Gould, S. E.: Pathology of the heart and blood vessels. Springfield, Ill.: Charles C. Thomas 1968.

Griffin, G. D. J., Essex, H. E.: Experimental production of interventricular septal defects—certain physiologic and pathologic effects. Surg. Gynec. Obstet **92**, 325–332 (1951).

Grover, R. F., Byrne-Quinn, E.: Attempted induction of pulmonary hypertension in the calf with anorexigens. Read at a Symposium on obesity, circulation and anorexigens. May 15, 16, Lucerne, Switzerland 1970.

Gurtner, H. P.: Ätiologie und Häufigkeit der primär vaskulären Formen des chronischen Cor pulmonale. Dtsch. med. Wschr. **94**, 850–852 (1969a).

Gurtner, H. P.: Pulmonary hypertension produced by ingestion of substances. Bull. physiopath. Resp. **5**, 435–441 (1969b).

Haddy, F. J., Ferrin, A. L., Hannon, D. W., Alden, J. F., Adams, W. L., Baronofsky, L. D.: Cardiac function in experimental mitral stenosis. Circulat. Res. **1**, 219–225 (1953).

Hamilton, W. F.: The physiology of the pulmonary circulation. J. Allergy **22**, 397–410 (1951).

Hannon, D. W., Ferrin, A., Haddy, F., Sprafka, J. L., Barnofsky, I. D.: Pulmonary artery changes in mitral stenosis. Surg. Forum **7**, 240–243 (1957).

Hardy, J. D., Eraslan, S., Dalton, M. L., Jr.: Autotransplantation and homotransplantation of the lung: further studies. J. thorac. cardiovasc. Surg. **46**, 606–615 (1963).

Harris, P.: Influence of acetylcholine on the pulmonary arterial pressure. Brit. Heart J. **19**, 272–276 (1957).

Harrison, C. V.: Experimental pulmonary arteriosclerosis. J. Path. Bact. **60**, 289–293 (1948).

Harrison, C. V.: Experimental pulmonary hypertension. J. Path. Bact. **63**, 195–200 (1951).

Hawe, A., Tsakiris, A. G., McGoon, D. C., Rastelli, G. G.: Experimental production of chronic graded mitral valve stenosis. J. thorac. cardiovasc. Surg. **60**, 559–564 (1970).

Hawley, J. G., Little, R. C., Feil, H.: Further studies of the cardiodynamics of experimental intraventricular communications. Circulation **1**, 321–328 (1950).

Hayek, H. v.: Über die funktionelle Anatomie der Lungengefäße. Verh. Dtsch. Ges. Kreisl.-Forsch. **17**, 17–26 (1951/2).

Heard, B. E.: An experimental study of thickening of the pulmonary arteries of rabbits produced by the organisation of fibrin. J. Path. Bact. **64**, 13–19 (1952).

Heath, D.: Pulmonary hypertension due to Crotalaria spectabilis. In: Pulmonary Circulation and Interstitial Space. **20**, 305–319 (1969).

Heath, D., Best, P. V.: The tunica media of the arteries of the lung in pulmonary hypertension. J. Path. Bact. **76**, 165–171 (1958).

Heath, D., Donald, D. E., Edwards, J. E.: Pulmonary vascular changes in a dog after aortopulmonary anastomosis for four years. Brit. Heart J. **21**, 187–196 (1959a).

Heath, D., Du Shane, J. W., Wood, E. H., Edwards, J. E.: The structure of the pulmonary trunk at different ages and in cases of pulmonary hypertension and pulmonary stenosis. J. Path. Bact. **77**, 443–456 (1959b).

Heath, D., Edwards, J. E.: The pathology of hypertensive pulmonary vascular disease. Circulation **18**, 533–547 (1958).

Heath, D., Helmholz, H. F., Jr., Burchell, H. B., Du Shane, J. W., Kirklin, J. W., Edwards, J. E.: Relation between structural changes in the small pulmonary arteries and the immediate reversibility of pulmonary hypertension following closure of ventricular and atrial septal defects. Circulation **18**, 1167–1174 (1958).

HEATH, D., KAY, J. M., SMITH, P.: A quantitative pathological study of the heart and pulmonary arteries of rats and dogs after prolonged feeding with Aminorex fumarate (Menocil). Uppsala: Proc. 12th Meeting Europ. Soc. for the Study of Drug Toxicity 1970.

HEATH, D., WHITAKER, W.: Hypertensive pulmonary vascular disease. Circulation **14**, 323–343 (1956).

HECHT, H. H., LANGE, R. L., CARNES, W. H., KNIDA, H., BLAKE, J. T.: Brisket disease. Trans. Ass. Amer. Phycns. **72**, 157–168 (1959).

HELLEMS, H. K., HAYNES, F. W., GOWDEY, J. F., DEXTER, L.: Pulmonary capillary pressure in man. J. Clin. Invest. **27**, 540 (1948).

HENNIGAR, G. R., FERGUSON, R. W. P.: Pulmonary vascular sclerosis as a result of Dirofilaria immitis infection in dogs. J. Amer. vet. med. Ass. **131**, 336–342 (1957).

HEPINSTALL, R. H.: The effects of high blood cholesterol. Brit. J. exp. Path. **38**, 438–449 (1957).

HERTZ, C. W.: Untersuchung über den Einfluß der alveolaren Gasdrucke auf die intrapulmonale Durchblutung beim Menschen. Klin. Wschr. **34**, 472–477 (1956a).

HERTZ, C. W.: Einseitige alveolare CO_2-Erhöhung und Durchblutungsgröße jeder Lungenseite beim Menschen. Klin. Wschr. **34**, 532–536 (1956b).

HICKHAM, J. B., CARGILL, W. H.: Effect of exercise on cardiac output and pulmonary arterial pressure in normal persons and in patients with cardiovascular disease and pulmonary emphysema. J. Clin. Invest. **27**, 10–23 (1948).

HOLMAN, E., BECK, C. S.: The physiological response of the circulatory system to experimental alterations. 1. The effect of intracardiac fistulae. J. exp. Med. **42**, 661–674 (1925).

JAMES, L. S., ROWE, R. D.: The pattern of response of pulmonary and systemic arterial pressures in newborn and older infants to short periods of hypoxia. J. Pediat. **51**, 5–11 (1957).

JAQUES, W. E., HYMAN, A. L.: Experimental supravalvular mitral stenosis in the dog. Arch. Path. **64**, 67–74 (1957a).

JAQUES, W. E., HYMAN, A. L.: Experimental pulmonary embolism in dogs. Arch. Path. **64**, 487–493 (1957b).

JORDAN, S. C., HICKEN, P., WATSON, D. A., HEATH, D., WHITAKER, W.: Pathology of the lungs in mitral stenosis in relation to respiratory function and pulmonary haemodynamics. Brit. Heart J. **28**, 101–107 (1966).

KABINS, S. A., FRIDMANN, J., NEUSTADT, J., ESPINOSA, G., KATZ, L. N.: Mechanisms leading to lung edema in pulmonary embolization. Amer. J. Physiol. **198**, 543–546 (1960).

KAHN, D. R., WILSON, W. S., TOLBERT, J. H., SLOAN, H.: Response of the reimplanted lung to hypoxia. Ann. thorac. Surg. **1**, 97–101 (1965).

KAINDL, F.: Primäre pulmonale Hypertension. Wien. Z. inn. Med. **50**, 451–453 (1969).

KAPANCI, I.: Hypertensive pulmonary vascular disease. Endothelial hyperplasia and its relations to intravascular fibrin precipitation. Amer. J. Path. **47**, 665–676 (1965).

KAY, J. M., HARRIS, P., HEATH, D.: Pulmonary hypertension produced in rats by ingestion of *Crotalaria spectabilis* seeds. Thorax **22**, 176–179 (1967).

KAY, J. M., HEATH, D., SMITH, P., BRAS, G., SUMMERELL, J.: Fulvine and the pulmonary circulation. Thorax **26**, 249–261 (1971a).

KAY, J. M., SMITH, P., HEATH, D.: Electron microscopy of crotalaria pulmonary hypertension. Thorax **24**, 511–526 (1969).

KAY, J. M., SMITH, F., HEATH, D.: Aminorex and the pulmonary circulation. Thorax **26**, 262–270 (1971b).

KAY, J. H., THOMAS, V., BLALOCK, A.: The experimental production of high interventricular septal defects. Surg. Gynec. Obstet. **96**, 529–535 (1953).

KENTERA, D., WALLACE, C. R., HAMILTON, W. F., ELLISON, L. T.: Hemodynamic response to hypoxia in dogs with chronic pulmonary hypertension. Amer. J. Physiol. **207**, 650–652 (1964).

KÖNN, G., STORB, R.: Über den Formwandel der kleinen Lungenarterien des Menschen nach der Geburt. Beitr. path. Anat. **123**, 212–250 (1960).

KRAUPP, O., STÜBLINGER, W., RABERGER, G., TURNHEIM, K.: Die Wirkung von Aminorex (Menocil®) auf die Hämodynamik des kleinen und großen Kreislaufs bei i.v. Darreichung am Hund. Naunyn-Schmiedebergs Arch. f. Pharmakologie u. exp. Pathologie. Pharmakol. **264**, 389–405 (1969)

KUX, M., MASSION, W. H.: Reflex changes in pulmonary hemodynamics resulting from microembolism. Europ. Surg. Res. **5**, 301–310 (1973).

LANG, E., HAUPT, E. J., KÖHLER, J. A., SCHMIDT, J.: Cor pulmonale durch Appetitzügler? Münch. med. Wschr. **111**, 405–412 (1969).

LAWRENCE, W., JR., ADAMS, W. E., CASSELS, D. E.: Constrictive pericarditis with obstruction of pulmonary veins. J. thorac. Surg. **17**, 832–840 (1948).

LEVY, S. E., BLALOCK, A.: Experimental observations on the effects of connecting by suture the left main pulmonary artery to the systemic circulation. J. thorac. Surg. **8**, 525–530 (1939).

LILJESTRAND, G.: Regulation of pulmonary arterial blood pressure. Arch. intern. Med. **81**, 162–172 (1948).

LILJESTRAND, G.: Chemical control of the distribution of the pulmonary blood flow. Acta physiol. scand. **44**, 216–240 (1958).

LITTLE, R. C., OPDYKE, D. F., HAWLEY, J. G.: Dynamics of experimental atrial septal defects. Amer. J. Physiol. **158**, 241–253 (1949).

LOGARAS, G.: Further studies of the pulmonary arterial blood pressure. Acta physiol. scand. **14**, 120–135 (1947).

LONGACRE, J. J., CARTER, B. N., QUILL, L. M.: An experimental study of some of the physiologic changes following total pneumonectomy. J. thorac. Surg. **6**, 237–249 (1937).

LOOGEN, P.: Der pulmonale Hochdruck bei angeborenen Herzfehlern mit hohem Stromvolumen. Arch. Kreisl.-Forsch. **28**, 1–55 (1958).

LÜLLMANN, H., PARWARESCH, M. R., SATTLER, M., SEILER, K. U., SIEGFRIEDT, A.: The effects of anorectic agents on the pulmonary pressure and morphology of rat lungs after chronic administration. Drug. Res. **22**, 2096–2099 (1972).

MACCALLUM, W. G., MCCLURE, R. D.: On the mechanical effects of experimental mitral stenosis and insufficiency. Bull. Johns Hopk. Hosp. **17**, 260–266 (1906).

MCGOON, D. C., SWAN, H. J. C., BRANDENBURG, R. O., CONALLY, D. C., KIRKLIN, J. W.: Arterial septal defect: factors affecting the surgical mortality rate. Circulation **19**, 195–200 (1958).

MCGUIRE, J., WESTCOTT, R. N., FOWLER, N. O.: Anoxia and human pulmonary vascular resistance. Trans. Ass. Amer. Phycns. **64**, 404–419 (1951).

MEISNER, H.: Zur Operationsindikation beim Vorhofseptumdefekt mit pulmonaler Hypertension. Thorax Chir. Vask. Chir. **14**, 546–551 (1966).

MÖNCKEBERG, J. G.: Über die genuine Arteriosklerose der Lungenarterie. Dtsch. med. Wschr. **33**, 1243–1246 (1907).

MOMMA, K., LINDE, L. M., FONKALSRUD, E. W., STEVENS, G. H., RANGEL, D. M., YAKEISHI, Y.: Hemodynamics and blood gas exchange in allografted canine lungs. Surgery **67**, 799–806 (1970).

MONGE, C.: High altitude disease. Physiol. Rev. **23**, 166–184 (1943).

MOSCHCOWITZ, E.: Hypertension of the pulmonary circulation; its cause, dynamics and relation to other circulatory states. Amer. J. med. Sci. **174**, 388–406 (1927).

MOTLEY, H. L., COURNAND, A., WERKÖ, L., HIMMELSTEIN, A., DRESDALE, D.: The influence of short periods of induced acute anoxia upon pulmonary artery pressures in man. Amer. J. Physiol. **150**, 315–320 (1947).

MUIRHEAD, E. E., MONTGOMERY, P. O. B.: Thrombo-embolic pulmonary arteritis and vascular sclerosis: its experimental production in rabbits by means of intravenously injected human amniotic fluid and autogenous blood clots. Arch. Path. **52**, 505–517 (1951).

MULLER, W. H., DAMMANN, J. F.: The treatment of certain congenital malformations of the heart by the creation of pulmonic stenosis to reduce pulmonary hypertension and excessive pulmonary blood flow. Surg. Gynec. Obstet. **95**, 213–219 (1952a).

MULLER, W. H., JR., DAMMANN, J. F., JR.: The surgical significance of pulmonary hypertension. Ann. Surg. **136**, 495–510 (1952b).

MULLER, W. H., DAMMANN, J. F., HEAD, W. H.: Changes in the pulmonary vessels produced by experimental pulmonary hypertension. Surgery **34**, 363–375 (1953).

NAKANA, J., FISHER, R. D.: Effects of aortico-pulmonary artery shunt on the cardiovascular dynamics. Cardiologia (Basel) **47**, 1–13 (1965).

NIGRO, S. L., EVANS, R. H., BENFIELD, J. R., GAGO, O., FRY, W. A., ADAMS, W. E.: Physiologic alterations of cardiopulmonary function in dogs living one and one-half years on only a reimplanted lung. J. thorac. cardiovasc. Surg. **46**, 598–605 (1963).

NISELL, O.: The influence of blood gases on the pulmonary vessels of the cat. Acta physiol. scand. **23**, 85–90 (1951a).

NISELL, O.: The influence of carbon dioxide on the respiratory movements of isolated perfused lungs. Acta physiol. scand. **23**, 352–360 (1951b).

OTTO, T. J., TRENKNER, M.: Homotransplantation of the lung in dogs with special reference to the circulation system in the transplant. Thorax **21**, 564–572 (1966).

OWEN, W. R., THOMAS, W. A., CASTLMAN, B., BLAND, E. F.: Unrecognized emboli to the lungs with subsequent cor pulmonale. New Engl. J. Med. **249**, 919–926 (1953).

PARASKOS, J., ADELSTEIN, S. J., SMITH, R., PICKMAN, F., DEXTER, L., DALEN, J.: Long-term follow-up of acute pulmonary embolism. Circulation **46** (Suppl. II), 49–57 (1972).

POSSELT, A.: Die Erkrankungen der Lungenschlagader. Ergebn. Path. **13**, 298–312 (1909).

PRICE, K. C., HATA, D., SMITH, J. R.: Pulmonary vasomotion resulting from miliary embolism of the lungs. Amer. J. Physiol. **182**, 183–190 (1955).

REEVES, J. T., LEATHERS, J. E.: Circulatory changes following birth of the calf and the effect of hypoxia. Circulat. Res. **15**, 343–354 (1964).

RHODES, E. L., O'ROURKE, P. T., LEE, R., STRAKER, J., KIRSCH, M. M.: The effect of levarterenol and phentolamine on the hypertensive pulmonary vasculature. Ann. thorac. Surg. **16**, 375–379 (1973).

RILEY, R. L., HIMMELSTEIN, A., MOTLEY, H. L., WEINER, H. M., COURNAND, A.: Studies of the pulmonary circulation at rest and during exercise in normal individuals and in patients with chronic pulmonary disease. Amer. J. Physiol. **152**, 372–382 (1948).

ROTTA, A., CANEPA, A., HURTADO, A., VELASQUEZ, T., CHAVES, R.: Pulmonary circulation at sea level and at high altitudes. J. appl. Physiol. **9**, 328–336 (1956).

RUDOLPH, A. M., DOORBAUGH, I. E., AULD, A. P. M., RUDOLPH, A. J., NADAS, A. S., SMITH, C. A., HUBELL, J. P.: Studies on the circulation in the new natal period. Pediatrics **27**, 551–566 (1961).

RUDOLPH, A. M., YUAN, S.: Response of the pulmonary vasculature to hypoxia and the hydrogen concentration changes. J. Clin. Invest. **45**, 399–411 (1966).

SABISTON, D. C., JR., WOLFE, W. G.: Experimental and clinical observations on the natural history of pulmonary ambolism. Ann. Surg. **168**, 1–15 (1968).

SCHILLING, J. A., HARVEY, R. B., BALKE, B., RATTUNDE, H. F.: Extensive pulmonary resection in dogs: altitude tolerance, work capacity, and pathologic-physiologic changes. Ann. Surg. **144**, 635–646 (1956).

SCHMIDT-HABELMANN, P., HORNUNG, J., PONTO, R., LOKEN, M. K., ZAMERA, R., CASTANEDA, A. R.: Pulmonary function studies with Xenon 133 after orthotopic cardiopulmonary autotransplantation in primates. Surg. Forum **23**, 277–279 (1972).

SCHOENMACKERS, J.: Pathologie der pulmonalen Hypertension. Veränderungen an Lungen-Bronchial-Lymphgefäßen. Thoraxchirurgie **14**, 465–480 (1966).

SCHWEIZER, W.: Die pulmonäre arterielle Hypertension. Schweiz. med. Wschr. **44**, 1055–1069 (1953).

SEBENING, F.: Zur Korrektur des Ventrikel-Septum-Defektes. Thoraxchirurgie **15**, 588–594 (1967).

SELDINGER, S. I.: Catheter replacement of the needle in percutaneous arteriography. Acta radiol. (Stockh.) **39**, 368–373 (1953).

SHAW, M. M., ADAMS, W. E., RASMUSSEN, R. A., HRIDINA, L. S., ARONSON, H. G.: Experimental production of insufficiency and stenosis of the heart valves in dogs. J. thorac. Surg. **12**, 322–330 (1943).

SHEPHERD, J. T., SEMLER, H. J., HELMHOLZ, H. F., WOOD, E. H.: Effects of infusion of acetylcholine on pulmonary vascular resistance in patients with pulmonary hypertension and congenital heart disease. Circulation **20**, 381–390 (1959).

SINGER, D., SALTZMAN, P. W., RIVERA-ESTRADA, C., PICK, R., KATZ, L. N.: Hemodynamic alterations following miliary pulmonary embolisation in relation to the pathogenesis of the consequent diffuse edema. Am. J. Physiol. **191**, 437–442 (1957).

SINGH, I., LAV, M., HOON, S., KHANNA, P. K., RAO, B. D. P.: High-altitude pulmonary hypertension. Lancet **2**, 146–150 (1965).

SLOAN, H., MORRIS, I. D., FIGLEY, M., LEE, R.: Temporary unilateral occlusion of the pulmonary artery in the preoperative evaluation of thoracic patients. J. thorac. Surg. **30**, 591–597 (1955).

SMITH, P., KAY, J. M., HEATH, D.: Hypertensive pulmonary vascular disease in rats after prolonged feeding with Crotalaria spectabilis seeds. The Journal of Pathology **102**, 97–106 (1970).

SMITH, W. M., KROOP, J. G.: Raynand's disease in primary pulmonary hypertension. J. Amer. med. Ass. **165**, 1245–1248 (1957).

STAEMMLER, M.: Die Thromboendarteritis obliterans der Lungenarterien. Klin. Wschr. **16**, 1669–1671 (1937).

STEINBERG, U.: Systematische Untersuchungen über die Arteriosklerose der Lungenschlagadern. II. Zur Frage der primären Pulmonalsklerose. Beitr. path. Anat. **82**, 443–463 (1929).

STEVENS, G. H., RANGEL, D. M., YAKEISHI, Y., FONKALSAND, E. W.: Technical problems in lung allotransplantation. Arch. Surg. **99**, 506–512 (1969).

STROUD, R. C., RAHN, H.: Effects of oxygen and carbon dioxide tensions upon resistance of pulmonary blood vessels. Amer. J. Physiol. **172**, 211–220 (1953).

THOMA, R.: Über die Histomechanik des Gefäßsystems und die Pathogenese der Angiosklerose. Virchows Arch. path. Anat. **204**, 1–74 (1911).

THOMAS, W. A., O'NEAL, R. M., LEE, K. T.: Experimental pulmonary hypertension and arteriosclerosis. Arch. Path. **62**, 56–61 (1956).

TRUMMER, M. J., BERG, P.: Lung transplantation. Springfield, Ill.: Charles C. Thomas 1968.

TURNER, J. H., LALICH, J. J.: Experimental cor pulmonale in the rat. Arch. Path. **79**, 409–418 (1965).

VALDIVIA, E.: Right ventricular hypertrophy in guinea pigs exposed to simulated high altitude. Circulat. Res. **5**, 612–616 (1957).

VASKO, J. S., ELKINS, R. C., FOGARTY, T. J., MORROW, A. G.: The experimental production of chronic mitral valvular obstruction. J. thorac. cardiovasc. Surg. **53**, 875–880 (1967).
VEITH, F. J., RICHARDS, K.: Mechanism and prevention of fixed high vascular resistance in autografted and allografted lungs. Science **163**, 699–701 (1969).
VILES, P. W., SHEPHERD, J. T.: Relationship between pH, PO_2 and PCO_2 in the pulmonary vascular bed of the cat. Amer. J. Physiol. **215**, 1170–1176 (1968).
VOGEL, J. H., BLOUNT, S. G.: The role of hydrogen ion concentration in the regulation of pulmonary arterial pressure. Circulation **32**, 788–796 (1965).
WAGENVOORT, C. A., HEATH, D., EDWARDS, J. E.: The pathology of the pulmonary vasculature. Springfield, Ill.: Charles C. Thomas 1964.
WALLACE, C. R., HAMILTON, W. F.: Study of spontaneous congestive heart failure in the dog. Circulat. Res. **6**, 301–314 (1962).
WARTMANN, W. A., JENNINGS, R. B., HUDSON, B.: Experimental arterial disease. The reaction of the pulmonary artery to minute emboli of blood clot. Circulation **4**, 747–755 (1951).
WEIDERANDERS, R. E., WHITE, S. M., SAICHEK, H. B.: The effect of pulmonary resection on pulmonary artery pressures. Ann. Surg. **160**, 889–896 (1964).
WEIDNER, M. G., LIGHT, R. A.: Role of the autonomic nervous system in the control of the pulmonary vascular bed. III. Further studies in experimental pulmonary embolism. Ann. Surg. **147**, 895–902 (1958).
WEISBERG, H., KLINE, I., JARTNER, R., ELLIS, A., KATZ, L. N.: The effect of starch embolisation on cardiac output of the dog. Circulation **28**, 823–829 (1963).
WERTHEIMER, M., MOLLER, J. H., CASTANEDA, A. R.: Pulmonary hypertension and congenital heart disease. Ann. thorac. Surg. **16**, 416–428 (1973).
WHITAKER, W., HEATH, D.: Idiopathic pulmonary hypertension: etiology, pathogenesis, diagnosis and treatment. Progr. cardiovasc. Dis. **1**, 380–396 (1959).
WILDEVOUUR, C. R. H., HEEMSTRA, H., TAMMELING, G. J., HILVERING, C., BOUMA, H. G. D., HOOR, F. TEN, SCHERPENISSE, L. A., KLEINE, J. W., ORIE, N. G. M., HEIDE, J. N. H. VAN D.: Long term observation of the changes in pulmonary arterial pressure after reimplantation of the canine lung. J. thorac. cardiovasc. Surg. **56**, 799–809 (1968).
WILL, D. H., ALEXANDER, A. F., REEVES, J. T., GRAVER, R. F.: High altitude induced pulmonary hypertension in normal cattle. Circulat. Res. **10**, 172–177 (1962).
WILLIAMS, M. H., JR.: Relationship between pulmonary artery pressure and blood flow in the dog's lung. Amer. J. Physiol. **179**, 243–245 (1954).
WILLIAMS, M. H., JR.: Mechanical versus reflex effects of diffuse pulmonary embolism in anesthetised dogs. Circulat. Res. **4**, 325–331 (1956).
WOOD, P.: An appreciation of mitral stenosis. Brit. med. J. **1**, 1051–1055 (1954).
WOOD, P.: Diseases of the Heart and Circulation. 2nd ed. London: Eyre Spottiswoode 1956.
WOOD, P.: Pulmonary hypertension with special reference to the vasoconstrictive factor. Brit. Heart J. **20**, 557–570 (1958).
WOOD, P.: Pulmonary hypertension. Mod. Conc. cardiov. Dis. **28**, 513–518 (1959).
WRIGHT, J. S., OSBORN, J. J., GERBODE, F.: Pulmonary vascular resistance in the young animal. J. cardiovasc. Surg. (Torino) **5**, 147–153 (1964).
YEH, T. J., ELLISON, L. T., ELLISON, R. G.: Functional evaluation of the autotransplanted lung in the dog. Amer. Rev. resp. Dis. **86**, 791–799 (1962).

Experimentally Induced Changes in Pulmonary Circulation[1]

M. S. ISLAM and W. T. ULMER

With 9 Figures

A. Introduction

The primary aim of this article is to review the changes in pulmonary circulation induced by various physicochemical and pharmacological agents. We feel, however, that a discussion of some aspects of the anatomical and physiological pattern of the pulmonary capillary system would also be helpful. Several excellent reviews of different aspects of pulmonary circulation have been published in recent years (AVIADO, 1965; FISHMAN, 1963), and only some salient features will be considered below.

"The pulmonary circulation is part of an elaborate tonometric system for external respiration; it exists for the perfusion of the lungs rather than for their nutrition" (AVIADO, 1965). Due to its unique position between the two sides of the heart, the system has to perform several important functions in addition to the main function of gas exchange. The pulmonary artery delivers the entire cardiac output to the capillaries for arterialization (KROGH, 1941). The system is responsible not only for maintaining the balance between the two sides of the heart under various stress conditions (RILEY et al., 1948), but also for coordinating the alveolar ventilation and pulmonary capillary circulation (RAHN et al., 1956; STRANDELL, 1970; ULMER et al., 1962, 1963; ULMER and REICHEL, 1963). Any consideration of pulmonary circulation without reference to the alveolar system would be incomplete.

Other functions performed by the system are:

1. A ready reservoir for the left ventricle, in that approximately 900 ml of blood are contained in the pulmonary vessels (COMROE, 1966), which are merely extensions of the left atrium. Fig. 1 presents the experimental recording of reservoir function of the pulmonary circulatory bed.

2. Control of the left ventricular output by varying the venous return (HAMILTON, 1940).

3. The pulmonary capillary system also functions as a filter bed for systemic venous particles of all kinds, including the normally formed elements of the blood (AMBRUS et al., 1954).

4. The walls of the pulmonary blood vessels can also neutralize certain endogenous noxae like serotonin and prevent them from damaging the heart (GADDUM et al., 1953).

5. The lungs have an additional arterial blood supply through the bronchial vessels of the systemic circulation (DOBIAS, 1970), which serve as the nutrient

[1] Aus dem Institut für Lungenfunktionsforschung Bochum in Verbindung mit der Westfälischen Wilhelms-Universität Münster (Chefarzt: Professor Dr. W. T. ULMER).

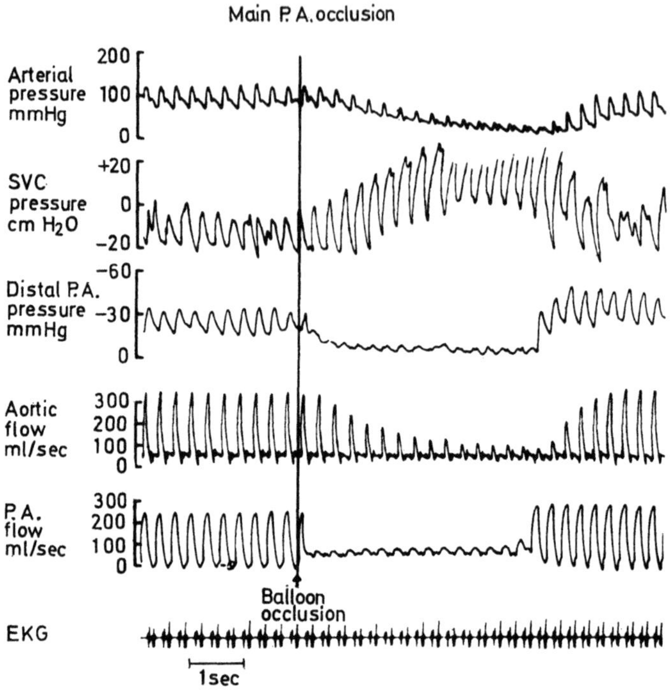

Fig. 1. Shows the reserve function of pulmonary circulation. Left ventricular stroke volume remained unchanged for 2 beats and then decreased for another 10 beats, even when the pulmonary artery was completely blocked by inflating a balloon. SVC—superior vena cava; P.A.—pulmonary artery (Adapted from Comroe, 1966)

vessels to the lungs. The pulmonary capillary system also controls water exchange by preventing bulk loss of fluid due to the oncotic pressure of the plasma (Chinard and Enns, 1954).

B. Morphology and Physiology of the Pulmonary Capillary System

From the time the lungs make their appearance in the early embryo, they become intimately associated with the primitive pulmonary arteries, and as the advancing lung buds begin to ramify, the vessels keep pace with their growth.

At the completion of lung development, each of the myriad airways is accompanied by corresponding ramifications of the pulmonary arteries (Krahl, 1962), whose branches closely parallel the ramifications of the airways. Pulmonary veins on the other hand pass from the periphery toward the hilus through planes of connective tissue that enclose lobules and segments of the lungs (Krahl, 1963). In the human lung approximately 300 million alveoli are juxtaposed to approximately the same number of capillary segments (Low, 1952; Weibel and Gomez, 1962). After the age of 8 years, an increase in size of the lung seems to involve an increase in the dimensions of existing alveolar capillary units rather than in their numbers (Low, 1952).

The pulmonary circulatory system is a low pressure system lacking an arteriolar network such as exists in the systemic circulation. Probably this anatomical arrangement facilitates the process of passively changing the caliber to accommodate a suitable amount of blood volume or vascular resistance to blood flow (AVIADO, 1960a; BATES et al., 1960; BERGOFSKY and HAAS, 1968; HEATH et al., 1959). The pulmonary artery rapidly subdivides into terminal branches which have thinner walls and wider bores than the corresponding branches of the systemic arterial tree. The media of the main pulmonary artery is one half as thick as that of aorta, with short elastic fibers that are arranged in a much less orderly manner than those in the aorta (HEATH et al., 1959). The structure of the large vessels seems better suited to varying their distensibility than does their geometry; nonetheless, it is possible that constriction of large vessels may also affect pulmonary vascular resistance to blood flow (EULER and LISHAJKO, 1958).

In the normal human lung the pulmonary arteries are end-arteries, continuing without branching to the level of the first alveoli in the walls of the respiratory bronchioles (MILLER, 1947; WEIBEL, 1959). The pulmonary veins are end-veins (WEIBEL, 1959), whose musculo-elastic components are more irregularly dispersed than those of the corresponding pulmonary arteries. The venous media contain more collagenous fibers. At the entry of the veins into the left arteria, extensions of cardiac muscles become incorporated into the venous walls. The suggestion has been made that under certain experimental conditions, these muscular extensions may act as "throttles" (BURCH and ROMNEY, 1954; ELIAKIM and AVIADO, 1961).

The pulmonary circulation with which we are concerned is a unique type of regional circulation, in that it supplies blood to a capillary system in intimate contact with the environmental condition. Spread out in the extremely thin walls of the pulmonary alveoli, the volume of which is cyclically modified, covering a surface area of approximately 70 square meters (CHIAND and ENNS, 1954; HEATH et al., 1959; LOW, 1952). The pulmonary capillary bed is the site of a fascinating interplay of physicochemical processes, whereby carbon dioxide diffuses out of the blood into the alveolar air in order to accommodate the incoming oxygen (EULER and LILJESTRAND, 1946; RAHN, 1949). Despite the fact that pulmonary flow equals systemic blood flow, the pulmonary vascular bed is a low pressure system, due mainly to the great distensibility of the walls of the main pulmonary artery and its branches, and to the very large capacity and deformity of the arteriolar, pre-capillary and capillary beds (FINLEY, 1961; WEST et al., 1961). It is believed that the blood flow takes the path of least resistance and may be shunted away from regions of the lungs where vascular resistance is increased (RAHN et al., 1956; REMINGTON and HAMILTON, 1947). The lung is equipped to operate very efficiently over a wide range of metabolic activities: the enormous expanse of alveolar capillary surface is capable of increasing during activity (RILEY et al., 1948), and the geometric distribution of airways and blood vessels favors the continued balance of alveolar ventilation and pulmonary capillary perfusion even during extreme conditions (BAINBRIDGE, 1931). Finally, governing the coordinated performance of this respiratory apparatus is a complicated system of ventilatory and circulatory controls; these succeed, despite the phasic and asynchronous nature of the ventilation and circulation, in stabilizing the gaseous composition of the alveolar gas and in ensuring adequate perfusion of the gas exchange surface.

I. Innervation

There is no doubt about either the existence of pulmonary vasomotor nerves or their ability to change pulmonary vascular calibers when appropriately stimulated (DALY and DALY, 1961; DALY and WRIGHT, 1957). Both vasodilatator and vasoconstrictor fibers have been identified in the upper sympathetic chain and in the vagus nerves (DALY, 1958; HARRIS, 1957; GADDUM et al., 1953). Because of the complicated intermingling of these fibers—not only with each other but also with bronchial and cardiac fibers—electrical stimulation often fails to separate vagal from sympathetic, and vasomotor from bronchomotor, effects (DALY, 1958). The large pulmonary arteries and veins are more richly innervated than their smaller counterparts (COLERIDGE et al., 1961). Nerve endings reach the medial and subendothelial layers of the large arteries and veins. EULER and LISHAJKO (1958) compared the concentration of norepinephrine in the central and in the peripheral portions of the human pulmonary vascular tree. They found a higher concentration of this substance in the larger pulmonary vessels, indicating that these vessels possess a more abundant sympathetic supply than their smaller counterparts. There is also evidence that the chemoreceptors of the aortic and carotid bodies, and possibly the baroreceptors, take part in reflex control of pulmonary circulation (DALY and DALY, 1961; DALY, 1958; PAINTAL, 1969, 1970).

II. Pressure-Flow Relationship

Flow ($\dot{Q}$) of a homogeneous fluid through a rigid tube is directly proportional to the pressure difference (P) and inversely proportional to the frictional resistance (R) offered by the system (FISHMAN, 1963):

$$\dot{Q} = \frac{P}{R}.$$

But the vascular bed is a non-linear, visco-elastic-frequency dependent system perfused by nonhomogenous fluid in which interconversion of energy becomes a relevant factor (FRY, 1959; MCDONALD, 1960) and in which the pressure-flow coordinate does not pass through the origin (BURTON, 1959; HADDY and CAMPBELL, 1953). Thus any factor that changes the pressure difference or frictional resistance would ultimately change the blood flow through the pulmonary bed.

COMROE (1966) reported that most of the resistance to flow is through the arterioles and capillaries since the venous system offers little resistance to flow. On the other hand WEST et al. (1961) reported from indirect measurements that the percentage of the total resistance residing in the pulmonary veins ranged from about 20% (CHINARD and ENNS, 1954) to 60% (AVIADO, 1965). Under certain stress conditions such as exercise, acute hypoxia and acute hypercapnia, heightened respiratory excursions complicate the precise measurement of pressures and of pulmonary blood flow. PERMUTT and co-workers (1961) stressed that in any situation in which alveolar pressure exceeds pulmonary venous pressure (by creating a discontinuity in pressure between the capillaries and the pulmonary veins), the use of pulmonary venous pressure for the calculation of total pulmonary vascular resistance is no longer valid (PERMUTT et al., 1961; ROSS et al., 1961). WEST et al. (1961) suggested that the distribution of the determinants of resistance to perfusion depending on the relationships of pulmonary arterial, left arterial and alveolar pressures in the different parts of the upright lung. Pulmonary resistance is therefore the indicator of a change in vascular diameter (BURTON, 1959; PIIPER, 1970); but, it may also indicate a change in parallel pathways or in blood viscosity (WHITTAKER and WINTON, 1933; LEVY et al., 1954; HAYNES and BURTON, 1959).

III. Veno-Arterial Shunt

The condition in which the mixed venous blood flows unaltered in terms of its gas composition into the left side of the heart, is called the venous-to-arterial

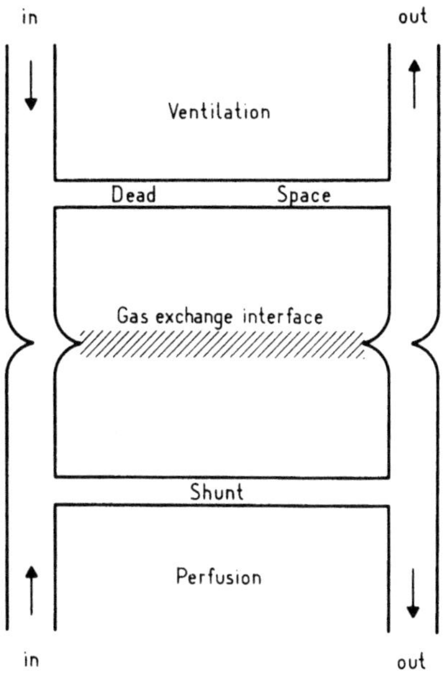

Fig. 2. Schematic representation of ventilation and perfusion with ventilatory dead space and left-right perfusion shunt

shunt. This situation may occur if mixed venous blood flows through the non-ventilated alveoli. In healthy lungs blood flow is distributed uniformly to each alveolus in proportion to its alveolar ventilation. Mixed venous blood entering each of the pulmonary capillaries has the same PO_2 and PCO_2 because of mixing in the heart. If the ratio of ventilation to perfusion is equal and uniform, then there should be no veno-arterial shunt. But, even in ideal conditions there is shunting, and this shunted volume in normal man and dog is about two per cent of the cardiac output (Bartels et al., 1955; Berggren, 1942; Ring et al., 1961). This small shunt volume is of interest from the anatomical point of view (Bostroem and Piiper, 1955; Rahn et al., 1952). A schematic presentation of alveolar air and pulmonary blood flow, not including gas exchange, is presented in Fig. 2.

Physiologically, the shunt is not significant; however in various pathological conditions, it increases tremendously, probably because of the inhomogeneous distribution of either alveolar ventilation or pulmonary blood flow (Comroe, 1966). Normal and extreme, disturbed perfusion/ventilation relationships are depicted in Fig. 3. The computation of shunt volume may be obtained as follows:

$$\frac{Qs}{Qt} = \frac{CaO_2 - CcO_2}{CvO_2 - CcO_2}$$

Qs = blood flow through the shunt
Qt = total blood flow
C = concentration (ml O_2/100 ml blood)
a = arterial blood
c = blood at the end of the pulmonary capillaries
v = mixed venous blood

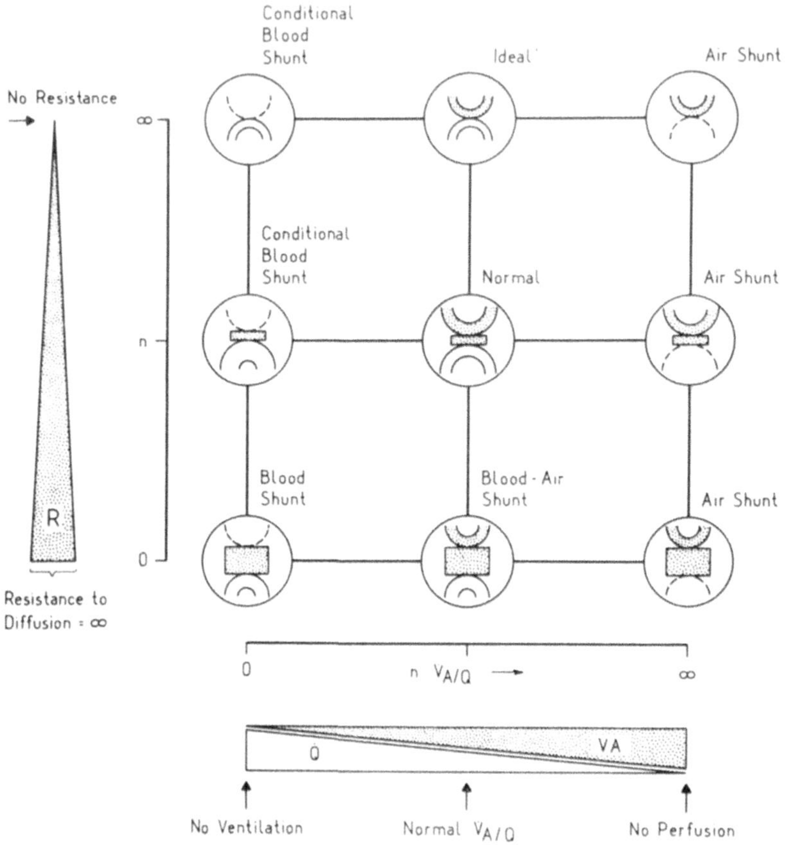

Fig. 3. Illustration of $\dot{V}A/\dot{Q}-D/\dot{Q}$ field concept relation. The $D/\dot{Q}$ ratio on the ordinate can be visualized as a resistance to the diffusion of O_2. The normal alveolus is in the center of the diagram. It must have a finite resistance to flow and a normal $\dot{V}A/Q$ ratio, or both; one can describe the deviation which in the extreme leads to blood shunts, air shunts and blood-air shunts (Adapted from PIIPER, 1961)

IV. Pulmonary Blood Volume

The pulmonary vasculature constitutes a distensible reservoir interposed between the two sides of the heart. The volume of blood contained in the lungs at any instant is determined passively by the balance between pulmonary inflow and outflow. It is also to a great extent influenced by the movements of the chest cage.

In isolated lung preparations or in thoracotomized animals, the pulmonary blood volume is available for direct measurement (MILNOR et al., 1960). Measurements under these conditions are not entirely reliable since surgical manipulation may drastically affect the caliber of the vessels and thus influence the blood volume. By far the most reliable technique for determining central pulmonary blood volume (peripheral vein, right atrium, pulmonary artery and peripheral artery, which is normally the sampling site) is the dye dilution technique. The volume of the fluid in a container can be calculated by adding a known quantity of dye and measuring the concentration of the dye after it has become evenly dispersed throughout the fluid. The volume is calculated as follows:

$$V = A/C$$

where V is the volume of fluid, A is the amount of dye added and C is the concentration of the dye in the fluid (STEWART, 1921; HAMILTON and REMINGTON, 1948). When the test substance is injected into a peripheral vein, the blood volume includes the whole cardiac blood volume. The central blood volume has been narrowed to pulmonary blood volume by the use of a catheterization (FORSSMANN, 1929; COURNAND et al., 1945, 1949; COURNAND and RANGES, 1941) technique.

Changes in the radioactivity in various portions of the lung field after the intravenous injection of radioactive tracers has been used to measure changes in pulmonary blood volume under various experimental conditions (LINDSEY and GUYTON, 1959; WEISSLER et al., 1959). The first step in narrowing the boudaries of the central blood volume was to inject the test substance into the pulmonary artery. In this way the blood volume obtained is approximately 10% of the total circulating blood volume (DOCK et al., 1961; JOHNSON, 1951; KUNIEDA, 1955). It is surprising how closely the indicator dilution value of 10% in intact man corresponds to the more direct measurements in animals (MILNOR et al., 1960). The indicator dilution technique value of 10% also agrees with the estimate based on the pulmonary vascular dimensions in animals.

Several factors can exert a positive or negative influence on pulmonary blood volume, for example, a change in pulmonary blood flow (HAMILTON, 1953; JOHNSON, 1951), pressure breathing and Valsalva's maneuver (BRAUNWALD et al., 1957; THOMAS et al., 1961), inflation of an antigravity suite (BONDURANT et al., 1960), change in body position (LAGERLÖF et al., 1951; SJÖSTRAND, 1953), systemic vasoconstriction or vasodilatation (FRITTS et al., 1960; SJÖSTRAND, 1953), immersion in water (HAMILTON and MAYO, 1944), stenosis of the pulmonary veins (DRINKER, 1945), and disorders of the left side of the heart (KOPELMAN and LEE, 1951). Obviously, too, any change in geometry of the pulmonary vascular system would influence its volume. But, it is very difficult to partition the blood volume shared by pulmonary arteries, capillaries and veins. Anatomical measurements in experimental animals showed that the capacity of the pre- and post-capillary segments is approximately the same and that the volume may be redistributed by means of various mechanical influences (PERMUTT et al., 1961; PIIPER, 1959).

PIIPER (1959, 1970) has reported more precise values for blood distribution, based on his experiments in isolated dog lungs: intrapulmonary artery—27%, capillary system—38% and intrapulmonary venous system—35%.

Knowledge of the size of the pulmonary capillary bed is of great interest. Since, however, it is not possible to measure it directly in the intact animal, its area can be, to a certain extent, approximated from measurements of the diffusing capacity for oxygen or carbon monoxide. One of the mechanisms involved in increasing the area of the pulmonary capillary bed is an increase in transmural pressure (ROSENBERG and FORSTER, 1960). The precise way in which this distending pressure is increased varies from circumstance to circumstance. Thus, in some conditions an increase in blood volume is involved, in others, prevascular pressure may decrease, at high lung volume capillaries may be passively stretched. A moderate change in pulmonary capillary blood flow does not influence the diffusing capacity (FORSTER, 1957; ROSS et al., 1959).

The pulmonary capillary blood volume is about 60 to 75 ml at rest (ROUGHTON, 1945; ROUGHTON and FORSTER, 1957), but it increases to around 100 ml during physical exercise (JOHNSON et al., 1960; ROUGHTON, 1945). Recent observations show that the volume is approximately 100 ml at rest (BATES et al., 1960), though it is not clear how much of this volume is artificial or due to biological differences (FORSTER, 1957; ROUGHTON and FORSTER, 1957). Anatomical measurements put the value at 1.2% of the total circulating blood.

WEIBEL (1969) found the value in human lung to be 150 to 200 ml or about 4% of the total circulating blood volume. This value is twice the value obtained by physiological measurements, and is probably due to the degree of lung inflation (WEIBEL, 1959).

V. Pulmonary Blood Flow

Under normal conditions, the pulmonary blood flow equals the output of each ventricle—the cardiac output. It is the usual practice to express the value of cardiac output per square meter of body surface area, which is termed the cardiac index. The accepted unit of cardiac output is liter/min/m^2 body surface area. Hence, the measurement of pulmonary blood flow is practically a measure of cardiac output. Several indirect and direct methods are available for the purpose of determining cardiac output: Because of the ease of application the indirect methods are more popular. Several methods have been proposed in the past for this purpose. They include calculation of changes in cardiac volume from the cardiac silhouette on roentgenographic plates (KJELLBERG et al., 1951; MEEK and EYSTER, 1923), from the pulse pressure contour and heart rate (HAMILTON and REMINGTON, 1947); ballistocardiographs were also used to determine cardiac ejection (DOCK and TAUBMAN, 1949; HAMILTON et al., 1945). All these methods, however, have serious limitations and are therefore seldom used for the regular determination of cardiac output.

The dye dilution technique has been used more successfully than the foregoing techniques. The volume is calculated according to the formula mentioned previously. STEWART (1921) demonstrated that this method can also be applied to fluid in motion, and several later studies confirmed the usefulness of this method (HAMILTON and REMINGTON, 1948; MOORE et al., 1929) and have used it for serial determinations. The most popular method for the determination of cardiac output is the Fick principle. The conventional expression of the Fick principle is:

$$\text{Cardiac output} = \frac{\text{oxygen consumption}}{\text{arteriovenous oxygen difference}}$$

The Fick principle has long been most commonly used for the determination of cardiac ejection of blood (AITKEN and SANFORD, 1970; COURNAND et al., 1945; BURKART, 1969). Even though it is the most widely used method, there are situations in which it gives erroneous results (NAHAS et al., 1953). The use of the Fick principle during hypoxia has been criticized by NAHAS et al. (1953), chiefly on the basis of the difficulties encountered in obtaining a steady state of oxygen consumption and of arterio-venous oxygen difference. Similar objections have also been raised by other authors (LEUSEN and DEMEESTER, 1954a, b) from their experiments on anesthetised dogs during hypoxia.

These indirect techniques are extensively used clinically and experimentally both in man and in animals. There are some reports of direct measurement of pulmonary blood flow in experimental animals by means of a rotameter inserted into the pulmonary artery, thus providing a more accurate estimation of blood flow changes (HÜRLIMANN and WIGGERS, 1953; AVIADO et al., 1957). This method is purely of theoretical interest and can only be used in animal experiments.

Krogh and Lindhard (1912) used an inert soluble gas to measure pulmonary capillary blood flow. But the use of inert gases to measure pulmonary capillary blood flow lagged once the direct Fick and Stewart-Hamilton methods became standardized, clinically useful techniques. However, it was revived when Lee and DuBois (1955) substituted the body plethysmograph for the spirometer to measure the rate of uptake of nitrous oxide. This modification promised not only to measure the rate of capillary blood flow but also the rate of flow at any instant (Lee and DuBois, 1955). Better instant flow results are obtained using the modified plethysmographic techniques (Bosman et al., 1961; Wasserman and Comroe, 1962) and electromagnetic flowmeter and cardiopneumonographic methods in the dog (Hamilton and Lombard, 1953; Morkin et al., 1962).

The nature of pulmonary capillary flow is one of the most conflicting areas in pulmonary hemodynamics. Knowledge of the pattern of pulmonary capillary flow is important for the understanding of both hemodynamics and gas (Forster, 1957; Piiper, 1961). As early as 1733, Stephan Hales (1769) observed for the first time in the frog that the pulmonary capillary flow is pulsatile. Later observations revealed that the capillary flow in mammals differed from that of amphibians (Wearn et al., 1934). However, indirect observations obtained with the plethysmograph in man (Bosman et al., 1961; Lee and DuBois, 1955; Linderholm et al., 1962; Wasserman and Comroe, 1962) are conclusively in favor of pulsatile flow of blood in the pulmonary capillary system. Nevertheless, the plethysmographic measurement is only valid as long as the airway resistance in different parts of the airways is relatively uniform.

VI. Distribution of Perfused Blood

The uniformity of blood perfusion to the various regions of the capillary system can be observed in different ways—by direct observation of the surface of the lung in the living animal (Bekauri et al., 1954; Dirken and Heemstra, 1948; Wearn et al., 1934), in excised lungs (Pritchard et al., 1954; Tuller et al., 1961) and also by the angiocardiographic technique.

Ventilation, perfusion and diffusion of the lung are precisely balanced in health (Finley, 1961; West et al., 1961) and become uneven in diseases (Aviado, 1960a) involving the pulmonary system. The pattern of change in the respiratory gas exchange ratio (Martin and Young, 1957; West et al., 1957) and the change in oxygen tension during O_2 breathing (Perkins et al., 1956; Finley, 1961) are used to relate ventilation to perfusion. The comparison of blood flow through different parts of the lungs has been studied either by bronchospirometry or by regional sampling of alveolar gas (Hertz, 1955; Fishman et al., 1955; Ulmer and Wenke, 1957). Bronchospirometric comparisons of oxygen uptake have disclosed that gravity rearranges the distribution of the blood flow within each lung (Mattson and Carlens, 1955). It is presupposed that all parts of the lungs breath the same inspired air; however, when different inspired mixtures are added to the inspirate, the procedure and calculations grow much more complex (Fishman et al., 1955; Venrath et al., 1952).

Hemodynamic measurements and analysis of the alveolar gas are consistent with bronchospirometric measurements (Lagerlöf et al., 1951). The oxygen tension decreases from the apex to the base of the lungs whereas the converse is true for carbon dioxide (Martin and Young, 1957; Rahn et al., 1956), and the respiratory quotient of the upper lobes is greater than that of the lower lobes (West et al., 1964). The perfusion/ventilation relationship is shown in Fig. 3.

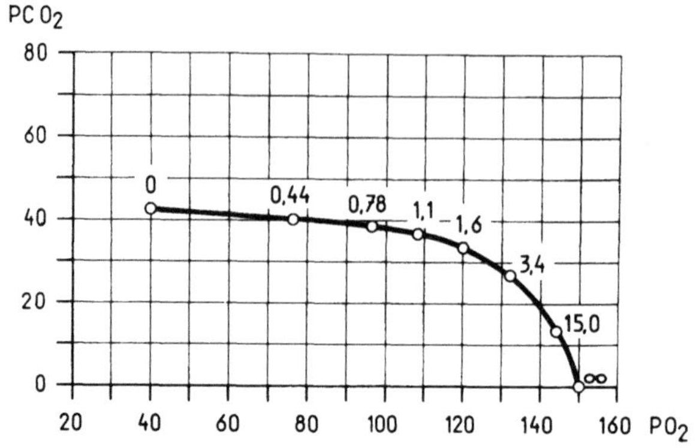

Fig. 4. Illustration of the ventilation-perfusion ratio or $\dot{V}A/Q$ curve. This line represents all possible gas combinations that can prevail as a result of the equilibration of mixed venous blood with inspired gas. The ratios of ventilation to perfusion responsible for various gas tensions are inducated. The ratios range from 0, representing the mixed venous blood gas tension to CO, representing the inspired gas tension (From RAHN et al., 1956)

Radioactive tracers have been used extensively in recent years to detect the distribution of inspired air as well as that of perfused blood (BOSMAN et al., 1961; DOLLERY and WEST, 1960; KNIPPING et al., 1955; WEST et al., 1961). It is an established fact that the normal lung itself is very inhomogenous. Due to this difficulty, a conceptual model of alveolo-capillary exchange has been used as a practical means of assessing pulmonary capillary perfusion. One such model is the homogenous "ideal lung", by means of which the inhomogenity may be demonstrated (LILIENTHAL et al., 1946; RAHN, 1949). The usual way to express deviations from homogenity in terms of their effect on the alveolar-arterial difference in oxygen tension, is commonly known as "A–a" gradient. From such a model one can visualize the inhomogenity of pulmonary capillary perfusion with respect to other gas exchanging parameters (BARTELS and RODEWALD, 1953; BERGGREN, 1942; BRIEHL and FISHMAN, 1960). Fig. 4 shows such ventilation/perfusion ratios. Other techniques are also in use to quantify the perfusion to gas exchange ratio (FINLEY, 1961; PIIPER, 1961).

C. Effect of Physical Agents

I. High Altitude

The negative effects of high altitude exposure on pulmonary circulation have been known for a long time and have been reviewed along with other manifestations of high altitude exposure by HULTGREN and LUNDBERG (1962). The acute form of pulmonary circulatory disorder is manifested as pulmonary edema (ARIAS-STELLA and KRUGER, 1963; FRED et al., 1962; HULTGREN et al., 1964). ALZAMARO-CASTRO et al. (1961), HULTGREN et al. (1962), MORALES GUZMAN (1962) and others (HOUSTON, 1960; STEWART, 1961) reported the occurrence of pulmonary edema among high altitude residents and mountaineers. FRED et al. (1962), using cardiac catheterization, measured high pulmonary arterial pressure and normal left arterial pressure in a patient with high altitude-induced pulmonary edema. They concluded that the syndrome resulted from a pulmonary vascular obstruction lying distally to the capillary bed and that the resultant increase of cardiac output may have been a contributing factor (MARTICORENA et al., 1962; TAPIA et al., 1962).

PENALOZA et al. (1962) reported high pulmonary pressures among natives and residents of Morococha, 4550 m above sea level with mean barometric pressure of 445 mm Hg and a tracheal PO_2 of about 80 mm Hg.

ROTTA et al. (1956), BANCHERO et al. (1962, 1963) and others (VOGEL et al., 1962; WILL et al., 1967) reported similar observations.

PENALOZA et al. (1962) indicated that acetylcholine or oxygen inhalation reduces high pulmonary pressure. This finding indicates that a certain degree of vasoconstriction is a cause of pulmonary pressure increase.

ARIAS-STELLA and SALDANA (1962), SALDANA and ARIAS-STELLA (1963a, b) considered that the muscular mass at the peripheral arterioles is more abundant among individuals residing at high altitudes than that of the sea level residents.

ALEXANDER (1962), ALEXANDER and JENSEN (1959) and co-workers presented evidence from their study on bovines that the pulmonary arteries and veins possess a muscular media with a diameter which can be as low as approximately 20 microns. This finding may explain the muscular hypertrophy in the small muscular arteries and arterioles of the lungs of clinical cases of high mountain disease and in experimental cattle with severe high altitude-induced pulmonary hypertension (GROVER et al., 1963; REEVES et al., 1963).

REEVES et al. (1963) and NAEYE (1962), NAEYE and BICKERMAN (1959) also observed hypertrophy of the smooth muscle of the pulmonary arteries in the lungs from residents of high altitudes.

Most of the studies on the effect of high altitude on the lesser circulation are carried out in relation to pulmonary hypertension and its probable causes. Direct data on pulmonary capillary blood volume and on the pattern of pulmonary capillary blood flow are very scanty. However an estimate of pulmonary capillary blood volume at high altitude can be obtained from the reports on pulmonary diffusing capacity. FORSTER (1957) and others (MCNEILL et al., 1958; LEWIS et al., 1958) showed a linear relationship between D_{LO_2} (ml/min/mm Hg) and $1/\emptyset$ (ml/min/mm Hg/ml/blood). BATES et al. (1960) reported that the differences in the rates of gas diffusion between individuals engaging in exercise at the same rate are mainly attributable to variations in the pulmonary capillary blood volume. In comparison, the reports of ROSENBERG and FORSTER (1959) and MCNEILL et al. (1958) indicated that the pulmonary diffusing capacity is independent of pulmonary capillary blood flow. On the basis of these reports, the measurement of pulmonary diffusion (carbon monoxide) capacity at high altitude may yield an idea of the pulmonary capillary bed.

There are several studies indicating a greater pulmonary diffusing capacity or reduced alveolo-arterial oxygen gradient among high altitude residents (REMMERS and MITHOEFER, 1969; VELASQUEZ, 1956). The recent studies of DEGRAFF et al. (1970) have provided data not only on pulmonary diffusion capacity but also on pulmonary capillary blood volume and flow at high altitude for native inhabitants and for sea-level dwellers who resided temporarily at high altitudes. It has been presumed that the increase in diffusing capacity resulted from increased membrane diffusing capacity and pulmonary capillary blood volume. An increase in membrane diffusing capacity is not significant when compared to values predicted from alveolar ventilation and pulmonary capillary blood flow. On the other hand pulmonary capillary blood volume is significantly greater than the predicted values regardless of the parameter used for prediction (REMMERS and MITHOEFER, 1969; VELASQUEZ, 1956; VELASQUEZ and FLORENTINI, 1966).

WEIL et al. (1968) found an 11% increase in total body blood volume among people residing at high altitudes for only two months. On the other hand, DEGRAFF et al. (1970) and WEST (1962a) observed no change in pulmonary capillary blood volume or diffusing capacity among temporary residents of high altitudes. But an increased diffusion capacity was observed by DEMPSEY et al. (1969) among long-term high-altitude residents.

The more recent study of WEISKOPF and SEVERINGHAUS (1972) is at variance with that of the previous workers (BEKAURI et al., 1954; BERGOFSKY and HAAS, 1968) in that they observed decreased diffusion capacity and pulmonary capillary blood volume in healthy subjects at high altitude. They argued that the abrupt change from hypoxia to hyperoxia at the start of the 10-sec breathholding may have resulted in dilatation of previously constricted pulmonary arterioles with the result that pulmonary capillary blood volume and therefore pulmonary diffusing capacity increase at high altitude.

II. Physical Exercise

HICKAM and CARGILL (1948) were among the pioneers who stressed the importance of lesser circulatory adjustment under physical exertion in health as well as in disease. They concluded from their study that the normal pulmonary vascular bed can accommodate large increases (twice the resting value) in the rate of blood flow, with little or no increase in mean pulmonary arterial pressure, in contrast to the significant increase in mean pulmonary pressures in patients with cardiopulmonary disorders with little or no increase in cardiac output. In the same year RILEY et al. (1948) reported similar results from their study on three normal subjects exercising in the erect position. DEXTER et al. (1951) and GLOGER (1972) observed a greater increase in arterial pressure than in wedge pressure in recumbent exercising subjects. The modified results of GLOGER are presented in Fig. 5.

On the other hand, ÖZCAN et al. (1952) and others (BARRATT-BOYES and WOOD, 1957; SANCETTA and KLEINERMAN, 1957; SANCETTA and RAKITA, 1957; SLONIM et al., 1954) noticed a fall in arterial resistance on the basis of arterial pressure alone in the recumbent position, and VARNAUSKAS (1955) obtained variable responses. The variability of intensity of the reduction of pulmonary vascular resistance is therefore related to the exercising position and is not entirely due to gravitational force (LAGERLÖF et al., 1951; O'DONNELL and MCILROY, 1962; RAO, 1963; SHIMOSATO and ETSTEN, 1963; SVANBERG, 1957). BÜHLMANN et al. (1955) obtained similar results of an insignificant rise in pulmonary arterial pressure in healthy subjects whereas patients with increased pulmonary arterial pressure showed greater increases under physical exertion. They also pointed out that in healthy individuals a steady state is reached within 8 to 10 min of exercise, but that in patients, reaching a steady state takes longer or never occurs at all. It is very difficult to draw a definite conclusion from such cases.

WIDIMSKY et al. (1963) studied the effect of repeated exercise on the lesser circulation of four healthy subjects and four patients with lung diseases. They found a fall in pulmonary arterial pressure during the second exercise period in all subjects studied, and normal or slightly increased wedge pressures.

In the pulmonary circulation large increments of blood flow may occur with relatively small increases of perfusion pressure, as has been found in perfusion experiments (BORST et al., 1956, 1957; CARLILL et al., 1957; LATEGOLA, 1958; MORET et al., 1961; WEIL et al., 1957). This must be due to increased distension

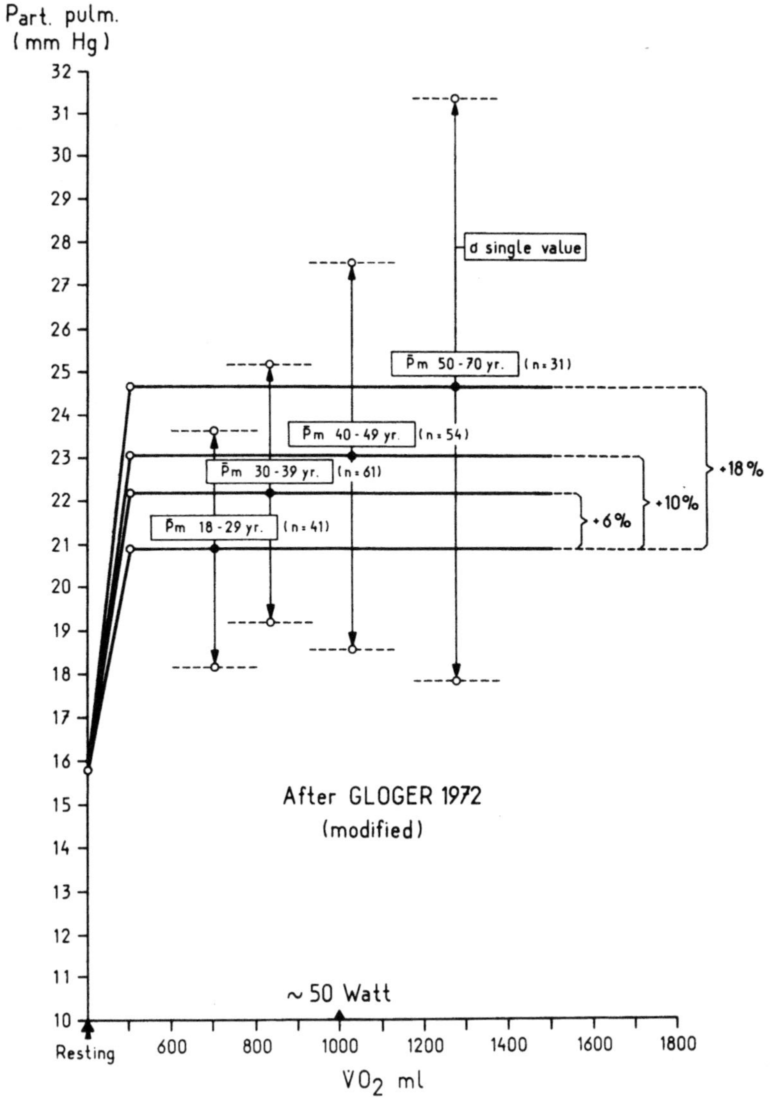

Fig. 5. Illustration of the relation of pulmonary arterial pressure and oxygen consumption at constant work load of about 50 watts in men of different age groups. Initial sharp increase in pressure occurred with initial rise in O_2 consumption and thereafter remained constant, though the O_2 consumption rose. Mean pressure increases in older subjects are greater than in the young

of the pulmonary vascular bed and to the opening up of previously closed channels, induced by the increased blood flow and the slight increase in perfusion pressure. If this passive distension occurs gradually, it could explain the gradual decline of pulmonary artery pressure during steady exercise and the corresponding increase in pulmonary capillary blood volume (BRAUNWALD and KELLY, 1960; CHAFFEE et al., 1963; FISHMAN, 1960).

Indirect evidence of passive distension of the vascular bed during exercise may be obtained from the study of diffusion capacity of the pulmonary bed under physical exertion. BATES et al. (1960) suggested that the increase in diffusion capacity during exercise may be accounted for by an increase in pulmonary capillary blood volume. In previous studies, ROSS et al. (1959) proposed that the increased diffusion capacity was due to increased ventilation during exercise. But, the reports of DEMUTH et al. (1965) and MILLER and JOHNSON (1966) support the view of BATES et al. (1960) in that the increase in pulmonary capillary blood volume is disproportionate to the increase in ventilation (DEMUTH et al., 1965; MILLER and JOHNSON, 1966).

III. Gravitational Force

It is an established fact that the distribution of gas and blood in the lung is to a great extent dependent on gravity (CLARKE et al., 1969; GLAISTER, 1967a, b; KANEKO et al., 1966; MILIC-EMILI et al., 1966; RAHN et al., 1956; WEST, 1962b; KATORIE et al., 1970), so that the respiratory ratios in the upper and lower regions of the lungs are different (MARTIN and YOUNG, 1957; VALENCA et al., 1971). BUSBY (1968) estimated that about 500 ml of the 650 ml blood usually pooled in the vascular bed of the leg are shifted to the thorax in the monkey, when the animal is changed from a vertical to a horizontal position. Forces that pool blood in the lower extremities are absent in the horizontal position as well as in weightlessness; hence, the distribution of blood in the two situations is similar (DONOMARCO and RIMINI, 1970; MEEHAN and RADER, 1971).

BRYAN et al. (1965, 1966), GLAISTER (1965, 1967) and HOPPIN et al. (1967) carried out acceleration studies on the distribution of pulmonary blood flow. HOPPIN et al. (1967) found no redistribution of blood flow in supine subjects exposed to a forward acceleration of 8 G (+Gx). However, these results were not confirmed by BRYAN et al. (1965, 1966) and GLAISTER (1965), who found a marked redistribution of blood flow during exposure to headward (+Gx) acceleration in seated subjects. GLAISTER (1970) concluded from his study that during +Gx, blood flow per alveolus rose at the back of the lung and then decreased over the last few centimeters. This zone of decreasing perfusion, which occurred despite a continuing rise in vascular pressure, is similar to that in isolated lung described by HUGHES et al. (1968a) and WEST et al. (1965), and to that in intact animals and man (HUGHES et al., 1968a, b). It has been attributed to an increase in resistance to flow from extravascular vessels, from resulting edema (WEST et al., 1965) or from the action of interstitial pressure (HUGHES et al., 1968a, b). Comparison of flow and ventilation curves, at +1 and +5 Gx (BRYAN et al., 1966), suggests that a common mechanism may be responsible for the reductions in blood flow and ventilation at the back of the lung. Though regional adjustment of perfusion has been demonstrated (ARBORELIUS, 1959; ATWELL et al., 1951), it appears to be a too insensitive and ineffective mechanism to account for the observed gross reduction in blood flow.

IV. Pressure Breathing

Rise in intrapulmonary air pressure causes a rise in pulmonary artery pressure. The increased pulmonary arterial pressure persists as long the elevated intrapulmonary pressure is maintained (SHARPEY-SCHAFER and BAIN, 1932). In the isolated perfused lung, positive inflation of the lung causes an increase in vascular resistance (CAPPS and LEWIS, 1907; EDWARDS, 1951). At normal rates of flow the dominant resistance in the pulmonary vascular bed is in the precapillary (DEBONO and CARO, 1963; DEXTER et al., 1951) segments. In the intact dog with open chest, the wedge arterial pressure usually drops at the institution of positive pressure breathing. WEBB and SMITH (1959) explained this fall as the outcome of the initial thrust of pressure against the bronchioles, which straightened and lengthened the pulmonary vasculature, thus enlarging the capillary bed (TSAGARIS and LANGE, 1964). There is also a reduction in shunt flow in the anesthetized dog, due to the opening of lung areas that have spontaneously collapsed (FINLEY et al., 1960). In anesthetized dogs, cardiac output is reduced under positive pressure breathing but there is no change in pulmonary vascular resistance (LINDE et al., 1961). In open chest animal experiments and in normal human study the pulmonary blood flow is influenced mainly by the level of positive intratracheal pressure but not by the presence or absence of a negative phase in the ventilative cycle (McDONALD et al., 1963; RONCORONI et al., 1962).

V. Hypovolemic Shock

Initially hypovolemia can cause a decrease in pulmonary arterial pressure, but persistent hypovolemia may lead to an increase in pulmonary arterial pressure (OPDYKE and WIGGERS, 1946; ROTHE and SELKURT, 1964; SARNOFF et al., 1954). ULMER (1968) and his associates (KILIAN et al., 1970) observed a similar trend in an experimental hypovolemic study in dogs. They found that the fall in pulmonary arterial pressure during the bleeding period and after 3 h of hypovolemia the pressure returned to almost pre-bleeding level. Reinfusion of various plasma expanders induced a significant increase in pulmonary arterial pressure (BURROWS and NIDEN, 1963; ENGSTEDT et al., 1967; MESSMER, 1968; VARNAUSKAS et al., 1965). Rise of pulmonary pressure may, perhaps, be due to centralization of circulatory blood volume under hypovolemia as mentioned by ULMER (1968). ROTHE and SELKURT (1964) considered these increases to be due to increased resistance offered by the vascular bed. Plugging up the small capillaries by agglutinated erythrocytes or by small blood clots may also play an important role in increasing the arterial pressure (HARDAWAY, 1962; SCHNEIDER, 1964). SCHMIDT and SCHMIER (1965) considered damage to the heart contractility as a pressure-increasing phenomenon, but KILIAN et al. (1970) did not obtain any evidence to support this idea. WIGGERS (1950) emphasized that myocardial insufficiency might play a part in shock complication, but not in all phases of shock. MESSMER (1968) wrote that the increase of flow resistance of the pulmonary circulation during reinfusion is dependent on the osmolarity of the infused solution.

In addition there are reports of increased viscosity and decreased suspension stability of the blood under hemorrhagic shock (GRUBER, 1968; NAVARRO and FERGUSON, 1968; GELIN, 1962). Perhaps these are the factors which initiate the process of cell aggregation.

The pulmonary perfusion/ventilation ratio is seriously disturbed in hypovolemic shock (BORDER et al., 1968; McLAUGHLIN et al., 1969; LUCAS et al., 1968). KILIAN et al. (1970) wrote that the decreasing pulmonary pressure at the initial phase of hypovolemia might induce collapse of the capillaries in the upper lung region. The results of BURROWS and NIDEN (1963) could explain the comments of KILIAN et al. (1970). They observed a decreased diffusion capacity in the upper lung region in hemorrhagic shock. Where the ventilation may remain as before and thereby increases the physiological dead space (KILIAN et al., 1970; ULMER, 1968). The increase of respiratory dead space has also been observed by others (FREEMAN and NUNN, 1959), but these authors found a decreased anatomic shunt. It is very difficult to reconcile the increased physiologic dead space with an unaltered or decreased shunt.

WAHRENBROCK et al. (1970) recently tried to clarify the mechanism of shunt in shock. They observed greater shunt volume in both induced atelectasis and shock together, and infusion of HCO_3 also augmented the shunt. They postulated that the mechanism involved is the combined effect of chemical, mechanical and reflex events.

VI. Pulmonary Emboli

Because the pulmonary circulation acts as a filter bed for the system (AMBRUS et al., 1954; GADDUM et al., 1953), it is accessible to various endo- and exogenous particles and chemicals which may cause embolic damage to the system. The effect of embolism on pulmonary circulation has been studied extensively (DAILY et al., 1966; HALMAGYI et al., 1964; HYMAN et al., 1964). When air was repeatedly injected into the pulmonary artery of rabbits, WRIGHT (1962) observed morphologic vascular changes similar to those in humans with pulmonary hypertension. NIDEN and AVIADO (1956) produced embolism with glass beads in anesthetized dogs and found an immediate sharp rise in pulmonary arterial pressure.

The most commonly offered explanation for the fatal increase in pulmonary arterial pressure is a reflex vasoconstriction. But DAILY et al. (1966) believe that a sufficient quantity of embolic material may result in a mechanical blockade capable of producing increased pulmonary arterial pressure. However, this idea has not been favored by others (HALMAGYI et al., 1964; HYMAN et al., 1964). HAGGARD and WALKER (1923) reported that the total cross-sectional area of the pulmonary artery and its branches must be reduced by more than 50% in dogs before any detectable changes in hemodynamics occur. The numbers necessary to achieve this effect in the dog vary, according to HYLAND and collaborators (1963), from 23 emboli with a diameter of 2.3 mm to 89845 emboli with a diameter of 0.17 mm. BERNTHAL et al. (1961) performed autoperfusion of the left lower lobe of the lung at a constant pressure and found that embolization with glass beads of a diameter of 0.075 mm resulted in a marked decrease of blood flow which gradually returned towards the normal level. This finding was interpreted as the occurrence of transient vasoconstriction. WILLIAMS (1926), on the other hand, produced emboli in the lungs of anesthetized dogs with 0.06 mm glass beads and found that pulmonary arterial pressure rose with each injection. This response was unaffected by denervation of the lobe or by administration of hexamethonium. Likewise BLOOR et al. (1970) perfused the lungs with autologus emboli and found an initial increase in pulmonary pressure and then a return to pre-emboli values within an hour. They pointed out that repeated embolizations produce a greater effect than the initial episode.

NIDEN and AVIADO (1956) carried out cross circulation studies in anesthetized dogs and found that pulmonary embolism produced with glass beads in one dog resulted in an increase in pulmonary pressure in the other. The effect was abolished by sectioning the vago-sympathetic trunks, and it was thought that the initial increase was due to a direct mechanical effect and that the late reaction might have been of a neurohumoral nature. The recent study of MASSION (1966) has provided a clearer picture of the mechanism of emboli-induced pulmonary hypertension. He performed studies in dogs which had one transplanted lung (i.e. denervated) and one intact lung. He found a significant increase in pulmonary arterial pressure when glass beads were applied to the intact side of the lung but observed little or no change when the same quantity of glass beads was introduced into the transplanted lung. The result of this study supports the conviction of the nervous involvement of emboli-induced pulmonary hypertension and corroborates the earlier work of SCHWIEGK (1935). MASSION (1966) also concludes from the study of HAMLIN and co-workers (1962) that 2 gm of glass beads cannot occlude more than 10 to 25% of one hemilung and that this is not sufficient to cause pulmonary hypertension.

There remains the question of whether the sympathetic or the vagal system is primarily involved. DALY and DALY (1961) showed that stimulation of the sympathetic chains at the levels of T_3 or T_4 often produced vasoconstrictive responses in the lung, while PRICE and associates (1955) were able to prevent death from pulmonary embolism by decerebration of the animal, indicating involvement of higher centers.

D. Effects of Chemical Agents

I. Hypoxia

In one of their earlier studies, VON EULER and LILJESTRAND (1946) described the increase in pulmonary arterial pressure in cats breathing air mixtures with low oxygen pressure. In the last two decades, hypoxia-induced pulmonary hypertension has been confirmed by many investigators both in animal (HAUGE, 1970; KAZEMI et al., 1972; REICHEL et al., 1965, 1966) and in human subjects (LOPEZ et al., 1967). Increase in cardiac output under moderate hypoxia has also been reported (FISHMAN et al., 1952; HERTZ, 1956). However there is inconsistent information regarding the volume of pulmonary capillary blood under hypoxic conditions (DURAND et al., 1970; GROVER et al., 1963, 1967; HANSEN et al., 1964). The increase in cardiac output under hypoxia obtained by REICHEL et al. (1965, 1966) and others (ENSON et al., 1964; WILL et al., 1962) lies in the range of 10% to 73% above the air breathing level. Therefore, it seems likely that hypoxia-induced pulmonary hypertension could occur as a result of vasoconstriction. The cause of this arterial vasoconstriction can be analyzed in a manner similar to that for analyzing changes in total resistance. The observation that hypoxia causes an increase in resistance whereas muscular exercise causes a decrease, indicates that the former is associated with active constriction, which is unrelated to increased blood flow (WILL et al., 1962; COURNAND et al., 1954; HERTZ, 1956; HIMMELSTEIN et al., 1958).

The increase in pulmonary arterial pressure may also occur as a result of elevated pressure in the left heart. The information regarding the effect of hypoxia on the left heart has been obtained mainly from animal experiments. During the inhalation of 2.5 to 13% oxygen, the left arterial pressure usually remained unchanged (LOGARAS, 1947; AVIADO et al., 1957; BERGOFSKY et al., 1962). A rise may occur if anoxia becomes so severe that cardiac failure occurs (GORLIN and LEWIS, 1954; WIGGERS, 1941). Otherwise, a rise in left arterial pressure may be disregarded as a cause for changes in pulmonary arterial pressure during hypoxia.

REICHEL et al. (1965) observed a greater increase of flow resistance of the pulmonary capillary system under moderate hypoxia (10 to 12% O_2 mixture) than under severe hypoxia (8% O_2 mixture). They explained this discrepancy as due to passive broadening of the capillaries under increased hydrostatic pressure and the greater blood flow through them. It is not unlikely that, under greater pressure, the dormant vessels may open up to receive the blood and thereby,

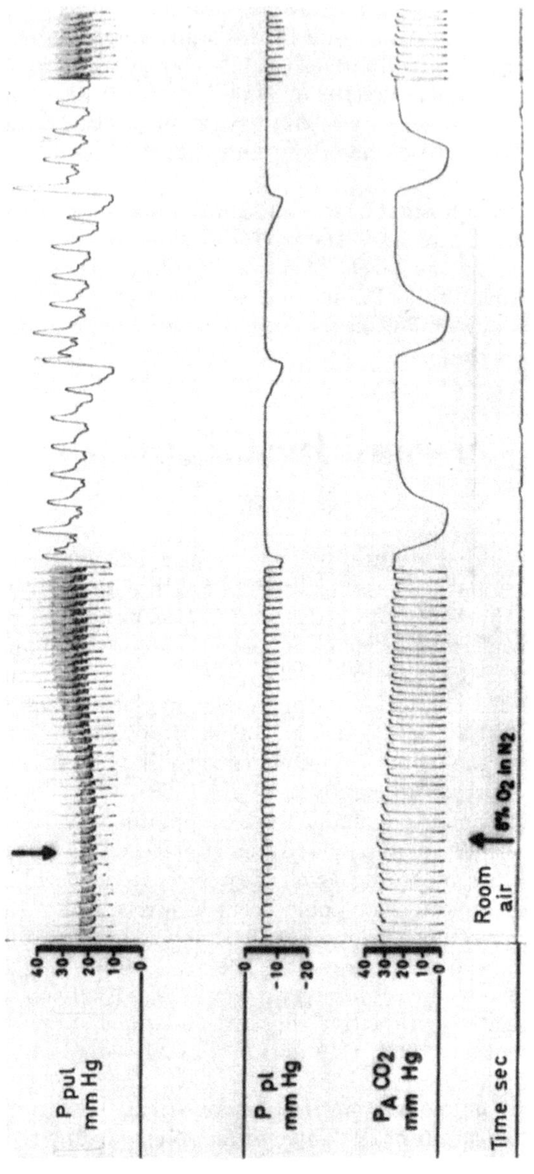

Fig. 6. Shows the original recording of pulmonary arterial pressure (P_{pul}), pleural pressure (P_{pl}) and alveolar CO_2 partial pressure (P_ACO_2), obtained from anesthetized dog exposed to low oxygen. Arrow marks when the animal was switched to low oxygen (8% O_2 in nitrogen) inspiratory gas mixture from room air breathing (From Reichel et al., 1965)

perhaps, reduce the flow resistance. An original recording of the influence of hypoxia (8% O_2) on pulmonary pressure is given in Fig. 6. The former is evident from the values of central blood volume and cardiac output obtained by these authors. The values obtained under moderate hypoxia are not much different from those obtained under air breathing, and the values increase only under severe hypoxia.

Von Euler and Liljestrand (1946) suggested that local hypoxia might play a role in controlling the distribution of pulmonary capillary blood flow. Himmelstein et al. (1958) reasoned that a local reduction in the alveolar oxygen pressure would constrict the vessels of the affected area, thereby diverting a portion of blood, passing through these channels, to better aerated parts of the lungs. A similar opinion has been expressed by HERTZ (1955, 1956), ROSSIER et al. (1958), BÜHLMAN et al. (1955) and others (ARBORELIUS, 1965; BERGOFSKY and HAAS, 1968). ULMER and WENKE (1957) reported that a decrease of oxygen pressure reduces the blood perfusion of the affected area within one minute, and they found no stagnation of blood flow even under severe hypoxia. KAZEMI et al. (1972) recently reported that there is a decrease of perfusion of 33% in the hypoxic lung and that the intensity of the response is inversely related to the alveolar oxygen pressure. In man and dog, an appreciable rise in pulmonary arterial pressure has been shown to occur when the arterial oxygen saturation drops below 80 to 85% (BORDEN et al., 1950; FISHMAN et al., 1952; MOUNSEY et al., 1952; VENRATH et al., 1955). REICHEL et al. (1965, 1966) observed an increase of pulmonary arterial pressure when the arterial oxygen pressure falls below 50 mm Hg. KAZEMI et al. (1972) confirmed the results of STROUD and RAHN (1953) and others (HAUGE and STAUB, 1969; SILOVE et al., 1968), that a significant reduction of pulmonary perfusion occurs with unilateral alveolar hypoxia, when alveolar oxygen pressure value falls below 63 mm Hg. Recent evidence presented by ULMER (1972) indicates that pulmonary hypertension occurs below 70 mm Hg of arterial oxygen pressure in patients with cor pulmonale. The greater effect of hypoxia in patients has been attributed to the structural change of the vascular system in chronic exposure.

VALENCA et al. (1971) found that pulmonary vasoconstriction response to alveolar hypoxia is significantly reduced in the immediate and early post operative periods in the re-implanted dog lung, but returns to normal between the second and third operative months. They suggested that an intact nervous connection along the bronchus and the major pulmonary vessels may be of importance in the hypoxic response. It has also been suggested that the vascular response is largely dependent upon the sympathetic system and does not require an intact vagal innervation (KAZEMI et al., 1972). A similar opinion has, previously, been expressed by STROUD and RAHN (1953) and AVIADO et al. (1957). However, our (ULMER et al., 1973) recent observations are at variance with the foregoing findings, since we observed marked hypoventilation and hypoxia and thus a significant increase of pulmonary arterial pressure in bilateral vago-sympathectomized dogs (ISLAM and ULMER, 1973a; ISLAM et al., 1974). The hypertension was reversed completely when the dogs breathed oxygen, thus providing indirect evidence to support the hypothesis that hypoxia-induced pulmonary hypertension is not mediated through the vago-sympathetic system but may follow some other path or is a result of some local mechanism. Our study does not exclude the possibility of left heart involvement under severe hypoxemia. There are also suggestions that local tissue acidosis (LILJESTRAND, 1958), local release of vasoactive substances (BARER, 1966; FISHMAN, 1963) or changes in the ionic composition of the vascular smooth muscle (BERGOFSKY and HOLTZMAN, 1967), play a significant role. In addition, there may also be a direct effect of hypoxia on the smooth muscle of the vessels. LLOYD (1964) found constriction of a strip of pulmonary arterial wall immersed in a fluorochemical medium with low oxygen pressure. HAUGE (HAUGE and MELMON, 1968; HAUGE and STAUB, 1969) and co-workers could inhibit the hypoxic pressure response in rats and cat lungs by pretreating with histamine-releasing agents.

SUSMANO and CARLETON (1971) could not completely reverse the hypoxic pulmonary hypertension with promethazine, a substance with strong antiserotonin properties. But they could completely reverse the effect with chlorpheniramine, a substance with only minimal antiserotonin properties.

II. Hyperoxia

The role of hyperoxia has been observed mainly in patients with either heart or lung disease. Very few reports are available on the effects of oxygen on pulmonary circulation in healthy subjects. Breathing of pure oxygen by dog (Harrison et al., 1927) or by man (Hamilton, 1940) is without appreciable effect on pulmonary arterial pressure or blood flow. Breathing oxygen instead of room air during physical exercise produces no change in either cardiac output or pulmonary arterial pressure. Smith et al. (1963) exposed dogs to 95 to 98% oxygen until they succumbed to respiratory failure. At autopsy the lungs were found to be red, hemorrhagic, edematous and congested. The blood-gas contents and cardiovascular parameters were maintained at essentially normal levels until approximately 2 to 3 h before death. On the other hand, pharmacological concentrations of oxygen cause a decrease in pulmonary arterial pressure (von Euler and Liljestrand, 1946; Logaras, 1947) and vascular resistance in isolated preparations (Duke, 1951; Nisell, 1950).

III. Hypercapnia

Von Euler and Liljestrand (1946) reported that hypercapnia can also produce an elevation of the pulmonary arterial pressure in cats. Subsequent studies have produced conflicting reports. Several investigators (Duke, 1951; Lopez-Majano, 1970; Nisell, 1950) have demonstrated carbon dioxide-induced pulmonary vasoconstriction in excised mammalian lungs, including those from dogs. Others, using either excised lungs (Hebb and Nimmo-Smith, 1948) or the whole animal (Stroud and Rahn, 1953), did not observe pulmonary vasoconstriction in the dog due to carbon dioxide breathing. Borst et al. (1957) observed an initial increase of vasoconstriction, but a return toward control values after 2 to 3 min of unilateral ventilation with carbon dioxide. They considered it to be due to the onset of vasoconstriction in the control lung as the pulmonary arterial and alveolar carbon dioxide concentrations increased on the control side.

Reichel et al. (1965) also failed to obtain any change in cardiac output, transmural pulmonary pressure or pulmonary vascular resistance in an anesthetized dog breathing a carbon dioxide-rich mixture, as shown in Fig. 7.

Similar observations in dogs as well as in human subjects have previously been made by Stroud and Rahn (1953) and Fishman et al. (1960). The findings of Bergofsky et al. (1959) show a different picture. He obtained a hypercapnic and metabolic acidosis dependent elevation of pulmonary arterial pressure and a change in left arterial pressure. But Shapiro et al. (1962) found a slight fall in left atrial pressure under metabolic acidosis at constant pulmonary pressure and heart minute volume. Therefore, it is difficult to accept the theory that metabolic acidosis induces an increase in pulmonary vascular resistance. The study of Bühlmann et al. (1955) illustrates this point. In a study on relaxed, artificially respired human subjects, they showed that the artificial hypoventilation of the alveolar space induced the expected increase of systolic and diastolic pulmonary arterial pressure with decreased oxygen saturation and increased carbon dioxide concentration in the blood. The pressure returned to normal when a 70% oxygen mixture was breathed, even though the carbon dioxide pressure remained at a higher concentration. The persistence of slightly elevated pressure could be due to increased cardiac minute volume. These authors obtained similar results from their study on

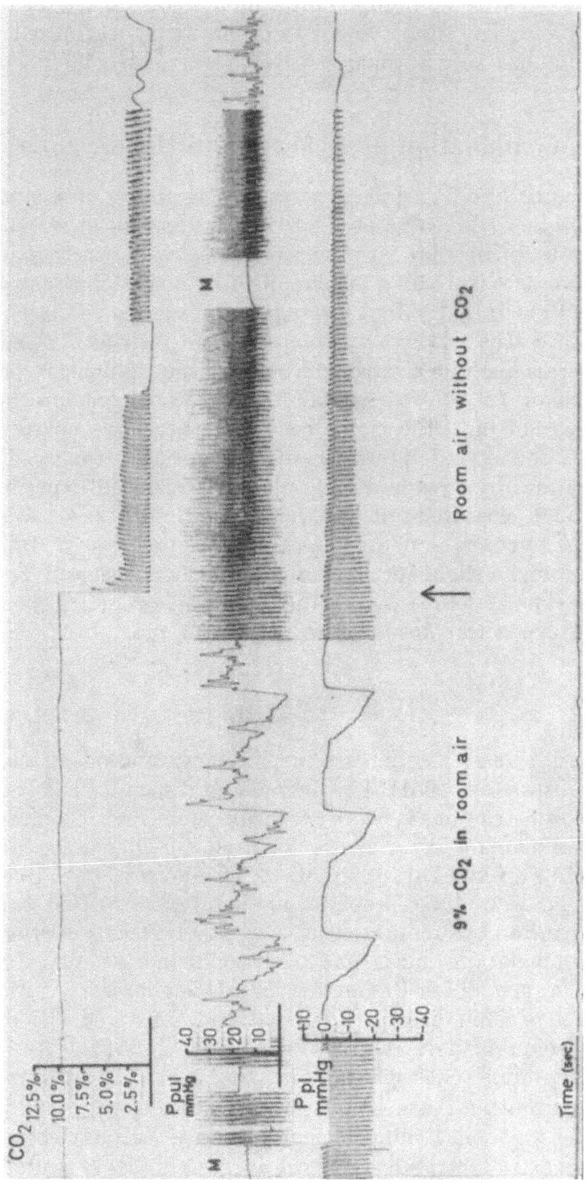

Fig. 7. Shows the original recording of alveolar CO_2 concentration (top) pulmonary arterial pressure (P_{pul}), (middle) and pleural pressure (P_{pl}) (bottom), obtained from anesthetized dog exposed to high CO_2 mixture. At arrow, the animal was returned to room air from high CO_2 (9%) gas mixture (From REICHEL et al., 1965)

artificially respired emphysema patients (BÜHLMANN et al., 1955). The enormous increase of ventilation under hypercapnia and its effect on the thorax might play a part in controlling the pulmonary circulation, which probably, in part, explains the conflicting reports on the effect of hypercapnia on pulmonary circulation. The exposure of dogs to a mixture high in carbon dioxide (9%) stimulates the ventilatory drive and thereby induces greater fluctuations on intrathoracic pressure. These pressure fluctuations are reflected in the pulmonary circulatory system. In such situations inspiration may induce a greater filling on the right atrium resulting in excess blood being pumped into the pulmonary bed during expiration (Reichel et al., 1965). The significance of ventilation synchronized with fluctuations in heart filling has been emphasized by Ulmer et al. (1966).

IV. Combination of Hypoxia and Hypercapnia

The occurrence of hypoxia and hypercapnia is almost inseparable in many heart and lung diseases (Baldwin et al., 1949; Bergofsky et al., 1959; Reichel et al., 1965; Ulmer, 1972). Clinical observations have shown that increased pulmonary arterial pressure is usually accompanied by a sudden rise of blood carbon dioxide tension (Yu et al., 1953). This indirectly suggests that chronic hypercapnia may reinforce the chronic hypoxic pressure response. Ulmer (1972) indicates that hypercapnia and acidosis may affect the right heart only when the pH value sinks below 7.2, at which point the left atrial pressure begins to rise. Acidosis influences not only the right heart but the entire heart (Daum et al., 1969), and thereby the hypoxic pressor response becomes stronger. The combined effects of hypoxia and hypercapnia have also been verified experimentally (Logaras, 1947) through closed circuit breathing, and no difference was obtained in the effect of either hypoxia alone or hypoxia with hypercapnia. Braun and collaborators (1958) found a slight increase of pulmonary pressure in 8 out of 13 dogs breathing 10% oxygen and 10% carbon dioxide in nitrogen, but the response was temporary and returned to control values within 15 min.

V. Anesthetics

Ether anesthesia causes an increase in pulmonary vascular resistance at the operational level (Johnson, 1951). This increase in resistance has been attributed to pulmonary vasoconstriction, as there are inconsistent reports on cardiac output. Intact animal and human experiments have shown increased cardiac output (Blalock, 1927; Fletcher et al., 1956; Malt, 1958; Vidt et al., 1959). However, investigations using heart-lung preparations showed decreased cardiac output following administration of subanesthetic or anesthetic levels of ether. The use of inhalative cyclopropane anesthesia has resulted in increased cardiac output in human subjects (Etsten, 1955; Patrick, 1957). It is not clear whether this effect is due to cyclopropane alone, because it is usually administered with other sedative drugs. However, some authors (Greisheimer et al., 1954; Jones et al., 1960) reported that cyclopropane caused a slight increase in cardiac output. The effect of halothane on cardiac output is also inconsistent (Deutsch et al., 1962; Kubota and Vandam, 1962; Payne et al., 1959). The small blood vessels have been shown to be sensitive to vasoconstrictors under general anesthesia (Baez and Orkin, 1963).

Leusen and Demeester (1953) reported that intravenous application of pentobarbital over a long period can induce pulmonary hypertension, whereas Price and Helrich (1955) found no significant increase in pulmonary vascular resistance in man with thiopental. We used pentothal (Islam and Ulmer, 1973 b; Islam et al., 1971, 1972) for about 6 to 8 h intravenously in our series of control experiments, and we observed very little or no change in pulmonary arterial pressure. Application of small doses of pentothal, within the observation period, induced a brief rise in pulmonary arterial pressure and a return to normal levels within a short period. Similar observations have previously been reported by other authors (Büttlmann and Hossli, 1956; Carbonera, 1955). The usual effect of anesthetic doses of thiopental in human subjects is a reduction of cardiac output (Elder et al., 1955;

Etsten and Li, 1955; Fieldman et al., 1955). In dogs thiopental causes either an increase (Greisheimer et al., 1956a, b) or a decrease (Davis et al., 1959) in cardiac output. In perfusion experiments with constant flow; thiopental causes a rise in pulmonary arterial pressure (Rittmeyer, 1962), which may be considered due to local pulmonary vasoconstriction.

E. Effects of Pharmacological Agents

I. Acetylcholine (ACH)

The drug is to some extent accepted as a vasodilating agent and is sometimes used to investigate the causative factors of vascular changes in pulmonary hypertension. Reduction in pulmonary vascular resistance by ACH is believed to be the result of vasoconstriction; otherwise, it is considered to be due to atherosclerosis or other organic obstruction (Comroe, 1966). But the definite role of ACH on pulmonary circulation is still conflicting and inconclusive. A large group of authors (Bjure et al., 1967; Dollery and Glazier, 1966; Glazier et al., 1968; Irnell and Nordgren, 1966; Söderholm and Widimsky, 1962; Söderholm, 1970) felt

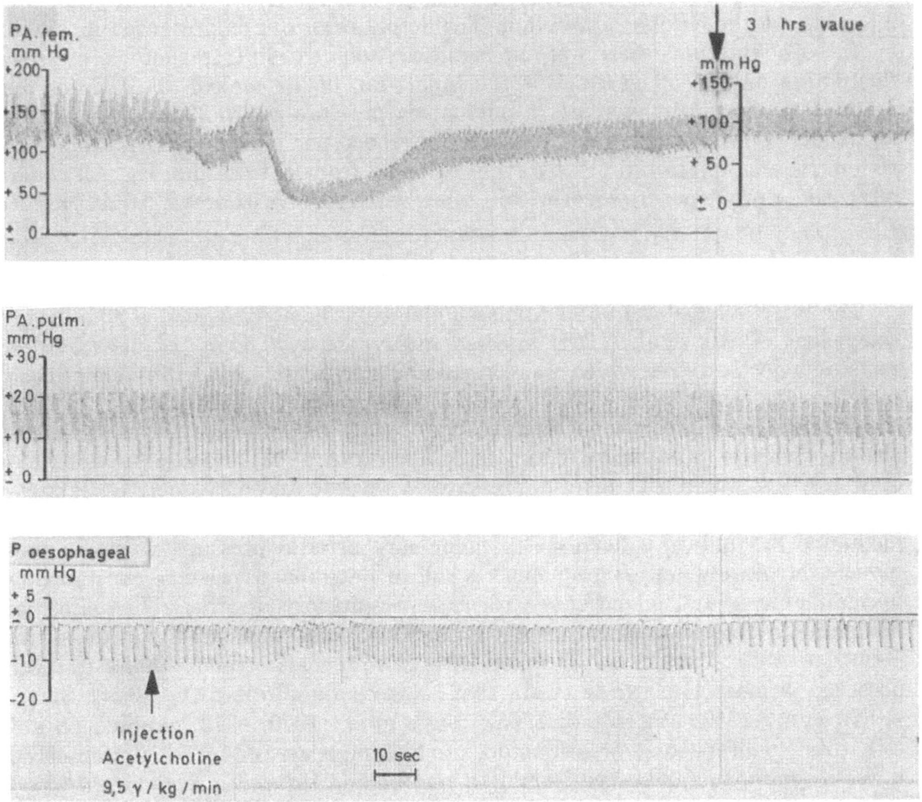

Fig. 8. Shows the original recording of femoral arterial pressure (P_{Afem}) (top), pulmonary arterial pressure (P_{Apul}) (middle) and esophageal pressure (P_{oes}) (bottom) from anesthetized dog. Arrow on the lower left hand side indicates the start of injection of acetylcholine into the right auricle. Arrow on the upper right hand side indicates the values obtained when the injection was continued for 3 h (From Kammler et al., 1970)

that ACH produced vasodilatation, whereas others considered the role of ACH to be vasoconstrictive (BISHOP et al., 1961; VON EULER, 1932; ROSE, 1957) or without definite action (HARRIS et al., 1956). The possible explanations for the different opinions are probably dependent on the status of the pulmonary vascular system prior to ACH application and on the amount of ACH applied (COLEBATCH et al., 1962; HARRIS et al., 1956; ROSE, 1957).

BEAN et al. (1951) observed an increase in pulmonary blood volume in response to ACH in isolated lobes of dog lung. They concluded that this is probably due to the simultaneous constriction of the small pulmonary veins and dilatation of small pulmonary arteries. In contrast, BORST et al. (1957) are of the opinion that ACH produces vasoconstriction in the intact dog. The effect of ACH on human pulmonary circulation is equally inconsistent and inconclusive (HARRIS et al., 1956). REICHEL (1969) reported that the influence of ACH on pulmonary circulation is complex due to its prominent dilatory action on systemic circulation and its constrictive effect on the bronchial system. Infusion of ACH induces bronchial obstruction with increased intrathoracic pressure fluctuation. Bronchoconstriction induces hypoxia and thereby vasoconstriction, which overshadows the vasodilatory effect of ACH. KAMMLER et al. (1970) injected ACH into the right atrium of anesthetized dogs and observed an increase of mean pulmonary arterial pressure of 12.5 mm Hg (12 to 13 mm Hg); no change was observed when the drug was injected into the carotis bifurcation. The actual recording is presented in Fig. 8.

In both situations there were no significant changes in intrathoracic pressure fluctuation and blood gases. But the inhalation of an aerosol of ACH for 6 h produced a significant increase in pulmonary pressure (14 to 23 mm Hg) as well as an increase in intrathoracic pressure difference per breath ranging from 4 to 19 mm Hg and an arterial blood oxygen decrease from 90 to 44 mm Hg. All values returned to pre-exposure level within a few minutes of withdrawal of ACH.

II. Histamine

The effect of histamine on human pulmonary hemodynamics is equally inconclusive. NEMIR et al. (1954) injected intravenously 0.55 mg of histamine in human subjects, a dose which was large enough to cause a fall in systemic blood pressure but which was without effect on the pulmonary circulation. Similar observations were reported by SPITZBARTH et al. (1957), whereas, others obtained either a decrease (HELANDER et al., 1962; WESTLING, 1963) or a rise (LAMBERTINI et al., 1960) in pulmonary arterial pressure. WESTLING and his associates (HELANDER et al., 1962; WESTLING, 1963) concluded from their observations in man that histamine can induce a decrease in pulmonary arterial pressure, a rise in pulmonary blood flow and consequently a fall in pulmonary vascular resistance in normal subjects and in patients with cardiorespiratory disorders. The effect of histamine in dogs (DELAUNOIS et al., 1959; FRIEDBERG et al., 1943; PAULET and BERNARD, 1963; PETERS and HORTON, 1944) also revealed trends similar to those observed in man (HELANDER et al., 1962; NAEYE and BICKERMAN, 1959; SPITZBARTH et al., 1957; WESTLING, 1963). ISLAM et al. (1970, 1972) exposed an anesthetized spontaneously breathing dogs to histamine aerosol for 6 h and observed a rise in pulmonary pressure from 12.2 to 19.5 mm Hg and a decrease in blood oxygen pressure from 97 to 70 mm Hg. The rise in pulmonary arterial pressure may be due to a direct effect of histamine or due to hypoxia following histamine inhalation.

The evidence supporting the local pulmonary vasoconstrictive effects of histamine are derived from perfusion experiments of lung (ALCOCK et al., 1935;

DALY, 1938; DALY et al., 1940; FOGGIE, 1937; GADDUM and HOLTZ, 1933; SIBUL, 1935). GREEFF and MOOG (1964) perfused guinea pig lungs with 0.2 µg and 1 µg histamine and observed a fall in perfusion flow from 7 ml/min to 4.5 and to less than 2 ml/min, respectively. GADDUM and HOLTZ (1933) obtained both arterial and venous histamine-induced vasoconstriction, whereas OKADA (1939) and SMITH and COXE (1951) demonstrated the greater sensitivity of the pulmonary vein than of the pulmonary artery to histamine. GILBERT et al. (1958) also observed a greater increase of venous resistance than of arterial resistance in isolated perfused dog lung, but direct observation of rabbit lung showed constriction of both arterioles and venules (IRWIN, 1960). AITKEN and SANFORD (1970) showed contraction of spiral strips of pulmonary artery in response to histamine. This response indicates the susceptibility of the pulmonary artery to histamine-induced constriction. AARSEN and ZEEGERS (1972) observed a progressively increased pulmonary arterial pressure in isolated perfused guinea pig lungs.

There are suggestions that the pressor effect of histamine is due to stimulation of the adrenal medulla and of the sympathetic system (TRENDELENBURG, 1957, 1961), and it is also believed that histamine is liberated by the sympathetic nerves. This suggestion is based on the detection of histamine in the pulmonary sympathetic nerves (VON EULER, 1949) and on the collection of histamine in the lung perfusate or in the circulating blood as a result of injection of epinephrine (KOCH and SZERB, 1950). Recently, OKPAKO (1972) reported that histamine caused a rise in perfusion pressure in isolated guinea pig lung perfused through the pulmonary artery. This effect was prevented and perfusion pressure decreased when mepyramine was administered prior to histamine; thus neither the pressor nor the depressor effect was modified by adrenoceptor blocking agents. The involvement of a cholinergic mechanism was also excluded since atropine failed to influence the effect of histamine. It is suggested that the pyrilamine-sensitive pressor and the pyrilamine-resistant depressor effects of histamine are mediated through different receptors.

III. 5-Hydroxytryptamine (5-HT)

Studies concerning the effect of 5-HT on pulmonary circulation in man are very scanty. REICHEL (1969) cited from the studies of the COURNAND (1950) group that the infusion of 5-HT in human subjects produced no change in the pulmonary circulation. The pulmonary vasoconstrictive effects of 5-HT have been obtained primarily from animal experiments (AARSEN and ZEEGERS, 1972; ALBERS and USINGER, 1956; AVIADO, 1960; OKADA, 1939).

GREEFF and MOOG (1964) observed a smaller decrease of perfusion flow in isolated perfused guinea pig lung produced by 5-HT than that produced by histamine. Similar results regarding the effectiveness of 5-HT action on isolated guinea pig lung have been presented by AARSEN and ZEEGERS (1972). Several authors (BHATTACHARYA, 1955; ROSE and LAZARO, 1958) have shown that various anti-5-HT substances can reverse the 5-HT-induced vasoconstriction. YOUNG et al. (1963) found an increase of pulmonary capillary blood volume of 6 to 13% in anesthetized dog given 5-HT. They found no change in left ventricular diastolic-systolic or airway pressure and concluded that 5-HT caused pulmonary venous constriction, which in turn leads to passive congestion of the pulmonary capillary bed. Previously MCGAFF and MILNOR (1962) observed a reduction of pulmonary capillary blood volume by 26%, which perhaps indicated generalized vasoconstriction. There are reports suggesting that continuous infusion of 5-HT caused an increase in pulmonary blood flow (RUDOLPH and PAUL, 1957; SHEPHERD et al.,

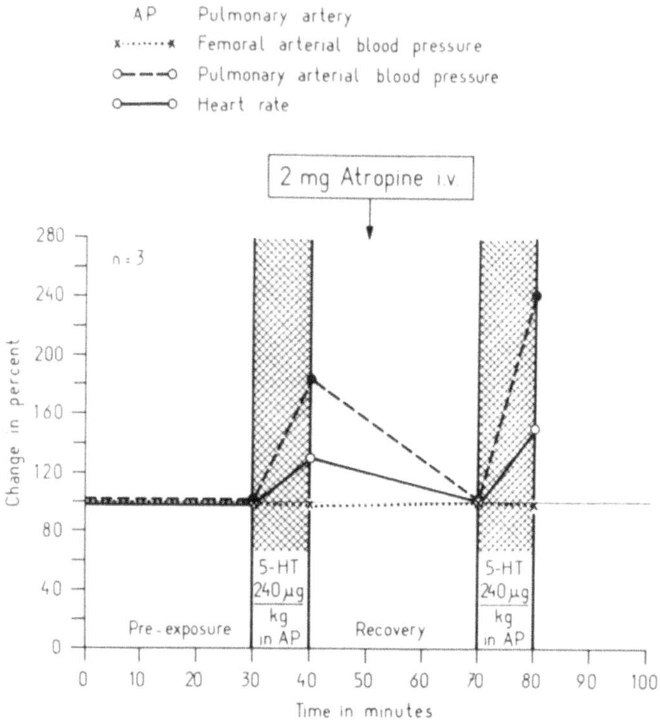

Fig. 9. Presents the per cent increase of pulmonary arterial pressure induced by 5-hydroxytryptamine (5-HT). 5-HT was injected directly into the pulmonary artery before and after intravenous injection of 2 mg of atropine. The increase in pulmonary arterial pressure is greater after the application of atropine

1959) and in pulmonary vascular resistance in dogs (CRUMPTON et al., 1959; McGAFF and MILNOR, 1962).

Continuous infusion of 5-HT caused increased pulmonary arterial pressure. AVIADO (1960) pointed out that this usually coincides with a rise in aortic blood pressure but that the duration of pulmonary arterial hypertension is longer. Previously, REID (1952) observed that when histamine was injected into the pulmonary artery of dogs, there was an immediate increase of pulmonary pressure, but when it was injected into the pulmonary venous side, no such immediate effect was evident. From our recent series (ISLAM et al., 1974) of experiments, we obtained an increase of pulmonary arterial pressure of about 40% above the resting value when 5-HT was given as aerosol inhalation and 80% when injected directly into the pulmonary artery. Systemic arterial pressure remained the same or was slightly decreased. Fig. 9 shows the effect of 5-HT on greater and lesser circulation before and after administration of atropine. Blood gases were also effected significantly in that oxygen tension decreased by 40% (77 to 45 mm Hg) and CO_2 increased by 30% (46 to 60 mm Hg).

A 10% fall in arterial blood oxygen saturation in anesthetized dog was reported previously by RUDOLPH and PAUL (1957). It has been concluded that this might be due to bronchoconstriction, increased blood flow or increased shunt. BORST et al. (1957) observed that reduction in flow of lung subjected to 5-HT was unaccompanied by changes in airway pressure. We (ISLAM et al., 1974) succeeded in blocking the bronchoconstrictive, but not the pulmonary arterial pressure, effects of 5-HT by intravenous application of atropine. Our results corroborate the findings of BORST et al. (1957) that 5-HT can induce pulmonary vasoconstriction without affecting the bronchial system. These findings are in disagreement with those of GREEFF and MOOG (1964), who reported that 5-HT is more a bronchoconstrictive than a vasoconstrictive agent.

IV. Bradykinin

Bradykinin is one of the most widely known endogenous peptides. Its action on pulmonary circulation is also inconsistent. Infusion of bradykinin in the anesthetized dog causes a fall in both systemic and pulmonary blood pressure (MAXWELL et al., 1962; ROWE et al., 1963).

FARITAS et al. (1964) studied the effect of bradykinin in 10 human subjects and concluded that there were no significant changes in pulmonary arterial or left atrial pressure but a definite rise in pulmonary blood flow and hence, a fall in pulmonary vascular resistance. The studies carried out in isolated organ preparations suggest that the action of bradykinin is pulmonary vasoconstrictive. AITKEN and SANFORD (1970) showed contraction of a spiral strip of pulmonary artery in response to bradykinin. GREEFF and MOOG (1964) infused isolated perfused guinea pig lung with 0.05 μg bradykinin and observed a fall of perfusion flow from 7 ml/min to about 2 ml/min. This fall is almost equal to that induced by 1 μg histamine. He concluded that bradykinin acts predominantly on the pulmonary vascular system rather than on the bronchial system. On the other hand, AARSEN and ZEEGERS (1972) found that bradykinin caused both broncho- and vasoconstriction in isolated perfused guinea pig lung.

V. Sympathomimetics

As early as 1951, VON EULER (1951) described that in general, the stimulation of the sympathetic system causes pulmonary vascular contraction and an increase in pulmonary blood pressure. He quoted from his earlier work that the stimulation of the sympathetic system caused a 40% increase of pulmonary pressure; this increase is almost equal to a pressure increase caused by completely blocking one lung artery. It is believed that the pressure effect of hypoxia is mediated through the sympathetic nervous system (BARER, 1966; BARWINSKY and REYES, 1966; BRUTSAERT, 1964; LLOYD, 1966; MCLAUGHLIN et al., 1966). These reports are generally based on the finding of small changes in pulmonary arterial pressure, and other reports have neither supported nor refuted the contention that catecholamines might be implicated in the response to acute hypoxia (HÜRLIMANN and WIGGERS, 1953). If endogenous norepinephrine is the mediator of increased pulmonary pressure in various situations, then the application of exogenous norepinephrine should also produce a similar effect. This hypothesis has been examined recently by SILOVE et al. (1968), who rapidly infused L-norepinephrine, isoproternol and epinephrine into the pulmonary artery of the lower lobe of the lung. They obtained increases ranging from 4 to 17 mm Hg at normal blood pH level in 5 out of 6 young calves with L-norepinephrine, significant reduction in pressure with isoproteronol, and a variable effect with epinephrine. Pulmonary pressure increases were also observed by GOLDRING et al. (1962) following infusion of norepinephrine in human subjects. They failed to obtain any increase in pulmonary vascular resistance and concluded that the pulmonary arterial pressure increase was due to back pressure from the left heart. These results contradict the findings of Silove et al. (1968), who showed an increase in pulmonary arterial pressure in the absence of an elevation of left atrial pressure. The pulmonary vasoconstrictive effects of norepinephrine have been shown previously by others (Barer, 1966; Nahas and MacDonald, 1959; Rose et al., 1955).

Various other sympathomimetic drugs, such as epinine, tyrmine, phenylephrine etc., induce pulmonary arterial hypertension in a manner similar to that of epinephrine in anesthetized animals. They act by inducing local pulmonary vasoconstriction and/or increased pulmonary blood flow (Dollery, 1970; Hyman, 1969; Tavares et al., 1972). Dopamine (3,4-dihydroxyphenyl-ethyl-amine) is a naturally occurring catecholamine and is a direct biochemical precursor to norepinephrine (Blaschko, 1957). Harrison et al. (1969) showed that infusion of dopamine causes a rise in pulmonary arterial pressure. Only at higher doses (25 and 30 μg/kg per min), however, was there evidence of a statistically significant pressor response. No change in vascular resistance was noted, which suggests a dopamine-induced increase in smooth muscle tension in the pulmonary vasculature (Harrison et al., 1969).

The changes in pulmonary circulation are caused primarily under experimental conditions or secondary to other diseases. In 1969, Smekal et al. (1970), Gahl and Greiser (1970) and Kummer (1970) reported a high incidence of primary pulmonary hypertension in patients who had taken aminorex or other appetite-reducing drugs for different periods of time.

In the biochemical sense amphetamine may stimulate noradrenaline release and hinder reabsorption. The pulmonary arterial hypertensive action of hydroxyamphetamine (Paredrine) in anesthetized dogs was noted by Friedberg et al. (1943). They concluded that the major cause for the hypertension is increased pulmonary blood flow and considered that the local effect is insignificant. Kraupp et al. (1970) studied the action of amphetamine and similar substances on the pulmonary circulation in anesthetized dogs and obtained an increase in pulmonary pressure of 18 to 22% above the initial values by slow infusion. In all cases light reduction of pulmonary capillary blood flow was observed. However, the increased transpulmonary pressure (pulmonary arterial pressure—left atrial pressure) was observed only with aminorex, whereas the pressure changes with noradrenaline, ephidrine and amphetamine were always accompanied by increased left atrial pressure.

References

Aarsen, P. N., Zeegers, A.: Effects of histamine, 5-hydroxytryptamine and bradykinin on the vascular system of isolated lungs of the guinea-pig and the influence of phenylbutazone on these effects. Brit. J. Pharmacol. **45**, 284–298 (1972).

Aitken, M. M., Sanford, J.: The effect of drugs on bovine tracheobronchial and pulmonary-vascular tissue. Brit. J. Pharmacol. **38**, 443–444 (1970).

Albers, C., Usinger, W.: Der Kreislauf des Hundes bei akutem Sauerstoffmangel. Pflügers Arch. ges. Physiol. **263**, 201–226 (1956).

Alcock, P., Berry, J. L., Daly, I. De B., Narayana, B.: The action on perfused lungs of drugs injected into the bronchial vascular system. Quart. J. exp. Physiol. **26**, 13–27 (1935).

Alexander, A. F.: The bovine lung: normal vascular histology and vascular lesions in high mountain disease. Med. thorac. **19**, 528–542 (1962).

Alexander, A. F., Jensen, R.: Gross cardiac changes in cattle with high mountain (brisket) disease and in experimental cattle maintained at high altitudes. Amer. J. vet. Res. **20**, 680–689 (1959).

Alzamora-Castro, V., Garrido-Lecca, G., Battilana, G.: Pulmonary edema of high altitude. Amer. J. Cardiol. **7**, 769–778 (1961).

AMBRUS, C. M., AMBRUS, J. L., JOHNSON, G. C., PACKMAN, E. W., CHERNICK, W. S., BACK, N., HARRISON, J. W. E.: Role of the lungs in regulation of the white blood cell level. Amer. J. Physiol. **178**, 33 (1954).

ARBORELIUS, M., JR.: Influence of unilateral hypoventilation on distribution of pulmonary blood flow in man. J. Appl. Physiol. **26**, 101–104 (1959).

ARBORELIUS, M., JR.: Influence of moderate hypoxia in one lung on the distribution of the pulmonary circulation and ventilation. Scand. J. clin. Lab. Invest. **17**, 257–259 (1965).

ARIAS-STELLA, J., KRUGER, H.: Pathology of high altitude pulmonary edema. Arch. Path. **76**, 147–157 (1963).

ARIAS-STELLA, J., SALDANA, M.: The muscular pulmonary arteries in people native to high altitude. Med. thorac. **19**, 484–493 (1962).

ATWELL, R. J., HICKAM, J. B., PHRYOR, W. W., PAGE, E. B.: Reduction of blood flow through the hypoxic lung. Amer. J. Physiol. **166**, 37–44 (1951).

AVIADO, D. M.: Effects of acute atelectasis on lobar blood flow. Amer. J. Physiol. **198**, 349 (1960a).

AVIADO, D. M.: Pulmonary venular responses to anoxia, 5-hydroxy-tryptamine and histamine. Amer. J. Physiol. **198**, 1032–1036 (1960b).

AVIADO, D. M.: The lung circulation. First ed. Oxford-London: Pergamon Press 1965.

AVIADO, D. M., LING, J. S., SCHMIDT, C. F.: Effects on anoxia on pulmonary circulation: Reflex pulmonary vasoconstriction. Amer. J. Physiol. **189**, 253–262 (1957).

BAEZ, S., ORKIN, L. R.: Effects of anesthetics on the response of the micro-circulation to circulating humors. Anesthesiology **24**, 568–579 (1963).

BAINBRIDGE, F. A.: The physiology of muscular exercise. 3rd ed. Rewritten by A. V. BOCK, D. B. DILL. London: Longmans, Green 1931.

BALDWIN, E. DE F., COURNAND, A., RICHARDS, D. W.: Pulmonary insufficiency; study of 122 cases of chronic pulmonary emphysema. Medicine (Baltimore) **28**, 201 (1949).

BANCHERO, N., SIME, F., PENALOZA, D., CRUZ, J., GAMBOA, R.: Effects of exercise on the heart and pulmonary circulation of the high altitudes. (Abstract.) Circulation 8, 686–687 (1963).

BANCHERO, N., SIME, F., PENALOZA, D., GAMBOA, R., CRUZ, J., MARTICORENA, E.: Pulmonary hypertension in children born and living in high altitudes. (Abstract.) Circulation **26**, 683 (1962).

BARER, G. R.: Reactivity of vessels of collapsed and ventilated lungs to drugs and hypoxia. Circulat. Res. **18**, 366–378 (1966).

BARRATT-BOYES, B. G., WOOD, E. H.: Hemodynamic response of healthy subjects to exercise in the supine position while breathing oxygen. J. appl. Physiol. **11**, 129–135 (1957).

BARTELS, H., BEER, R., FLEISCHER, E., HOFFHEINZ, H. J., KRALL, J., RODEWALD, G., WENNER, J., WITT, I.: Bestimmung von Kurzschlußblutung und Diffusionskapazität der Lunge bei Gesunden und Lungenkranken. Pflügers Arch. ges. Physiol. **261**, 99 (1955).

BARTELS, H., RODEWALD, G.: Die alveolar-arterielle Sauerstoffdruckdifferenz und das Problem des Gasaustausches in der menschlichen Lunge. Pflügers Arch. ges. Physiol. **258**, 163 (1953).

BARWINSKY, J., REYES, H.: Study of the effects of alphaadrenergic blockade with phenooxybenzamine on pulmonary vascular resistance. Circulation 34 (Suppl. 3), 50 (1966).

BATES, D. V., VARIS, C. J., DONEVAN, R. E., CHRISTIE, R. V.: Variations in the pulmonary capillary blood volume and membrane diffusion component in health and disease. J. clin. Invest. **39**, 1401–1412 (1960).

BEAN, J. B., PORTER, W., MAYO, W. P., O'DONNELL, P., GRAY, G. W.: Vascular response in dog lung induced by alterations in pulmonary arterial CO_2 tension and by acetylcholine. Amer. J. Physiol. **166**, 723 (1951).

BEKAURI, N. V., IL'INA, A. I., TONKIKH, A. V.: Concerning the physiology of the plumonary circulation. Direct visualization of the pulmonary circulation in warm blooded animals. Fiziol. Zhr. **40**, 295 (1954).

BERGGREN, S. M.: The oxygen deficit of arterial blood caused by nonventilating parts of the lung. Acta physiol. scand. **4**, Suppl. 11 (1942).

BERGOFSKY, E. H., HAAS, F.: An investigation of the site of pulmonary vascular response to hypoxia. Bull. physiopath. resp. **4**, 91–103 (1968).

BERGOFSKY, E. H., HOTZMAN, S.: Mechanism involved in pulmonary arterial pressor response to hypoxia. Circulation Res. **20**, 506–519 (1967).

BERGOFSKY, E. H., LEHR, D. E., FISHMAN, A. P.: The effect of changes in hydrogen ion concentration on the pulmonary circulation. J. clin. Invest. **41**, 1492–1502 (1962).

BERGOFSKY, E. H., TURINO, G. M., FISHMAN, A. P.: Cardiorespiratory failure in kyphoscoliosis. Medicine (Baltimore) **38**, 263 (1959).

BERNTHAL, T., HORRES, A. D., TAYLOR, J. T.: Pulmonary vascular obstruction in graded tachypneagenic diffuse embolism. Amer. J. Physiol. **200**, 279–286 (1961).

BHATTACHARYA, B. K.: A pharmacological study on the effect of 5-hydroxytryptamine and its antagonists on the bronchial musculature. Arch. int. Pharmacodyn. **103**, 357–369 (1955).
BISHOP, J. M., HARRIS, P., BATEMAN, M., DAVIDSON, L. A. G.: The effect of acetylcholine upon respiratory gas exchange in mitral stenosis. J. clin. Invest. **40**, 105 (1961).
BJURE, J., HELANDER, E., LINDELL, S.-E., SÖDERHOLM, B., WESTLING, H.: Effect of acetylcholine and histamine on the pulmonary circulation in normal men and women. Scand. J. Resp. Dis. **48**, 214–226 (1967).
BLALOCK, A.: Cardiac output in the dog during ether anesthesia. I. The effect of ether anesthesia on the cardiac output. Arch. Surg. **14**, 732–751 (1927).
BLASCHKO, H.: Formation of catecholamines in the animal body. Brit. med. Bull. **13**, 162–165 (1957).
BLOOR, C. M., SOBEL, B. E., HENRY, P. D.: Autologous pulmonary embolism in the intact, unanesthetized dog. J. appl. Physiol. **29**, 670–674 (1970).
BONDURANT, S., MEAD, J., COOK, C. D.: A re-evaluation of effects of acute central congestion on pulmonary compliance in normal subjects. J. appl. Physiol. **15**, 875 (1960).
BORDEN, C. W., WILSON, R. H., EBERT, R. V., WELLS, H. S.: Pulmonary hypertension in chronic pulmonary emphysema. Amer. J. Med. **8**, 701 (1950).
BORDER, J. R., TIBBETTS, J. C., SCHENK, W. G.: Hypoxic hyperventilation and acute respiratory failure in the severely stressed patient: massive pulmonary arteriovenous shunts? Surgery **64**, 710–719 (1968).
BORST, H. G., BERGLUND, E., MCGREGOR, M.: Effects of pharmacologic agents on the pulmonary circulation in the dog. Studies on epinephrine, norepinephrine, 5-hydroxytryptamine, acetylcholine, histamine and aminophylline. J. clin. Invest. **36**, 669 (1957).
BORST, H. G., BERGLUND, E., WHITTENBERGER, J. L., MEAD, J., MCGREGOR, M., COLLIER, C.: The effect of pulmonary vascular pressures on the mechanical properties of the lungs of anesthetized dogs. J. clin. Invest. **36**, 1708–1714 (1957).
BORST, H. G., MCGREGOR, M., WHITTENBERGER, J. L., BERGLUND, E.: Influence of pulmonary arterial and left atrial pressures on pulmonary vascular resistance. Circulat. Res. **4**, 393–399 (1956).
BORST, H. G., WHITTENBERGER, J. L., BERGLUND, E., MCGREGOR, M.: Effects of unilateral hypoxia and hypercapnia on pulmonary blood flow distribution in the dog. Amer. J. Physiol. **191**, 446–452 (1957).
BOSMAN, R., HONOUR, A. J., LEE, G. DE J., MARSHALL, R. M., STOTT, F. D.: Instantaneous pulmonary blood flow measurement in man. J. Physiol. (Lond.) **159**, 15 (1961).
BOSTROEM, B., PIIPER, J.: Über arterio-venöse Anastomosen und Kurzschlußdurchblutung in der Lunge. Pflügers Arch. ges. Physiol. **261**, 165 (1955).
BRAUN, K., ROSENBERG, S. Z., ELIAKIM, M., STERN, S.: Effect of simultaneous hypoxia and hypercapnia on the pulmonary arterial pressor of the dog. Arch. int. physiol. et biochem. **66**, 515 (1958).
BRAUNWALD, E., BINION, J. T., MORGAN, W. L., JR., SARNOFF, S. J.: Alterations in central blood volume and cardiac output induced by positive pressure breathing and counteracted by metaraminol (Aramine). Circulat. Res. **5**, 670 (1957).
BRAUNWALD, E., KELLY, E. R.: The effects of exercise on central blood volume in man. J. clin. Invest. **39**, 413 (1960).
BRIEHL, R. W., FISHMAN, A. P.: Principles of the Bohr integration procedure and their application to measurement of diffusing capacity of the lung for oxygen. J. appl. Physiol. **15**, 337 (1960).
BRUTSAERT, D.: Influence of reserpine and of adrenolytic agents on the pulmonary arterial pressor response to hypoxia and catecholamines. Arch. int. Physiol. **72**, 395–412 (1964).
BRYAN, A. C., MACNAMARA, W. D., SIMPSON, J., WAGNER, H. N.: Effect of acceleration on the distribution of pulmonary blood flow. J. appl. Physiol. **20**, 1129–1132 (1965).
BRYAN, A. C., MILIC-EMILI, J., PENGELLY, D.: Effect of gravity on the distribution of pulmonary ventilation. J. appl. Physiol. **21**, 778–784 (1966).
BÜHLMANN, A., SCHAUB, F., LUCHSINGER, P.: Die Hämodynamik des Lungenkreislaufes während Ruhe und körperlicher Arbeit beim Gesunden und bei den verschiedenen Formen der pulmonalen Hypertonie. Schweiz. med. Wschr. **85**, 253 (1955).
BÜTTLMANN, A., HOSSLI, G.: Hämodynamische Untersuchungen bei akuter Hypoventilation. Schweiz. med. Wschr. **86**, 681–684 (1956).
BURCH, G. E., ROMNEY, R. B.: Functional anatomy and "throttle valve" action of the pulmonary veins. Amer. Heart J. **47**, 58 (1954).
BURKART, F.: The exercise test in patients with obstructive pulmonary hypertension. Int. Symp. on Pulmonary Circulation. Progr. Resp. Res. **5**, 395–399 (1969).
BURROWS, B., NIDEN, A. H.: Effects of anemia and hemorrhagic shock on pulmonary diffusion in the dog lung. J. appl. Physiol. **150**, 123 (1963).

BURTON, A. C.: The relation between pressure and flow in the pulmonary bed. In: Pulmonary circulation. New York: Grune & Stratton 1959.
BUSBY, D. E.: Space clinical medicine. Dordrecht, Holland: Reidal 1968.
CAPPS, J. A., LEWIS, P. D.: Observations upon certain blood pressure lowering reflexes that arise from irritation of inflamed pleura. Amer. J. med. Sci. **134**, 868–894 (1907).
CARBONERA, D.: L'insufficienza cardio-polmonale acuta (sindrome die Condorelli) durante l'anesthesia. Rif. med. **69**, 957–960 (1955).
CARLILL, S. D., DUKE, H. N., JONES, M.: Some observations on pulmonary haemodynamics in the cat. J. Physiol. (Lond.) **136**, 112–121 (1957).
CHAFFEE, W. R., SMULYAN, H., KEIGHLEY, J. F., EICH, R. H.: The effect of exercise in pulmonary blood volume. Amer. Heart J. **66**, 657–663 (1963).
CHINARD, F. P., ENNS, T.: Transcapillary pulmonary exchange of water in the dog. Amer. J. Physiol. **178**, 197 (1954).
CLARKE, S. W., JONES, J. G., GLAISTER, D. H.: Changes in pulmonary ventilation in different postures. Clin. Sci. **37**, 357–369 (1969).
COLEBATCH, H. J. H., OLSEN, C. R., NADEL, J. A.: Pulmonary arterial blood supply to peripheral airways: Effect of acetylcholine, serotonin and histamine. Circulation **26**, 700 (1962).
COLERIDGE, J. C. G., KIDD, C., SHARP, J. A.: The distribution, connexions and histology of baroreceptors in the pulmonary artery, with some observations on the sensory innervation of the ductus arteriosus. J. Physiol. (Lond.) **156**, 591 (1961).
COMROE, J. H., JR.: Physiology of Respiration. Chicago: Year Book Med. Pub. Inc. 1966.
COURNAND, A.: Some aspects of the pulmonary circulation in normal man and in chronic cardio-pulmonary disease. Circulation **2**, 641 (1950).
COURNAND, A., BALDWIN, J. S., HIMMELSTEIN, A.: Cardiac catheterization in congenital heart disease. New York: The Commonwealth Fund 1949.
COURNAND, A., MITCHELL, A., FISHMAN, A. P.: Applicability of direct Fick method to measurement of pulmonary blood flow during induced acute hypoxia. Fed. Proc. **13**, 31 (1954).
COURNAND, A., RANGES, H. A.: Catheterization of right auricle in man. Proc. Soc. Exp. Biol. (N.Y.) **46**, 462–466 (1941).
COURNAND, A., RILEY, R. L., BREED, E. S., BALDWIN, DE F., RICHARDS, D. W.: Measurement of cardiac output in man using technique of catheterization of right auricle or ventricle. J. clin. Invest. **24**, 106–116 (1945).
CRUMPTON, C. W., CASTILLO, C. A., ROWE, G. G., MAXWELL, G. M.: Serotonin and the dynamics of the heart. Ann. N.Y. Acad. Sci. **80**, 960–968 (1959).
DAILY, P. O., GRIFFIN, A., BLACKSTONE, E., MOULDER, P. V.: The hemodynamic effects of localized pulmonary embolism. Surg. Gynec. Obstet. **123**, 765–773 (1966).
DALY, I. DE B.: Observations on the blood-perfused lungs of the dog, guinea-pig, and macacus rhesus, with special reference to "spontaneous" lung movements. Quart. J. exp. Physiol. **28**, 357–403 (1938).
DALY, I. DE B.: Intrinsic mechanisms of the lung. Quart. J. Exp. Physiol. **43**, 2 (1958).
DALY, I. DE B., DALY, M. DE B.: The nervous control of the pulmonary circulation. In: Problems of Pulmonary Circulation. Ciba Foundation Study Group No. 8. Boston: Little, Brown 1961.
DALY, I. DE B., FOGGIE, P., HEBB, C. O.: An experimental analysis of the action of adrenaline and histamine on different parts of pulmonary vascular bed. Quart. J. exp. Physiol. **30**, 21–44 (1940).
DALY, M. DE B., WRIGHT, P. G.: The effects of anticholinesterases upon pulmonary vascular resistance in the dog. J. Physiol. (Lond.) **139**, 273–293 (1957).
DAUM, S., KROFTA, K., DRAB, K., NIKODÝMOVÁ, L., SVORČIK, S., JÁHN, J.: Die Lungenzirkulation während der akuten Hyperkapnie und hyperkapnischen Acidose. Verh. Ges. Lungen-Atmungsforschg. **2**, 122 (1969).
DAVIS, F., NASH, C. B., WOODBURY, R. A.: Cardiovascular effects of anesthetic doses of thiopental sodium. Anesth. Analg. Curr. Res. **38**, 222–228 (1959).
DE BONO, E. F., CARO, G. G.: Effect of lung-inflating pressure on pulmonary blood pressure and flow. Amer. J. Physiol. **205**, 1178–1186 (1963).
DEGRAFF, A. C., JR., GROVER, R. F., JOHNSON, R. L., JR., HAMMOND, J. W., JR., MILLER, J. M.: Diffusing capacity of the lung in Caucasians native to 3,100 m. J. appl. Physiol. **29** (1), 71–76 (1970).
DELAUNOIS, A. L., KORDECKI, R., POLET, H., RYZEWSKI, J.: Cardiac output, arterial blood pressure and pulmonary arterial pressure in histamine shock. Arch. int. Pharmacodyn. **120**, 114–119 (1959).
DEMPSEY, J., BIRNBAUM, M., RANKIN, J.: Exercise pulmonary gas exchange under varying duration of hypoxic exposure. (Abstract.) Fed. Proc. **28**, 593.(1969).
DEMUTH, G. R., HOWATT. W. F., HILL, B. M.: The growth of lung function. Pediatrics **35** 161–218 (1965).

Deutsch, S., Linde, H. W., Dripps, R. D., Price, H. L.: Circulatory and respiratory actions of halothane in normal man. Anesthesiology **23**, 631–638 (1962).

Dexter, L., Whittenberger, J. L., Haynes, F. W., Goodale, W. T., Gorlin, R., Sawyer, C. G.: Effect of exercise on circulatory dynamics of normal individuals. J. appl. Physiol. **3**, 439–453 (1951).

Dirken, M. N. J., Heemstra, H.: The adaptation of the lung circulation to ventilation. Quart. J. exp. Physiol. **34**, 213 (1948).

Dobiáš, J.: Morphology of bronchopulmonary anastomoses, their occurrence and importance. Int. Symp. on Pulmonary Circulation, Prague, 1969. Progr. Resp. Res. **5**, 412–420 (1970).

Dock, D. S., Kraus, W. L., McGuire, L. B., Hyland, J. W., Haynes, F. W., Dexter, L.: The pulmonary blood volume in man. J. clin. Invest. **40**, 317 (1961).

Dock, W., Taubman, F.: Some technics for recording the ballisto-cardiogram directly from the body. Amer. J. Med. **7**, 751–755 (1949).

Dollery, C. T.: Effects of vasodilator drugs on the pulmonary circulation. Int. Symp. on Pulmonary Circulation, Prague, 1969. Progr. Resp. Res. **5**, 105–112 (1970).

Dollery, C. T., Glazier, J. M. B.: Pharmacological effects of drugs on the pulmonary circulation in man. Clin. Pharmacol. Ther. **7**, 807–818 (1966).

Dollery, C. T., West, J. B.: Regional uptake of radioactive oxygen, carbon monoxide and carbon dioxide in the lungs of patients with mitral stenosis. Circulat. Res. **8**, 765 (1960).

Donomarco, J. R., Rimini, R.: Venous pressure of man in space. Aerospace Med. **41**, 175–178 (1970).

Drinker, C. K.: Pulmonary edema and inflammation. Cambridge: Harvard Univ. Press 1945.

Duke, H. N.: Pulmonary vasomotor responses of isolated perfused cat lungs to anoxia and hypercapnia. Quart. J. exp. Physiol. **36**, 75 (1951).

Durand, J., Leroy Ladurie, M., Ranson-Bitker, B.: Effects of hypoxia and hypercapnia on the repartition of pulmonary blood flow in supine subjects. Int. Symp. on Pulmonary Circulation, Prague, 1969. Progr. Resp. Res. **5**, 156–165 (1970).

Edwards, W. S.: The effects of lung inflation and epinephrine on pulmonary vascular resistance. Amer. J. Physiol. **167**, 756–762 (1951).

Elder, J. D., Jr., Nagano, S. M., Eastwood, D. W., Harnagel, D.: Circulatory changes associated with thiopental anesthesia in man. Anesthesiology **16**, 394–400 (1955).

Eliakim, M., Aviado, D. M.: Effects of nerve stimulation and drugs on the extrapulmonary portion of the pulmonary vein. J. Pharmacol. exp. Ther. **133**, 304 (1961).

Engstedt, L., Freyschuss, U., Kaijser, L., Asen, P.: Hemodynamic findings in patients with intravascular red cell aggregation. Acta med. scand. **182**, 68 (1967).

Enson, Y., Giuntini, C., Lewis, M. L., Morris, T. Q., Ferrer, M. I., Harvey, R.: The influence of hydrogen ion concentration and hypoxia on the pulmonary circulation. J. clin. Invest. **40**, 1146 (1964).

Etsten, B., Li, T. H.: Hemodynamic changes during thiopental anesthesia in humans: cardiac output, stroke volume, total peripheral resistance, and intrathoracic blood volume. J. clin. Invest. **34**, 500–510 (1955).

Etsten, B., Reynolds, R. N., Li, T. H.: The effects of controlled respiration on circulation during cyclopropane anesthesia. Anesthesiology **16**, 365–374 (1955).

Euler, U. S. von: A vaso-constrictor action of acetylcholine on the rabbit's pulmonary circulation. J. Physiol. (Lond.) **74**, 271 (1932).

Euler, U. S. von: Histamine as a specific constituent of certain autonomic nerve fibres. Acta physiol. scand. **19**, 85–93 (1949).

Euler, U. S. von: Physiologie des Lungenkreislaufs. Verh. dtsch. Ges. Kreisl.-Forsch. **17**, 8 (1951).

Euler, U. S. von, Liljestrand, G.: Observations on the pulmonary arterial blood pressure in the cat. Acta physiol. scand. **12**, 301 (1946).

Euler, U. S. von, Lishajko, F.: Catecholamines in the vascular wall. Acta physiol. scand. **42**, 33 (1958).

Faritas, F. M. de, Faraco, E. Z., Azevedo, D. F. de: General circulatory alterations induced by intravenous infusion of synthetic bradykinin in man. Circulation **29**, 66–70 (1964).

Fieldman, E. J., Ridley, R. W., Wood, E. H.: Hemodynamic studies during thiopental sodium and nitrous oxide anesthesia in humans. Anesthesiology **16**, 473–489 (1955).

Finley, T. N.: The determination of uneven pulmonary blood flow from the arterial oxygen tension during nitrogen washout. J. clin. Invest. **40**, 1727 (1961).

Finley, T. N., Lenfant, C., Haab, P., Piiper, J., Rahn, H.: Venous admixture in the pulmonary circulation of anesthetized dogs. J. appl. Physiol. **15**, 418–424 (1960).

Fishman, A. P.: Dynamics of the pulmonary circulation. Handbook of Physiology. Sec. 2: Circulation II. Baltimore: Waverly Press 1963.

Fishman, A. P., Fritts, H. W., Jr., Cournand, A.: Effects of breathing carbon dioxide upon the pulmonary circulation. Circulation **22**, 220–225 (1960).

FISHMAN, A. P., HIMMELSTEIN, A., FRITTS, H. W., JR., COURNAND, A.: Blood flow through each lung in man during unilateral hypoxia. J. clin. Invest. **34**, 637 (1955).
FISHMAN, A. P., MCCLEMENT, J., HIMMELSTEIN, A., COURNAND, A.: Effects of acute anoxia on the circulation and respiration in patients with chronic pulmonary disease studied during the steady state. J. clin. Invest. **31**, 770 (1952).
FLETCHER, G., PENDER, J. W., WOOD, E. H.: Hemodynamic effects of ether anesthesia and surgery in 11 cases. Anesth. Analg. Curr. Res. **35**, 18–32 (1956).
FOGGIE, P.: The action of adrenaline, acetylcholine, and histamine on the lungs of the rat. Quart. J. exp. Physiol. **26**, 225–233 (1937).
FORSSMANN, W.: Probing of the right heart. Klin. Wschr. 8, 2085–2087 (1929).
FORSTER, R. E.: Exchange of gases between alveolar air and pulmonary capillary blood: pulmonary diffusing capacity. Physiol. Rev. **37**, 391 (1957).
FRED, H. L., SCHMIDT, A. M., BATES, T., HECHT, H. H.: Acute pulmonary edema of altitude. Circulation **25**, 929–937 (1962).
FREEMAN, J., NUNN, J. F.: Ventilation-perfusion relationships after hemorrhage on pulmonary circulation and gas exchange. J. clin. Invest. **38**, 524–537 (1959).
FRIEDBERG, L., KATZ, L. N., STEINITZ, F. S.: The effect of drugs on the pulmonary and systemic arterial pressures in the trained unanesthetized dog. Renin, angiotonin, adrenalin, pitressin, paredrine, digitalis, acetylcholine, papaverine, histamine, amyl nitrite and aminophyllin. J. Pharmacol. exp. Ther. **77**, 80–106 (1943).
FRITTS, H. W., JR., ODELL, J. E., HARRIS, P., BRAUNWALD, E. W., FISHMAN, A. P.: Effects of acute hypoxia on the volume of blood in the thorax. Circulation **22**, 216 (1960).
FRY, D. L.: Methods of flow estimation by pressure sensing techniques. IRE Trans. Med. Electronics ME-**6**, 264 (1959).
GADDUM, J. H., HEBB, C. O., SILBER, A., SWAN, A. A.: 5-hydroxytryptamine pharmacological action and destruction in perfused lungs. Quart. J. exp. Physiol. **38**, 255 (1953).
GADDUM, J. H., HOLTZ, P.: The localization of the action of drugs on the pulmonary vessels of dogs and cats. J. Physiol. (Lond.) **77**, 139–158 (1933).
GAHL, K., GREISER, E.: Erfahrungen einer klinisch-epidemiologischen Studie zum Problem der primär vaskulären pulmonalen Hypertonie. Schweiz. med. Wschr. **100**, 2154–2157 (1970).
GELIN, L. E.: Flüssigkeitsersatz im Schock. In: Schock, Pathogenese und Therapie. Berlin: Springer 1962.
GILBERT, R. P., HINSHAW, L. B., KUIDA, H., VISSCHER, M. B.: Effects of histamine, 5-hydroxytryptamine and epinephrine on pulmonary hemodynamics with particular reference to arterial and venous segment resistances. Amer. J. Physiol. **194**, 165–170 (1958).
GLAISTER, D. H.: Regional ventilation and perfusion in the lung during positive acceleration measured with ^{133}Xe. J. Physiol. (Lond.) **177**, 73–74 (1965).
GLAISTER, D. H.: The effect of posture on the distribution of ventilation and blood flow in the normal lung. Clin. Sci. **33**, 391–398 (1967a).
GLAISTER, D. H.: A flat beam collimator for radioisotope scanning of the lung. Brit. J. Radiol. **40**, 670–675 (1967b).
GLAISTER, D. H.: The effect of positive centrifugal acceleration upon the distribution of ventilation and perfusion within the human lung, and its relation to pulmonary arterial and intraoesophageal pressures. Proc. roy. Soc. B **168**, 311–334 (1967c).
GLAISTER, D. H.: Distribution of pulmonary blood flow and ventilation during forward ($+G_X$) acceleration. J. appl. Physiol. **29**, 432–439 (1970).
GLAZIER, J. B., DOLLERY, C. T., HUGHES, J. M. B.: Effects of acetylcholine on regional pulmonary blood flow in patients with mitral stenosis. Circulation **38**, 136–143 (1968).
GLOGER, K.: Die Altersabhängigkeit des Pulmonalarteriendruckes während stufenweise gesteigerter Ergometerarbeit. Kreisl.-Forsch. **61**, 728 (1972).
GOLDRING, R. M., TURINO, G. M., COHEN, G., JAMESON, A. G., BASS, B. G., FISHMAN, A. P.: The catecholamines in the pulmonary arterial pressor response to acute hypoxia. J. clin. Invest. **41**, 1211–1221 (1962).
GORLIN, R., LEWIS, B. M.: Circulatory adjustments to hypoxia in dogs. J. appl. Physiol. **7**, 180–185 (1954).
GREEFF, K., MOOG, E.: Vergleichende Untersuchungen über die bronchoconstrictorische und gefäßconstrictorische Wirkung des Bradykinins, Histamins und Serotonins an isolierten Lungenpräparaten. Naunyn-Schmiedebergs Arch. exp. Path. Pharmak. **248**, 204–215 (1964).
GREISHEIMER, E. M., ELLIS, D. W., STEWART, G., MAKARENKO, L., OLEKSYSHYN, N., THOMPSON, K. T.: Cardiac output by the dye dilution technique under thiopental sodium oxygen and ether anesthesia. Amer. J. Physiol. **186**, 101–104 (1956a).
GREISHEIMER, E. M., ELLIS, D. W., STEWART, G., MAKARENKO, L., OLEKSYSHYN, N., THOMPSON, K. T.: Cardiovascular responses to several ultrashort acting barbiturates. Anesthesiology **17**, 385–390 (1956b).

Greisheimer, E. M., Ellis, D. W., Webber, D. L., Baier, H. N., Lynch, P. R.: Cardiac output by cuvette oximeter under cyclopropane-oxygen anesthesia. Amer. J. Physiol. **177**, 489–492 (1954).

Grover, R. F., Reeves, J. T., Will, D. H., Blount, S. G., Jr.: Pulmonary vasoconstriction in steers at high altitude. J. appl. Physiol. **18**, 567–574 (1963).

Grover, R. F., Saltin, B., Hartley, L. H., Johnson, R. L., Jr.: Decreased stroke volume during maximal exercise in man at high altitude. Fed. Proc. **26**, 665 (1967).

Gruber, U. F.: Blutersatz. Berlin: Springer 1968.

Guzmán, A.: Thirty-five cases of high altitude pulmonary edema. (Abstract.) The IV World Congress of Cardiology (Mexico City) 246, 1962.

Haddy, F. J., Campbell, G. S.: Pulmonary vascular resistance in anesthetized dogs. Amer. J. Physiol. **172**, 747 (1953).

Haggard, G. E., Walker, A. M.: The physiology of pulmonary embolism as disclosed by quantitative occlusion of the pulmonary artery. Arch. Surg. **6**, 764 (1923).

Hales, S.: Statistical Essays: Haemostatics, 1733. 3rd ed. London: Wilson and Nicol 1769.

Halmagyi, D. F. J., Starzecki, B. Horner,, G. J.: Humoral transmission of cardiorespiratory changes in experimental lung embolism. Circulat. Res. **14**, 546–554 (1964).

Hamilton, W. F.: Pressure relations in the pulmonary circuit in blood, heart and circulation. Publ. Amer. Ass. Adv. Sci. **13**, 324 (1940).

Hamilton, W. F.: The physiology of the cardiac output. Circulation **8**, 527 (1953).

Hamilton, W. F., Dow, P., Remington, J. W.: The relationship between the cardiac ejection curve and the ballistocardiographic forces. Amer. J. Physiol. **144**, 557–570 (1945).

Hamilton, W. F., Lombard, E. A.: Intrathoracic volume changes in relation to the cardiopneumogram. Circulat. Res. **1**, 76 (1953).

Hamilton, W. F., Mayo, J. P.: Changes in the vital capacity when the body is immersed in water. Amer. J. Physiol. **141**, 51 (1944).

Hamilton, W. F., Remington, J. W.: The measurement of the stroke volume from the pressure pulse. Amer. J. Physiol. **148**, 14–24 (1947).

Hamilton, W. F., Remington, J. W.: Comparison of the time concentration curves in arterial blood of diffusible and nondiffusible substances when injected at a constant rate and when injected instantaneously. Amer. J. Physiol. **148**, 35–39 (1948).

Hamlin, R. L., Marsland, W. P., Smith, C. R., Sapirstein, L. A.: Fractional distribution of right ventricular output in the lungs of dogs. Circulat. Res. **10**, 763–766 (1962).

Hansen, J. T., Page, N., Barnstein, N. F.: Cardiovascular changes at high altitude. In: The Physiological Effects of High Altitude. New York: Macmillan 1964.

Hardaway, R. M.: The role of intravascular clotting in the etiology of shock. Ann. Surg. **155**, 325 (1962).

Harris, P.: Influence of acetylcholine on the pulmonary arterial pressure. Brit. Heart J. **19**, 272 (1957).

Harris, P., Fritts, H. W., Jr., Clauss, R. H., Odell, J. E., Cournand, A.: Influence of acetylcholine on man pulmonary circulation under normal and hypoxic conditions. Proc. Soc. exp. Biol. (N.Y.) **93**, 77–79 (1956).

Harrison, D. C., Pirages, S., Robison, S. C., Wintroub, B. U.: The pulmonary and systemic circulatory response to dopamine infusion. Brit. J. Pharmacol. **37**, 618–626 (1969).

Harrison, T. R., Wilson, C. P., Neighbors, D. E. W., Pilcher, C.: Regulation of circulation. VII. Effects of anoxemia of mild degree on the cardiac output of unnarcotized dogs. Amer. J. Physiol. **83**, 275 (1927).

Hauge, A.: The pulmonary vasoconstrictor response to acute hypoxia. Studies on mechanism and site of action. Int. Symp. on Pulmonary Circulation, Prague, 1969. Progr. Resp. Res. **5**, 145–155 (1970).

Hauge, A., Melmon, K. L.: Role of histamine in hypoxic pulmonary hypertension in the rat. II. Depletion of histamine, serotonin and catecholamines. Circulat. Res. **44**, 385–392 (1968).

Hauge, A., Staub, N. C.: Prevention of hypoxia vasoconstriction in cat lung by histamine-releasing agent 48/80. J. appl. Physiol. **26**, 693–699 (1969).

Haynes, R. H., Burton, A. C.: Role of the non-Newtonian behavior of blood in hemodynamics. Amer. J. Physiol. **197**, 943 (1959).

Heath, D., Du Shane, J. W., Wood, E. H., Edwards, J. E.: The structure of the pulmonary trunk at different ages and in cases of pulmonary hypertension and pulmonary stenosis. J. Path. Bact. **77**, 443 (1959).

Hebb, C. O., Nimmo-Smith, R. H.: Pulmonary vasoconstriction in response to inhalation of CO_2 in the isolated perfused lungs of Macacus rhesus. Quart. J. exp. Physiol. **34**, 159 (1948).

Helander, E., Lindell, S. E., Söderholm, B., Westling, H.: Observations on the pulmonary circulation during induced bronchial asthma. Acta allerg. (Kbh.) **17**, 112–129 (1962).

HERTZ, C. W.: Die Durchblutungsgröße hypoventilierter Lungenbezirke. Verh. dtsch. Ges. Kreisl.-Forsch. **21**, 447 (1955).
HERTZ, C. W.: Untersuchungen über den Einfluß der alveolaren Gasdrucke auf die intrapulmonale Durchblutungsverteilung beim Menschen. Klin. Wschr. **34**, 472 (1956).
HICKAM, J. B., CARGILL, W. H.: Effect of exercise on cardiac output and pulmonary arterial pressure in normal persons and in patients with cardiovascular disease and pulmonary emphysema. J. clin. Invest. **27**, 10–23 (1948).
HIMMELSTEIN, A., HARRIS, P., FRITTS, H. W., JR., COURNAND, A.: Effect of severe unilateral hypoxia on the partition of pulmonary blood flow in man. J. thorac. Surg. **36**, 369 (1958).
HOPPIN, F. G., KUHL, D. E., HYDE, R. W.: Distribution of pulmonary blood flow as affected by transverse ($+G_X$) acceleration. J. appl. Physiol. **22**, 469–474 (1967).
HOUSTON, C. S.: Acute pulmonary edema of high altitude. New Engl. J. Med. **263**, 478–480 (1960).
HÜRLIMANN, A., WIGGERS, C. J.: The effects of progressive general anoxia on the pulmonary circulation. Circulat. Res. **1**, 230–237 (1953).
HUGHES, J. M. B., GLAZIER, J. B., MALONEY, J. E., WEST, J. B.: Effect of extra-alveolar vessels on distribution of blood flow in the dog lung. J. appl. Physiol. **25**, 701–712 (1968a).
HUGHES, J. M. B., GLAZIER, J. B., MALONEY, J. E., WEST, J. B.: Effect of lung volume on the distribution of pulmonary blood flow in man. Resp. Physiol. **4**, 58–72 (1968b).
HULTGREN, H. N., LOPEZ, C. E., LUNDBERG, E., MILLER, H.: Physiologic studies of pulmonary edema at high altitudes. Circulation **29**, 393–408 (1964).
HULTGREN, H. N., LUNDBERG, E.: Medical problems of high altitude. Mod. Conc. cardiov. Dis. **31**, 719–724 (1962).
HULTGREN, H., SPICKARD, W., LOPEZ, C.: Further studies of high altitude pulmonary oedema. Brit. Heart J. **24**, 95–102 (1962).
HYLAND, J. W. G., SMITH, T., MCGUIRE, L. B., HARRISON, D. C., HAYNES, F. W., DEXTER, L.: Effect of selective embolization of various sized pulmonary arteries in dogs. Amer. J. Physiol. **204**, 619–625 (1963).
HYMAN, A. L.: The direct effects of vasoactive agents on pulmonary veins. Studies or responses to acetylcholine, serotonin, histamine and isoproterenol in intact dogs. J. Pharmacol. exp. Ther. **168**, 96–105 (1969).
HYMAN, A. L., MYERS, W. D., MEYER, A.: The effect of acute pulmonary embolus upon cardiopulmonary hemodynamics. Amer. Heart J. **67**, 313–323 (1964).
IRNELL, L., NORDGREN, L.: Effects of acetylcholine infusion on the pulmonary circulation in patients with bronchial-asthma. Acta med. scand. **179**, 385 (1966).
IRWIN, J. W.: The pulmonary microcirculation. R. I. med. J. **43**, 522–527 (1960).
ISLAM, M. S., KAMMLER, E., KILIAN, J., WALTER, F., WELLER, W., ULMER, W. T.: Der Einfluß biogener Amine auf die Atmung und den kleinen Kreislauf. II. Mitteilung: Verhalten von Atmung und Kreislauf bei Histamininhalation und nachfolgender Antihistamingabe. Pneumonologie **143**, 336 (1970).
ISLAM, M. S., MELVILLE, G. N., ULMER, W. T.: Role of atropine in antagonising the effect of 5-hydroxytryptamine (5-HT) on bronchial and pulmonary vascular system. Respiration **31**, 47 (1974).
ISLAM, M. S., RASCHE, B., VASTAG, E., ULMER, W. T.: Empfindlichkeitssteigerung der Bronchialmuskulatur durch proteolytische Fermente im Sputum. Pneumonologie **146**, 232 (1971).
ISLAM, M. S., RASCHE, B., VASTAG, E., ULMER, W. T.: Über den Wirkungsmechanismus von Histamin in den Atemwegen. Respiration **29**, 538 (1972).
ISLAM, M. S., ULMER, W. T.: Der Wirkungsmechanismus von Serotonin (5-Hydroxytryptamin) und Histamin bei der Atemwegsobstruktion. Respiration **30**, 360 (1973a).
ISLAM, M. S., ULMER, W. T.: Über die Rolle von Serotonin als Bronchokonstriktor. Pneumonologie **148**, 135 (1973b).
ISLAM, M. S., VASTAG, E., ULMER, W. T.: Sulphur-dioxide induced bronchial hyperreactivity against acetylcholine. Int. Arch. Arbeitsmed. **29**, 221 (1972).
JOHNSON, R. L., SPICER, W. S., BISHOP, J. M., FORSTER, R. E.: Pulmonary capillary blood volume, flow and diffusing capacity during exercise. J. appl. Physiol. **15**, 893 (1960).
JOHNSON, S. R.: The effect of some anaesthetic agents on the circulation in man: with special reference to the significance of pulmonary blood volume for the circulatory regulation. Acta chir. scand. 102: Suppl. **158**, 5–137 (1951).
JONES, R. E., GULDMANN, N., LINDE, H. W., DRIPPS, R. D., PRICE, H. L.: Cyclopropane anesthesia. III. Effects of cyclopropane on respiration and circulation in normal man. Anesthesiology **21**, 380–393 (1960).
KAMMLER, E., WELLER, W., ISLAM, M. S., SELL, R., ULMER, W. T.: Der Einfluß biogener Amine auf die Atmung und den kleinen Kreislauf. I. Wirkung von Acetylcholin bei Inhalation und Injektion in den rechten Vorhof und den Truncus bicaroticus. Pneumonologie **142**, 67–82 (1970).

Kaneko, K., Milic-Emili, J., Dolovich, M. B., Dawson, A., Bates, D. V.: Regional distribution of ventilation and perfusion as a function of body position. J. appl. Physiol. **21**, 767–777 (1966).

Katorie, R., Amorim, D. de S., Theye, R. A., Wood, E. H.: Influence of body position on regional pulmonary arterial-venous shunts in intact dogs. J. appl. Physiol. **29**, 288–296 (1970).

Kazemi, H., Bruecke, P. E., Parsons, E. F.: Role of the autonomic nervous system in the hypoxic response of the pulmonary vascular bed. Resp. Physiol. **15**, 245–254 (1972).

Kilian, J., Islam, M. S., Vatter, J., Weller, W., Ulmer, W. T.: Kreislauf, Atmung und Nierenfunktion im hämorrhagischen Schock und nach Infusion verschiedener Lösungen. Anaesthesist **19**, 280–289 (1970).

Kjellberg, S. R., Lonroth, H., Rudhe, U.: The effect of various factors on the roentgenological determination of the cardiac volume. Acta radiol. (Stockh.) **35**, 413–427 (1951).

Knipping, H. W., Bolt, W., Venrath, H., Valentin, H., Ludes, H., Endler, P.: Eine neue Methode zur Prüfung der Herz- und Lungenfunktion. Die regionale Funktionsanalyse in der Lungen- und Herzklinik mit Hilfe des radioaktiven Edelgases Xenon 133 (Isotopen-Thorakographie). Dtsch. med. Wschr. **80**, 1146 (1955).

Koch, J., Szerb, J.: Liberation of histamine by adrenaline from isolated lung. Arch. int. Pharmacodyn. **81**, 91–98 (1950).

Kopelman, H., Lee, G. de J.: The intrathoracic blood volume in mitral stenosis and left ventricular failure. Clin. Sci. **10**, 383 (1951).

Krahl, V. E.: Relationships of peripheral pulmonary vessels to the respiratory areas of the lung. Med. Thorac. **19**, 194–207 (1962).

Krahl, V. E.: A method of studying the living lung in the closed thorax, and some preliminary observations. Angiology **14**, 149–159 (1963).

Kraupp, O., Stühlinger, W., Turnheim, K.: Vergleichende Untersuchungen über die Wirkung von Aminorex, Ephedrin, Noradrenalin, Amphetamin und N. Chlorpropylamphetamin auf die Hämodynamik des großen und kleinen Kreislaufs an Hunden. Schweiz. med. Wschr. **100**, 2154 (1970).

Krogh, A.: The comparative physiology of respiratory mechanism. Philadelphia: Univ. Pennsylvania Press 1941.

Krogh, A., Lindhard, J.: Measurements of the blood flow through the lungs of man. Scand. Arch. Physiol. **27**, 100 (1912).

Kubota, Y., Vandam, L. D.: Circulatory effects of halothane in patients with heart disease. Clin. Pharmacol. Ther. **3**, 153–162 (1962).

Kummer, F.: Appetite depressants and pulmonary hypertension. Int. Symp. on Pulmonary Circulation, Prague, 1969. Progr. Resp. Res. **5**, 33–35 (1970).

Kunieda, T.: Determination of pulmonary blood volume in patients with mitral valve disease by T-1824 dye method. Kokyu to Junkan **3**, 510 (1955).

Lagerlöf, H., Eliasch, H., Werkö, L., Berglund, E.: Orthostatic changes of the pulmonary and peripheral circulation in man. Scand. J. clin. Lab. Invest. **3**, 85 (1951).

Lambertini, A., Lanari, A., Lanari Zubiaur, F.: La presión arterial pulmonar en ataques de asma espontáneos e inducidos por histamina. Medicina (B. Aires) **20**, 93–96 (1960).

Lategola, M. T.: Pressure-flow relationships in the dog lung during acute subtotal pulmonary vascular occlusion. Amer. J. Physiol. **192**, 613–619 (1958).

Lee, G. de J., Dubois, A. B.: Pulmonary capillary blood flow in man. J. clin. Invest. **34**, 1380 (1955).

Leusen, I., Demeester, G.: Pulmonary vascular resistance in anesthetized dogs. Exp. Med. Surg. **11**, 217–221 (1953).

Leusen, I., Demeester, G.: De invloed van de hypoxia op de pulmonaire ciculatie van de hond. Verh. Vlaam. Akad. Geneesk. Belg. **16**, 231–254 (1954a).

Leusen, I., Demeester, G.: La résistance pulmonaire dans l'hypoxemie aiguë. Arch. int. Pharmacodyn. **96**, 490–492 (1954b).

Levy, M. N., Brind, S. H., Brandlin, F. R., Phillips, F. A., Jr.: The relationship between pressure and flow in the systemic circulation of the dog. Circulat. Res. **2**, 372 (1954).

Lewis, B. M., Lin, T. H., Noe, F. E., Komisaruk, R.: The measurement of pulmonary capillary blood volume and pulmonary membrane diffusing capacity in normal subjects: the effects of exercise and position. J. clin. Invest. **37**, 1061 (1958).

Lilienthal, J. L., Jr., Riley, R. L., Proemmel, D. D., Franke, R. E.: An experimental analysis in man of the oxygen pressure gradient from alveolar air to arterial blood during rest and exercise at sea level and at altitude. Amer. J. Physiol. **147**, 199 (1946).

Liljestrand, G.: Chemical control of the distribution of the pulmonary blood flow. Acta physiol. scand. **44**, 216–240 (1958).

Linde, L. M., Simmons, D. H., Ellman, E. L.: Pulmonary hemodynamics during positive-pressure breathing. J. appl. Physiol. **16**, 644–646 (1961).

LINDERHOLM, H., KIMBEL, P., LEWIS, D. H., DUBOIS, A. B.: Pulmonary capillary blood flow during cardiac catheterization. J. appl. Physiol. **17**, 135 (1962).
LINDSEY, A. W., GUYTON, A. C.: Continuous recording of pulmonary blood volume: pulmonary pressure and volume changes. Amer. J. Physiol. **197**, 959 (1959).
LLOYD, T. C., JR.: Effects of alveolar hypoxia on pulmonary vascular resistance. J. appl. Physiol. **19**, 1086–1094 (1964).
LLOYD, T. C., JR.: Role of nerve pathways in the hypoxic vasoconstriction of lung. J. appl. Physiol. **21**, 1351–1355 (1966).
LOGARAS, G.: Further studies of the pulmonary arterial blood pressure. Acta physiol. scand. **14**, 120–135 (1947).
LOPEZ-MAJANO, V.: Regulation of the pulmonary circulation. Int. Symp. on Pulmonary circulation, Prague, 1969. Progr. Resp. Res. **5**, 188–202 (1970).
LOPEZ-MAJANO, V., WAGNER, N. H., JR., TWINNING, R. H., CHERNICK, V.: Time factor in the shifting of blood produced by unilateral hypoxia. Amer. Rev. resp. Dis. **96**, 1190–1198 (1967).
LOW, I. N.: Electron microscopy of the rat lung. Anat. Rec. **113**, 437 (1952).
LUCAS, C., ROSS, M., WILSON, R. F.: Physiologic shunting in the lungs in shock or trauma. Surg. Forum **19**, 35–36 (1968).
MALT, R. A.: Depressant effect of ether on the heart: a study with the ultralow-frequency force ballistocardiograph. Amer. Heart J. **55**, 572–581 (1958).
MARTICORENA, E., TAPIA, F., DYER, J., HELLRIEGEL, K., SEVERINE, J., GAMBOA, R., BANCHERO, N., PEÑALOZA, D.: Acute pulmonary edema by ascending to high altitudes. (Abstract.) The IV World Congress of Cardiology (Mexico City) 229, 1962.
MARTIN, C. J., YOUNG, A. C.: Ventilation-perfused variations within the lung. J. appl. Physiol. **11**, 371 (1957).
MASSION, W. H.: The role of reflex hypotension in pulmonary embolism. Pflügers Arch. ges. Physiol. **288**, 109–117 (1966).
MATTSON, S. B., CARLENS, E.: Lobar ventilation and oxygen uptake in man. J. thorac. Surg. **30**, 676 (1955).
MAXWELL, G. M., ELLIOTT, R. B., KNEEBONE, G. M.: Effects of bradykinin on the systemic and coronary vascular bed of the intact dog. Circulat. Res. **10**, 359–363 (1962).
MCDONALD, D. A.: Blood flow in arteries. London: Arnold 1960.
MCDONALD, K. E., CAMP, F. A., SCHENK, W. G., JR.: A comparison of three mechanical ventilators. Effects on pulmonary blood flow. Arch. Surg. **87**, 796–800 (1963).
MCGAFF, C. J., MILNOR, W. R.: Effects of serotonin on pulmonary blood volume in the dog. Amer. J. Physiol. **202**, 957–959 (1962).
MCLAUGHLIN, J. S., BUCKLEY, M. J., BERY, W. B., MORROW, A. G.: Pulmonary vascular dynamics during acute hypoxia: modification by reserpine pretreatment or adrenalectomy. Surgery **59**, 1031–1036 (1966).
MCLAUGHLIN, J. S., SUDDHIMONDALA, C., MECH, K., JR., LLACER, R. L., HOUSTON, J., BLIDE, R., ATTAR, S., COWLEY, R. A.: Pulmonary gas exchange in shock in humans. Ann. Surg. **169**, 42–56 (1969).
MCNEILL, R. S., RANKIN, J., FORSTER, R. E.: The diffusing capacity of the pulmonary membrane and the pulmonary capillary blood volume in cardiopulmonary disease. Clin. Sci. **17**, 465 (1958).
MEEHAN, J. P., RADER, R. D.: Cardiovascular observations of the Macaca nemestrina monkey in biosatellite III. Aerospace Med. **42**, 322–336 (1971).
MEEK, W. J., EYSTER, J. A. E.: Cardiac size and output in man during rest and moderate exercise. Amer. J. Physiol. **63**, 400–401 (1923).
MESSMER, K.: Die Wirkung hypertoner Lösungen bei Ratten im irreversiblen Schock. Anaesthesist **17**, 295 (1968).
MILIC-EMILI, J., HENDERSON, J. A. M., DOLOVICH, M. B., TROP, D., KANEKO, K.: Regional distribution of inspired gas in the lung. J. appl. Physiol. **21**, 749–759 (1966).
MILLER, J. M., JOHNSON, R. L., JR.: Effect of lung inflation on pulmonary diffusing capacity at rest and exercise. J. clin. Invest. **45**, 493–500 (1966).
MILLER, W. S.: The Lung. Springfield, Ill.: Thomas 1947.
MILNOR, W. R., JOSE, A. D., MCGAFF, C. J.: Pulmonary vascular volume, resistance and compliance in man. Circulation **22**, 130 (1960).
MOORE, J. W., KINSMAN, J. M., HAMILTON, W. F., SPURLING, R. G.: Studies on the circulation. II. Cardiac output determinations; comparison of the injection method with the direct Fick procedure. Amer. J. Physiol. **89**, 331–339 (1929).
MORET, P. R., PATTAY, J., MEGEVAND, R.: Circulation pulmonaire. I. Relations entre débit, pression et résistance. Etude expérimentale. Acta cardiol. (Brux.) **16**, 557–583 (1961).
MORKIN, E., LEVINE, O. R., BOWMAN, F. O., FISHMAN, A. P.: The nature of pulmonary capillary blood flow and gas exchange. J. clin. Invest. **41**, 1386 (1962).

Mounsey, J. P. D., Ritzmann, L. W., Selverstone, N. J., Briscoe, W. A., McLemore, G. A.: Circulatory changes in severe pulmonary emphysema. Brit. Heart J. **14**, 153 (1952).
Naeye, R. L.: Hypoxemia effects on the pulmonary vascular bed. Med. thorac. **19**, 302–309 (1962).
Naeye, R. L., Bickerman, H. A.: The effects of hypoxemia on the pulmonary arterial bed of humans and rats. (Abstract.) Fed. Proc. **18**, 497 (1959).
Nahas, G. G., MacDonald, I.: Effects of norepinephrine and 5-hydroxytryptamine on the pulmonary circulation of the spinal dog. Amer. J. Physiol. **196**, 1045–1048 (1959).
Nahas, G. G., Visscher, M. B., Haddy, F. J.: Discrepancies in cardiac output measurements by two applications of the direct Fick principle. J. appl. Physiol. **6**, 292–296 (1953).
Navarro, R. U., Ferguson, C. C.: Treatment of experimental hemorrhagic shock by the combined use of hyperbaric oxygen and low molecular weight dextran. Surgery **63**, 775 (1968).
Nemir, P., Jr., Stone, H. H., Mackrell, T. N., Hawthorne, H. R.: Studies on pulmonary embolism utilizing the method of controlled unilateral pulmonary artery occlusion. Surg. Forum **5**, 210–214 (1954).
Niden, A. H., Aviado, D. M.: Effects of pulmonary embolism on the pulmonary circulation with special reference to arteriovenous shunts in the lung. Circulat. Res. **6**, 67–73 (1956).
Nisell, O.: Action of oxygen and carbon dioxide on the bronchioles and vessels of the isolated perfused lungs. Acta physiol. scand. **21**, Suppl. 73 (1950).
O'Donnell, T. V., McIlroy, M. B.: The circulatory effects of squatting. Amer. Heart J. **64**, 347–356 (1962).
Özcan, R., Harmanci, N., Bassipahi, M.: Study on the hemodynamics of the pulmonary circulation at rest and after effort in normal and patients with chronic pulmonary disease. Istanbul Contrib. Clin. Sci. **2**, 27–55 (1952).
Okada, S.: Pharmacological studies of smooth muscle of lung blood vessels and of the bronchial muscles. II. The action of histamine, adrenaline and piuitrin upon the exposed and circulated lung, with special reference to their interrelations on the occurrence. (In Japanese.) Nippon Naibunpi Gakkai Zasshi **15**, 919–933 (1939).
Okpako, D. T.: A dual action of histamine on guinea-pig lung vessels. Brit. J. Pharmacol. **44**, 311–321 (1972).
Opdyke, D. F., Wiggers, C. J.: Studies of right and left ventricular activity during hemorrhagic hypotension and shock. Amer. J. Physiol. **147**, 270 (1946).
Paintal, A. S.: Mechanism of stimulation of type J pulmonary receptors. J. Physiol. (Lond.) **203**, 511 (1969).
Paintal, A. S.: The mechanism of excitation of type J receptors, and the J reflex. In: Breathing: Hering-Breuer, Centenary Symposium. Ciba Foundation Symposium. 59–76, 1970.
Patrick, R. T.: Relationship of anesthetic agents to hypotension. Ann. N.Y. Acad. Sci. **66**, 983–987 (1957).
Paulet, G., Bernard, J. P.: Debit cardiaque et masse sanguine centrale au cours d'une perfusion veineuse d'histamine. J. Physiol. (Paris) **55**, 315–317 (1963).
Payne, J. P., Gardiner, D., Verner, I. R.: Cardiac output during halothane anaesthesia. Brit. J. Anaesth. **31**, 87–90 (1959).
Penaloza, D., Sime, F., Banchero, N., Gamboa, R.: Pulmonary hypertension in healthy man born and living at high altitudes. Med. thorac. **19**, 449–460 (1962).
Perkins, J. F., Jr., Adams, W. E., Flores, A.: Arterial oxygen saturation vs. alveolar oxygen tension as a measure of venous admixture and diffusion difficulty in the lung. J. appl. Physiol. **8**, 455 (1956).
Permutt, S., Howell, J. B. L., Proctor, D. F., Riley, R. L.: Effect of lung inflation on static pressure-volume characteristics of pulmonary vessels. J. appl. Physiol. **16**, 64 (1961).
Peters, G. A., Horton, B. T.: Continuous intravenous administration of histamine: effect on the electrocardiogram and serum potassium. Amer. Heart J. **27**, 845–857 (1944).
Piiper, J.: Größe des Arterien-, des Capillar- und des Venenvolumens in der isolierten Hundelunge. Pflügers Arch. ges. Physiol. **269**, 182 (1959).
Piiper, J.: Variations of ventilation and diffusing capacity to perfusion determining the alveolar-arterial O_2 difference: theory. J. appl. Physiol. **16**, 507 (1961).
Piiper, J.: Attempts to determine volume, compliance and resistance to flow of pulmonary vascular compartments. Int. Symp. on Pulmonary Circulation, Prague, 1969. Progr. Resp. Res. **5**, 40–52 (1970).
Price, H. L., Helrich, M.: The effect of cyclopropane, diethyl ether, nitrous oxide, thiopental, and hydrogen ion concentration on the myocardial function of the dog heart-lung preparation. J. Pharmacol. exp. Ther. **115**, 206–216 (1955).
Price, K. C., Hata, D., Smith, J. R.: Pulmonary vasomotion resulting from miliary embolism of the lungs. Amer. J. Physiol. **182**, 183–190 (1955).

PRITCHARD, M. M. L., DANIEL, P. M., ARDRAN, G. M.: Peripheral ischemia of the lung. Brit. J. Radiol. **27**, 93 (1954).
RAHN, H.: A concept of mean alveolar air and the ventilation-blood flow relationships during pulmonary gas exchange. Amer. J. Physiol. **158**, 21 (1949).
RAHN, H., SADOUL, P., FARHI, L. E., SHAPIRO, J.: Distribution of ventilation and perfusion in the lobes of the dog's lung in the supine and erect position. J. appl. Physiol. **8**, 417–426 (1956).
RAHN, H., STROUD, R. C., TOBIN, C. E.: Visualization of arteriovenous shunts by cinefluorography in the lungs of normal dogs. Proc. Soc. exp. Biol. (N.Y.) **80**, 239 (1952).
RAO, S.: Cardiovascular responses to headstand posture. J. appl. Physiol. **18**, 987–990 (1963).
REEVES, J. T., GROVER, E. B., GROVER, R. F.: Circulatory responses to high altitude in the cat and rabbit. J. appl. Physiol. **18**, 575–579 (1963).
REICHEL, G.: Ursachen pulmonalen Hochdrucks. Verh. Ges. Lungen-Atmungsforsch. Band 2. Berlin: Springer 1969.
REICHEL, G., REIF, E., WELLER, W.: Über die Bedeutung der alveolärgasabhängigen funktionellen Faktoren für die Entstehung der pulmonalen Hypertonie. Verh. Dtsch. Ges. Kreislaufforsch. **31**, 77 (1965).
REICHEL, G., WELLER, W., REIF, E.: Der Einfluß der alveolären Hypoventilation auf den kleinen Kreislauf und das Herz. Med. thorac. **23**, 197–224 (1966).
REID, G.: Circulatory effects of 5-hydroxytryptamine. J. Physiol. (Lond.) **118**, 435–453 (1952).
REMINGTON, J. W., HAMILTON, W. F.: The evaluation of the work of the heart. Amer. J. Physiol. **150**, 292 (1947).
REMMERS, J. E., MITHOEFER, J. C.: The carbon monoxide diffusing capacity in permanent residents at high altitudes. Resp. Physiol. **6**, 233–244 (1969).
RILEY, R. L., HIMMELSTEIN, A., MOTLEY, H. L., WEINER, H. M., COURNAND, A.: Studies of the pulmonary circulation at rest and during exercise in normal individuals and in patients with chronic pulmonary disease. Amer. J. Physiol. **152**, 372–382 (1948).
RING, G. C., BLUM, A. S., KURBATOV, T., MOSS, W. G., SMITH, W.: Size of microspheres passing through pulmonary circuit in the dog. Amer. J. Physiol. **200**, 1191 (1961).
RITTMEYER, P.: Experimentelle Untersuchungen über die Wirkung vasopressorischer Substanzen auf den kleinen Kreislauf. Anaesthesist **11**, 359–361 (1962).
RONCORONI, A. J., AGREST, A., ROEHR, E., GRZESKO, S.: Hemodynamics during mechanical ventilation. Amer. Heart J. **64**, 207–220 (1962).
ROSE, J. C.: Active constriction and dilatation in pulmonary circulation in response to acetylcholine. Proc. Soc. exp. Biol. (N.Y.) **94**, 734 (1957).
ROSE, J. C., FREIS, E. D., HUFNAGEL, C. A., MASULLO, E. A.: Effect of epinephrine and norepinephrine in dogs studied with mechanical left ventricle. Amer. J. Physiol. **182**, 197–202 (1955).
ROSE, J. C., LAZARO, E. J.: Pulmonary vascular responses to serotonin and effects of certain serotonin antagonists. Circulat. Res. **6**, 283–288 (1958).
ROSENBERG, E., FORSTER, R. E.: Relative importance of intravascular pressure and blood flow in determining the diffusing capacity of isolated perfused cat lung. Fed. Proc. **18**, 130 (1959).
ROSENBERG, E., FORSTER, R. E.: Changes in diffusing capacity of isolated cat lungs with blood pressure and flow. J. appl. Physiol. **15**, 883 (1960).
ROSS, A., THOMAS, L. J., JR., NAGEL, E. L., PROMMAS, D. C.: Pulmonary vascular resistance as determined by lung inflation and vascular pressures. J. appl. Physiol. **16**, 77 (1961).
ROSS, J. C., FRAYSER, R., HICKAM, J. B.: A study of the mechanism by which excercise increases the pulmonary diffusing capacity for carbon monoxide. J. clin. Invest. **38**, 916 (1959).
ROSSIER, P. H., BÜHLMANN, A., WIESINGER, K.: Physiologie und Physiopathologie der Atmung. Berlin: Springer 1958.
ROTHE, C. F., SELKURT, E. E.: Cardiac and peripheral failure in hemorrhagic shock in the dog. Amer. J. Physiol. **207**, 203 (1964).
ROTTA, A., CÁNEPA, A., HURTADO, A., VELAŚQUEZ, T., CHÁVEZ, R.: Pulmonary circulation at sea level and at high altitudes. J. appl. Physiol. **9**, 328–336 (1956).
ROUGHTON, F. J. W.: The average time spent by the blood in the human lung capillary and its relation to the rates of CO uptake and elimination in man. Amer. J. Physiol. **143**, 621 (1945).
ROUGHTON, F. J. W., FORSTER, R. E.: Relative importance of diffusion and chemical reaction rates in determining rate of exchange of gases in the human lung, with special reference to true diffusing capacity of pulmonary membrane and volume of blood in the lung capillaries. J. appl. Physiol. **11**, 290 (1957).
ROWE, G. G., AFONSO, S., CASTILLO, C. A., LIOY, F., LUGO, J. E., CRUMPTON, C. E.: The systemic and coronary hemodynamic effect of synthetic bradykinin. Amer. Heart J. **65**, 656–663 (1963).

RUDOLPH, A. M., PAUL, M. H.: Pulmonary and systemic vascular response to continuous infusion of 5-hydroxytryptamine (Serotonin) in the dog. Amer. J. Physiol. **189**, 263–268 (1957).

SALDANA, M., ARIAS-STELLA, J.: Studies on the structure of the pulmonary trunk. I. Normal changes in the elastic configuration of the human pulmonary trunk at different ages. Circulation **27**, 1086–1093 (1963a).

SALDANA, M., ARIAS-STELLA, J.: Studies on the structure of the pulmonary trunk. II. The evolution of the elastic configuration of the pulmonary trunk in people native to high altitudes. Circulation **27**, 1094–1100 (1963b).

SANCETTA, S. M., KLEINERMAN, J.: Effect of mild, steady state exercise on total pulmonary resistance of normal subjects and those with isolated aortic valvular lesions. Amer. Heart J. **53**, 404–414 (1957).

SANCETTA, S. M., RAKITA, L.: Response of pulmonary artery pressure and total pulmonary resistance of untrained, convalescent man to prolonged mild steady state exercise. J. clin. Invest. **36**, 1138–1149 (1957).

SARNOFF, S. J., CASE, R. B., WAITHE, P. E., ISAACS, J. P.: Insufficient coronary flow and myocardial failure as a complicating factor in late hemorrhagic shock. Amer. J. Physiol. **176**, 439 (1954).

SCHMIDT, H. D., SCHMIER, J.: Kontraktilitätsschäden des Herzens im frühen hämorrhagischen Schock. Pflügers Arch. ges. Physiol. **285**, 241 (1965).

SCHNEIDER, M.: Zur Pathophysiologie des Schocks. In: Schock und Plasmaexpander, S. 1. Berlin: Springer 1964.

SCHWIEGK, H.: Der Lungenentlastungsreflex. Pflügers Arch. ges. Physiol. **236**, 206–219 (1935).

SHAPIRO, B. J., SIMMONS, D. H., LINDE, L. M.: Pulmonary hemodynamics in acute metabolic acidosis. Fed. Proc. **21**, 109 (1962).

SHARPEY-SCHAFER, E., BAIN, W. A.: The effects of changes in intrapulmonary air-pressure on the pulmonary and aortic circulation of the dog. Quart. J. exp. Physiol. **22**, 101–147 (1932).

SHEPHERD, J. T., DONALD, D. E., LINDER, E., SWAN, H. J. C.: Effect of small doses of 5-hydroxytryptamine (Serotonin) on pulmonary circulation in the closed-chest dog. Amer. J. Physiol. **197**, 963–967 (1959).

SHIMOSATO, S., ETSTEN, B.: Performance of digitalized heart during halothane anesthesia. Anesthesiology **24**, 41–50 (1963).

SIBUL, I.: Über das Verhalten von Histamin in der Lunge. Pflügers Arch. ges. Physiol. **235**, 742–755 (1935).

SILOVE, E. D., INOUE, T., GROVER, R. F.: Comparison of hypoxia, pH and sympathomimetic drugs on bovine pulmonary vasculature. J. appl. Physiol. **24**, 355–365 (1968).

SJÖSTRAND, T.: Volume and distribution of blood and their significance in regulating the circulation. Physiol. Rev. **33**, 202 (1953).

SLONIM, N. B., RAVIN, A., BALCHUM, O. J., DRESSLER, S. H.: The effect of mild exercise in the supine position on the pulmonary arterial pressure of five normal human subjects. J. clin. Invest. **33**, 1022–1030 (1954).

SMEKAL, P. V., STANDFUSS, K., RAU, G.: Incidence of primary pulmonary hypertension after intake aminorexfumarat (Menocil). Regulation of respiration in primary pulmonary hypertension. Int. Symp. on Pulmonary Circulation, Prague, 1969. Progr. Resp. Res. **5**, 22–29 (1970).

SMITH, C. W., LEHAN, P. H., MONKS, J. J.: Cardiopulmonary manifestations with high O_2 tension at atmospheric pressure. J. appl. Physiol. **18**, 849–853 (1963).

SMITH, D. J., COXE, J. W.: Reactions of isolated pulmonary blood vessels to anoxia, epinephrine, acetylcholine and histamine. Amer. J. Physiol. **167**, 732–737 (1951).

SÖDERHOLM, B.: Effect of drugs on pulmonary circulation in normal man and patients with cardiopulmonary disease. Int. Symp. on Pulmonary Circulation, Prague, 1969. Progr. Resp. Res. **5**, 113–118 (1970).

SÖDERHOLM, B., WIDIMSKY, J.: The effect of acetylcholine infusion on the pulmonary circulation in cases of impaired ventilation. Acta med. scand. **172**, 219 (1962).

SPITZBARTH, H., GERSMEYER, E. F., WEYLAND, H., GASTEYER, K. H.: Der Pulmonalarteriendruck des Menschen bei Kreislaufveränderungen im Phenothiazinschlaf. Klin. Wschr. **35**, 87–91 (1957).

STEWART, G. N.: The output of the heart in dogs. Amer. J. Physiol. **57**, 27–50 (1921).

STEWART, L. R.: Acute pulmonary oedema of high altitude. N. Z. med. J. **60**, 79–80 (1961).

STRANDELL, T.: Pulmonary blood flow and pressure in old age effect of body position, exercise and physical training. Int. Symp. on Pulmonary Circulation, Prague 1969. Progr. Resp. Res. **5**, 356–364 (1970).

STROUD, R. C., RAHN, H.: Effect of O_2 and CO_2 tensions upon the resistance of pulmonary blood vessels. Amer. J. Physiol. **172**, 211–220 (1953).

Susmano, A., Carleton, R. A.: Prevention of hypoxic pulmonary hypertension by chloropheniramine. J. appl. Physiol. **31**, 531–535 (1971).
Svanberg, L.: Influence of posture on the lung volumes, ventilation and circulation in normals. A spirometric-bronchospirometric investigation. Scand. J. clin. Lab. Invest. **9** (Suppl. 25), 1–195 (1957).
Tapia, F., Marticorena, E., Dyer, J., Severino, J., Gamboa, R., Banchero, N., Penaloza, D.: Acute pulmonary edema caused by ascending to high altitudes. (Abstract.) Circulation **26**, 794 (1962).
Tavares, P., Martinelli, J. G., Lisboa, C., Teixeira, D. S.: Effects of isoproterenol on the pulmonary circulation of the canine lung. Bull. physio.-path. resp. 8, 937–946 (1972).
Thomas, L. J., Jr., Griffo, Z. J., Roos, A.: Effect of negative-pressure inflation of the lung on pulmonary vascular resistance. J. appl. Physiol. **16**, 451 (1961).
Trendelenburg, U.: Stimulation of sympathetic centers by histamine. Circulat. Res. **5**, 105–110 (1957).
Trendelenburg, U.: The pressor response of the cat to histamine and pilocarpine. J. Pharmacol. exp. Ther. **131**, 65–72 (1961).
Tsagaris, T. J., Lange, R. L.: Effect of airway pressure on postarteriolar pulmonary vessels. (Abstract.) Fed. Proc. **23**, 418 (1964).
Tuller, M. A., Lehr, D. E., Fishman, A. P.: Induced alterations in the distribution of pulmonary blood flow. Fed. Proc. **20**, 106 (1961).
Ulmer, W. T.: Atmung und Kreislauf im Schock. Therapiewoche **18**, 1918–1924 (1968).
Ulmer, W. T.: Hypertrophie des rechten Herzens aus der Sicht des Klinikers. Verh. dtsch. Ges. Kreisl.-Forsch. **38**, 102 (1972).
Ulmer, W. T., Dorsch, J., Iravani, J., Schüler, K.-G., Stempel, G., Vastag, E.: Anticholinergika als Bronchodilatatoren. Arzneimittel-Forsch. **23**, 468 (1973).
Ulmer, W. T., Hertle, F., Krauss, L., Malikiosis, X. Ap.: Untersuchungen über die interalveoläre Ventilation und über die Lageabhängigkeit des Ventilations/Perfusionsverhältnisses in der Lunge. Pflügers Arch. ges. Physiol. **275**, 628 (1962).
Ulmer, W. T., Hertle, F., Reichel, G.: Die Abhängigkeit des exspiratorisch alveolär/arteriellen Kohlensäuredruckgradienten von Körperlage und Lebensalter. Poumon **10**, 1305 (1963).
Ulmer, W. T., Reichel, G.: Untersuchungen über die Altersabhängigkeit der alveolären und arteriellen Sauerstoff- und Kohlensäuredrucke. Klin. Wschr. **41**, 1 (1963).
Ulmer, W. T., Reif, E., Weller, W.: Die obstruktiven Atemwegserkrankungen. In: Pathophysiologie des Kreislaufes, der Ventilation und des Gasaustausches. Stuttgart: Thieme 1966.
Ulmer, W. T., Wenke, A.: Bronchospirometrische Untersuchungen zur Frage der gasspannungsabhängigen Durchblutungsregulation der Alveolarkapillaren. Arch. Kreisl.-Forsch. **26**, 256 (1957).
Valenca, L. M., Lincoln, J. C. R., Strieder, D. J., Kazemi, H.: Hypoxic pulmonary vascular response of reimplanted dog lung. J. thorac. cardiovasc. Surg. **61**, 857–862 (1971).
Varnauskas, E.: Studies in hypertensive cardiovascular disease with special reference to cardiac function. Scand. J. clin. Lab. Invest. **7**, Suppl., 5–117 (1955).
Varnauskas, E., Korsgren, M., Houk, P., Prerovsky, J.: Hemodynamic effects of Rheomacrodex. Scand. J. clin. Lab. Invest. **17**, 81 (1965).
Velasquez, T.: Maximal diffusing capacity of the lungs at high altitude. USA school of Aviation medicine. Report No. **56**–108, 1–9 (1956).
Velasquez, T., Florentini, E.: Maxima capacidad de difusion del pulmon en nativos de la altura. Arch. Inst. Biol. Andina **1**, 179–187 (1966).
Venrath, H., Lechtenbörger, H., Valentin, H., Bolt, W.: Das Verhalten von Atmung und Kreislauf bei uni- und bilateraler Sauerstoffmangelatmung; ein Beitrag zur Kompensation akuter Hypoxie durch Kreislaufumstellung. Z. Kreisl.-Forsch. **44**, 544 (1955).
Venrath, H., Rotthof, R., Valentin, H., Bolt, W.: Bronchospirographische Untersuchungen bei Durchblutungsstörungen im kleinen Kreislauf. Beitr. Klin. Tuberk. **107**, 291 (1952).
Vidt, D. G., Bredemeyer, A., Sapirstein, E., Sapirstein, L. A.: Effect of ether anesthesia on the cardiac output, blood pressure, and distribution of blood flow in the albino rat. Circulat. Res. **7**, 759–764 (1959).
Vogel, J. H. K., Weaver, W. F., Rose, R. L., Blount, S. G., Jr., Grover, R. F.: Pulmonary hypertension in children born and living in high altitudes. (Abstract.) Circulation **26**, 683 (1962).
Wahrenbrock, E. A., Carrico, C. J., Amundsen, D. A., Trummer, M. J., Severinghaus, J. W.: Increased atelectatic pulmonary shunt during hemorrhagic shock in dogs. J. appl. Physiol. **29**, 615–621 (1970).

WASSERMAN, K., COMROE, J. H., JR.: A method for estimating instantaneous pulmonary capillary blood flow in man. J. clin. Invest. **41**, 410 (1962).

WEARN, J. T., ERNSTENE, A. C., BROMER, A. W., BARR, J. S., GERMAN, W. J., ZSCHIESCHE, L. J.: The normal behavior of the pulmonary blood vessels with observations on intermittence of the flow of blood in the arterioles and capillaries. Amer. J. Physiol. **106**, 236 (1934).

WEBB, W. R., SMITH, J. R.: Pulmonary hemodynamics as affected by varying levels of respiratory pressure. Surg. Forum **9**, 371–374 (1959).

WEIBEL, E.: Die Blutgefäßanastomosen in der menschlichen Lunge. Z. Zellforsch. **50**, 653 (1959).

WEIBEL, E. R., GOMEZ, D. M.: The architecture of the human lung. Science **137**, 3530 (1962).

WEIL, J. V., JAMIESON, G., BROWN, D. W., GROVER, R. F.: The red cell mass-arterial oxygen relationship in normal man; application to patients with chronic obstructive airway disease. J. clin. Invest. **47**, 1626–1639 (1968).

WEIL, P., SALISBURY, P. F., STATE, D.: Physiological factors influencing pulmonary artery pressure during separate perfusion of systemic and pulmonary circulations in the dog. Amer. J. Physiol. **191**, 453–460 (1957).

WEISKOPF, R. B., SEVERINGHAUS, J. W.: Diffusing capacity of the lung for CO in man during acute acclimation to 14,246f. J. appl. Physiol. **32**, 285 (1972).

WEISSLER, A. M., MCCRAW, B. H., WARREN, J. V.: Pulmonary blood volume determined by a radioactive tracer technique. J. appl. Physiol. **14**, 531 (1959).

WEST, J. B.: Diffusing capacity of the lung for carbon monoxide at high altitude. J. appl. Physiol. **17**, 421–426 (1962a).

WEST, J. B.: Regional differences in gas exchange in the lung of erect man. J. appl. Physiol. **17**, 893–898 (1962b).

WEST, J. B., DOLLERY, C. T., HEARD, B. E.: Increased pulmonary vascular resistance in the dependent zone of the isolated dog lung caused by perivascular edema. Circulat. Res. **17**, 191–206 (1965).

WEST, J. B., DOLLERY, C. T., HUGH-JONES, P.: The use of radioactive carbon dioxide to measure regional blood flow in the lungs of patients with pulmonary disease. J. clin. Invest. **40**, 1 (1961).

WEST, J. B., DOLLERY, C. T., NAIMARK, A.: Distribution of blood flow in isolated lung; relation to vascular and alveolar pressures. J. appl. Physiol. **19**, 713–724 (1964).

WEST, J. B., FOWLER, K. T., HUGH-JONES, P., O'DONNELL, T. V.: The measurement of the inequality of ventilation and of perfusion in the lung by the analyses of single expirates. Clin. Sci. **16**, 549 (1957).

WESTLING, H.: Effect of histamine on the pulmonary circulation in man. Proc. 1st Int. Pharmacol. Mtg. Pergamon Press **9**, 117–124 (1963).

WHITTAKER, S. R. F., WINTON, F. R.: Apparent viscosity of blood flowing in isolated hindlimb of dog and its variation with corpuscular concentration. J. Physiol. (Lond.) **78**, 339 (1933).

WIDIMSKY, J., BERGLUND, E., MALMBERG, R.: Effect of repeated exercise on the lesser circulation. J. appl. Physiol. **18**, 983–986 (1963).

WIGGERS, C. J.: Cardiac adaptations in acute progressive anoxia. Ann. intern. Med. **14**, 1237–1247 (1941).

WIGGERS, C. J.: Physiology of shock. New York: The Commonwealth Fund 1950.

WILL, D. H., ALEXANDER, A. F., REEVES, J. T., GROVER, R. F.: High altitude induced pulmonary hypertension in normal cattle. Circulat. Res. **10**, 172 (1962).

WILLIAMS, H. M.: Mechanical vs. reflex effects of diffuse pulmonary embolism in anesthetized dogs. Circulat. Res. **4**, 325–331 (1926).

WRIGHT, R. R.: Experimental pulmonary hypertension produced by recurrent air emboli. Med. thorac. **19**, 423–427 (1962).

YOUNG, R. C., JR., NAGANO, H., VAUGHAN, T. R., STAUB, N. C.: Pulmonary capillary blood volume in dog: effects of 5-hydroxytryptamine. J. appl. Physiol. **18**, 264–268 (1963).

YU, P. N. G., LOVEJOY, F. W., JR., JOOS, H. A., NYE, R. E., JR., MCCANN, W. S.: Studies of pulmonary hypertension. I. Pulmonary circulatory dynamics in patients with pulmonary emphysema at rest. J. clin. Invest. **32**, 130 (1953).

Genetic Induction of a Cardiomyopathy

K. Lossnitzer

With 11 Figures

A. Introduction

I. General Aspects of Myocardial Cell Damage with Special Reference to the Term Cardiomyopathy

Coronary sclerosis, hypertension, bacteria, and viruses have been regarded as the main causes of myocardial disease. Recently, great interest has been focused on other factors, especially hormones and toxic substances that may produce myocardial cell damage. Very often it is difficult to evaluate their extra-cardiac etio-pathogenesis with respect to the myocardial damage. Therefore, Buechner (1957) established, from the pathologist's point of view, the concept of cellular hypoxydosis (blocking of the oxidative process) as the general pathogenic basis for cellular damage. Hypoxydosis may be due to hypoxia, lack of substrate, alterations of the enzymes assisting substrate utilization or oxidative phosphorylation. On the other hand, Fleckenstein (1969) favored the more general idea of a deficiency of high-energy phosphates or a blockage prohibiting their utilization as the ultimate principle of cell death. Deficiency can arise through increased consumption and or decreased production.

The clinical term cardiomyopathy was introduced by Brigden (1957); he used it to denote diseases of the heart muscle of unknown and unusual etiology and pathogenesis. The interest in this group of diseases has increased since then (CIBA FOUNDATION SYMPOSIUM, 1964; CIBA FOUNDATION STUDY GROUP No. 37, 1971; Edington et al., 1968, Fejfar, 1968; Goodwin, 1970 and 1974; Grosse-Brockhoff, 1971; Korb, 1973; Kuebler et al., 1973; WHO, 1969). It must be emphasized that the term cardiomyopathy covers not only cardiac degeneration, but also cardiac hypertrophy and myocardial dysfunction (loss of power or loss of compliance) leading to cardiac insufficiency. The interrelationship between these clinical, morphological, and functional phenomena is not yet fully understood. Many models of degenerative lesions of cardiac muscle have been developed within the field of experimental cardiology. Extensive information is available in the publications of Hecht (1970), Morin and Côte (1972), Rona (1971), Selye (1970), and Wenzel (1967). It has become increasingly evident that disturbance of the interplay of several modifiable cellular functions may lead to irreversible damage, i.e. necrosis. Selye (1961) described the electrolyte-steroid cardiopathy characterized by hyalinization (ESCH), the electrolyte-steroid cardiopathy with necroses (ESCN), and the electrolyte-steroid cardiopathy characterized by calcification (ESCC). The names of the prototypes of cardiomyopathy indicate their multicausal origin, and also the essence of the microscopic damage to the myocardium. It must be emphasized, however, that these various myocardial lesions are not provoked exclusively by the combined administration of certain electrolytes and steroids, but also by a number of other interventions, some single, which most probably interfere with the myocardial electrolyte metabolism. BAJUSZ (1967a) differentiated between primary (metabolic), secondary (occlusive), and transitional forms of necrotizing cardiomyopathies with respect to the manner of their induction and attempted to give an outline of the comparative morphogenesis and enzyme histogenesis of these induced lesions. BAJUSZ (1963) and SELYE (1958) stressed the fact that most of the pathogens are "potential" factors. They clearly demonstrated the existence of factors that can significantly influence (increase or decrease) the resistance of the cardiac cells to conditions that are usually harmful, so modifying their response, i.e. the development of structural and functional abnormalities. In accordance with this concept, RONA and DUSEK (1972) demonstrated that myocardial necrosis following coronary artery ligation induced a significant increase in the resistance of the remaining noninfarcted myocardium against the harmful insult, in their case the necrotizing effect of isoproterenol. The genetic induction of myocardial damage might represent a special case where the myocardial cellular resistance is endogenously lowered to such a degree that even physiological living conditions are harmful to the heart.

II. Development of Cell Death: Theoretical Analysis

Any noxious stimulus attacking the cardiac cell is assumed to initially cause a cellular response of the same kind (morphological, mechanical, electrical, or biochemical). Depending on the sensitivity of the applied observation methods, one may also be able to detect immediately the ensuing mechanical, structural, electrical or biochemical changes. However, the different methodological sensitivities are still puzzling. Thus far it has been very difficult, in fact nearly impossible, to establish a complete sequence of action–reaction relationships among various pathogenetic phenomena. On the other hand, in many instances it is unclear whether certain conditions or substances interfere directly with one or simultaneously with several cellular sites, or whether they act indirectly through complex extracellular and extracardiac mechanisms, or even in a heterogeneous manner. Therefore, it seems reasonable to place more emphasis on an attempt to outline a general, crucial pattern of effects occurring in myocardial cells resulting from a variety of different influences, than to analyze a detailed pathogenetic chain of specific events. Especially under hypoxic and ischemic conditions, the course of such effects can be followed up with an electron microscope (BUECHNER and ONISHI, 1968; CAULFIELD and KLIONSKY, 1959; FERRANS and ROBERTS, 1971/72; HATT and MORAVEC, 1971/72; JENNINGS et al., 1969; KORB and TOTOVIĆ, 1969) and by biochemical methods (CASE, 1972; FLECKENSTEIN, 1969; GUDBJARNASON, 1972; JENNINGS et al., 1965; OLSON et al., 1971/72; OPIE and OWEN, 1973; SHEN and JENNINGS, 1972b; SPIECKERMANN, 1971/72; WOLLENBERGER et al., 1971/72). These investigations demonstrated the existence of both reversible and irreversible changes. The reversible changes eventually return to normal if the noxious influence is abolished or counteracted, whereas the irreversible "prenecrotic" changes progress irretrievably to necrosis (structural cell death) and to complete loss of high-energy phosphates (metabolic cell death). The borderline between reversible and irreversible changes, however, seems to be vague.

III. The Purpose Inducing Experimental Myocardial Lesions

A primary reason for producing cardiac lesions is to obtain information about substances or conditions which have a harmful effect on the heart as well as to analyze the factors which sensitize or desensitize the heart muscle cells in reaction to these influences. A more precise aspect of this approach is to define permissable limits for the viability of cardiac cells. The study of the pathogenesis of cardiac lesions of different origins will provide a large amount of information through which structural, mechanical, electrical, and biochemical phenomena can be correlated and the sequence of alterations substantiated. In addition, it may be possible to differentiate between reversible and irreversible changes, as has already been accomplished under ischemic and hypoxic conditions, respectively (BUECHNER and ONISHI, 1968; BRACHFELD, 1972; FLECKENSTEIN, 1964; SHEN and JENNINGS, 1972a). Furthermore, it is highly interesting to discriminate between specific and stereotypic or non-specific myocellular reactions. The stereotypic reactions are obviously the important ones, since they may represent a common terminal pathway of different pathological processes that comprise a general pattern of cellular pathology. To find a counter-balance to a reversible, common pathogenetic step would be of immense significance.

IV. The Significance of Genetically Induced Myocardial Degeneration

The main purpose of genetically inducing myocardial lesions is to prove that they can be induced by this method and that they are inheritable. If the disease is hereditary, the presence of a defective gene cannot be excluded from all the other tissue cells. However, as these cells do not degenerate, either adaptive mechanisms come into play within them or the special aberrated gene-linked processes do not become effective after cellular differentiation. Moreover, if the myocardial cells exhibit the genetic defect and if other extracardiac abnormalities are excluded, then one can assume that endogenous myocellular factors are responsible for the decrease in myocardial resistance to normal environmental influences. If, in addition, a certain pathogenic step occurs within genetically defective cells that is known to occur in cardiac conditions of various etiology, and this step can be beneficially influenced, this would support the idea that there may be a common terminal pathway of cellular degeneration. This stage in the pathway, still being reversible, would be the decisive one in the process of necrotization (see A, Section III).

An experimental model of such a hereditary cardiomyopathy should stimulate the search for a similar condition in humans, especially because of the growing awareness of a great number of human heart diseases from unusual or unknown origins. If one could succeed in finding a similar condition in humans or a great number of parallels to human conditions—for instance to hypertrophic cardiomyopathy, cardiac involvement within muscular dystrophy, or Friedreich's disease—the experimental model would provide a unique opportunity for extensive, clinically relevant investigations. The results of these investigations might aid in early diagnosis in man and may possibly lead to an effective therapy.

B. Cardiomyopathy of the Syrian Hamster

I. Genetic Background

In addition to hereditary myopathy in the mouse with about 3% involvement of the myocardium (MICHELSON et al., 1955; JASMIN and BAJUSZ, 1962), a morphologically similar process was described in Syrian hamsters by HOMBURGER et al. (1962, 1966) and by BAJUSZ et al. (1966a). Animals of both sexes exhibit degenerative lesions of the striated musculature and the myocardium with a 100% incidence. The myopathic strain designated BIO 14.6 was the first to be derived

Table 1. Facets in various stages of hereditary

"Prenecrotic" Phase (until the 5th week of life)	Progressive Myocardial Necrotization (from the 5th until the 10–12th week)	Cardiac Hypertrophy (beginning in the 4th week and ranging far beyond the 120th day of life)
Contractile resp. hemodynamic changes		
No depressed dp/dt_{max}, but prolonged time to peak height of developed tension and reduced tension development within the length–tension curve (Langendorff perfusion, strain BIO 14.6)	Reduced dp/dt_{max}, V_{CE}, and V_{max}. Normal end-diastolic and systolic pressures (*in vivo*, strain BIO 8262).	Depressed peak height of contraction, tension time index, tension time per min. Decreased stress relaxation (Langendorff perfusion, strain BIO 14.6). Normal right and left ventricular end-diastolic pressures, normal stroke volume; slightly decreased cardiac output (*in vivo*, strain BIO 14.6).
Gross pathologic changes		
None	Yellowish-white plaques and streaks that follow the direction of the heart muscle fibers (strains BIO 14.6 and BIO 8262).	Increased ratio heart weight/body weight (strain BIO 14.6). Increase of heart weight associated with increase in solid constituents (strain BIO 14.6). Sometimes subaortic thickening of intraventricular septum (strain BIO 14.6).
Light microscopic changes		
Accumulation of intracellular lipid droplets (strain BIO 8262)	Intracellular edema, focal myolysis with eosinophilia, granular disintegration of myoplasma, infiltration with round cells. Calcification of myocardial cells. Calcifying myocardial giant cells. Fibroblasts and beginning replacement fibrosis (strains BIO 14.6 and BIO 8262).	Myocardial fiber enlargement (strain BIO 14.6). Replacement fibrosis (strains BIO 14.6 and BIO 8262).
Electron microscopic changes		
(studies performed only in strain BIO 8262) Appearance of cardiomyoblasts with poorly developed and partly unarranged myofilament. Increased number of mitochondria; cristolysis of mitochondria. "Partial necroses", i.e. contraction bands with homogenization and lysis of filaments. Partial dissolution of nuclear membrane and escape of nuclear portions into sarcoplasm. Increased numbers of polysomes. Hyperplasia of the Golgi system and endoplasmic reticulum. Progressive widening of triads.	"Partial necroses". Mitochondrial swelling and condensed forms of mitochondria. Multiple electron dense irregular particles. Loss of cell membrane and associated basement membrane. Calcification of sarcomeres. Dehiscence of intercalated discs.	Increased numbers of polysomes. Hyperplasia of the Golgi system and endoplasmic reticulum. Splitting of Z-lines. Hypertrophy of myofibrils through addition of more filaments. Increased number of myofibrils and mitochondria.

Overt Heart Failure (after the 200th day of life)	Literature
Depressed dp/dt_{max}, peak height of contraction, tension time per min.. Prolonged time to peak height of developed tension. Decreased stress relaxation. Reduced tension development within length–tension curve (Langendorff perfusion, strain BIO 14.6). Absence of Bowditch phenomenon (myocardium of congested BIO 14.6 hamsters). Elevation of end-diastolic pressures of both ventricles; decrease in left, increase in right ventricular systolic pressure; decreased dp/dt_{max} in both ventricles. Increased stroke volume. Normal to slightly increased cardiac output. Increased compliance (*in vivo*, strain BIO 14.6). Depressed dp/dt_{max}, V_{CE}, V_{max}, decrease in left ventricular systolic pressure (*in vivo*, strain BIO 8262).	ABELMANN et al., 1972 ABELMANN et al., 1973 BRINK and LOCHNER, 1967 BRINK and LOCHNER, 1969 HAJDU and POSNER, 1971 JEFFREY et al., 1970 LOCHNER et al., 1970 STAUCH and LOSSNITZER, 1972 STAUCH and LOSSNITZER, 1974
Dilated and flabby hearts, sometimes with mural thrombi (strains BIO 14.6 and BIO 8262). Cyanosis, distended neck veins, pulmonary and liver congestion. Hydrothorax, hydropericardium, ascites, and subcutaneous edema (strain BIO 14.6).	ALOUSI and BEARDS, 1972 BAJUSZ, 1969a BAJUSZ et al., 1966a BAJUSZ et al., 1967b BAJUSZ and LOSSNITZER, 1968 BAJUSZ et al., 1969a FEDELESOVA and DHALLA, 1971 GERTZ et al., 1972 MCCOLLUM et al., 1970
Scar formation and interstitial calcium deposits. Patchy myocardial atrophy. Only little myolytic changes (strains BIO 14.6 and BIO 8262). Marked edema of intimal layer of auricles and valves (strain BIO 14.6).	BAJUSZ, 1969b BAJUSZ et al., 1966a BAJUSZ and LOSSNITZER, 1968 BAJUSZ et al., 1969a MOHR and LOSSNITZER, 1972 MOHR and LOSSNITZER, 1974
Again "partial necroses", degeneration of mitochondria. Disappearance of glycogen. Accumulation of lipid droplets and lipochrome pigment. Intracellular edema. Dehiscence of intercalated discs. Activation of collagen formation.	BAJUSZ et al., 1969b BUECHNER, 1971 BUECHNER and ONISHI, 1970 NADKARNI et al., 1972 NAKAO et al., 1970 ONISHI et al., 1970

Table 1

"Prenecrotic" Phase (until the 5th week of life)	Progressive Myocardial Necrotization (from the 5th until the 10–12th week)	Cardiac Hypertrophy (beginning in the 4th week and ranging far beyond the 120th day of life)
Biochemical changes		
Accelerated norepinephrine synthesis and binding in myocardial tissue (strain BIO 14.6). Elevated mitochondrial calcium levels (strain BIO 14.6). Slightly elevated myocardial calcium content (only in strain BIO 14.6). Latent disturbance of myocardial calcium metabolism (strain BIO 8262). Elevated hydroxybutyric dehydrogenase serum values (strain BIO 8262).	Decreased activity of pH 5 enzyme fraction, selective deficiency of labeling in heavy polysomes in cell-free system of myocardium (strain BIO 14.6). Increased myocardial norepinephrine content (strain BIO 14.6). Pronounced increase of myocardial calcium content (strains BIO 14.6 and BIO 8262) and net uptake of ^{45}Ca (strain BIO 8262).	Increased DNA-dependent RNA-polymerase activity. Elevated cardiac protein and RNA-content. Equivocal incorporation of amino acids into heart protein. Increase in cardiac norepinephrine stores and norepinephrine formation. Depression of calcium binding, uptake and release of myocardial sarcoplasmic reticulum. Reduced myocardial calcium oxalate capacity (strain BIO 14.6). Equivocal depression of oxidative phosphorylation. Enhanced glucose metabolism.

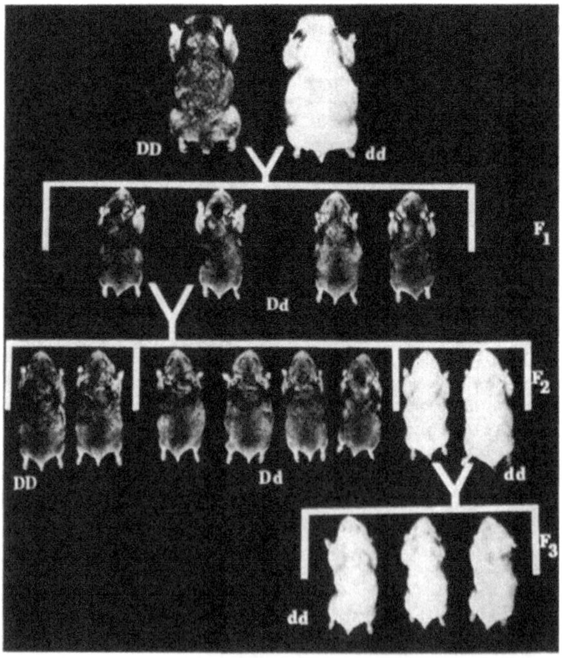

Fig. 1. The cardiomyopathy of the BIO 14.6 strain is transmitted by an autosomal recessive gene. New cardiomyopathic lines, such as strain BIO 8262 and BIO 4054, were obtained by crossbreeding between healthy (DD) and BIO 14.6 (dd) hamsters. The carriers (Dd) in the F_1 and F_2 generation do not exhibit disease manifestations. In the F_3 generation a 100% incidence of the cardiomyopathic lesions is reached. (From BAJUSZ and LOSSNITZER, 1968)

(continued)

Overt Heart Failure (after the 200th day of life)	Literature
Inhibition and uncoupling of oxidative phosphorylation. Reduced content of high-energy phosphates. Reduced "calcium pumping" of sarcoplasmic reticulum and mitochondria. Elevated myocardial cholesterol/phospholipid ratio. Decreased myocardial norepinephrine content (strain BIO 14.6). Increased myocardial calcium content (strains BIO 14.6 and BIO 8262).	ALOUSI and BEARDS, 1972 ANGELAKOS et al., 1972 ANGELAKOS et al., 1973b BESTER et al., 1973 FEDELESOVA and DHALLA, 1971 GERTZ et al., 1970b GERTZ et al., 1972 LINDENMAYER et al., 1970 LOCHNER et al., 1968 LOCHNER et al., 1970 LOSSNITZER and BAJUSZ, 1974 LOSSNITZER et al., 1974a LOSSNITZER et al., 1974b MCCOLLUM et al., 1970 MOHR and LOSSNITZER, 1972 NAIR and UMALI, 1970 OWENS et al., 1972 SCHWARTZ et al., 1968 SULHAKE and DHALLA, 1971 WROGEMANN and BLANCHAER, 1974

from inbred lines of *Mesocricetus auratus* and was developed through brother–sister mating from 1956 onward. This line has been intensively investigated and was, inbred for well over 20 generations, when new myopathic lines (BIO 8262, BIO 4054, UM-X 7.1) were developed. The BIO 8262 line, for instance, was derived from cross breeding females of the BIO 14.6 line with healthy males of the randomly bred BIO RB line. Previous genetic studies clearly indicated transmission of the disease by an autosomal recessive gene (HOMBURGER et al., 1966) (Fig. 1). Thus, mating myopathic hamsters with healthy animals will produce in the F_3-generation, with 100% incidence, a new (sub-)line suffering from myopathy and cardiomyopathy. The new BIO 8262 animals were also inbred for more than 20 generations. In comparison to the BIO 14.6 line, which is recommended as a model for congestive heart failure (BAJUSZ, 1967a; BAJUSZ et al., 1969a) and cardiac hypertrophy (BAJUSZ et al., 1969b; ONISHI et al., 1970), the BIO 8262 animals obviously do not suffer from congestion (STAUCH and LOSSNITZER, 1972) (Table 1). However, the BIO 14.6 hamsters suffered from at least two other accompanying and possibly interfering diseases—the Schwartz-Bartter syndrome and secondary hyperaldosteronism (CANTIN and BAJUSZ, 1968; CANTIN et al., 1972; HORVATH et al., 1972; LOSSNITZER and BAJUSZ, 1974); the BIO 8262 line does not seem to be afflicted with these conditions which are associated with disturbances of the water and electrolyte balance, respectively (LOSSNITZER et al., 1974b). This provides evidence for the predominance of the genetic aberration with respect to special processes restricted to the striated musculature. Thus, in accordance to the classification suggested by FEJFAR (1968), GROSSE-BROCKHOFF (1971) and ROBERTS and FERRANS (1973) in humans the cardiomyopathy of the hamsters should be labelled as a secondary one.

II. Clinical Course and Gross Pathology

Degenerative lesions occur in all striated muscles, but with particular consistence and intensity in the heart. BAJUSZ (1969a) stressed that viral and other infectious agents, as well as nutritional factors (e.g. vitamin E, selenium, thiamine, potassium, and magnesium deficiencies), do not play a part in its etiology.

Lesions of the skeletal musculature, which are similar to those in the heart, were observed as early as within the first week after birth in both the BIO 14.6 and BIO 8262 strains (HOMBURGER et al., 1966; MOHR and LOSSNITZER, 1972, 1974). Cardiac lesions, however, arise in BIO 14.6 female hamsters about the 30th day of life and about 10 days later in males (BAJUSZ et al., 1966a). In strain BIO 8262 the cardiac lesions develop after the 5th week of life (MOHR and LOSSNITZER, 1972, 1974). Myopathic hamsters cannot be differentiated from healthy animals by their outward appearance at this stage of life. BIO 14.6 hamsters become increasingly congested after the 100th postnatal day, showing overt left and right heart failure with hyperpnea, pulmonary congestion, subcutaneous edema, ascites, liver congestion, hydrothorax, and hydropericardium. BIO 8262 hamsters do not exhibit such signs of congestion (see Table 1). With age they show distinct signs of muscular dystrophy, especially of the limb girdle, and die from as yet unknown causes between the 200th and 400th day of life. Their death occurs later than that of BIO 14.6 hamsters, which do not usually survive more then 300 days, whereas normal hamsters have a life span of about two to three years.

Gross pathological signs are discernable in the heart with the naked eye in 50-day-old hamsters of the BIO 14.6 and BIO 8262 strains and become even more pronounced in older animals. The myocardium presents yellowish-white longitudinal streaks (Fig. 2). Cross sections display no preference in the localization of

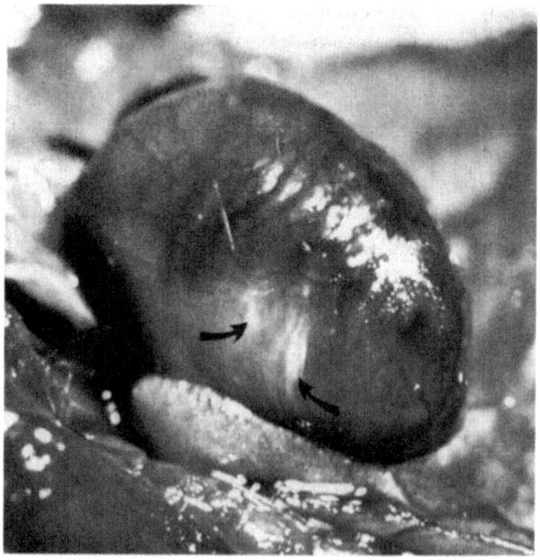

Fig. 2. Heart *in situ* of a 205-day-old cardiomyopathic female hamster, strain BIO 8262. In the middle part of the left ventricular wall yellowish-white scars appear as plaques and streaks and follow the direction of the muscle fibers (arrows)

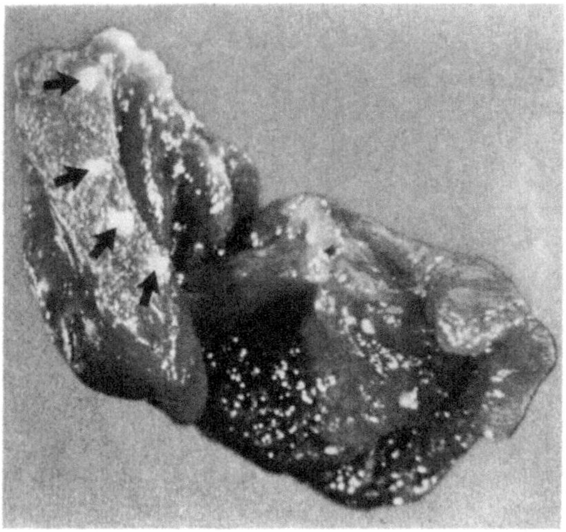

Fig. 3. Cross section of the intraventricular septum of the heart from a 153-day-old cardiomyopathic male hamster, strain BIO 8262. Four demarcated areas of scarring are located in the subendocardial layer to the left ventricle (arrows)

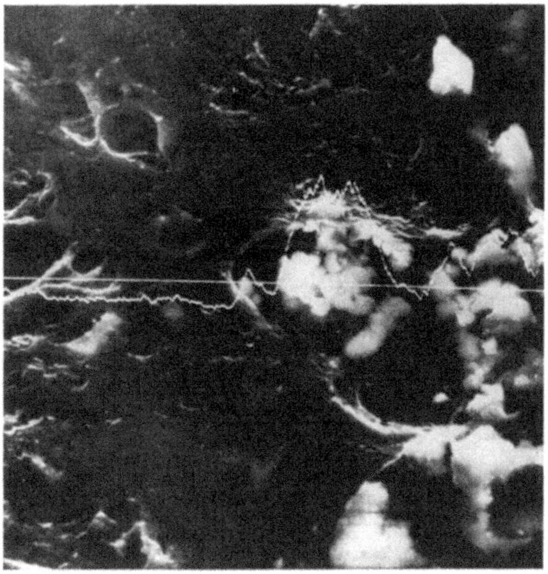

Fig. 4. Energy-dispersive X-ray microanalysis of cardiomyopathic myocardium from a BIO 8262 hamster. Electron microscopic picture and line scan: in areas of mineral salt deposits—visible by light microscopy—a high counting rate for calcium and phosphate can be detected. The counting rates for calcium are demonstrated in this picture. (From MOHR et al., 1973)

the streaks, which may sometimes lie close to the subendocardial region (Fig. 3) or at other times, in the middle of the myocardial wall or in the subepicardial layers. X-ray micro analysis revealed calcium and phosphate deposits in these areas (MOHR et al., 1973) (Fig. 4). In 80- to 130-day-old cardiomyopathic hamsters

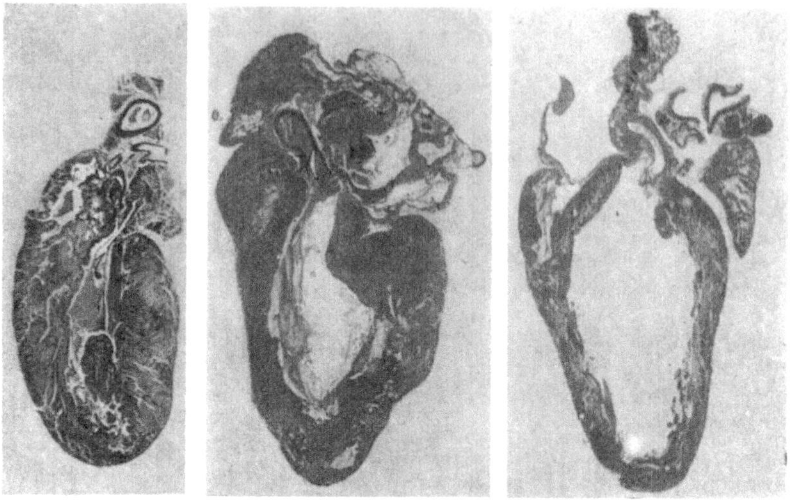

Fig. 5. The development of cardiomyopathy of the hamsters passes through 3 stages, which can be distinctly differentiated in strain BIO 14.6. Left: development of focal myocardial lesions. Middle: cardiac hypertrophy and dilation. Right: extended myocardial dilation. Hearts from 62-, 88-, and 105-day-old male hamsters of strain BIO 14.6. (From BAJUSZ and LOSSNITZER, 1968)

of strain BIO 14.6, hypertrophy of the ventricles becomes macroscopically evident (Fig. 5). The heart weight/body weight ratio was found to be increased in over 200-day-old cardiomyopathic hamsters of strains BIO 14.6, BIO 8262, and BIO 4054 as compared with controls (ALOUSI and BEARDS, 1972; FEDELESOVA and DHALIA, 1971; MCCOLLUM et al., 1970). Studies of GERTZ et al. (1972) revealed that beginning sometime after 120 days, the increase of heart weight of BIO 14.6 hamsters is associated with an increase in the solid constituents, not primarily with edema formation. Old cardiomyopathic hearts, which are dilated and flabby, sometimes contain mural thrombi. However in 8 out of 653 myopathic BIO 14.6 hamsters examined at autopsy, asymmetric left ventricular hypertrophy resembling muscular subaortic stenosis was observed (BAJUSZ, 1967b). This appearance can be labelled without any doubt with the clinical term hypertrophic obstructive cardiomyopathy as outlined by GOODWIN (1970). Concurrent long-term administration of norepinephrine (0.8 mg/kg body weight, s.c.) and thyroxine (0.5 mg/kg body weight, s.c.)—known to induce cardiac hypertrophy (MCCALLISTER and PAGE, 1973)—twice daily for eight weeks, initiated during the prenecrotic phase of the cardiomyopathy, elicited subaortic stenosis, with predominant thickening of the upper half of the free wall of the left ventricle and the interventricular septum, in 60% of the hamsters (BAJUSZ, 1967b). Spontaneous ventricular aneurysms and cardiac rupture occurring during the advanced stages of the cardiomyopathy were also reported (BAJUSZ, 1969a).

III. Hemodynamic Function and Electrocardiogram

Hemodynamic studies by JEFFREY et al. (1970) and ABELMANN et al. (1972) in congested old BIO 14.6 hamsters exhibited increased end-diastolic pressure in both ventricles. There was a decrease in left and an increase in right ventricular systolic pressure as well as a depression of dp/dt_{max} in both ventricles. The stroke volume was significantly increased whilst the vascular resistance was decreased. STAUCH and LOSSNITZER (1972) were unable to find increased end-diastolic pressure in the non-congested BIO 8262 hamsters of a similar age, but they measured a lowered left ventricular systolic pressure with depressed dp/dt_{max}. The recent experiments of STAUCH and LOSSNITZER (1974) performed on 70- and over 200-day-old BIO 8262 hamsters disclosed in both age groups considerably reduced contractility as measured by dp/dt_{max} as well as by V_{CE} and V_{max} of the left ventricle. According to the viewpoint of KATZ (1972), reduced dp/dt reflects a depressed rate of delivery of calcium ions to the contractile proteins, and depressed V_{max} represents a decreased rate of mechanochemical transformation of energy by the contractile proteins. Thus, disturbed myocardial calcium metabolism and an altered state of the contractile proteins are likely to exist in the cardiomyopathic hearts. Interestingly, LOCHNER et al. (1970), studying the mechanical activity of cardiomyopathic hearts from strain BIO 14.6 in a modified Langendorff perfusion system, did not find a depressed dp/dt_{max}, but prolonged time to peak height of developed tension in 5- to 6-week-old and 3-month-old animals, respectively. However, comparison of length-tension curves from normal and myopathic hearts showed that after a certain lengthening tension development decreased in cardiomyopathic hearts as increments of lengthening increased. Cardiomyopathic animals older than 5 months exhibited significantly reduced tension development and contractility, as well as a pattern of reduced systolic tension development for increments in lengthening from the onset in their length-tension curves (BRINK and LOCHNER, 1969; LOCHNER et al., 1970). Decreased distensibility found in the hearts of these hamsters is considered one causal factor for the reduction in tension development and contractility, which eventually leads to heart failure.

Hemodynamic in vivo studies by ABELMANN et al. (1973) in old pre-edematous and edematous BIO 14.6 hamsters, which included a study of the effect of methoxamine in the latter, revealed that the cardiac condition initially causes a "hypokinetic" circulatory state, which is later transformed into a "hyperkinetic" one. These authors postulated that subsequent extracardiac factors in edematous animals, such as water retention and vasodilatation, induce increased pre-load of the heart and decreased after-load, respectively, thus converting the initially "hypokinetic" state of low output failure into a "hyperkinetic" state of high output failure. Compliance studies in hearts of the congested hamsters showed —contrary to the studies of BRINK and LOCHNER (1967), BRINK et al. (1969) and LOCHNER et al. (1970)—increased distensibility, which is thought to invoke progressive cardiac dilatation.

Electrocardiographic studies performed by ANGELAKOS (1968) and ANGELAKOS et al. (1973a) showed notching and slurring of the QRS-complex concomitant with the development of myocardial fibrosis. A decreased heart rate, as found by ABELMANN et al. (1972) in old BIO 14.6 hamsters, could not be discovered in the BIO 8262 hamsters of a similar age (STAUCH and LOSSNITZER, 1972, 1974).

IV. Serum Enzymes and Electrolytes

Increased activities of the serum enzymes CPK, GOT, and LDH were found in 30-day-old hamsters of strains BIO 14.6 and BIO 8262 and in older animals of both strains (HOMBURGER et al., 1966; BAJUSZ and LOSSNITZER, 1968; WROGEMANN and BLANCHAER, 1968; LOSSNITZER et al., unpublished). This increase can be attributed to the degeneration of the myocardium as well as to that of the skeletal musculature. Elevated values for HBDH (hydroxybutyric dehydrogenase) in 30-day-old BIO 8262 hamsters reported by MOHR and LOSSNITZER (1972), however, are likely to result exclusively from altered myocardial cells. This indicates a severe defect of the myocardial plasma membranes as early as during the light-microscopic "prenecrotic" stage of the cardiomyopathy.

The elevated serum calcium concentration discovered in young BIO 14.6 hamsters (CANTIN et al., 1972; LOSSNITZER and BAJUSZ, 1974) obviously does not contribute to the development of the muscular degeneration as previously speculated, since it could not be found in BIO 8262 animals (LOSSNITZER et al., 1974b) suffering from the same muscle disease. The decreased potassium and increased sodium levels which were found only in serum of over-250-day-old and congested BIO 14.6 hamsters were attributed to secondary aldosteronism (LOSSNITZER and BAJUSZ, 1974).

V. Histopathology

Several histopathological phenomena were observed with the light microscope. Their occurrence was subsequent as well as partly overlapping (see Table 1).

1. Lipid Droplets

During the prenecrotic phase, accumulation of intracellular lipid droplets (BAJUSZ and LOSSNITZER, 1968), is the sole myocardial abnormality of BIO 14.6 hamsters. Cytoplasmic accumulation of fat droplets, however, is a rather nonspecific phenomenon, since its presence has been reported in different conditions such as acute infectious processes; poisoning with phosphorus, arsenic, chloroform, and ether; malignancy; ischemia; and hypoxemia (BRACHFELD, 1972; BUECHNER, 1957; MEESSEN and POCHE, 1963). Increased numbers of lipid droplets were also found in hearts of rats with alloxan-induced diabetes (UNGAR et al., 1955) and as one of the earliest alterations in myocardial cells of animals treated with sympathomimetic amines such as norepinephrine (FERRANS et al., 1972; HOAK et al., 1969; SCHENK and MOSS, 1966), epinephrine (FERRANS et al., 1970; HIGHMAN et al., 1965; LEHR et al., 1969; SHIMAMOTO and HIRAMOTO, 1966), and isoproterenol CSAPO et al., 1972; FERRANS et al., 1964; HIOTT, 1969; MARUFFO, 1967; RONA et al., 1959). In progressively degenerating myocardial cells from BIO 14.6 hamsters, lipid droplets could no longer be observed. Hence, the accumulation of lipid droplets in the prenecrotic myocardial cells must be regarded as a reversible phenomenon and clearly differentiated from fatty degeneration. It could indicate a transitory increased myocardial extraction of fatty acids and/or a disturbance of the Krebs cycle indicating mitochondrial alteration.

2. Myocytolysis and Coagulation Necrosis

Observations of BAJUSZ et al. (1969a) on strain BIO 14.6 revealed that the earliest histologically detectable abnormality is intracellular edema followed by focal myolysis (Fig. 6a). Fiber disintegration was marked by dissolution of myofibrils with the cytosol becoming filled with a relatively amorphous material. The myofibrils eventually disappeared, and the sarcolemmal remnants were often indistinguishable from endomysial connective tissue.

MOHR and LOSSNITZER (1972, 1974), reported the light microscopic changes in the myocardium of BIO 8262 hamsters. They observed intensive eosinophilia with granular disintegration of myoplasm (Fig. 6b). Coagulation necrosis was followed by mononuclear cell infiltration (Fig. 6c) and resorption of the necrotic material with replacement fibrosis (Fig. 6d). Such changes were also found by BAJUSZ et al. (1969a) in BIO 14.6 hamsters, however, usually in large degenerating areas.

In the BIO 14.6 strain, the lesions are randomly distributed throughout the walls of both ventricles and auricles, the interventricular septum apparently being the least affected (BAJUSZ et al., 1969a), whereas in the BIO 8262 strain, the interventricular septum and left ventricle were predominantly, and the right ventricle only rarely, involved; auricles were not studied (MOHR and LOSSNITZER, 1974).

Disseminated myocardial lesions—also labeled as spotty or multifocal—can be recognized under various conditions. BUECHNER (1957) ascribed them as being primarily due to hypoxidotic conditions. They could be induced through the administration of catecholamines such as isoproterenol (RONA et al., 1959), epinephrine (VEITH, 1940), and norepinephrine (SCHENK and MOSS, 1966). POCHE (1957) described a similar myocardial necrotization after administration of triiodothyronine. The electrolyte-steroid cardiopathy with necroses described by SELYE (1961) in rats treated with mineralocorticoids and Na_2HPO_4 displays again this pattern of multifocal coagulation necrosis. Potassium, magnesium, or chloride deficiencies (SELYE, 1961) are additional conditions that may be accompanied by the same pattern of myocardial necrosis. Interestingly, in humans with hypertrophic as well as idiopathic dilated-type (congestive) cardiomyopathy, such necrotic foci could only be detected rarely in the cardiac walls (ROBERTS and FERRANS, 1973; OLSEN, 1973; VAN NOORDEN et al., 1971). In both cardiomyopathic hamster strains (BIO 14.6 and BIO 8262) the appearance of newly formed lesions decreases with age, the necrotizing process only being progressive for about 40 days, as was demonstrated in the BIO 14.6 hamsters (BAJUSZ et al., 1969a). Proliferation of fibroblasts with *de novo* formation of connective tissue fibers was observed in the final stage of the disease. These late findings resemble, at least to some extent, the light microscopic picture of the dilated-type idiopathic cardiomyopathy in humans. Thus, like in hamsters, in human heart disease there may also exist only a transient necrotizing period, which during the progressively necrotizing phase is clinically without serious symptoms. Necropsy findings in humans could supposedly only reflect the terminal stage of a previously necrotizing cardiomyopathy. Electron microscopic findings reported by ROBERTS and FERRANS (1973) such as cellular edema, accumulation of lipid droplets and lysosomes, myofibrillar damage and mitochondrial swelling with cristolysis, considered as degenerative and derived from biopsies of living people with idiopathic cardiomegaly, seem to prove this assumption.

3. Myocardial Calcification and Giant Cells

During the earliest stage of necrotization, myocardial calcification was usually absent within the lesions of the cardiomyopathic hamsters. When it did occur, it was generally seen in deteriorated areas (BAJUSZ, 1969b; BAJUSZ et al., 1969a; MOHR and LOSSNITZER, 1974). In the BIO 14.6 strain it appeared in two different forms: either deposited in degenerating muscle fibers only, or also involving the surrounding connective tissue. Since in BIO 8262 hamsters the serum calcium level was normal (LOSSNITZER et al., 1974b) and in both hamster strains (BIO 14.6 and BIO 8262) the blood vessels were free of any pathological findings and the calcium salts were deposited in individual myocardial cells, the calcification in the cardiomyopathic hamster hearts can be labeled as "dystrophic". Contrary to the myocardium of the BIO 14.6 hamsters, animals of the BIO 8262 strain developed calcification of myocardial cells in foci often separated from necrotic areas. In younger animals these calcified muscle cells appeared mainly as multinucleated giant cells (Fig. 6d); in old animals they disappeared and calcium phosphate was then located between collagen fibers (MOHR and LOSSNITZER, 1974). The calcifying giant cells are taken as further evidence of a slowly progressive degeneration process possibly resulting from a regenerating attempt of altered individual cardiac cells.

Precipitation of calcium in necrotic muscle fibers was reported in the electrolyte-steroid cardiopathy with necroses, in the papain cardiopathy, and under the conditions of potassium, magnesium, or chloride deficiency, whereas little or no calcification was found to occur in necrotic muscle fibers induced by plasmoid, epinephrine, norepinephrine, and isoproterenol (SELYE, 1961). On the other hand, BLOOM and DAVIS (1972) and MORETTI et al. (1973) showed by atomic absorption spectrophotometric tissue analysis that administration of adrenergic amines such as isoproterenol, epinephrine, and norepinephrine provoked almost immediate myocardial calcium accumulation. MEESSEN and POCHE (1963) mentioned calcified heart muscle cells in infarcted areas of human hearts. ROBERTS and FERRANS (1973) also observed focal calcific deposits in myocardial cells of patients who died after periods of prolonged shock, of renal failure, and after cardiac operations. Hence, the calcification of myocardial cells in the cardiomyopathic hamsters seems to be a general phenomenon of cell injury like lipid accumulation and disseminated coagulation necrosis. These three phenomena may be interrelated. Formation of myogenic giant cells with calcific deposits, however, appears to be rather specific.

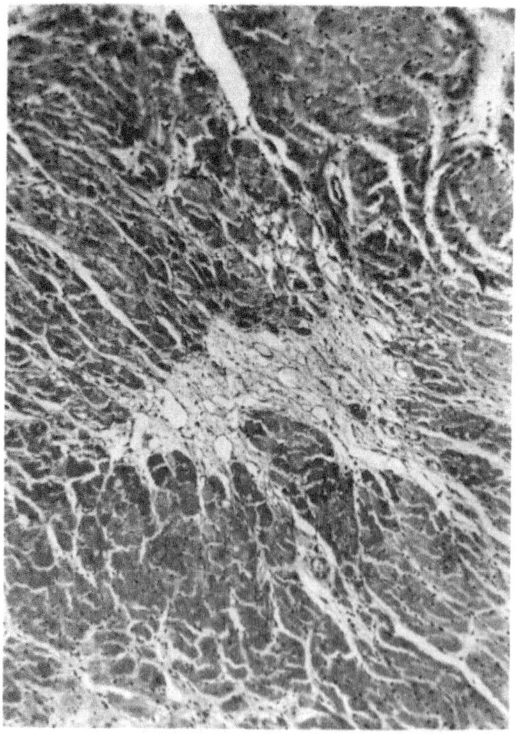

Fig. 6a

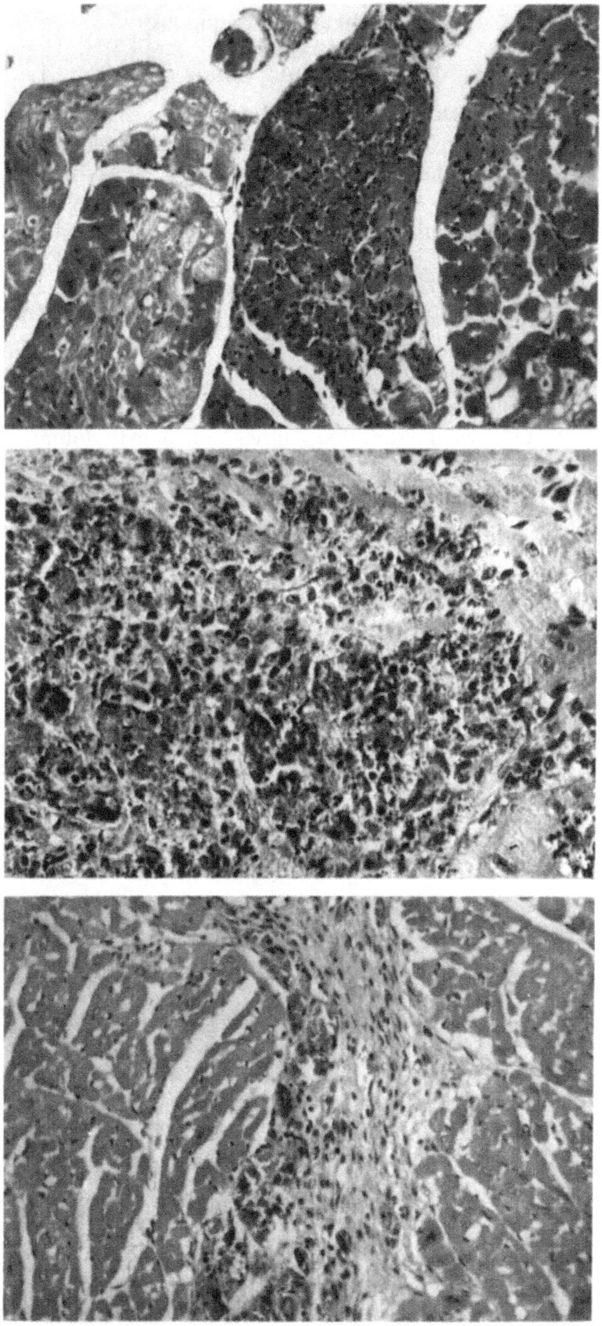

b

c

d

Fig. 6. (a) Focal myolysis with minimal cellular reaction. Sarcolemmal remnants. Myocardium of a 50-day-old male BIO 14.6 hamster. Hematoxylin–eosin. ×120. (From Bajusz and Lossnitzer, 1968.) (b) Beginning coagulation necrosis in the papillary muscle. Myocardium of a 63-day-old male BIO 8262 hamster. Hematoxylin–eosin. ×220. (c) Coagulation necrosis with infiltration of mononuclear cells. Myocardium of a 70-day-old female BIO 8262 hamster. Hematoxylin–eosin. ×220. (d) Small myocardial scar with remnants of calcification partially located in myogenic giant cells. Myocardium of a 72-day-old male BIO 8262 hamster. Hematoxylin–eosin. ×220

VI. Electron Microscopy

1. Cardiomyoblasts

As yet, electron microscopic investigations have been performed only in strain BIO 14.6 of the myopathic hamsters. The studies disclosed abnormalities as early as in the "prenecrotic" phase of the heart disease. BUECHNER and ONISHI (1970) and ONISHI et al. (1970) described irregularly shaped primitive cardiac muscle cells referred to as cardiomyoblasts, intermingled with normal cardiomyocytes in young cardiomyopathic hamsters. These cells are very similar to those found by MARKWALD (1973) in hamster embryos between 8 to 12 days *post coitum.* They can be detected up to about the 20th day of life, exhibit strikingly poor cytoplasmic structure and appear more translucent than normal cardiocytes. Until the 10th day of life they display undeveloped sarcomeres with only small, unarranged filament groups, half sarcomeres, and sometimes after sarcoplasmic condensation thin elementary fibrils with expanded Z-lines and poorly delimited thin and thick filaments (Fig. 7). Thus, BUECHNER and ONISHI (1970) suggested a genetically determined enzyme defect leading to disturbed formation of actomyosin. As HOLTZER et al. (1957) assume a priming effect of the sarcolemma for the correct arrange-

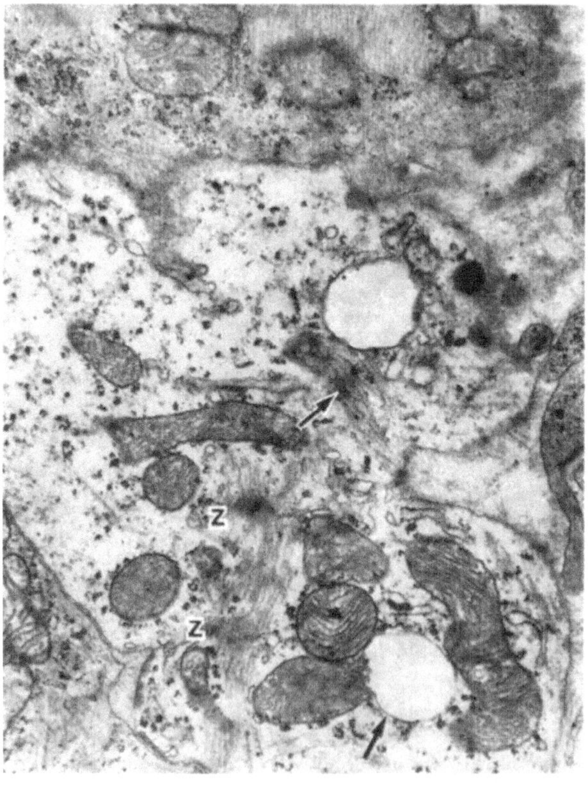

Fig. 7. Part of a cardiomyoblast in the left ventricle of a 10-day-old BIO 14.6 hamster. Dense amorphous Z-line material (arrow in the middle of the picture), so-called sarcoplasmic condensation with insertion of free filaments. Formation of half sarcomeres. Arrangement of a sarcomeric structure between two primitive Z-bands. Many polysomes (dark dots); mitochondria, at the lower part of the picture with adhering vesicle (arrow). ×20000. (From BUECHNER, 1971)

ment of myofilaments it is not too speculative to think of an early failure in this structure of the cardiomyopathic cells. However, abnormal arrangement of myofibrils, which often run in several directions, and muscle bundles arranged in disorderly fashion interspersed with tracts of connective tissue, as observed in patients with obstructive hypertrophic cardiomyopathy (FERRANS et al., 1973; VAN NOORDEN et al., 1971), could not be detected in the cardiomyopathic hamsters.

2. Progressive Changes

Specifically enhanced activity of the nuclei, which reaches a maximum on the 20th postnatal day, is manifested by partial dissolution of the nuclear membranes and by escape of nuclear portions into the sarcoplasm (Fig. 8). In addition, intense augmentation of polysomes surrounding the nucleus becomes evident as well as a large number of ergastoplasmic structures with and without ribosome-carrying membranes and hyperplasia of the Golgi apparatus. These changes could also be seen after aortic constriction in dogs (ONISHI et al., 1969; BUECHNER and ONISHI, 1970) and in humans with hypertrophic obstructive cardiomyopathy (FERRANS et al., 1973) as well as idiopathic cardiomegaly of the dilated type (ROBERTS and FERRANS, 1973). Rats treated with norepinephrine exhibited hypertrophy of the Golgi zone, and the numbers of ribosomes in cardiac muscle cells were also increased (FERRANS et al., 1972). The accumulation of ribosomes is related to an

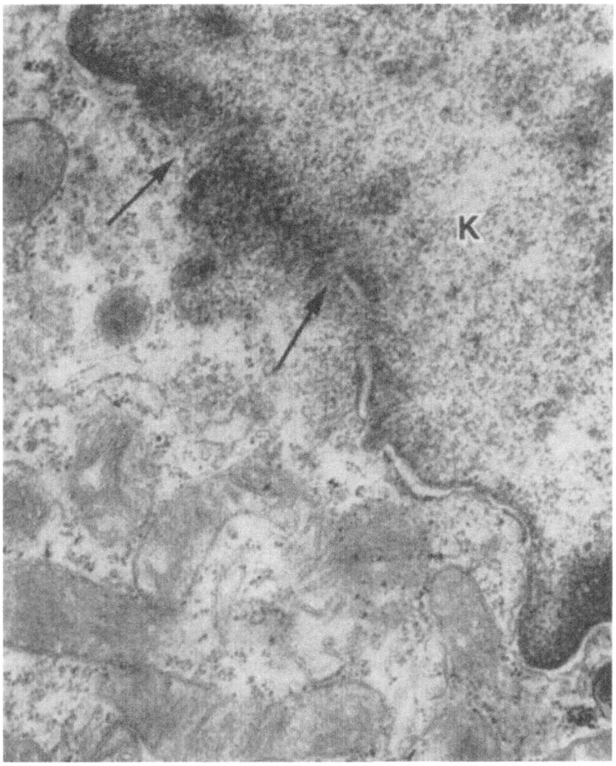

Fig. 8. Portion of a myocardial cell from the left ventricle of a 5-day-old BIO 14.6 hamster. A wide gap (arrows) of the outer and inner membrane of the nucleus (K). Prolapse of RNA-granules into the cytoplasm. ×37500. (From ONISHI et al., 1970)

increase in protein synthesis. As in all of these conditions, an increased number of mitochondria (mitochondriosis) with a dense pattern of cristae mitochondriales can also be detected in the cardiomyopathic hamsters. All the changes together are described as "progressive" and are thought to result from the retarded development of the myofilaments with subsequent accelerated protein synthesis in the early life of the hamsters (BUECHNER, 1971). Since a progressive increase of the number and thickening of elementary fibrils becomes evident as early as at the 20th day, and later on is combined with a splitting of the Z-lines—phenomena also observed in humans with idiopathic obstructive and non-obstructive cardiomyopathies (FERRANS et al., 1973)—the stimulated protein synthesis is thought to provoke surplus-hypertrophy (BAJUSZ et al., 1969b; BUECHNER and ONISHI, 1970; BUECHNER, 1971). Cardiac hypertrophy induced by thyroxine (McCALLISTER and PAGE, 1973) and provoked by isoproterenol (PFITZER et al., 1972) also exhibited an increase of myofibrillar volume and mitochondria with densely packed cristae or the formation of new myofilaments and augmentation of mitochondria and ribosomes, respectively. However, alterations of other subcellular structures differed from those in the cardiomyopathic hamster myocardiocytes. Progressive alterations, especially the development of ergastoplasmic structures, persist in the hearts of these hamsters for the rest of their lifes. Occasionally, cotton-plug-like filamentous clusters, globular formations of irregularly arranged fine filaments, can also be seen in the vicinity of the Golgi system.

3. Regressive Changes

On the other hand, so-called "regressive" changes in the light microscopic "prenecrotic" hearts of BIO 14.6 hamsters were also noticed (BUECHNER and ONISHI, 1970; NADKARNI et al., 1972; NAKAO et al., 1970; ONISHI et al., 1970). Mitochondria, elementary fibrils, and the intercalated discs seem to be particularly involved. Cristolysis occurs first, followed by vacuolization and swelling of mitochondria with their matrix becoming clarified. These abnormalities can be detected as early as the 5th and 10th postnatal days. On the 10th day, so-called "contraction bands" appear together with homogenization of the filaments, i.e. condensation of blurring Z-bands and especially disappearance of the I-band region secondary to lysis of filamentous material (Fig. 9). BUECHNER (1971) speaks of "partial necrosis". Furthermore, dehiscence of the intercalated discs is frequently seen. The changes are similar to those observed under hypoxic conditions (BUECHNER, 1971), after administration of large doses of thyroxine (SUSIN and HERDSON, 1967) and after administration of isoproterenol (BLOOM and CANCILLA, 1969; FERRANS et al., 1964; CSAPÓ et al., 1972). However, ischemia with reperfusion (SHEN and JENNINGS, 1972a), aortic constriction (BUECHNER and ONISHI, 1970), norepinephrine (DAVID et al., 1968; FERRANS et al., 1972), epinephrine (FERRANS et al., 1970), small doses of thyroxine as well as dinitrophenol (POCHE, 1962), magnesium deficiency (HEGGTVEIT et al., 1964; SUSIN and HERDSON, 1967), and vitamin B_1-deficiency (SUZUKI, 1967) induced similar non-specific mitochondrial changes and contraction bands with lysis of filamentous material, whereas dehiscence of the intercalated discs was not reported. Similar mitochondrial and myofibrillar changes could also be detected in humans with left ventricular hypertrophy due to organic obstruction (OLSEN, 1973), with hypertrophic cardiomyopathy with obstruction (FERRANS et al., 1973; OLSEN, 1973; PEARSE, 1964; VAN NOORDEN et al., 1971), with idiopathic cardiomegaly of the dilated type (FERRANS et al., 1973; VAN NOORDEN et al., 1971), and with alcoholic cardiomyopathy (ALEXANDER, 1968).

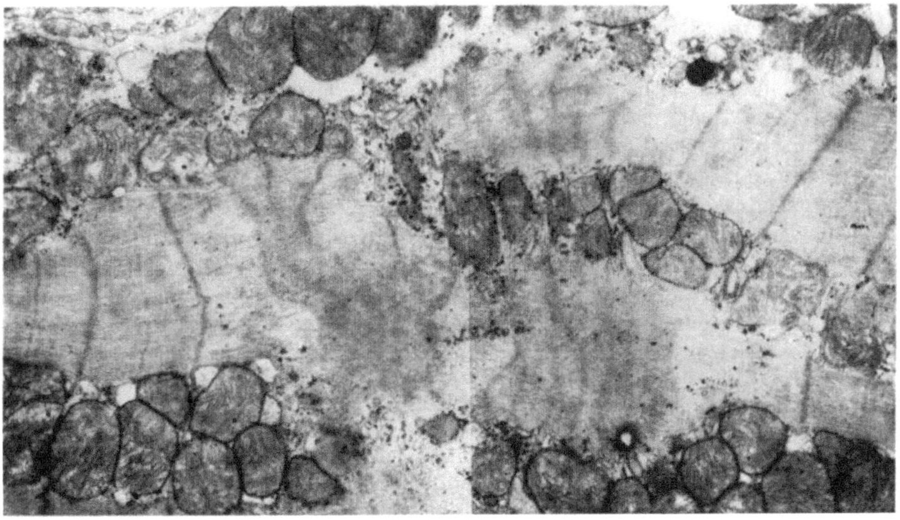

Fig. 9. Part of a myocardial cell from the left ventricle of a 30-day-old BIO 14.6 hamster. Contraction bands with homogenization of filaments and blurring Z-bands. ×16000. (From BUECHNER, 1970)

These prenecrotic regressive changes of the mitochondria and of the contractile system—being considered non-specific and remaining unresolved by the light microscope—suggest a disturbance in energy generation (mitochondria) as well as in energy utilization by excitation–contraction coupling (contractile system). From the studies, it could not be clarified which of the two is primary. It must be pointed out that the electron microscopic survey in myocardial cells of the BIO 14.6 hamsters did not reveal unequivocal results with respect to the sarcoplasmic tubular system, another important partner of the excitation–contraction coupling system. With the exception of human obstructive hypertrophic cardiomyopathy (PEARSE, 1964; FERRANS et al., 1973), all of the foregoing conditions showed swelling and dilation of the sarcotubular system. While NAKAO et al. (1970) observed a loss of the cell membranes and found evidence of morphological change in the T-system, with widening and dilation of the intercalated discs and triads, ONISHI et al. (1970) were unable to discover changes in the sarcolemma and T-system in the myocardial cells of hamsters with hereditary cardiomyopathy.

NAKAO et al. found that the subcellular focal lesions in the cardiomyopathic hamster myocardium later often contained multiple electron-dense irregular particles, presumably disintegrated intracellular organelles. However, whether they consist of mitochondrial particles containing calcium (NAKAO et al., 1970) or of myolytic changes together with calcification of sarcomeres (BUECHNER, 1971) remains controversial. In contrast to humans with hypertrophic (asymmetric) and dilated-type cardiomyopathy (OLSEN, 1973; PEARSE, 1964; ROBERTS and FERRANS, 1973; VAN NOORDEN et al., 1971), in which the myocardial glycogen content seemed to be distinctly increased, the cardiomyopathic hamsters exhibited no such changes (NADKARNI et al., 1972; ONISHI et al., 1970).

The alterations of the mitochondria, filaments, and intercalated discs became less prominent with age; however, in the final stage of the disease, coinciding with the onset of cardiac insufficiency, they apparently regain importance.

VII. Biochemistry

Thus far, biochemical, clinical, hemodynamic, and morphological studies carried out in the diseased hamsters disclosed several important changes of their cardiomyopathy which subsequently become evident (Table 1). Their relationships remain to be clarified. Biochemical alterations during the "prenecrotic" phase of the cardiomyopathy must be considered particularly important, because they precede myocardial necrosis and provide a base for this process. Most of the studies, however, were made on necrotizing myocardium or on hearts suffering from severe cardiac failure. The results are very difficult to evaluate, since they may represent either the cause or the consequence of these various processes. Nevertheless, they must not be neglected. Either they will disclose similarities or differences when compared with cardiomyopathies induced by other means, thus pointing to a more general pattern of cardiomyopathy or to specific alterations interlinked with the hereditary cardiomyopathy of the hamsters.

1. Myocardial Protein Synthesis

Protein synthesis is a prerequisite for the maintenance of the structural elements and the enzymes of the cells and thus for their correct functioning and restitution after injury. BESTER et al. (1973) found in cell-free systems of heart and skeletal muscles of 2- and 6-month-old BIO 14.6 hamsters decreased activity of the pH 5 enzyme fraction in the synthesis of proteins directed by endogenous mRNA and a selective deficiency of labeling in heavy polysomes into a polypeptide synthesizing system. These findings clearly indicate a disturbance in muscular protein synthesis. Since it is known from the work of HEYWOOD et al. (1967) that heavy polysomes participate in the synthesis of myosin, a disturbance in the development of this contractile protein is likely. Depressed V_{max}, which is found in BIO 8262 hamsters as young as 70 days old (STAUCH and LOSSNITZER, 1974), may also be related to disturbed myosin production.

To correlate the defect in the pH 5 enzyme fraction and in the labeling in the heavy polysomes with the development of myocardial necrosis appears highly speculative, since thesed isturbances were even more pronounced in 6-month-old cardiomyopathic hamsters in which only very few newly formed lesions could be seen (BAJUSZ et al., 1969a). On the other hand, the findings of BUECHNER and ONISHI (1970) showing cardiomyoblasts with delayed development of myofilaments in prenecrotic hearts as well as cells with a dense pattern of free polysomes within the perinuclear region seem to agree to some extent with the foregoing metabolic findings. Before drawing any conclusions, however, biochemical studies should be extended to the "prenecrotic" cardiomyopathic heart.

Increased protein synthesis, as assumed from electron microscopic findings showing nuclear hyperactivity, augmentation of polysomes and cardiac hypertrophy, can be correlated with increased DNA-dependent RNA polymerase activity, which reached its peak in 40-day-old cardiomyopathic hamsters and which declined thereafter (NAIR and UMALI, 1970). BUECHNER (1971) suggested a compensatory mechanism, which may be provoked by delayed filament ripening seen in the cardiomyoblasts (see B., Section VI–1). LOCHNER et al. (1971), however, were unable to detect elevated myocardial protein synthesis at this stage of the cardiomyopathy from measurements of the *in vitro* incorporation of lysin and leucine into a soluble protein fraction and into actomyosin of 60- to 90-day-old BIO 14.6 hamsters. On the other hand, these authors found an enhanced incorporation of these amino acids into cardiomyopathic hearts of 180- to 240-day-old hamsters that correlated well with myocardial hypertrophy. No collagen proliferation was observed during this phase (GERTZ et al., 1970a). ALOUSI and BEARDS (1972) observed reduced incorporation of alanine and uridine into both heart protein and RNA in the 8- to 9-month-old cardiomyopathic hamsters; however, the cardiac protein and RNA contents were elevated.

Although the findings on myocardial protein synthesis are still equivocal, they may have some bearing upon the clarification of the contractile insufficiency and cardiac hypertrophy which could be detected in the cardiomyopathic hamsters. It must be emphasized, however, that contractile insufficiency and hypertrophy are complex, interrelated entities. Further experiments are needed in order to clarify these interrelationships.

2. Myocardial Norepinephrine Content and Synthesis

The study of the behavior of myocardial norepinephrine revealed some promising aspects which seemed to contribute to the elucidation of the etio-pathogenesis of the myocardial lesions in this hereditary cardiomyopathy.

ANGELAKOS et al. (1972, 1973b) reported that normal myocardial norepinephrine content in 1-month-old cardiomyopathic hearts of BIO 14.6 hamsters increased concomitantly with the development of necrosis. Later, during the stage of macroscopically evident hypertrophy and myocardial scarring, the norepinephrine content (μg/g tissue) decreased, in spite of increased fluorescence intensity of adrenergic nerve terminals in undamaged areas (ALOUSI and BEARDS, 1972; ANGELAKOS et al., 1972). Moreover, microspectrofluorometric measurements (ANGELAKOS et al., 1973b) revealed that, in mature controls, adrenergic terminal fluorescence was higher in the cardiac apex than in the base. Such a difference did not exist in the diseased hamsters, in which in all parts of the heart the fluorescence was higher than in the controls. In addition, accelerated norepinephrine synthesis as well as avid binding of H^3-norepinephrine were found in the "prenecrotic" cardiomyopathic hearts (ANGELAKOS et al., 1973b). Histochemical and electron microscopic findings of PEARSE (1964), who studied human hearts with obstructive cardiomyopathy, revealed proliferation of sympathetic nerve fibers with consequent and demonstrable noradrenosis (increased myocardial catecholamine content). These findings somewhat resemble those observed in cardiomyopathic hamsters. Furthermore, it is known from experimental cardiology that multifocal myocardial lesions similar to those seen in cardiomyopathic hamsters can be induced by i.v. infusions of norepinephrine (0.1 to 4.0 μg/kg/min) into cats, dogs, and rabbits (HOAK et al., 1969; SCHENK and MOSS, 1966; SZAKÁCS and CANNON, 1958) as well as by individual s.c. doses of 4 and 2 mg/kg, respectively, into rats (DAVID et al., 1968; FERRANS et al., 1972).

ANGELAKOS et al. (1973b) believe that this hereditary disease of hamsters represents an adrenergic cardiomyopathy, which might be provoked by an endogenously increased activity of the sympathetic nervous system. It must be emphasized, however, that the heart rate was found to be decreased or unchanged, and dp/dt_{max} and the peripheral vascular resistance reduced (ABELMANN et al., 1972; STAUCH and LOSSNITZER, 1972, 1974). Yet, it may be that locally augmented cardiac norepinephrine metabolism is secondary to a disturbed synthesis of the contractile proteins with impaired contractile function. At present, it does not seem too important whether the increased cardiac norepinephrine content is primary or secondary in nature, because its necrotizing effect is known, and a good correlation was demonstrated between its increased content and synthesis of cardiac norepinephrine stores and intensity of myocardial necrosis in the hamster.

However, in order to substantiate the increased influence of norepinephrine on the myocardium of the hamsters, the relatively specific metabolic effects of this adrenergic hormone have to be demonstrated.

3. Myocardial Calcium Metabolism in Prenecrotic and Necrotizing Hearts

The well-established metabolic effects of the adrenergic hormones, including norepinephrine, such as increased cardiac adenylcyclase activity with increase in cyclic AMP (BENFEY, 1971; EPSTEIN et al., 1970; KOHRMAN, 1973; MURAD et al., 1962), increased activity of lipoprotein lipase (MALLOV and CERRA, 1967), and of phosphorylase (DHALLA, 1966; HORNBROOK and CABRAL, 1972; MCNEILL and BRODY, 1969) have not yet been examined in the prenecrotic or early necrotizing myocardium of cardiomyopathic hamsters. It is also known from the experiments of REGAN et al. (1967) that triglyceride accumulates in the myocardium under the influence of norepinephrine; however, no such accumulation could be discovered in 65- to 70-day-old BIO 14.6 hamsters by SZOLLÁR et al., (1973).

Norepinephrine (MORETTI et al., 1973) like isoproterenol (FLECKENSTEIN, 1971b; BLOOM and DAVIES, 1972) can induce accumulation of calcium in rat hearts and increase the density of hypothetic divalent cation channels available in the sarcolemma of chick hearts, thereby increasing the inward Ca^{2+}-current into the myocardial cells (SHIGENOBU and SPERELAKIS, 1973). LOSSNITZER and BAJUSZ (1974) and LOSSNITZER et al. (1974b) found that both the slightly elevated and normal myocardial calcium content in "prenecrotic" hearts of BIO 14.6 and BIO 8262 hamsters, respectively, were markedly increased in necrotizing myocardium of both strains of hamsters. Thus, the myocardial calcium accumulation in the cardiomyopathic hamsters seems to correlate well with their increased myocardial norepinephrine content (see B., Section VII–2).

It is known from the studies of REUTER (1965), FLECKENSTEIN (1971b) and SHIGENOBU and SPERELAKIS (1972) that not only norepinephrine, but also epinephrine and isoproterenol produce a rapid augmentation of calcium conductivity of myocardial plasma membranes. The order of effectiveness is isoproterenol $>$ epinephrine $\geq$ norepinephrine. Furthermore, it was estabiished by FLECKENSTEIN (1971a, b) that catecholamine-induced calcium overload of the myocardial cytosol, in particular, results in potentiation of the calcium-dependent excitation–contraction coupling with increased ATP-consumption, myocardial tension development, and oxygen demand leading to myocardial fiber necrosis. In this respect it was important that KATZ (1967) and LUCHI and KRITCHER (1967) were unable to demonstrate that norepinephrine and various other agents known to alter cardiac contractility had any direct action on cardiac myosin and actomyosin.

CHIMOSKEY and GERGELY (1968) proved that norepinephrine by itself did not affect calcium uptake of cardiac sarcoplasmic reticulum. KATZ and REPKE (1973) demonstrated a cyclic AMP-dependent protein kinase which regulates its calcium uptake. However, since in 10- and 60-day-old cardiomyopathic hamster hearts the calcium uptake, binding, and capacity of sarcoplasmic reticulum were normal (GERTZ et al., 1970b), myocardial calcium accumulation can be assumed to take place in mitochondria and in the cytosol.

WROGEMANN and BLANCHAER (1974) actually found elevated mitochondrial calcium levels in hearts of 22-day-old BIO 14.6 hamsters by density gradient centrifugation. Contraction bands, observed even in "prenecrotic" hearts of BIO 14.6 hamsters by BUECHNER and ONISHI (1970), which were labeled as "partial necrosis" when homogenization and lysis of myofibrillar structures occurred, point strongly to the existence of overload with functionally active calcium in the cytosol. Since it is well accepted that interaction of calcium ions with troponin —a modulator protein of the contraction process which is attached to the contractile protein actin (HASSELBACH, 1971; OLSON, 1971)—initiates the interaction between actin and myosin (KATZ et al., 1971; KATZ and REPKE, 1973; LEGATO and LANGER, 1969), contraction bands indicate not only the functional activity but also the site of action of the myocellular calcium overload. It should be stressed, however, that the appearance of contraction bands is a very common phenomenon in the pathogenesis of myocardial cell damage (see B., Section VI–3).

BAJUSZ et al. (1966b) demonstrated that s.c. injections of epinephrine (4 mg/kg twice daily for two consecutive days), unlike norepinephrine, produced within two days severe calcifying necrosis in "prenecrotic" myocardium of 25-day-old cardiomyopathic BIO 14.6 hamsters, whereas no such changes appeared in healthy controls. However, in 50-day-old cardiomyopathic hamsters exhibiting mild to moderate degrees of spontaneous necrosis, the same dose of both catecholamines greatly aggravated the heart muscle pathology. Increasing sensitivity of the cardiomyopathic heart muscle cells to exogenous catecholamines with respect to their calcium uptake seems to exist.

Recent experiments of LOSSNITZER et al. (1974a) demonstrated a latent disturbance of the calcium metabolism in "prenecrotic" hearts of cardiomyopathic BIO 8262 hamsters when the animals were exposed to a fairly low dose of isoproterenol (1 mg/kg body weight, s.c.). The myocardial calcium content and net uptake of ^{45}Ca of untreated cardiomyopathic hamsters did not differ from those of healthy control animals. However, after injection of isoproterenol the calcium content became distinctly elevated 6 hours later in cardiomyopathic animals but remained unchanged in healthy controls (Fig. 10). Although isoproterenol induced an elevated myocardial net uptake of ^{45}Ca in both strains, that of the cardiomyopathic hearts was distinctly greater (Fig. 11). These facts indicate potential imbalance of myocardial calcium turnover in prenecrotic cardiomyopathic hamsters. Despite a good correlation between myocardial norepinepinephrine and calcium accumulation in spontaneously necrotizing hearts of the cardiomyopathic hamsters a strict linkage between both processes appears therefore still uncertain. Since a greater susceptibility to catecholamines of the membranes of the cardiomyopathic heart muscle cells as the sole cause of calcium accumulation seems on the other hand also questionable supposedly limited capacities of cardiac bio-membranes for calcium turnover in combination with increasing stimulation by catecholamines might be the underlying processes for the development of myocardial calcium accumulation.

It was outlined by FLECKENSTEIN (1971a, b) that increased influx of calcium ions through the plasma membranes into cells is a decisive "prenecrotic" factor in the chain of pathogenetic events of their necrotization which can be beneficially influenced. Simultaneous application of isoproterenol and of the so-called "calcium-antagonistic" compound verapamil, known to decrease the calcium conductivity of myocellular plasma membranes (FLECKENSTEIN, 1971a; KOHLHARDT et al., 1972) without blocking adrenergic β-receptors (NAYLER et al., 1968; ROBAK and GRYGLEWSKI, 1970), resulted in inhibition of isoproterenol-stimulated calcium accumulation in "prenecrotic" cardiomyopathic hearts of the BIO 8262 hamsters (LOSSNITZER et al., 1974a). Long-term application of this compound starting on the 30th day of life was fully effective in preventing the effect of myocardial calcium overload as well as the occurrence of myocardial necroses and degeneration seen in untreated cardiomyopathic litter mates of the cardiomyopathic hamsters (BAJUSZ and JASMIN, 1974; LOSSNITZER and MOHR, 1973). These findings clearly demonstrate that not so much the still questionable overstimula-

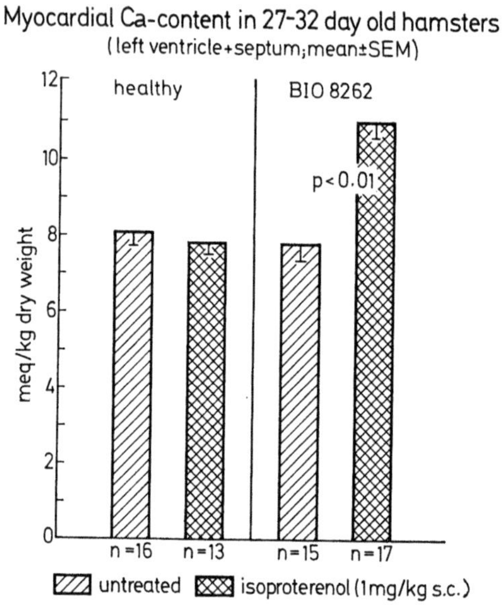

Fig. 10. Myocardial calcium content of left ventricular muscle 6 hrs after s.c. administration of 1 mg/kg body weight isoproterenol. The calcium content remains unchanged in healthy control hamsters, whereas it is significantly increased in "prenecrotic" cardiomyopathic myocardium of BIO 8262 hamsters. (From LOSSNITZER et al., 1974a)

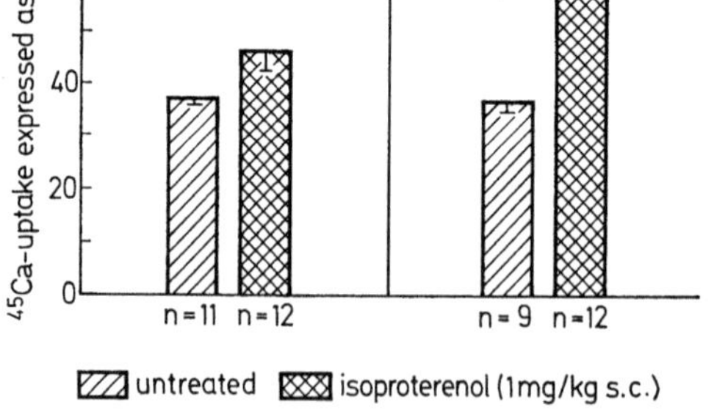

Fig. 11. Myocardial net ^{45}Ca uptake 6 hrs after s.c. administration of 1 mg/kg body weight isoproterenol. A slight increase can be seen in healthy control myocardium. However, the "prenecrotic" left ventricular muscle, in which the multifocal coagulation necroses will occur later, exhibits a much higher actual content of ^{45}Ca. (Modified from LOSSNITZER et al., 1974a)

tion of β-receptors but overload of the myocardial cells with calcium ions is the decisive factor in the chain of pathogenetic steps leading to necrosis in this cardiomyopathy of hamsters. For the first time it was demonstrated in a spontaneously occurring cardiac condition that altered myocellular permeability to harmful overload with calcium ions can be influenced by pharmacological means. Functionally disturbed myocardial plasma membranes seem to represent a decreased resistance of the myocardial cells, i.e. a preceding prenecrotic pathogenetic step. In this respect, findings of RONA et al. (1974) are significant; following norepinephrine infusion, they demonstrated permeability changes in cardiac muscle cell membranes that precede myofilament and mitochondrial alterations.

4. The "Calcium Pump" of the Myocardial Sarcoplasmic Reticulum and Mitochondria

Since in excitation–contraction coupling—the process which modulates myocardial contractility—not only an interaction between calcium and the plasma membrane (BEELER and REUTER, 1970; CORABOEUF, 1971; MASCHER and PEPER, 1969; NAYLER and MERRILLEES, 1971; NAYLER, 1973; REUTER, 1967; REUTER and BEELER, 1969) as well as the contractile proteins (EBASHI et al., 1968; HONIG, 1968; HONIG and REEDY, 1973; JENNY, 1968; KATZ et al., 1971; WEBER et al., 1964), but also a calcium interaction with the sarcoplasmic reticulum (ENTMAN, 1970; KATZ and REPKE, 1973; NAYLER and MERRILLEES, 1971; SCHWARTZ, 1971; SHINEBOURNE and WHITE, 1970; SULHAKE and DHALLA, 1970) and, of minor significance, with the mitochondria (DHALLA, 1969; HARIGAYA and SCHWARTZ, 1969; HAUGAARD et al., 1969; KUEBLER and SHINEBOURNE, 1971; LEHNINGER, 1970; PATRIARCA and CARAFOLI, 1968) could be demonstrated, a variety of studies were performed on the cardiomyopathic hamsters hearts with respect to the loss of their contractile function and in order to elucidate the interrelationship between calcium and the sarcoplasmic reticulum as well as the mitochondria.

Reduced "calcium pumping" of the sarcoplasmic reticulum (GERTZ et al., 1970b, 1972; MCCOLLUM et al., 1970; SULHAKE and DHALLA, 1971) and of the mitochondria (SCHWARTZ et al., 1968; LINDENMAYER et al., 1970; SULHAKE and DHALLA, 1971) as well as the absence of the Bowditch phenomenon (HAJDU and POSNER, 1971) could be shown in over 200-day-old cardiomyopathic hamsters of strain BIO 14.6. However, no difference in the total Ca^{2+}–Mg^{2+}-stimulated ATPase activities of heavy microsomes (= enriched preparation of sarcoplasmic reticulum) and mitochondria were observed in hearts between control and cardiomyopathic hamsters 225 days of age (SULHAKE and DHALLA, 1971). Since a lipid dependency has been demonstrated for the calcium flux and calcium-stimulated ATPase of sarcoplasmic reticulum by MACLENNAN et al. (1971) and MARTONOSI et al. (1971), and a cholesterol lecithin monolayer will not interact with calcium ions when the molar ratio is increased above 0.25 (SHAH et al., 1967), the failure of the "calcium pump" was related to altered lipid composition of myocardial bio-membranes or membrane lipid-dependent enzymes by OWENS et al. (1972). They found an elevated cholesterol/phospholipid ratio in the myocardium of 230-day-old but not in 30-day-old BIO 14.6 hamsters. An increased proportion of mitochondria or sarcolemmal membranes, which are rich in cholesterol in relation to sarcoplasmic reticulum could be ruled out. GERTZ et al. (1970b) also found a markedly reduced calcium oxalate capacity in hearts of 200- to 300-day-old cardiomyopathic hamsters. Nevertheless, calcium oxalate capacity per unit sarcoplasmic reticulum was unchanged, suggesting a dilution of the sarcoplasmic reticulum in the hypertrophied hearts. Hypertrophy of the cardiomyopathic hearts was determined by macroscopic and electron microscopic investigations (see Table 1). In accordance with the conception of ENTMAN (1970), the absence of the Bowditch phenomenon as well as the lowered quantity of sarcoplasmic reticulum in hypertrophied heart muscle cells accompanied by the defective "calcium pump" should be related to contractile insufficiency detected in the cardiomyopathic hamsters (see Table 1).

However, these factors can only be considered at the utmost as contributory, since depressed contractility was found in 70-day-old non-congested cardiomyopathic hamsters (STAUCH and LOSSNITZER, 1974), when the biochemical aberrations could not be detected. GERTZ et al. (1970b, 1972) were unable to find abnormal calcium binding, uptake, and capacity of sarcoplasmic reticulum in 10- and about 60-day-old cardiomyopathic hearts, respectively. The quantity of sarcoplasmic reticulum of the myocardium was also not lowered during this age range. Mitochondrial calcium binding was not studied in "prenecrotic" and progressively necrotizing hearts. LINDENMAYER et al. (1970) only detected slightly depressed mitochondrial calcium binding in cardiomyopathic hearts of 140- to 160-day-old hamsters of strain BIO 14.6.

From all these findings it can be concluded that the reduced contractility of the cardiomyopathic hamster hearts is a highly complex problem arising from alterations of the contractile proteins (see B., Section III), hypertrophy, and the defective "calcium pump" of the sarcoplasmic reticulum and mitochondria, i.e. of the subcellular membranes. Moreover, the failure of the "calcium pump" can hardly be attributed to the necrotizing processes, as it was not seen during the development of necrotization. Cardiac necrotization, in turn, does not appear secondary to failure of the sarcoplasmic or mitochondrial "calcium pump", because this change became obvious when newly formed lesions were minimal or no longer present.

5. Oxidative Phosphorylation, High-Energy Phosphates, and Substrate Metabolism

VARGO et al. (1972) speculated, after observing significant respiratory stimulation of the myocardium in over-100-day-old BIO 4054 hamsters in response to ouabain, that the defective "calcium pump" of the sarcoplasmic reticulum might be responsible for the uncoupling and ensuing inhibition of oxidative phosphorylation in cardiomyopathic hamsters. Since an interaction between calcium and mitochondria is also known for the myocardium (KUEBLER and SHINEBOURNE, 1971; LEHNINGER, 1970), the failing "calcium pump" of the sarcoplasmic reticulum could expose mitochondria to higher calcium concentrations, which subsequently would induce energy-linked mitochondrial accumulation of calcium as an alternative to oxidative phosphorylation (LEHNINGER, 1970). WROGEMANN and BLANCHAER (1974) recently reported slightly elevated calcium levels in mitochondria of hearts from BIO 14.6 hamsters as early as 22 days old. They postulated that an abnormal population of small mitochondria with high calcium levels exists in the prenecrotic myocardium. Since defective plasma membranes could induce the flooding of the cytosol with calcium ions (see Section VII-3), they seem to be indirectly responsible for the mitochondrial calcification at this phase of the disease, when no disturbance of the sarcoplasmic functions with respect to calcium could be evidenced (GERTZ et al., 1970b, 1972). On the other hand, normal oxidative phosphorylation was found in myocardial mitochondria of 5- to 6-week-old (LOCHNER et al., 1970) and 97- to 124-day-old (WROGEMANN and BLANCHAER, 1968) cardiomyopathic hamsters of strain BIO 14.6. This indicates the methodological difficulties that hamper the unveiling of possibly discrete functional aberrations restricted to a small number of cells. In this respect it is important to note that only about 5 to 10% of the myocardial cells will become necrotic, while the remaining tissue will partly exhibit hypertrophy of myocardial cells as well as contractile insufficiency.

Since (1) no depression of oxidative phosphorylation could be detected in progressively necrotizing hearts of the cardiomyopathic hamsters (LOCHNER et al., 1970; WROGEMANN and BLANCHAER, 1968); (2) an equivocal depression of oxidative phosphorylation was seen in cardiomyopathic hearts up to 160 days of age (LINDENMAYER et al., 1970; LOCHNER et al., 1968; LOCHNER et al., 1970; WROGEMANN and BLANCHAER, 1968); and (3) a distinct depression of oxidative phosphorylation with reduced oxygen uptake could only be seen in over-200-day-old cardiomyopathic hearts (LINDENMAYER et al., 1970; LOCHNER et al., 1970; SCHWARTZ et al., 1968), which exhibited signs of severe congestive heart failure but no apparent necrotization, with some precaution it can be concluded that depression of oxidative phosphorylation is probably not involved in the causation of the myocardial necrosis. In addition, it also does not seem to be responsible for the reduced myocardial contractility because this was apparent much earlier in life. However, defective oxidative phosphorylation could possibly aggravate cardiac insufficiency. Reduced mitochondrial calcium accumulation in the final stage of the disease (LINDENMAYER et al., 1970; SCHWARTZ et al., 1968; SULHAKE and DHALLA, 1971) definitely indicates deterioration of mitochondria with impaired electron transport.

Obviously secondary to mitochondrial deterioration with reduced high-energy phosphate production, the high-energy phosphates were unequivocally reduced in over-200-day-old BIO 14.6 hamsters, as was shown by FEDELESOVA and DHALLA (1971) in hearts *in vivo* and by LOCHNER et al. (1970) in perfused hearts. In 90- to 140-day-old cardiomyopathic hearts *in vivo* no change in ATP content and only a slight reduction of creatine phosphate were observed (LOCHNER et al., 1968; LOCHNER, 1970). KELLEY (1968) measured depressed oxidation of octanoic acid in slices from hypertrophic cardiomyopathic hearts of congested hamsters with unspecified age, confirming the impaired mitochondrial function seen in over-200-day-old cardiomyopathic hamsters. BRINK and LOCHNER (1967), however, demonstrated normal oxidation of palmitate in 90-day-old perfused hearts with affected oxidative phosphorylation of questionable significance. On the other hand, the glucose metabolism of heart slices from cardiomyopathic hamsters of the same age was undoubtedly enhanced with increased oxygen uptake, lactate- and carbon dioxide production, while the pyruvate metabolism was unchanged (LOCHNER et al., 1968). The results were referred to accelerated glycolysis. Increased oxygen uptake and carbon dioxide production, only seen when glucose was metabolized, is thought to be due to de-inhibition of rate-limiting steps since—with the exception of lactate dehydrogenase, which surprisingly was reduced—the *in vitro* activities of the glycolytic enzymes were not altered. The cause of such a speculative de-inhibition remains unknown. Whether these metabolic aberrations also exist during the "prenecrotic" phase of the cardiomyopathy has not yet been investigated.

C. Summary and Conclusions

Hereditary cardiomyopathy in Syrian golden hamsters provides a unique disease model in which pathological processes, such as myocardial necrotization, hypertrophy, contractile failure, and possibly conduction defects can be closely followed up and interrelated. Thus far a great deal of information has been compiled—though sometimes controversial—by morphological, functional, and biochemical studies. However, no interrelating of the various phenomena had been attempted; in particular, no serious effort was made to correlate the main cardiac conditions: necrotization, hypertrophy, and failure. Some confusion seems to have arisen due to the existence of several strains of cardiomyopathic hamsters that show distinct variations in the course of the disease.

Although the cardiomyopathy can be experimentally induced by inbreeding, it is a spontaneous disease that occurs consistently. Since it is accompanied by skeletal muscular dystrophy it must be termed secondary cardiomyopathy. Clinically it resembles a condition that also can usually be seen in humans afflicted with muscular dystrophy. Four distinct stages that partly overlap could be detected in its course: the prenecrotic, progressively necrotizing, hypertrophy, and congestive phases (see Table 1). The clinical picture of overt heart failure with congestion was only seen in strain BIO 14.6 but not in strain BIO 8262, which is also well described. The reason for this difference in behavior is not known. By comparing these two strains of cardiomyopathic hamsters, interrelationships between contractile and circulatory failure with its consequences could possibly be established.

A disturbance in the embryonic development of muscle cells may underlie the disease with cardiocytes in different stages of postnatal maturity. Delay of filament ripening seems to be one of the earliest detectable features. It remains to be clarified whether supposedly contractile failure of such cells is a stimulus in a feedback mechanism for increasing adrenergic activity found in the cardiomyopathic hearts (ANGELAKOS et al., 1972 and 1973b).

Latent disturbance of myocardial calcium metabolism could be noted during the prenecrotic phase of the disease. This conditioning, together with increasing sympathetic activity, appears to be the metabolic background for myocardial necrotization, since calcium overload and necrotization of myocardium induced by catecholamines has been well established. It seems plausible that the increased activity of the cardiac sympathetic nervous system may easily lead to manifestation of that formerly latent electrolyte disturbance with concomitant calcium overload, loss of high energy phosphates, and degeneration of certain cardiocytes in these hamsters. This is based on the fact that a good correlation was demonstrated between augmented norepinephrine content and intensity of necrotization in their myocardium. In addition, by application of a so-called calcium-antagonistic compound, which decreases transmembrane calcium conductivity but does not block β-receptors, cardiac necrotization was fully prevented in these hamsters. Hence the hypothesis of myocardial calcium overload as a decisive and nonspecific factor for myocardial necrotization, derived from pharmacological experiments on the isoproterenol-treated rat by FLECKENSTEIN (1969, 1971a, b), could for the first time be successfully proven in a spontaneous and hereditary heart disease. Since there is also evidence of disturbed myocardial calcium metabolism in many other cardiac conditions (see LOSSNITZER et al., 1974b), the concept of calcium overload as a determining factor for cardiac necrotization (i.e. that factor which converts reversible into irreversible self-perpetuating processes) gains greater significance. Furthermore, symptomatic therapy against cardiac necrotization using calcium-antagonistic compounds seems to be a promising subject for research on various other cardiac conditions.

As yet cardiac hypertrophy in the hamster has not been sufficiently described and defined in relation to the patterns of human pathology. However, we can say that it certainly does not resemble human hypertrophic obstructive cardiomyopathy. Histological findings, the clinical course in the majority of the hamsters, and hemodynamic studies are against such an assumption. BUECHNER (1971) suggests surplus hypertrophy resulting from retarded development of filaments, with a subsequently accelerated myofibrillar protein synthesis. It remains to be determined whether increased sympathetic activity in response to initially reduced contractile power represents the metabolic stimulus or whether other metabolic processes are significantly involved. It is not absurd to speculate that the degree of susceptibility to catecholamine stimuli or the strength of the stimulus itself determines whether cardiocytes develop necrosis or hypertrophy; this would then be the switch for determining the outcome of these two morphological processes.

Disturbed protein synthesis and contractile failure were demonstrated in young hamsters with necrotizing hearts. It is now important that these disturbances will also be demonstrated in as yet prenecrotic hamster hearts. This would provide a promising starting-point for studies through which metabolic disorders of myocardial protein synthesis, calcium metabolism, and adrenergic activity could be interlinked with functional and morphological features of contractile failure, necrosis, and hypertrophy. However, it was revealed, as for most of the cardiac conditions, that the different processes neither start simultaneously nor progress synchronously and uniformly in all cells of the same myocardium. This intriguing finding in particular presents great difficulties in obtaining unequivocal results and final conclusions. Information on the differentiating factors would be of immense value.

Nevertheless, there is no doubt that hereditary cardiomyopathy of the Syrian hamsters has opened up numerous research possibilities and has already contributed a large amount of information to experimental cardiology. It is unique in that it provides a model of a spontaneous disease although it was experimentally induced by brother-sister mating.

References

Abelmann, W. H., Jeffrey, F. E., Wagner, R.: Hemodynamics of the hereditary cardiomyopathy of Syrian hamsters. In: Recent advances in studies on cardiac structure and metabolism, vol. 1: Myocardiology. Baltimore-London-Tokyo: University Park Press 1972.

Abelmann, W. H., Wagner, R. L., Bajusz, E.: Serial hemodynamic observations in hereditary cardiomyopathy of the Syrian hamster. In: Recent advances in studies on cardiac structure and metabolism, vol. 2: Cardiomyopathies. Baltimore-London-Tokyo: University Park Press 1973.

Alexander, C. S.: The concept of alcoholic myocardiopathy. Med. Clin. N. Amer. **52**, 1183–1191 (1968).

Alousi, A. A., Beards, J. A.: Catecholamine, protein, and RNA content in advanced congestive heart failure in the Syrian hamster. In: Recent advances in studies on cardiac structure and metabolism, vol. 1: Myocardiology. Baltimore-London-Tokyo: University Park Press 1972.

Angelakos, E. T.: Electrocardiographic (ECG) changes and cardiac catecholamine concentrations in the dystrophic hamster strain (BIO 14.6 line) at various ages. Trans. N.Y. Acad. Sci. **30**, 955–596 (1968).

Angelakos, E. T., Carballo, L. C., Daniels, J. B., King, M. B., Bajusz, E.: Adrenergic neurohumors in the heart of hamsters with hereditary myopathy during cardiac hypertrophy and failure. In: Recent advances in studies on cardiac structure and metabolism, vol. 1: Myocardiology. Baltimore-London-Tokyo: University Park Press 1972.

Angelakos, E. T., Daniels, J., Robinson, S., Bajusz, E.: Electrocardiographic changes during a progressive focal myocardiopathy in hamsters. In: Recent advances in studies on cardiac structure and metabolism, vol. 2: Cardiomyopathies. Baltimore-London-Tokyo: University Park Press 1973a.

Angelakos, E. T., King, M. B., Carballo, L.: Cardiac adrenergic innervation in hamsters with hereditary myocardiopathy: chemical and histochemical studies. In: Recent advances in studies on cardiac structure and metabolism, vol. 2: Cardiomyopathies. Baltimore-London-Tokyo: University Park Press 1973b.

Bajusz, E.: Conditioning factors for cardiac necroses. Basel-New York: S. Karger 1963.

Bajusz, E.: Experimental pathology and histochemistry of heart muscle. In: Methods and achievments in experimental pathology. Basel-New York: S. Karger 1967a.

Bajusz, E.: Experimental muscular subaortic stenosis (hypertrophic obstructive cardiomyopathy). Amer. J. Cardiol. **19**, 117–118 (1967b).
Bajusz, E.: Hereditary cardiomyopathy: a new disease model. Amer. Heart J. **77**, 686–696 (1969a).
Bajusz, E.: Dystrophic calcification of myocardium as conditioning factor in genesis of congestive heart failure. Amer. Heart J. **78**, 202–210 (1969b).
Bajusz, E., Baker, J. R., Nixon, C. W.: Effects of catecholamines upon cardiac and skeletal muscles of dystrophic hamsters. Fed. Proc. **25**, 475 (1966a).
Bajusz, E., Baker, J. R., Nixon, C. W., Homburger, F.: Spontaneous, hereditary myocardial degeneration and congestive heart failure in a strain of Syrian hamsters. Ann. N.Y. Acad. Sci. **156**, 105–129 (1969a).
Bajusz, E., Buechner, F., Onishi, S., Rickers, K.: Hypertrophie des Herzmuskels bei erbbedingter Myopathie. Naturwissenschaften **56**, 568–569 (1969b).
Bajusz, E., Homburger, F., Baker, J. R., Opie, L. H.: The heart muscle in muscular dystrophy with special reference to involvement of the cardiovascular system in the hereditary myopathy of the hamster. Ann. N.Y. Acad. Sci. **138**, 213–229 (1966b).
Bajusz, E., Jasmin, G.: Prevention of myocardial degeneration in hamsters with hereditary cardiomyopathy. In: Recent advances in studies on cardiac structure and metabolism, vol. 5: Myocardial cell damage. (In press.) Baltimore-London-Tokyo: University Park Press 1974.
Bajusz, E., Lossnitzer, K.: Ein neues Krankheitsmodell: Erbliche nichtvaskuläre Myokarddegeneration mit Herzinsuffizienz. Münch. med. Wschr. **31**, 1756–1768 (1968).
Beeler, G. W., Reuter, H.: The relation between membrane potential, membrane currents and activation of contraction in ventricular myocardial fibers. J. Physiol. (Lond.) **207**, 211–229 (1970).
Benfey, B. G.: Lack of relationship between myocardial cyclic AMP concentration and inotropic effects of sympathomimetic amines. Brit. J. Pharmacol. **43**, 757–763 (1971).
Bester, A. J., Gevers, W., Hawtrey, A. O.: A possible defect in protein synthesis underlying inherited cardiomyopathy of Syrian hamsters. In: Recent advances in studies on cardiac structure and metabolism, vol. 2: Cardiomyopathies. Baltimore-London-Tokyo: University Park Press 1973.
Bloom, S., Cancilla, P. A.: Myocytolysis and mitochondrial calcification in rat myocardium after low doses of isoproterenol. Amer. J. Path. **54**, 373–391 (1969).
Bloom, S., Davis, D. L.: Calcium as mediator of isoproterenol-induced myocardial necrosis. Amer. J. Path. **69**, 459–470 (1972).
Brachfeld, N.: The pathogenesis of myocardial cell death. In: Recent advances in studies on cardiac structure and metabolism, vol. 1: Myocardiology. Baltimore-London-Tokyo: University Park Press 1972.
Brigden, W.: Uncommon myocardial diseases. Lancet **1957 II**, 1179–1184, 1243–1249.
Brink, A. J., Lochner, A.: Work performance of the isolated perfused beating heart in the hereditary myocardiopathy of the Syrian hamster. Circulat. Res. **21**, 391–401 (1967).
Brink, A. J., Lochner, A., Kotze, J. C. N.: Contractility and tension development of the myopathic hamster (BIO 14.6) heart. Cardiovasc. Res. **3**, 453–458 (1969).
Buechner, F.: Die Pathologie der cellulären und geweblichen Oxydationen. Die Hypoxydosen. In: Handbuch der allgemeinen Pathologie. Berlin-Heidelberg-New York: Springer 1957.
Buechner, F.: Qualitative morphology of heart failure: light and electron microscopic characteristics of acute and chronic heart failure. In: Methods and achievments in experimental pathology. Basel: S. Karger 1971.
Buechner, F., Onishi, S.: Der Herzmuskel bei akuter Koronarinsuffizienz im elektronenmikroskopischen Bild. Munich-Berlin-Vienna: Urban & Schwarzenberg 1968.
Buechner, F., Onishi, S.: Herzhypertrophie und Herzinsuffizienz in der Sicht der Elektronenmikroskopie. Munich-Berlin-Vienna: Urban & Schwarzenberg 1970.
Cantin, M., Bajusz, E.: Changes in the juxtaglomerular apparatus and adrenal cortex of cardiomyopathic (BIO 14.6) hamsters. Trans. N.Y. Acad. Sci. **30**, 957–959 (1968).
Cantin, M., Leone, A., Bajusz, E.: Participation of renal electrolytes in the mechanism of edema in congestive heart failure: studies on cardiomyopathic hamsters. In: Recent advances in studies on cardiac structure and metabolism, vol. 1: Myocardiology. Baltimore-London-Tokyo: University Park Press 1972.
Case, R. B.: Myocardial potassium loss during ischemia. In: Recent advances in studies on cardiac structure and metabolism, vol. 1: Myocardiology. Baltimore-London-Tokyo: University Park Press 1972.
Caulfield, J. B., Klionsky, B.: Myocardial ischemia and early infarction. An electron microscopic study. Amer. J. Path. **35**, 489–523 (1959).
Chimoskey, J. E., Gergely, J.: Effect of norepinephrine, ouabain, and pH on cardiac sarcoplasmic reticulum. Arch. int. Pharmacodyn. **176**, 289–297 (1968).

CIBA FOUNDATION STUDY GROUP No. 37: Hypertrophic obstructive cardiomyopathy. London: J. & A. Churchill 1971.
CIBA FOUNDATION SYMPOSIUM: Cardiomyopathies. London: J. & A. Churchill 1964.
CORABOEUF, E.: Membrane ionic permeabilities and contractile phenomena in myocardium. Cardiovasc. Res., Suppl. I, 55–63 (1971).
CSAPÓ, Z., DUSEK, J., RONA, G.: Early alterations of the cardiac muscle cells in isoproterenol-induced necrosis. Arch. Path. **93**, 356–365 (1972).
DAVID, H., HECHT, A., UERLINGS, I.: Noradrenalinbedingte Feinstrukturveränderungen des Herzmuskels der Ratte. Beitr. path. Anat. **137**, 1–18 (1968).
DHALLA, N. S.: Studies on the phosphorylase activity in isolated perfused rat heart. Arch. int. Physiol. **74**, 476–488 (1966).
DHALLA, N. S.: Excitation-contraction coupling in heart. I. Comparison of calcium uptake by the sarcoplasmic reticulum and mitochondria of the rat heart. Arch. int. Physiol. Biochem. **77**, 916–933 (1969).
EBASHI, S., KODAMA, A., EBASHI, F.: Troponin: I. Preparation and physiological function. J. Biochem. **64**, 465–477 (1968).
EDINGTON, G. M., HUTT, M. S. R., PARRY, E. H. O., ANTIA, A. U.: Idiopathic cardiomegaly. Cardiologia (Basel) **52**, 33–43 (1968).
ENTMAN, M. L.: Calcium and cardiac contractility. Amer. J. med. Sci. **259**, 164–167 (1970).
EPSTEIN, S. E., SKELTON, C. L., LEVEY, G. S., ENTMAN, M.: Adenyl cyclase and myocardial contractility. Ann. intern. Med. **72**, 561–578 (1970).
FEDELESOVA, M., DHALLA, N. S.: High energy phosphate stores in the hearts of genetically dystrophic hamsters. J. molec. cell. Cardiol. **3**, 93–102 (1971).
FEJFAR, Z.: Cardiomyopathies—An international problem. Cardiologia (Basel) **52**, 9–19 (1968).
FERRANS, V. J., HIBBS, R. G., BLACK, W. C., WEILBAECHER, D. G.: Isoproterenol-induced myocardial necrosis. A histochemical and electron microscopic study. Amer. Heart J. **68**, 71–90 (1964).
FERRANS, V. J., HIBBS, R. G., CIPRIANO, P. R., BUJA, L. M.: Histochemical and electron microscopic studies of norepinephrine-induced myocardial necroses in rats. In: Recent advances in studies on cardiac structure and metabolism, vol. 1: Myocardiology. Baltimore-London-Tokyo: University Park Press 1972.
FERRANS, V. J., HIBBS, R. G., WEILY, H. S., WEILBAECHER, D. G., WALSH, J. J., BURCH, G. E.: A histochemical and electron microscopic study of epinephrine-induced myocardial necrosis. J. molec. cell. Cardiol. **1**, 11–22 (1970).
FERRANS, V. J., MASSUMI, R. A., SHUGOLL, G. I., ALI, N., ROBERTS, W. C.: Ultrastructural studies of myocardial biopsies in 45 patients with obstructive or congestive cardiomyopathy. In: Recent advances in studies on cardiac structure and metabolism, vol. 2: Cardiomyopathies. Baltimore-London-Tokyo: University Park Press 1973.
FERRANS, V. J., ROBERTS, W. C.: Myocardial ultrastructure in acute and chronic hypoxia. Cardiology **56**, 144–160 (1971/72).
FLECKENSTEIN, A.: Die Bedeutung der energiereichen Phosphate für Kontraktilität und Tonus des Myokards. Verh. dtsch. Ges. inn. Med. **70**, 81–99 (1964).
FLECKENSTEIN, A.: Myokardstoffwechsel und Nekrose. In: Herzinfarkt und Schock. Stuttgart: Georg Thieme 1969.
FLECKENSTEIN, A.: Neuere Ergebnisse zur Physiologie, Pharmakologie und Pathologie der elektromechanischen Koppelungsprozesse im Warmblütermyokard. In: Vorträge der Erlanger Physiologentagung 1970. Berlin-Heidelberg-New York: Springer 1971a.
FLECKENSTEIN, A.: Specific inhibitors and promotors of calcium action in the excitation-contraction coupling of heart muscle and their role in the prevention or production of myocardial lesions. In: Calcium and the heart. London-New York: Academic Press 1971b.
GERTZ, E. W., STAM, A. C., BAJUSZ, E., SONNENBLICK, E. H.: A biochemical defect in the function of the sarcoplasmic reticulum in the hereditary cardiopathy of the Syrian hamster. In: Recent advances in studies on cardiac structure and metabolism, vol. 1: Myocardiology. Baltimore-London-Tokyo: University Park Press 1972.
GERTZ, E. W., STAM, A. C., SONNENBLICK, E. H.: Dissociation of collagen proliferation from hypertrophy and experimental cardiomyopathy. Amer. J. Cardiol. **26**, 634–635 (1970a).
GERTZ, E. W., STAM, A. C., SONNENBLICK, E. H.: A quantitative and qualitative defect in the sarcoplasmic reticulum in the hereditary cardiomyopathy of the Syrian hamster. Biochem. biophys. Res. Commun. **40**, 746–753 (1970b).
GOODWIN, J. F.: Congestive and hypertropic cardiomyopathies. Lancet **1970 I**, 731–739.
GOODWIN, J. F.: Prospects and predictions for the cardiomyopathies. Circulation **50**, 210–219 (1974).
GROSSE-BROCKHOFF, F.: Zur Klassifizierung, Ätiologie und Pathogenese der Myokardiopathien. Dtsch. med. Wschr. **96**, 659–663 (1971).

GUDBJARNASON, S.: Inhibition of energy transfer in ischemic heart muscle. In: Recent advances in studies on cardiac structure and metabolism, vol. 1: Myocardiology. Baltimore-London-Tokyo: University Park Press 1972.

HAJDU, S., POSNER, C. J.: Absence of Bowditch-phenomenon in the ventricular muscle of hamsters with hereditary cardiomyopathy. Amer. Heart J. **81**, 781–789 (1971).

HARIGAYA, S., SCHWARTZ, A.: The rate of calcium binding and uptake in normal animals and failing cardiac muscle: membrane vesicles ("relaxing system") and mitochondria. Circulat. Res. **25**, 781–794 (1969).

HASSELBACH, W.: Die chemomechanische Koppelung im contractilen System des Myokards. Verh. dtsch. Ges. inn. Med. **77**, 13–19 (1971).

HATT, P. Y., MORAVEC, J.: Acute hypoxia of the myocardium. Ultrastructural changes. Cardiology **56**, 73–84 (1971/72).

HAUGAARD, N., HAUGAARD, E. S., LEE, N. H., HORN, R. S.: Possible role of mitochondria in regulation of cardiac contractility. Fed. Proc. **28**, 1657–1662 (1969).

HECHT, A.: Einführung in experimentelle Grundlagen moderner Herzmuskelpathologie. Jena: VEB Gustav Fischer 1970.

HEGGTVEIT, H. A., HERMAN, L., MISHRA, R. K.: Cardiac necrosis and calcification in experimental magnesium deficiency. A light and electron microscopic study. Amer. J. Path. **45**, 757–782 (1964).

HEYWOOD, S. M., DOWBEN, R. M., RICH, A.: The identification of polyribosomes synthesizing myosin. Proc. nat. Acad. Sci. (Wash.) **57**, 1002–1009 (1967).

HIGHMAN, B., ALTLAND, P. D., GARBUS, J.: Pathological and serum-enzyme changes after epinephrine in oil and adrenergic blocking agent. Arch. Path. **80**, 332–344 (1965).

HIOTT, D. W.: Ultrastructural changes in heart muscle after hemorrhagic shock and isoproterenol infusions. Arch. int. Pharmacodyn. **180**, 206–216 (1969).

HOAK, J. C., WARNER, E. D., CONNOR, W. E.: New concept of levaterenol-induced acute myocardial necrosis. Arch. Path. **87**, 332–338 (1969).

HOLTZER, H., MARSHALL, J. M., FINCK, H.: An analysis of myogenesis by the use of fluorescent antimyosin. J. biophys. biochem. Cytol. **3**, 705–725 (1957).

HOMBURGER, F., BAKER, J. R., NIXON, C. W., WILGRAM, G.: New hereditary disease of Syrian hamsters. Primary, generalized polymyopathy and cardiac necrosis. Arch. intern. Med. **110**, 660–662 (1962).

HOMBURGER, F., NIXON, C. W., EPPENBERGER, M., BAKER, J. R.: Hereditary myopathy in Syrian hamster: studies on pathogenesis. Ann. N.Y. Acad. Sci. **138**, 14–27 (1966).

HONIG, C. R.: Effect of catecholamine analogs on the utilization of calcium by cardiac actomyosin systems. In: Heart failure. Pathophysiological and clinical aspects. Stuttgart: Georg Thieme 1968.

HONIG, C. R., REDDY, Y. S.: Effect of catecholamine analogs on control of actomyosin by native tropomyosin and calcium: the nature of the negative inotropic reception. J. Pharmacol. exp. Ther. **184**, 330–338 (1973).

HORNBROOK, K. R., CABRAL, A.: Enhancement by thyroid hormone treatment of norepinephrine-induced phosphorylase activation in the rat heart. Biochem. Pharmacol. **21**, 897–907 (1972).

HORVATH, E., BAJUSZ, E., KOVACS, K.: Study of the hypothalamic-hypophyseal system in hereditary cardiomyopathic hamsters. In: Recent advances in studies on cardiac structure and metabolism, vol. 1: Myocardiology. Baltimore-London-Tokyo: University Park Press 1972.

JASMIN, G., BAJUSZ, E.: Myocardial lesions in strain 129 dystrophic mice. Nature (Lond.) **193**, 181–182 (1962).

JEFFREY, F. E., WAGNER, R., ABELMANN, W. H.: Left and right ventricular pressures in the normal and the cardiomyopathic Syrian hamster (Mesocricetus auratus) (35175). Proc. Soc. exp. Biol. (N.Y.) **135**, 940–943 (1970).

JENNINGS, R. B., KALTENBACH, J. P., SOMMERS, H. M.: Cell death: electrolyte alteration in injured and dying myocardial cells. In: Electrolytes and cardiovascular diseases. Basel-New York: S. Karger 1965.

JENNINGS, R. B., SOMMERS, H. M., HERDSON, P. B., KALTENBACH, J. P.: Part II. Cardiopathies and factors influencing myocardial degeneration. Ischemic injury of myocardium. Ann. N.Y. Acad. Sci. **156**, 61–78 (1969).

JENNY, E.: Die physikalischen Eigenschaften der kontraktilen Proteine bei suffizientem und insuffizientem Myokard. In: Heart failure. Pathophysiological and clinical aspects. Stuttgart: Georg Thieme 1968.

KATZ, A. M.: Absence of direct actions of norepinephrine on cardiac myosin and cardiac actomyosin. Amer. J. Physiol. **212**, 39–42 (1967).

KATZ, A. M.: The force-velocity curve. A biochemist's view-point. Cardiology **57**, 2–10 (1972).

KATZ, A. M., GOODHARDT, P. J., GOODHARDT, H. L.: Calcium and the cardiac contractile proteins. In: Calcium and the heart. London-New York: Academic Press 1971.

KATZ, A. M., REPKE, D. I.: Calcium-membrane interactions in the myocardium: Effects of ouabain, epinephrine and 3',5'-cyclic adenosine monophosphate. Amer. J. Cardiol. **31**, 193–201 (1973).

KELLEY, T. F.: Altered lipoprotein lipase and lipid metabolism in the myocardium of BIO 14.6 myopathic hamsters. Trans. N.Y. Acad. Sci. **30**, 960–961 (1968).

KOHLHARDT, M., BAUER, B., KRAUSE, H., FLECKENSTEIN, A.: Differentiation of the transmembrane Na and Ca channels in mammalian cardiac fibers by the use of specific inhibitors. Pflügers Arch. **335**, 309–322 (1972).

KOHRMAN, A. F.: Patterns of development of adenyl cyclase activity and norepinephrine responsiveness in the rat. Pediat. Res. **7**, 575–581 (1973).

KORB, G.: Heart diseases of unknown etiology: problems of terminology and classification. In: Recent advances in studies on cardiac structure and metabolism, vol. 2: Cardiomyopathies. Baltimore-London-Tokyo: University Park Press 1973.

KORB, G., TOTOVIĆ, V.: Electron microscopic studies on experimental ischemic lesions of the heart. Ann. N.Y. Acad. Sci. **156**, 48–60 (1969).

KUEBLER, W., KUHN, H., LOOGEN, F.: Die Kardiomyopathien. Ihre Einteilung nach ätiologischen und klinischen Gesichtspunkten. Z. Kardiologie **62**, 3–22 (1973).

KUEBLER, W., SHINEBOURNE, E. A.: Calcium and the mitochondria. In: Calcium and the heart. London-New York: Academic Press 1971.

LEGATO, M. J., LANGER, G. A.: The subcellular localization of calcium ion in mammalian myocardium. J. Cell Biol. **41**, 401–423 (1969).

LEHNINGER, A. L.: Mitochondria and calcium ion transport. The fifth jubilee lecture. Biochem. J. **119**, 129–138 (1970).

LEHR, D., KRUKOWSKI, M., CHAU, R.: Acute myocardial injury produced by sympathomimetic amines. Israel J. med. Sci. **5**, 519–524 (1969).

LINDENMAYER, G. E., HARIGAYA, S., BAJUSZ, E., SCHWARTZ, A.: Oxidative phosphorylation and calcium transport of mitochondria isolated from cardiomyopathic hamster hearts. J. molec. cell. Cardiol. **1**, 249–259 (1970).

LOCHNER, A., BRINK, A., BRINK, A. J.: Protein synthesis in the myocardiopathy and muscular dystrophy of the Syrian hamster. Clin. Sci. **40**, 89–94 (1971).

LOCHNER, A., BRINK, A. J., WALT, J. J. VAN DER: The significance of biochemical and structural changes in the development of the myocardiopathy in the Syrian hamster. J. molec. cell. Cardiol. **1**, 47–64 (1970).

LOCHNER, A., OPIE, L. H., BRINK, A. J., BOSMAN, A. R.: Defective oxidative phosphorylation in hereditary myocardiopathy in the Syrian hamster. Cardiovasc. Res. **3**, 297–307 (1968).

LOSSNITZER, K., BAJUSZ, E.: Water and electrolyte alterations during the life course of the BIO 14.6 Syrian golden hamster. A disease model of a hereditary cardiomyopathy. J. molec. cell. Cardiol. **6**, 163–177 (1974).

LOSSNITZER, K., JANKE, J., HEIN, B., STAUCH, M., FLECKENSTEIN, A.: Disturbed myocardial calcium metabolism — A possible pathogenic factor in the hereditary cardiomyopathy of the Syrian hamster. In: Recent advances in studies on cardiac structure and metabolism, vol. 5: Myocardial cell damage. (In press.) Baltimore-London-Tokyo: University Park Press 1974a.

LOSSNITZER, K., MOHR, W.: Prevention of myocardial necroses in myopathic hamsters. J. IRCS **1**, 14 (1973).

LOSSNITZER, K., STEINHARDT, B., GREWE, N., STAUCH, M.: Charakteristische Elektrolytveränderungen bei der erblichen Myopathie mit Kardiomyopathie des Syrischen Goldhamsters (Stamm BIO 8262). Basic Res. Cardiol., in press (1974b).

LUCHI, R. J., KRITCHER, E. M.: Drug effects on cardiac myosin adenosine triphosphatase activity. J. Pharmacol. exp. Ther. **158**, 540–545 (1967).

MACLENNAN, D. H., SEEMAN, P., ILES, G. H., YIP, C. C.: Membrane formation by the adenosine triphosphatase of sarcoplasmic reticulum. J. biol. Chem. **246**, 2702–2710 (1971).

MALLOV, S., CERRA, F.: Effect of ethanol intoxication and catecholamines on cardiac lipoprotein lipase activity in rats. J. Pharmacol. exp. Ther. **156**, 426–444 (1967).

MARKWALD, R. R.: Distribution and relationship of precursor Z material to organizing myofibrillar bundles in embryonic rat and hamster ventricular myocytes. J. molec. cell. Cardiol. **5**, 341–350 (1973).

MARTONOSI, A., DONLEY, J. R., PUCELL, A. G., HALPIN, R. A.: Sarcoplasmic reticulum XI. The mode of involvement of phospholipids in the hydrolysis of ATP by sarcoplasmic reticulum membranes. Arch. Biochem. **144**, 529–540 (1971).

MARUFFO, C. A.: Fine structural study of myocardial changes induced by isoproterenol in Rhesus monkeys (Macaca mulatta). Amer. J. Path. **50**, 27–37 (1967).

Mascher, D., Peper, K.: Two components of inward current in myocardial muscle fibers. Pflügers Arch. **307**, 190–203 (1969).
McCallister, L. P., Page, E.: Effects of thyroxin on ultrastructure of rat myocardial cells: a stereological study. J. Ultrastruct. Res. **42**, 136–155 (1973).
McCollum, W. B., Crow, C., Harigaya, S., Bajusz, E., Schwartz, A.: Calcium binding by cardiac relaxing system isolated from myopathic Syrian hamsters (strain 14.6, 8262, and 4054). J. molec. cell. Cardiol. **1**, 445–457 (1970).
McNeill, J. H., Brody, T. M.: The effect of d- and l-norepinephrine on rat cardiac phosphorylase activation. J. Pharmacol. exp. Ther. **165**, 97–101 (1969).
Meessen, H., Poche, R.: Pathomorphologie des Myokards. In: Das Herz des Menschen. Stuttgart: Georg Thieme 1963.
Michelson, A. M., Russell, E. S., Harman, P. J.: Dystrophia muscularis: a hereditary primary myopathy in the house mouse. Proc. nat. Acad. Sci. (Wash.) **41**, 1079–1084 (1955).
Mohr, W., Hersener, J., Lossnitzer, K.: Der Nachweis von Calcium-Phosphat in der Herzmuskulatur mittels Röntgenmikroanalyse. Virchows Arch. Abt. A **358**, 259–264 (1973).
Mohr, W., Lossnitzer, K.: Morphologische und klinische Manifestationen der hereditären Myopathie beim Syrischen Goldhamster (BIO 8262). Verh. dtsch. Ges. Path. **56**, 645 (1972).
Mohr, W., Lossnitzer, K.: Morphologische Untersuchungen an Hamstern des Stammes BIO 8262 mit erblicher Myopathie und Kardiomyopathie. Beitr. Path. **153**, 178–193 (1974).
Moretti, A., Arcari, G., Laterza, L., Suchowsky, G. K.: The effect of catecholamines and adrenergic blocking agents on the calcium and glycogen content in the rat heart. Farmaco, Ed. sci. **28**, 3–7 (1973).
Morin, Y., Cote, G.: Toxic agents and cardiomyopathies. Cardiovasc. Clin. **4**, 245–267 (1972).
Murad, F., Chi, Y. M., Rall, T. W., Sutherland, E. W.: Adenyl cyclase. III. The effect of catecholamines and choline esters on the formation of adenosine 3′,5′-phosphate by preparations from cardiac muscle and liver. J. biol. Chem. **237**, 1233–1238 (1962).
Nadkarni, B. B., Hunt, B., Heggtveit, H. A.: Early ultrastructural and biochemical changes in the myopathic hamster heart. In: Recent advances in studies on cardiac structure and metabolism, vol. 1: Myocardiology. Baltimore-London-Tokyo: University Park Press 1972.
Nair, K. G., Umali, T.: Increased RNA polymerase activity in the cardiomyopathy of the Syrian hamster. Circulation **42**, Suppl. III–61 (1970).
Nakao, K., Oka, M., Chen, C., Bajusz, E., Angrist, A.: Studies of the spontaneous myocardiopathy in the BIO 14.6 strain of hamster. Path. et Microbiol. (Basel) **35**, 118–124 (1970).
Nayler, W. G.: An effect of ouabain on the superficially located stores of calcium in cardiac muscle cells. J. molec. cell. Cardiol. **5**, 101–110 (1973).
Nayler, W. G., McInnes, I., Swann, J. B., Price, J. M., Carson, V., Race, D., Lowe, T. E.: Some effects of iproveratril (Isoptin) on the cardiovascular system. J. Pharmacol. exp. Ther. **161**, 247–261 (1968).
Nayler, W. G., Merrillees, N. C. R.: Cellular exchange of calcium. In: Calcium and the heart. London-New York: Academic Press 1971.
Noorden, S. van, Olsen, E. G. J., Pearse, A. G. E.: Hypertrophic obstructive cardiomyopathy, a histological, histochemical, and ultrastructural study of biopsy material. Cardiovasc. Res. **5**, 118–131 (1971).
Olsen, E. G. J.: Pathology of hypertrophic obstructive cardiomyopathy. In: Recent advances in studies on cardiac structure and metabolism, vol. 2: Cardiomyopathies. Baltimore-London-Tokyo: University Park Press 1973.
Olson, R. E.: Introduction to calcium and the heart. In: Calcium and the heart. London-New York: Academic Press 1971.
Olson, R. E., Dhalla, N. S., Sun, C. N.: Changes in energy stores in the hypoxic heart. Cardiology **56**, 114–124 (1971/72).
Onishi, S., Bajusz, E., Buechner, F., Rickers, K.: Herzmuskelhypertrophie bei erbbedingter Myopathie des syrischen Hamsters nach elektronenmikroskopischen Untersuchungen. Beitr. path. Anat. **140**, 119–141 (1970).
Onishi, S., Buechner, F., Zittel, R., Therman, M.: Das elektronenmikroskopische Bild der Herzmuskelzelle des Hundes bei experimenteller Herzhypertrophie in der Anpassungsphase. Beitr. path. Anat. **139**, 94–114 (1969).
Opie, L. H., Owen, P.: Glycolysis in acute experimental myocardial infarction: pathways of metabolism and preliminary results. In: Recent advances in studies on cardiac structure and metabolism, vol. 2: Cardiomyopathies. Baltimore-London-Tokyo: University Park Press 1973.
Owens, K., Weglicki, W. B., Sonnenblick, E. H., Gertz, E. W.: Phospholipid and cholesterol content of ventricular tissue from the cardiomyopathic Syrian hamster. J. molec. cell. Cardiol. **4**, 229–236 (1972).

PATRIARCA, P., CARAFOLI, E.: A study of intracellular transport of calcium in rat heart. J. Cell Physiol. **72**, 29–38 (1968).

PEARSE, A. G. E.: The histochemistry and electron microscopy of obstructive cardiomyopathy. In: CIBA-Foundation Symposium on Cardiomyopathies. London: J. & A. Churchill 1964.

PFITZER, P., KNIERIEM, H.-J., DIETRICH, H., HERBERTZ, G.: Hypertrophie des Rattenherzens nach Isoproterenol (morphometrische, elektronenmikroskopische, autoradiographische, cytophotometrische und biochemische Befunde). Virchows Arch. Abt. B **12**, 22–38 (1972).

POCHE, R.: Das submikroskopische Bild der Herzmuskelveränderungen nach Überdosierung von Schilddrüsenhormon. Beitr. path. Anat. **118**, 407–420 (1957).

POCHE, R.: Über den Einfluß von Dinitrophenol und Thyroxin auf die Ultrastruktur des Herzmuskels bei der Ratte. Virchows Arch. path. Anat. **335**, 282–297 (1962).

REGAN, T. J., MOSCHOS, C. B., OLDEWURTEL, H. A., WEISSE, A. B., ASOKAN, S. K.: Dominance of lipid metabolism in the myocardium under the influence of l-norepinephrine. J. Lab. clin. Med. **70**, 221–228 (1967).

REUTER, H.: Über die Wirkung von Adrenalin auf den cellulären Ca-Umsatz des Meerschweinchenvorhofs. Naunyn-Schmiedebergs Arch. exp. Path. Pharmak. **251**, 401–412 (1965).

REUTER, H.: The dependence of slow inward current in Purkinje fibres on the extracellular calcium concentration. J. Physiol. (Lond.) **192**, 479–492 (1967).

REUTER, H., BEELER, G. W.: Calcium current and activation of contraction in ventricular myocardial fibers. Science **163**, 399–401 (1969).

ROBAK, J., GRYGLEWSKI, R.: The influence of propranolol, inpea, iproveratril and some l-naphthylethyl-amine derivates on the myocardial phosphorylase activity. Biochem. Pharmacol. **19**, 1221–1227 (1970).

ROBERTS, W. C., FERRANS, V. J.: Morphologic observations in the cardiomyopathies. In: Myocardial disease. New York: Grune & Stratton 1973.

RONA, G.: Cardiac adaptation to insult. In: Papers from the Symposium on Metabolism and Disease presented by the Food and Drug Directorate in Ottawa, Canada, June 10 and 11, 1971, p. 50–59. Health and Welfare Canada 1971.

RONA, G., BOUTET, M., HUETTNER, I.: Membrane permeability alterations as manifestations of early cardiac muscle cell injury. In: Recent advances in studies on cardiac structure and metabolism, vol. 5: Myocardial cell damage. (In press.) Baltimore-London-Tokyo: University Park Press 1974.

RONA, G., CHAPPEL, C. I., BALAZS, T., GAUDRY, R.: An infarct-like myocardial lesion and other toxic manifestations produced by isoproterenol in the rat. Arch. Path. **67**, 443–455 (1959).

RONA, G., DUSEK, J.: Studies on the mechanism of increased myocardial resistance. In: Recent advances in studies on cardiac structure and metabolism, vol. 1: Myocardiology. Baltimore-London-Tokyo: University Park Press 1972.

SCHENK, E. A., MOSS, A. J.: Cardiovascular effects of sustained norepinephrine infusions. II. Morphology. Circulat. Res. **18**, 605–615 (1966).

SCHWARTZ, A.: Calcium and the sarcoplasmic reticulum. In: Calcium and the heart. London-New York: Academic Press 1971.

SCHWARTZ, A., LINDENMAYER, G. E., HARIGAYA, S.: Respiratory control and calcium transport in heart mitochondria from the cardiomyopathic Syrian hamster. Trans. N.Y. Acad. Sci. **30**, 951–954 (1968).

SELYE, H.: The chemical prevention of cardiac necrosis. New York: The Ronald Press Company 1958.

SELYE, H.: The pluricausal cardiopathies. Springfield, Ill.: Charles C. Thomas 1961.

SELYE, H.: Experimental cardiovascular diseases, part 1. Berlin-New York-Heidelberg: Springer 1970.

SHAH, D. O., SCHULMAN, J. H.: Influence of calcium, cholesterol, and unsaturation on lecithin monolayers. J. Lipid Res. **8**, 215–226 (1967).

SHEN, A. C., JENNINGS, R. B.: Myocardial calcium and magnesium in acute ischemic injury. Amer. J. Path. **67**, 417–434 (1972a).

SHEN, A. C., JENNINGS, R. B.: Kinetics of calcium accumulation in acute myocardial ischemic injury. Amer. J. Path. **67**, 441–452 (1972b).

SHIGENOBU, K., SPERELAKIS, N.: Calcium current channels induced by catecholamines in chick embryonic hearts whose fast socium channels are blocked by tetrodotoxin or elevated potassium. Circulat. Res. **31**, 932–952 (1972).

SHIMAMOTO, T., HIRAMOTO, Y.: Electron microscopic observations on edematous myocardial response to epinephrine. In: Prevention of ischemic heart disease: principles and practice. Springfield, Ill.: Charles C. Thomas 1966.

SHINEBOURNE, E., WHITE, R.: Cyclic AMP and calcium uptake of the sarcoplasmic reticulum in relation to increased rate of relaxation under the influence of catecholamines. Cardiovasc. Res. **4**, 194–200 (1970).

SPIECKERMANN, P. G.: Relation between ultrastructural lesions and changes in the content of energy-rich phosphates in the ischemic myocardium. Cardiology **56**, 369–370 (1971/72).

STAUCH, M., LOSSNITZER, K.: Druck und Kontraktilität des linken Ventrikels unter verschiedenen Bedingungen beim syrischen Goldhamster mit hereditärer Kardiomyopathie. Verh. dtsch. Ges. Kreisl.-Forsch. **38**, 142–146 (1972).

STAUCH, M., LOSSNITZER, K.: Left ventricular function in Syrian hamsters of different age with hereditary cardiomyopathy. In: Recent advances in studies on cardiac structure and metabolism, vol. 5: Myocardial cell damage. (In press.) Baltimore-London-Tokyo: University Park Press 1974.

SULHAKE, P. V., DHALLA, N. S.: Excitation-contraction coupling in heart. III. Evidence against the involvement of adenosine cyclic 3′,5′-monophosphate in calcium transport by sarcotubular vesicles of canine myocardium. Molec. Pharmacol. **6**, 659–666 (1970).

SULHAKE, P. V., DHALLA, N. S.: Excitation-contraction coupling in heart. VII. Calcium accumulation in subcellular particles in congestive heart failure. J. clin. Invest. **50**, 1019–1027 (1971).

SUSIN, M., HERDSON, P. B.: Fine structural changes in rat myocardium induced by thyroxine and by magnesium deficiency. Arch. Path. **83**, 86–98 (1967).

SUZUKI, T.: Electron microscopic study on myocardial lesions in thiamine-deficient rats. Tohoku J. exp. Med. **91**, 249–259 (1957).

SZAKÁCS, J. E., CANNON, A.: l-norepinephrine myocarditis. Amer. J. clin. Path. **30**, 425–434 (1958).

SZOLLAR, L., PUCSOK, J., SZELENYI, I., SOS, J.: Lipid composition of serum, heart, and liver of hereditary myocardiopathic hamsters (BIO 14.6). In: Recent advances in studies on cardiac structure and metabolism, vol. 2: Cardiomyopathies. Baltimore-London-Tokyo: University Park Press 1973.

UNGAR, J., GILBERT, M., SIEGEL, A.: Studies on myocardial metabolism in diabetes. Amer. J. Med. **18**, 385–396 (1955).

VARGO, T. A., WOOD, J. M., SCHWARTZ, A.: An effect of ouabain on isolated heart tissue from cardiomyopathic Syrian hamsters. J. molec. cell. Cardiol. **4**, 495–506 (1972).

VEITH, G.: Experimentelle Untersuchungen zur Wirkung von Adrenalin auf den Herzmuskel. Arch. Kreisl.-Forsch. **6**, 335–360 (1940).

WEBER, A., HERZ, R., REISS, I.: The regulation of myofibrillar activity by calcium. Proc. roy. Soc. B **160**, 489–501 (1964).

WENZEL, D. G.: Drug-induced cardiomyopathies. J. pharm. Sci. **56**, 1209–1224 (1967).

WOLLENBERGER, A., ONNEN, K., HINTERBERGER, K., RABITZSCH, G., KLEITKE, B.: Myocardial protein synthesis in acute myocardial hypoxia and ischemia. Cardiology **56**, 48–64 (1971/72).

WORLD HEALTH ORGANIZATION (WHO). International work in cardiovascular diseases, 1959–1969. Genf 1969.

WROGEMANN, K., BLANCHAER, M. C.: Respiration and oxidative phosphorylation by muscle and heart mitochondria of hamsters with hereditary myocardiopathy and polymyopathy. Canad. J. Biochem. **46**, 323–329 (1968).

WROGEMANN, K., BLANCHAER, M. C.: On the role of the mitochondria in the hereditary cardiomyopathy of the Syrian hamster. In: Recent advances in studies on cardiac structure and metabolism, vol. 5: Myocardial cell damage. (In press.) Baltimore-London-Tokyo: University Park Press 1974.

Basic Actions of Ions and Drugs on Myocardial High-Energy Phosphate Metabolism and Contractility[1]

A. FLECKENSTEIN, H. J. DÖRING, J. JANKE, and Y. K. BYON

With 49 Figures

A. Introduction

It is generally assumed that the mechanical activity of contractile tissues is closely linked to the metabolism of high-energy phosphates, particularly adenosine triphosphate (ATP) and creatine phosphate (CP). The splitting of ATP is believed to be the primary source of contraction energy, ATP being instantaneously restored at the expense of CP. Subsequently, ATP and CP are resynthetized by a long chain of rapid recovery reactions which conserve, in the form of high-energy phosphate bonds, the free energy available from the aerobic and anaerobic substrate breakdown. As to heart muscle, contractility as well as cellular integrity clearly depend on an undisturbed oxygen supply. This led to the suggestion that contractile failure in general as well as structural damage of the myocardium might basically originate from hypoxic high-energy phosphate deficiency.

To obtain a more direct insight into the interrelationship between high-energy phosphate metabolism and myocardial contractility, extensive research work has been done over the past 3 decades, particularly with animal experiments. However, despite considerable effort, the biochemical background of contractile failure remained for some time rather obscure because the decrease in contractile force could obviously not be related to unidirectional changes in the myocardial organophosphate concentrations. Thus in certain forms of cardiac incompetence the expected exhaustion of the ATP and CP stores was easily detectable, whereas in other cases even elevated levels of the myocardial high-energy phosphate compounds were observed.

In this conflicting situation we decided, 20 years ago, to reinvestigate the problem by an exact analysis of a wide variety of experimentally produced disorders of cardiac contractility. The study was successful in that it led to a classification of acute experimental heart failure into two distinct types:

1. *The first type shows a reduction of cardiac contractility resulting from a true exhaustion of the high-energy phosphate stores.* The loss of contractility produced in this way is associated with a decrease of the CP fraction by 80 to 90%. This deficiency can be due to anoxia, coronary occlusion, carbon monoxide inhalation, or intravenous administration of metabolic poisons such as cyanide, fluoroacetate, or 2,4-dinitrophenol (FLECKENSTEIN, JANKE, and GERLACH, 1959; FLECKENSTEIN, 1960, 1963b; DÖRING and KAMMERMEIER, 1963).

---
[1] From the Physiological Institute, University of Freiburg, Federal Republic of Germany.

2. *The second type of heart incompetence, on the other hand, shows a reduction of cardiac contractility produced by a deficient utilization of high-energy phosphates.* In this case the synthesis of energy-rich phosphates is not impaired so that their concentrations may even be increased above the normal level. But the energy conserved in the form of ATP and CP cannot be channelled into the contraction process (FLECKENSTEIN, 1963a, b, 1964, 1965, 1967, 1968, 1970/71a, b, 1974; FLECKENSTEIN, DÖRING, and KAMMERMEIER, 1966, 1967, 1968, 1968a).

Needless to say that in both types of cardiac incompetence the energetic state is essentially identical as far as the amount of phosphate-bond energy, which is available to the contractile system, becomes insufficient. Therefore, in both types of cardiac incompetence the acute reactions of the contractile machinery are quite uniform, consisting of contractile weakness and ventricular dilation. The situation is comparable to a motorcar which stops if the gasoline tank is empty or if the utilization of the gasoline is blocked by some interference with internal combustion.

The aim of the present article is:

a) To summarize the experimental data on which this classification of contractile failure is based.

b) To accumulate further evidence for the function of ATP and CP as fundamental energy sources of systolic contractility and diastolic tone, and

c) to shed more light into the mechanism of action of a considerable number of drugs and poisons with inotropic heart effects.

B. Experimental Procedures

Most of the results to be discussed in the following chapters originate from studies carried out in our own laboratories. Thus some introductory remarks on the general methods used throughout these investigations are given.

Hearts in situ. Our observations were made on a total of more than 900 open chest preparations of guinea pigs and on 30 cats under artificial respiration. Throughout the experiments arterial and venous blood pressures were measured with suitable Statham elements of different sensitivity. In addition, new mechano-electronic methods were developed for a continuous registration of the systolic and diastolic heart diameter [KAMMERMEIER and DÖRING: Pflügers Arch. ges. Physiol. **273**, 311 (1961)], and for ultrasensitive recordings of the heart rate [KRAUSE: Z. Kreisl.-Forsch. 52, 128 (1963)]. Furthermore, in a smaller number of experiments, the concomitant changes in arterial oxygen tension were analyzed using an oxygen electrode [CARLSON, BRINK, and BRONK: Rev. of Sci. Inst. **21**, 923 (1950)]. Supplementary observations were also carried out on 200 *heart-lung preparations* of guinea pigs with a bubble flow meter to determine the systemic output of the failing hearts under strictly controlled conditions of arterial and venous blood pressure.

Isolated myocardium. For measurements of isometric tension transducer valves (RCA 5734) were applied on 420 electrically driven isolated rabbit atria and on about 600 isolated papillary muscles of guinea pigs, cats, and monkeys (*M. rhesus*). In most experiments on papillary muscles, single fiber action potentials or respiration rates were also recorded together with the mechanical activity. For this purpose intracellular microelectrodes and oxygen electrodes were used.

Chemical analysis. To investigate changes in the phosphate fractions of the myocardium, the ventricles of 440 guinea pigs, 200 rats, and 30 cats as well as 420 rabbit atria were frozen at different stages of contractile insufficiency. This was achieved either by immersion in liquid nitrogen, propanol, or isopentane or, in the case of isolated atria, by rapid compression of the tissue between 2 blocks of

Table 1. Concentrations of high-energy phosphate compounds in the left ventricular myocardium of hearts *in situ* (cat, rat, guinea pig) and heart–lung preparations (guinea pig). The figures represent the absolute concentrations (μM/g tissue wet weight) and the relative contents expressed as percentages of total acid-soluble phosphorus. Values shown are means ± standard error of the mean

	N	ATP		ADP		AMP		Ratio ATP/ADP	Creatine phosphate		Inorganic phosphate		
		μM/g	%	μM/g	%	μM/g	%		μM/g	%	μM/g	%	
Cat ventricle	6	4.3 ±0.21	34.7 ±0.80	0.8 ±0.03	4.5 ±0.22	0.5 ±0.03	1.3 ±0.04	5.4 ±0.15	7.6 ±0.03	20.3 ±0.09	3.8 ±0.09	10.2 ±0.09	Hearts *in situ*
Rat ventricle	32	4.7 ±0.06	43.2 ±0.40	1.0 ±0.04	6.1 ±0.20	0.6 ±0.04	1.8 ±0.10	4.9 ±0.13	6.4 ±0.11	19.9 ±0.30	3.1 ±0.11	9.4 ±0.30	Hearts *in situ*
Guinea pig ventricle	8	4.7 ±0.06	37.9 ±0.56	0.9 ±0.04	4.9 ±0.28	0.6 ±0.04	1.5 ±0.14	5.7 ±0.26	8.6 ±0.35	23.0 ±0.93	3.2 ±0.26	8.8 ±0.76	Hearts *in situ*
Guinea pig ventricle	12	4.6 ±0.12	37.6 ±0.72	0.8 ±0.02	4.3 ±0.11	0.6 ±0.02	1.6 ±0.07	5.7 ±0.17	7.9 ±0.22	21.2 ±0.44	4.4 ±0.11	11.8 ±0.26	Heart–lung preparations

Table 2. Influence of different tissue freezing techniques on the myocardial ATP, creatine phosphate, and inorganic phosphate concentrations of normal control hearts of guinea pigs. Values shown are means ± standard error of the mean

	ATP		Creatine phosphate		Inorganic phosphate	
	μM/g	%	μM/g	%	μM/g	%
Excision of heart under artificial respiration. Rapid immersion in liquid N_2	4.8 ±0.17	36.9 ±2.14	8.5 ±0.73	23.3 ±1.37	3.1 ±0.31	8.0 ±0.94
Excision of heart *without* artificial respiration. Rapid immersion in liquid N_2	3.1 ±0.14	33.4 ±1.13	1.4 ±0.22	5.2 ±0.84	8.0 ±0.92	29.3 ±3.31
Freezing of heart *in situ* with propanol (−95° C) under artificial respiration	5.0 ±0.10	41.0 ±1.76	6.9 ±0.61	18.0 ±1.41	3.7 ±0.34	9.3 ±1.13
Freezing of heart *in situ* with petroleum ether (−150° C) under artificial respiration	4.6 ±0.04	37.2 ±1.02	7.9 ±0.23	21.2 ±0.25	3.3 ±0.22	8.8 ±0.50

deeply cooled aluminium [WOLLENBERGER, RISTAU, and SCHOFFA: Pflügers Arch. ges. Physiol. **270**, 399 (1960)]. Then the frozen tissue, thoroughly cleaned from ventricular blood with a dental whirl, was ground and extracted with ice-cold 0.3 M perchloric acid. After neutralizing the extracts, the separation and purification of the most prominent phosphate compounds, e.g. ATP, ADP, AMP, CP, and inorganic phosphate, was carried out by means of paper chromatography[2] followed by a quantitative determination according to a modification [GERLACH and DEUTICKE: Biochem. Z. **337**, 477 (1963)] of the method of BARTLETT: J. Biol. Chem. **234**, 466 (1959). The analytical figures were calculated for blood-free ventricular tissue if the intramural blood content exceeded 8% of the fresh weight.

It is to be noted that the analytical data of the "normal" control values of ATP and CP in the myocardium will only reflect the "true" intracellular levels if the imminent hydrolysis of these very labile compounds is sufficiently inhibited by careful experimental techniques. This requires not only suitable procedures of tissue freezing, extract neutralization, and separation on paper, but also the prevention of a hypoxic high-energy phosphate breakdown during the preceding experimental stages (thoracotomy; excision of the hearts). As pointed out by FLECKENSTEIN, JANKE, and GERLACH (1959a), it seems to be primarily due to inadequate treatment of the cardiac tissue that, in the past, most of the classical data concerning the "normal" ATP and CP concentrations of the intact ventricular myocardium were definitely too low (EGGLETON and EGGLETON, 1927; LE PAGE, 1946; MOMMAERTS, 1951; COPER, HERKEN, and SENFT, 1958; MICHAL, NAEGLE, DANFORTH, BALLARD, and BING, 1959; SCHMITZ, 1961; and others). The higher figures obtained in our own experiments are listed in Table 1. With adequate methods even the myocardial high-energy phosphate contents of heart–lung preparations are nearly equal to those of normal guinea pig hearts *in situ*. This indicates that heart–lung preparations are also suitable for the studies concerned.

[2] For more technical details see FLECKENSTEIN and JANKE: Pflügers Arch. ges. Physiol. **258**, 177 (1953); **265**, 237 (1957); GERLACH and JANKE: Biochem. Z. **330**, 565 (1958); FLECKENSTEIN, JANKE and GERLACH: Klin. Wschr. **37**, 451 (1959); SCHILDBERG and FLECKENSTEIN: Pflügers Arch. ges. Physiol. **283**, 137 (1965).

The most important technical improvement probably consists of taking out the hearts under artificial air respiration. Interestingly enough, in such experiments the CP content of normal left ventricular myocardium of guinea pigs was approximately 5–6 times greater than that of another group of animals in which the respiration pump was stopped during this operation for about 10 sec (Table 2). Conversely, the different freezing techniques with liquid nitrogen, propanol (−95° C), petroleum ether (−150° C), or isopentane (−170° C) did not produce specific changes in the ATP and CP concentrations.

C. Contractile Failure as a Result of Cardiac High-Energy Phosphate Exhaustion

I. Myocardial High-Energy Phosphate Breakdown in Anoxia or Ischemia

Many authors have shown that anoxia or ischemia leads to a rapid drop in myocardial CP and ATP (FAWAZ, HAWA, and TUTUNJI, 1957; FLECKENSTEIN, JANKE, and GERLACH, 1959; THORN, HEIMANN, MÜLDENER, ISSELHARD, and GERCKEN, 1959; SZEKERES and SCHEIN, 1959; ISSELHARD, 1960; LAMPRECHT, MICHAL, and NÄGLE, 1961; DÖRING and KAMMERMEIER, 1961; BENSON, EVANS, HALLAWAY, PHIBBS, and FREIER, 1961; FEINSTEIN ,1962; NÄGLE, HOCKERTS, and BÖGELMANN, 1964). Accordingly, in our experiments on thoracotomized guinea pigs, rats, and cats, creatine phosphate was reduced in the myocardium of the left ventricle by about 80 to 90% after artificial respiration had been stopped for 1 min. ATP decreases more slowly so that only about one-third of the normal

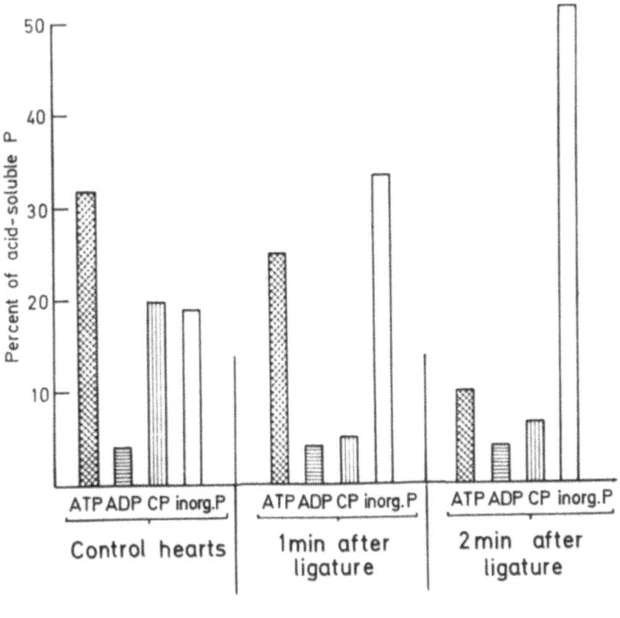

Fig. 1. Breakdown of CP and ATP within 1 and 2 min, respectively, following the ligature of both coronary arteries. Analytical data obtained from the apical region of the left ventricular myocardium of 2 cats (FLECKENSTEIN, JANKE, and GERLACH, 1959)

ATP content of the myocardium was lost within 3 min. Inorganic phosphate changes in the opposite direction. Practically identical results were obtained in the ischemic myocardial tissue of cats after coronary occlusion or if pure nitrogen was administered by the respiration pump (FLECKENSTEIN, JANKE, and GERLACH, 1959). Fig. 1 demonstrates the acute CP and ATP breakdown in the apical region of 2 cat hearts within 1 and 2 min, respectively, after ligature of both coronary arteries. Due to fibrillation, contractility of the hearts had nearly ceased when the tissue was frozen in liquid nitrogen. Although the myocardial CP is always more rapidly exhausted than the ATP fraction, the degradation of the ATP fraction also becomes nearly complete when the duration of asphyxia or ischemia is extended to 10 or 15 min (Fig. 3). But if, on the other hand, air respiration is resumed with a delay of no longer than 3 to 4 min the recovery of CP is nearly as quick as its breakdown. The restoration of the ATP concentration was usually somewhat retarded.

II. Time Correlation between Creatine Phosphate Loss and Ventricular Dilation

The characteristic changes in the high-energy phosphate content, particularly in the CP supply, are closely associated with alterations in cardiac contractility. Most obvious—amongst other symptoms of cardiac failure—is an acute increase of the diastolic volume of both ventricles (Fig. 2). This dilation is partly due to the reduction of systolic output. But apart from this, the deficiency of high-energy phosphates clearly affects the diastolic tonus. The acute dilation of anoxic or asphytic hearts has been described by many authors (MATHISON, 1910; FÜHNER and STARLING, 1913; ZONDEK, 1919; GREMELS and STARLING, 1926; JARISCH and WASTL, 1926; BARCROFT, 1927; TAKEUCHI, 1925; LOEWY and MAYER, 1926; STRUGHOLD, 1930; RUSHMER, 1961; BÜCHNER and IIJIMA, 1961). According to TAKEUCHI's results

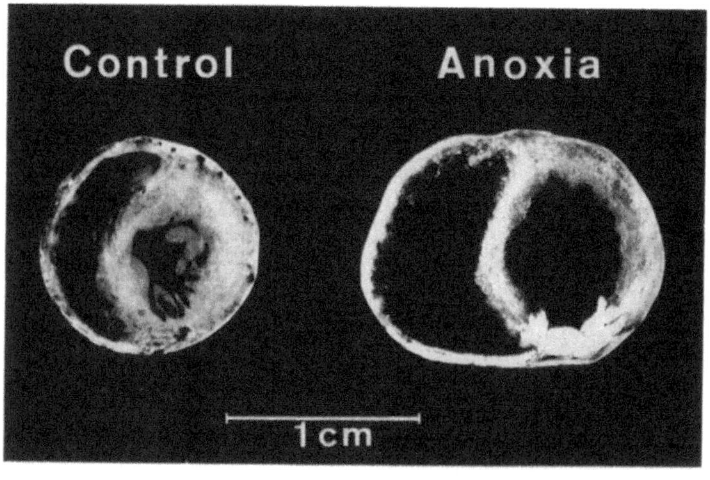

Fig. 2. Acute anoxic dilation of a guinea pig heart due to artificial respiration with pure nitrogen for 3 min. The dry weight of the dilated heart corresponds with that of the control. Furthermore, the body weights of the 2 animals were identical (Observations of FLECKENSTEIN, DÖRING, KAMMERMEIER, and HILDEBRANDT; see FLECKENSTEIN: Proceedings 6th Internat. Congr. Internal Med., pp. 37–51. Basel: Benno Schwabe, 1960)

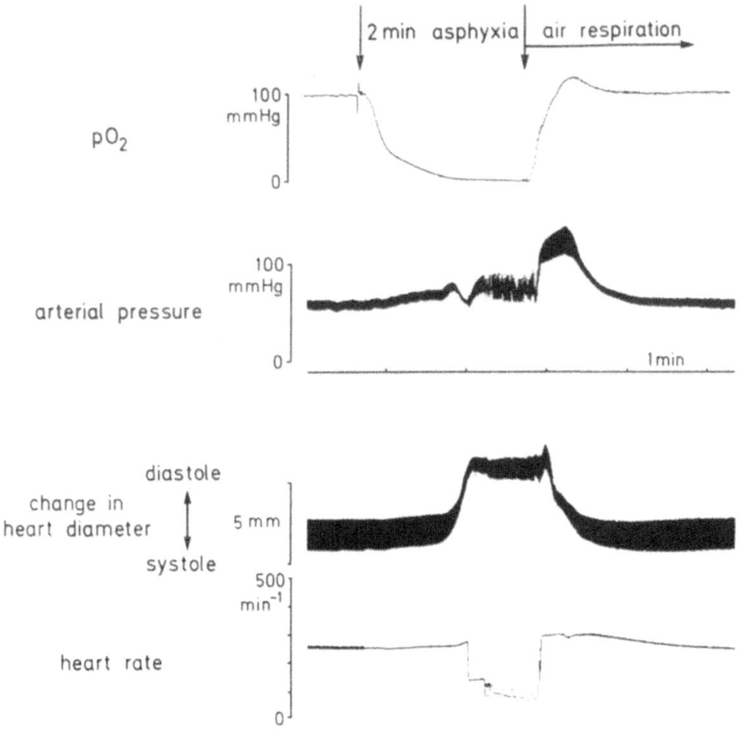

Fig. 3. Time correlation between some hemodynamic parameters such as arterial pressure heart diameter, contraction amplitude, cardiac frequency, and the arterial oxygen content (pO_2) during acute asphyxia of 2 min. The experiment was carried out on a guinea pig (open chest preparation with the pericardium removed). Each increase in heart diameter (diastole, ventricular dilation) produces an upward deflection of the recording system whereas each downward movement means a decrease in heart diameter (systole, restoration of cardiac tone). The pO_2 was measured with an oxygen electrode in the carotid artery. Severe cardiac incompetence developed at a pO_2 of approximately 10 mm Hg. The rise in arterial blood pressure is caused by a concomitant increase in sympathetic activity. However, the maximum blood pressure response to the liberated sympathetic transmitters is postponed until contractile force recovers upon readmission of air. At the peak of cardiac dilation the heart rate dropped to less than one half of the normal due to a partial block of AV-conduction

and our own observations, the maximum ventricular expansion is reached when the oxygen saturation of the blood falls to almost zero (Fig. 3). OPITZ and SCHNEIDER (1950) reported dilation at a venous pO_2 of 12 mm Hg. As to the critical oxygen saturation of the arterial blood at which contractile failure develops, the figures differ more widely: 50% according to JARISCH and WASTL (1926) and ALLELA (1958); 40% according to GREMELS and STARLING (1926); 30% according to BRETSCHNEIDER (1958); and 10 to 20% according to GORLIN and LEWIS (1954) and MERKER (1943). Probably with regard to these largely scattered data no serious attempt has been made by these authors to correlate the development of cardiac incompetence with definite alterations in myocardial metabolism.

The first reports about the surprisingly close interrelation-ship between myocardial CP content and diastolic ventricular volume were presented by FLECKENSTEIN (1960), DÖRING and KAMMERMEIER (1963) and FLECKENSTEIN (1964). Fig. 4 shows the striking time correlation between the mechanical behavior of a

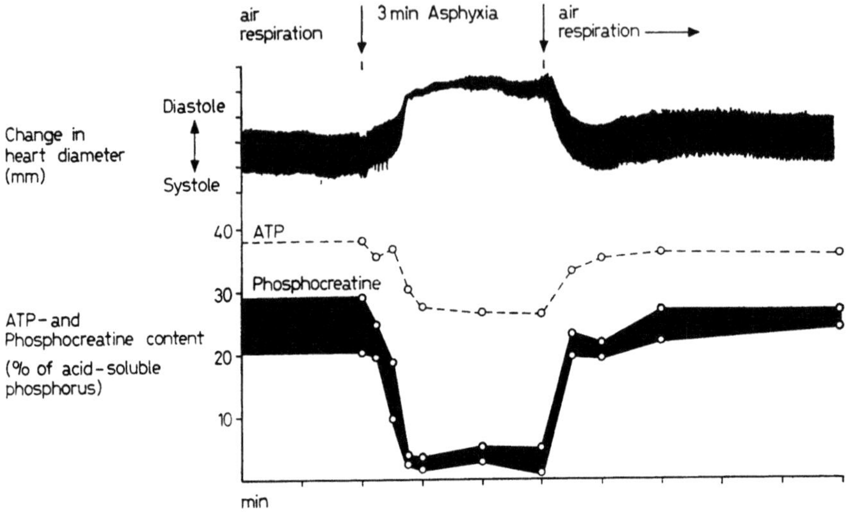

Fig. 4. Time correlation between mechanical activity and changes in the high-energy phosphate content of the guinea pig myocardium in a state of asphyxia, and thereafter, during post-asphyctic recovery. Obviously the acute ventricular dilation and the reduction in contraction amplitude during the 1st min of asphyxia coincide completely with the drop in creatine phosphate (CP). Accordingly, contractility and heart diameter return to normal as soon as the CP supply is restored after resuming respiration. The concentrations of CP, ATP, and inorganic P were analyzed in 32 asphyctic or postasphyctic left ventricles (open chest preparations). The values are expressed as per cent of the total acid-soluble phosphorus of the blood-free cardiac tissue. The absolute control values obtained on 32 non-asphyxiated hearts were as follows: ATP 4.6 (± 0.1); CP 8.3 (± 0.25); inorganic P 3.2 (± 0.1) μM/g. All values shown are means $\pm$ S.E. of the mean

beating guinea pig heart *in situ* and the changes in the high-energy phosphate content of the myocardium both in the state of asphyxia and, thereafter, during post-asphyctic recovery. As indicated by the steep upward deflection of the upper curve, the acute dilation of the ventricles reaches its maximum within 60 sec together with the breakdown of the CP fraction. This rapid loss of diastolic tone clearly precedes the loss of systolic contractility, because in the case of prolonged anoxia or asphyxia the asystolic arrest of the hearts does not occur earlier than with a delay of at least 6 min (Fig. 5). If, on the other hand, anoxia or asphyxia is limited to 3 to 4 min both contractility and heart diameter return to normal as soon as the CP supply is restored after resuming respiration.

Anoxic ventricular dilation is most obvious in hearts with the pericardium removed. Such ventricles are often so largely expanded that within 1 min of anoxia, the tricuspidal valve becomes insufficient. If, however, in our experiments on guinea pigs the degree of dilation was restricted by the surrounding intact pericardium, not more than about 60% of the maximum heart diameter could be measured in full anoxia. Under these circumstances anoxic valvular dysfunction was less frequent. Another common side effect of myocardial anoxia or asphyxia is a sudden drop in cardiac frequency to about one half or less, just at the peak of dilation (Fig. 3). The reason is an impairment of AV-conduction due to oxygen lack; but additional inhibitory influences due to anesthesia or anoxic hyperkaliemia are not excluded. As can be seen from Fig. 6, the anoxic reduction in heart rate is not a regular phenomenon, and by no means responsible for the

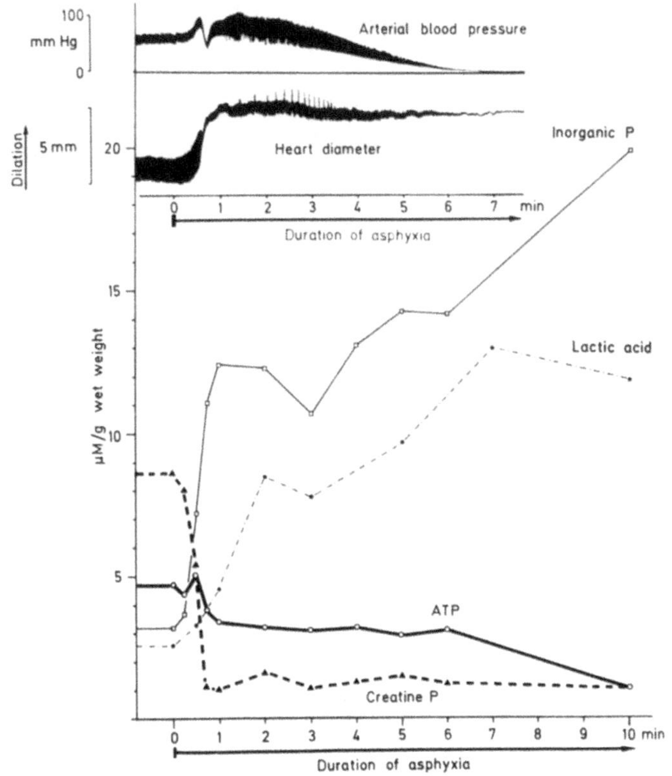

Fig. 5. Concentration changes of the most prominent acid-soluble phosphate fractions of the guinea pig myocardium during the course of prolonged asphyxia. The rise in lactic acid concentration roughly parallels that of inorganic P. The time correlation between rapid CP exhaustion and ventricular dilation (within 60 sec) is again obvious. Complete loss of systolic contractility and drop of arterial blood pressure to zero takes place within 6 min

augmentation of diastolic heart volume because in this experiment anoxia produces massive ventricular dilation without any chronotropic influence. Additional observations were also made on a considerable number of heart–lung preparations with constant heart rates and stabilized arterial and venous blood pressures. The principal result was essentially the same as on hearts *in situ*: Anoxic ventricular dilation neither depends on a reduction of cardiac frequency nor on changes in blood pressure but merely on the loss of contractile diastolic tone which, in turn, results from high-energy phosphate deficiency. Obviously the hearts are dilated as long as the CP concentration is lowered to an insufficient level. Further observations have shown that an acute ventricular dilation can also be produced by other factors which exhaust the CP store, e.g. carbon monoxide respiration or metabolic inhibitors (NaCN, fluoroacetate, 2,4-dinitrophenol). Fig. 7 represents experiments in which, after previous treatment with these poisons, the hearts were frozen for the chemical analysis just at the peak of ventricular dilation (Döring, Kammermeier, and Byon, 1962). The data demonstrate that again, in all these cases, the breakdown of CP was most closely related to the sudden increase in heart diameter.

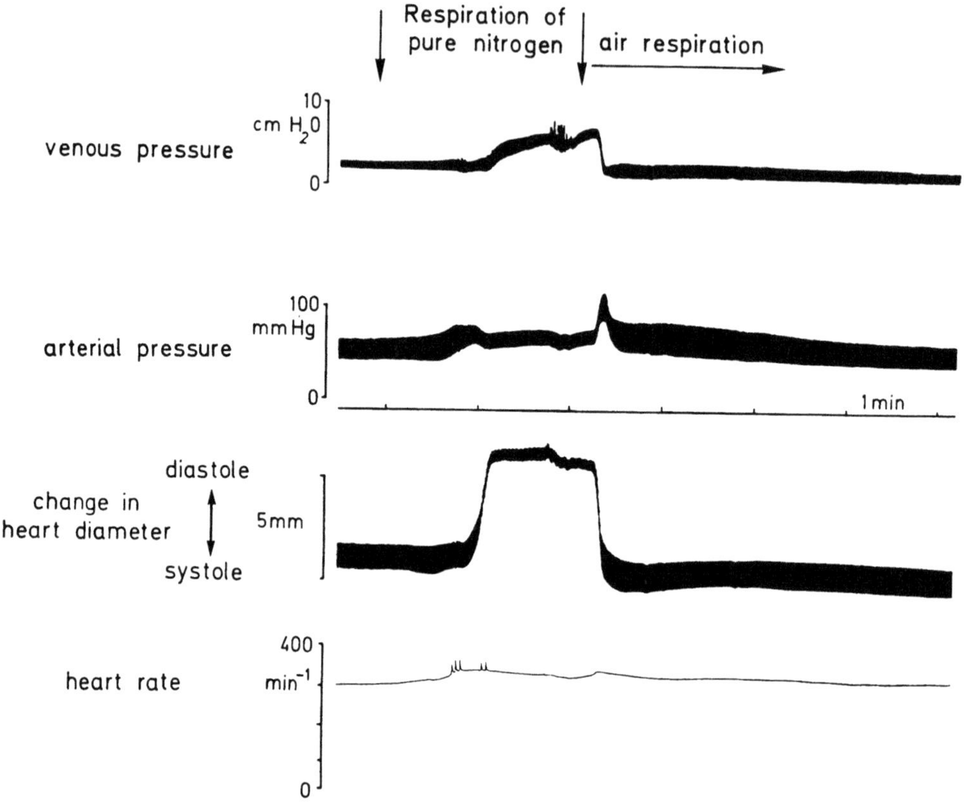

Fig. 6. Acute dilation of a guinea pig heart due to artificial respiration of the animal with pure nitrogen. Recovery of cardiac tone upon return to air respiration. Exposure to nitrogen for 134 sec. The increase in heart diameter is obviously not related to the usual anoxic drop in heart rate (prolongation of the diastolic filling time) because, in the present experiment, cardiac frequency remains constant

III. Degradation of ATP and Other Nucleotides — a Limiting Factor in the Reanimation of Anoxic or Ischemic Hearts

In contrast to CP, the ATP concentration seems to be less critical. Thus, during postasphyctic recovery after prolonged periods of cardiac standstill, we were able to show that complete restoration of the strength of contraction requires a full CP supply, whereas ATP concentration may remain considerably below normal. Nevertheless, this ATP reduction can become a limiting factor in reviving the anoxic hearts if more than 50 to 60% of the original ATP has definitely disappeared (KAMMERMEIER, 1964). With the use of our techniques the adenosine nucleotides of the normal and asphyctic myocardium can be easily visualized in ultraviolet light of 260 mμ after separation on paper. As can be seen from Fig. 8 a large amount of ATP is broken down during prolonged asphyxia since the large spot which represents ATP in the chromatogram of the control heart is reduced to about $^1/_5$ of the normal size after an oxygen lack of 15 min at 37° C. This breakdown goes beyond the step of ADP and AMP. As shown in our laboratory by GERLACH, DEUTICKE, and DREISBACH (1963) the progressive degradation of ATP in anoxic hearts rapidly leads to the formation of adenosine, inosine, hypoxan-

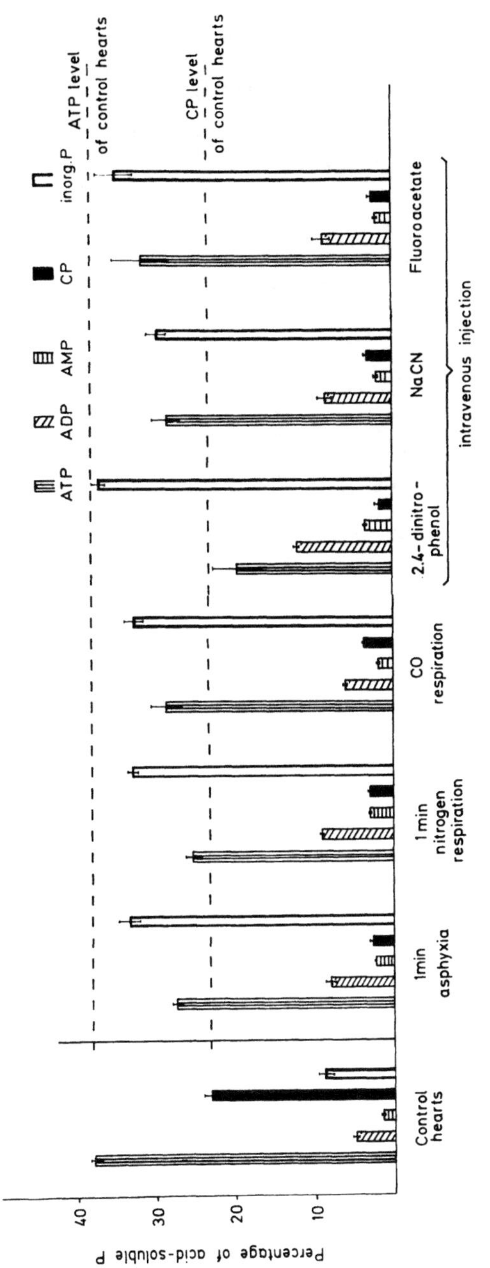

Fig. 7. Exhaustion of CP and decrease in ATP at the peak of ventricular dilation produced by asphyxia, respiration of pure nitrogen, respiration of air with 4 vol-% CO, or i.v. injection of 30 mg/kg 2,4-dinitrophenol, 9 mg/kg NaCN, 25 mg/kg fluoroacetate. Values shown are means ± S.E. of the mean (From DÖRING, KAMMERMEIER, and BYON, 1962)

thine, and xanthine (Table 3). But, apart from ADP and AMP, only adenosine is suitable for rapid ATP resynthesis in the postasphyctic recovery period whereas the formation of inosine, hypoxanthine, or xanthine signifies a practically irreversible ATP-loss. The minimum amount of ATP which has to be resynthetized from residual ADP, AMP, and adenosine, when myocardial contractility should reappear, is approximately 40% of the original ATP content. Therefore, the

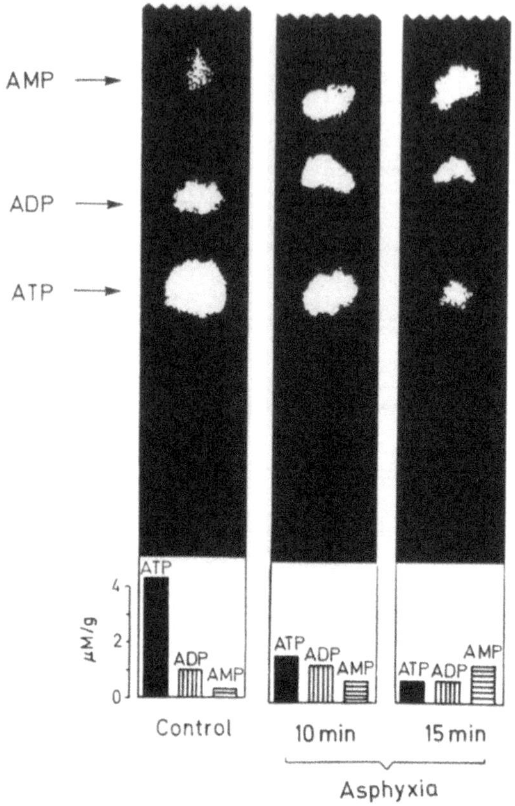

Fig. 8. Progressive breakdown of myocardial ATP produced by asphyxia of a duration of 15 min. After separation on paper, the ultraviolet-absorbing nucleotides ATP, ADP, and AMP were visualized by the photoprint technique of MARKHAM and SMITH [Biochemic. J. **45**, 294 (1949)] at a wave length of 260 mμ. Obviously, the big ultraviolet-absorbing spot in the control chromatogram, which represents ATP, decreases more and more in the chromatograms of asphyctic hearts. In addition, the total amount of adenosine nucleotides diminishes due to further degradation (FLECKENSTEIN, 1963b)

possibility of reanimation of an anoxic or ischemic heart becomes progressively worse as the degradation of the nucleotides procedes towards the useless end-products. A similar anoxic breakdown has also been found for the guanine nucleotides which again leads to the appearance of xanthine and for the uridine nucleotides which are eventually degraded to uracil (GERLACH, DEUTICKE, and DREISBACH, 1963).

In summarizing our observations it is to be stressed that the contractile failure in cases of asphyxia, anoxia, ischemia, after ligature of the coronary arteries or under the influence of inhibitors of glycolysis, respiration or phosphorylation clearly has a biochemical basis. In fact any interruption of the high-energy phosphate supply, as indicated by an exhaustion of CP, leads to almost immediate disorders of cardiac contractility. Interestingly enough phosphate-bond energy is not only utilized by the contractile system to cover the expenses of systolic work but also to maintain cardiac diastolic tone. The correlation between changes in diastolic tone and myocardial CP content is particularly evident. The changes in

Table 3. Pathways of myocardial nucleotide degradation in asphyxia (GERLACH, DEUTICKE, and DREISBACH 1963)

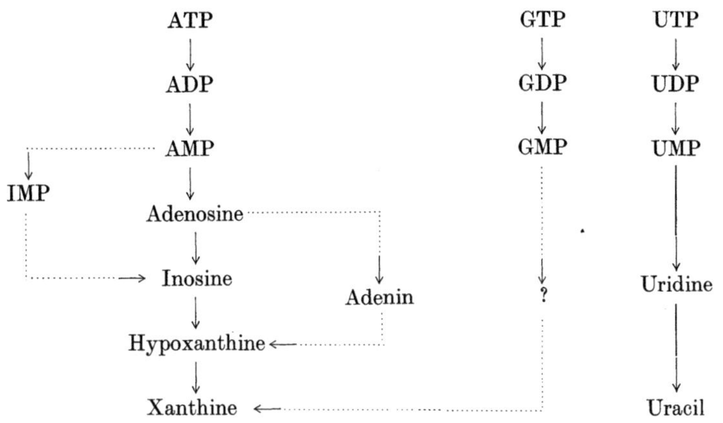

ATP, on the other hand, do not exhibit such a close connection with the mechanical events. But this can be explained:

1. By the fact that ATP, being the immediate energy source for contraction, is instantaneously restored at the expense of CP, and

2. by the assumption that only a minor fraction of ATP, probably amounting to about $^1/_5$ to $^1/_4$ of the total ATP content of the myocardium, is directly concerned with contraction and, consequently, equilibrates with CP.

Apart from contractile function, structural integrity cannot be maintained when the high-energy phosphate pools are empty. Therefore, all factors which interfere with the high-energy phosphate supply also produce cellular destruction. The involvement of high-energy phosphates in myocardial cell regeneration and maintenance of structural integrity are discussed in Chapter E of this article.

D. Contractile Cardiac Failure Produced by Deficient Utilization of High-Energy Phosphates

I. Selective Loss of Myocardial Contractility upon Ca Withdrawal

There is overwhelming evidence that during excitation of mammalian myocardial fibers two kinds of extracellular cations enter the cell: Na ions, which are responsible for the creation of the action potential, and Ca ions, which are needed for the activation of the contractile machinery. In addition (simultaneously with the transmembrane Ca influx) Ca is also liberated from certain intracellular stores. This rapid rise in the cytoplasmic free Ca concentration during excitation initiates the splitting of ATP by the Ca-dependent ATPase of the myofibrils so that phosphate-bond energy is transformed into mechanical work. This means, in other words, that the Ca ions act as mediators in excitation–contraction coupling between the bioelectric events at the sarcolemma membrane and the intracellular biochemical processes which utilize ATP for contraction (see reviews of HASSELBACH and WEBER, 1965; EBASHI and ENDO, 1968; KATZ, 1970; FLECKENSTEIN, 1970/71a, b). Therefore contractility is lost in a Ca-deficient medium.

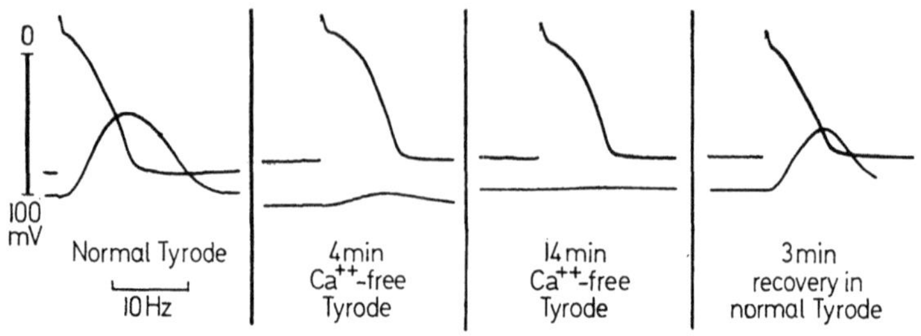

Fig. 9. Complete loss of contractility of an isolated rabbit papillary muscle in a Ca-free Tyrode solution at 37° C. Rapid recovery in ordinary Tyrode solution. Rate of stimulation: 3 shocks/min. Potentials were measured with intracellular microelectrodes of conventional type. Isometric tensions were recorded with a transducer valve (RCA 5734)

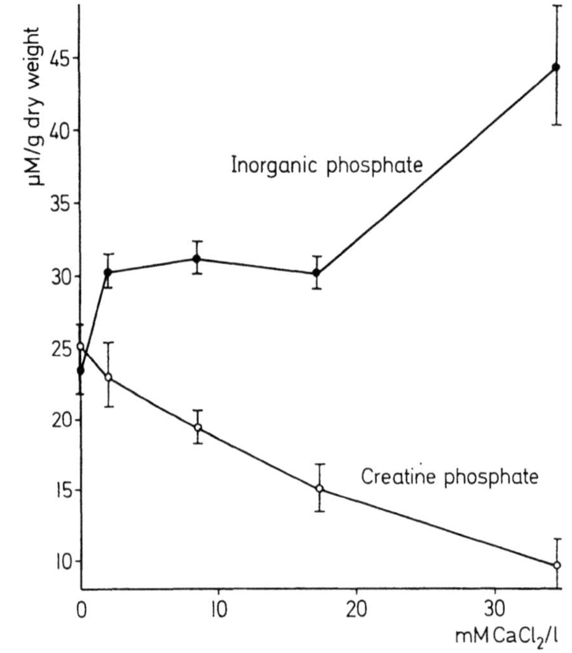

Fig. 10. Influence of increasing extracellular Ca on the creatine phosphate and inorganic phosphate content of the atrial myocardium (32 isolated rabbit auricles) at a constant rate of stimulation of 200 shocks/min. Simultaneously with CP, the ATP concentration was also reduced from a maximum of 15.3 ($\pm$0.7) μM/g dry weight at zero Ca to 9.0 ($\pm$0.9) μM/g in the Ca-rich Tyrode solution with 34.6 mM Ca/l. Temperature: 30° C (From SCHILDBERG and FLECKENSTEIN, 1965)

Fig. 9 shows some kind of fundamental experiment in which an electrically stimulated rabbit papillary muscle was put into a Ca-free Tyrode solution. Single fiber action potentials and isometric mechanograms were continuously recorded. As expected, isometric peak tension falls to almost zero within 14 min in a Ca-free environment, whereas the action potentials do not change appreciably. However, the mechanical function of the cardiac fibers is rapidly restored on return to a normal Ca-containing medium. Biochemically, Ca withdrawal produces a striking insufficiency of the contractile system to split high-energy phosphate compounds

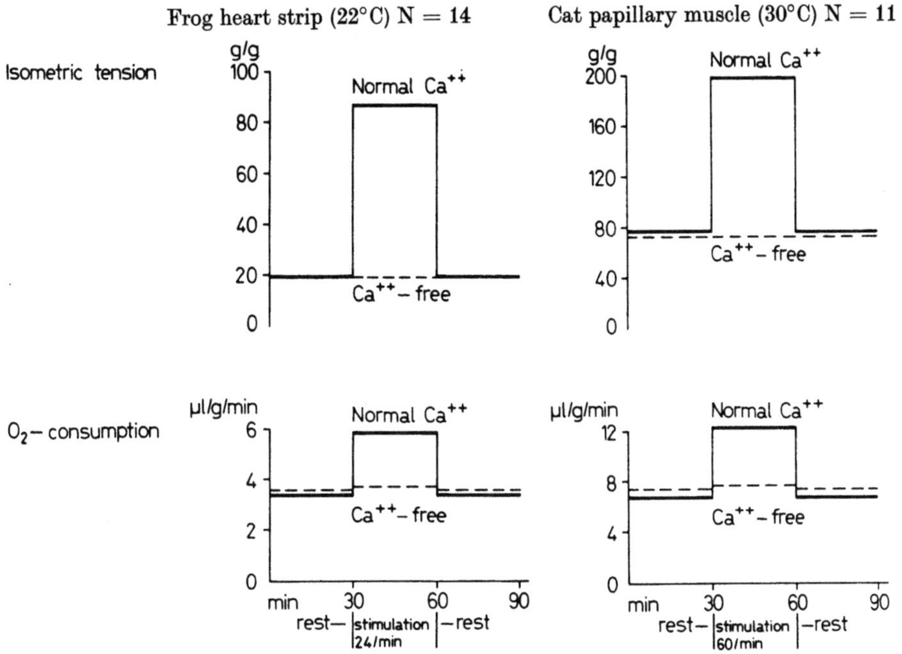

Fig. 11. Mean O_2-consumption of 14 isolated frog ventricular strips and 11 cat papillary muscles at rest and during activity both in ordinary Ringer's solution and in a Ca-free medium. The rates of O_2-consumption were calculated from O_2-tension measurements in the surrounding fluid using a platinum electrode. Simultaneously, the mechanical activity was registered by recording the isometric tension with an inductive force transducer. The contractility of the Ca-deprived preparations was negligible during the stimulation period whereas electrical excitability persisted [Byon and Fleckenstein: Pflügers Arch. ges. Physiol. **283**, R 15 (1965); see Fleckenstein, 1963a; Fleckenstein, Döring, and Kammermeier, 1966/67]

in the state of excitation (Fleckenstein, Schwoerer, and Janke, 1961; Flekkenstein and Schwoerer, 1961; Fleckenstein,1963; Schildberg and Flekkenstein, 1965). But after addition of Ca, the high-energy phosphate utilization is normalized. If, on the other hand, the extracellular Ca concentration is increased above normal, more Ca is taken up by the beating heart so that both splitting of high-energy phosphates and contractility are potentiated. Fig. 10 demonstrates, for instance, the stepwise decline of CP and the opposite change in orthophosphate due to an increase in the extracellular Ca concentration. The experiments were carried out on isolated rabbit auricles at a constant stimulation rate of 200/min. Isometric tension was also increased by the rise in Ca up to a maximum of about 10 mM/l, a value fivefold above normal. Ca concentrations, which were still higher than that value, activated the splitting of high-energy phosphates even more but failed to produce a proportional augmentation of tension. This drop in efficiency signifies the beginning of exhaustion and seems to be a natural consequence of the progressive consumption of CP.

All these observations clearly show that Ca ions not only trigger the contractile process but also quantitatively control the output of mechanical tension in regulating the amount of ATP which is metabolized during activity. These findings on intact myocardial fibers agree with the results obtained on subcellular muscle constituents such as isolated myofibrils or contractile proteins, which were also found to require the addition of Ca for superprecipitation and maximum ATPase activity (Mommaerts, 1950; Weber and Winicur, 1961; Weber and

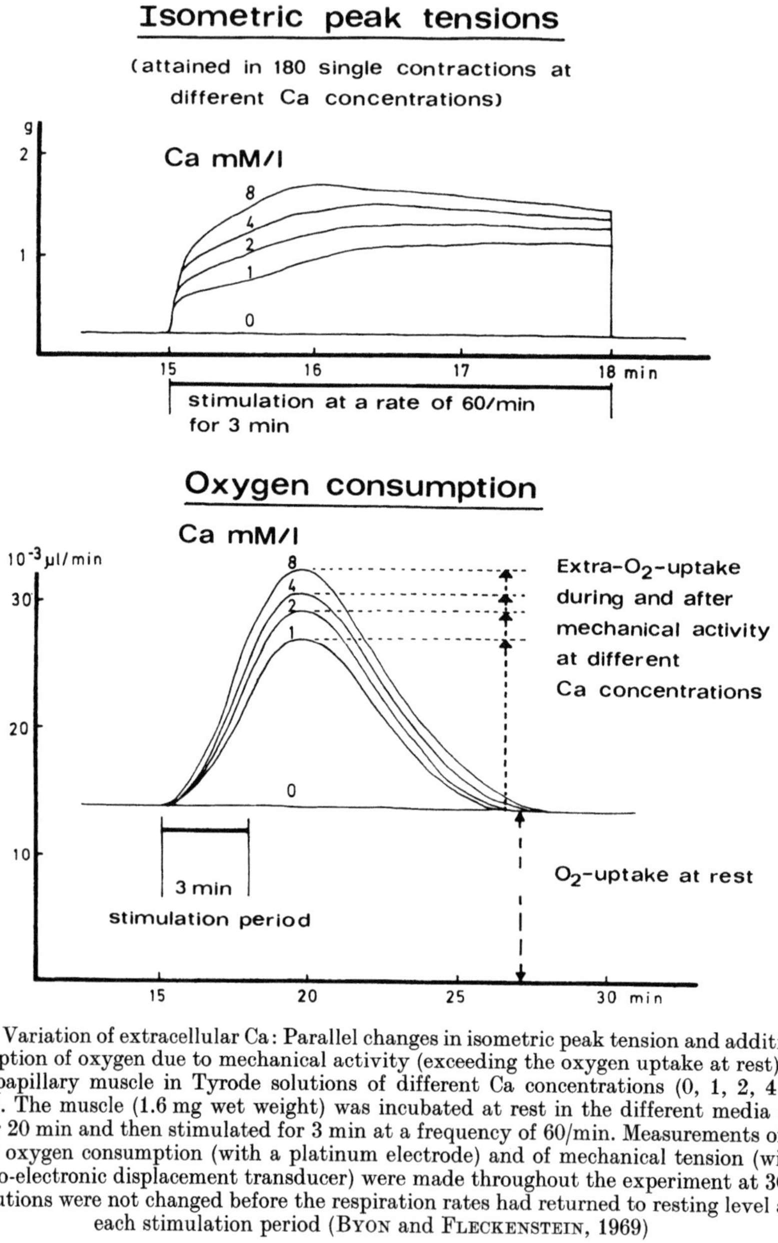

Fig. 12. Variation of extracellular Ca: Parallel changes in isometric peak tension and additional consumption of oxygen due to mechanical activity (exceeding the oxygen uptake at rest) of a rabbit papillary muscle in Tyrode solutions of different Ca concentrations (0, 1, 2, 4 and 8 mM/l). The muscle (1.6 mg wet weight) was incubated at rest in the different media each time for 20 min and then stimulated for 3 min at a frequency of 60/min. Measurements of the rates of oxygen consumption (with a platinum electrode) and of mechanical tension (with a mechano-electronic displacement transducer) were made throughout the experiment at 30° C. The solutions were not changed before the respiration rates had returned to resting level after each stimulation period (BYON and FLECKENSTEIN, 1969)

HERZ, 1963; SEIDEL and GERGELY, 1963). In resting heart muscle the free sarcoplasmic Ca concentration is in the range of 10^{-7} M. This is below the level at which interaction between actin and myosin occurs. In order to obtain a maximum contractile response during excitation, the sarcoplasmic Ca concentration must increase by approximately 100 times up to 10^{-5} M. About 80% of this Ca (needed for full activation of the contractile system) seems to be released from intracellular storage sites, whereas about 20% enters the excited myocardial cell from the extracellular space through the depolarized sarcolemma membrane. Conversely,

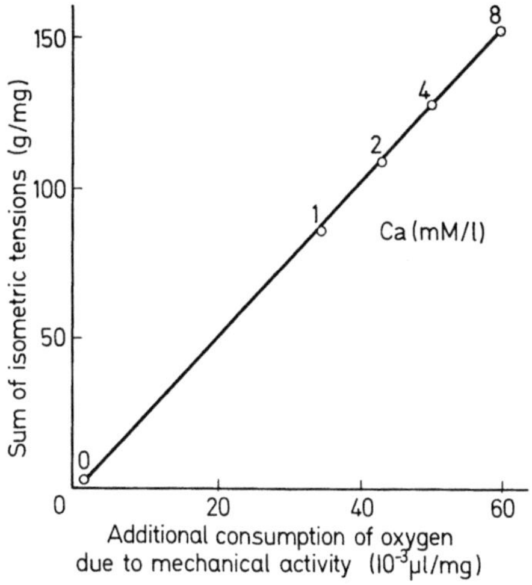

Fig. 13. Variation of extracellular Ca: Linear correlation between isometric tension and the additional consumption of oxygen (due to mechanical activity) of a rabbit papillary muscle in Tyrode solutions of different Ca concentrations (0, 1, 2, 4, and 8 mM/l). The graph shows the sum of the isometric peak tensions produced during each stimulation period (3 min) plotted against the corresponding additional consumptions of oxygen during and after stimulation. Fig. 13 represents an evaluation of the experiment shown in Fig. 12 (BYON and FLECKENSTEIN, 1969)

relaxation is initiated by removal of free Ca ions from the myofibrils. This is mainly achieved by the active re-absorption of Ca into the intracellular stores with the help of an ATP-driven Ca pump (HASSELBACH and MAKINOSE, 1961; EBASHI and LIPMANN, 1962; FANBURG, FINKEL, and MARTONOSI, 1964). The specific sites of the re-uptake of Ca are probably the longitudinal compartments of the sarcoplasmic reticulum and, perhaps, the mitochondria. In other words this means that during the contraction cycle, Ca ions not only activate the myofibrillar ATPase in order to produce mechanical tension, but also stimulate intracellular Ca transport ATPases in order to initiate the subsequent relaxation.

It is a well-known fact that the breakdown of high-energy phosphates in the cell will also give rise to intensified glycolytic and oxidative reactions. So it is not surprising that the rate of formation of lactic acid and, particularly, the rate of oxygen consumption in active heart muscle are also highly "Ca-sensitive". Fig. 11 demonstrates the rates of oxygen consumption of isolated frog ventricular strips and of cat papillary muscles at rest and during stimulation, both in ordinary Ringer solution and in a Ca-free medium. Obviously, oxygen consumption at rest does not differ appreciably whether or not the surrounding fluid contains Ca. But if stimulation occurs, the oxygen consumption rises sharply, but only in presence of Ca, whereas it remains more or less at resting level in the Ca-deprived myocardium, which responds electrically but not mechanically to stimulation. If, on the other hand, the Ca concentration is increased above normal, the activity metabolism will be further intensified. In the concentration range between 0 and 8 mM/l there is a strictly linear relationship between isometric tension development of rabbit papillary muscles and the concomitant increase in oxygen uptake (BYON and FLECKENSTEIN, 1969; Figs. 12 and 13). The maximum tension development was reached at a Ca concentration of about 10 mM/l.

The data show that Ca ions, in regulating the amount of ATP consumed during contraction (and relaxation), also determine, as a result of this, the rate of oxidative processes which subsequently have to reconstitute the high-energy phosphate stores. In quiescent heart muscle, on the other hand, resting tension and basic oxygen consumption are rather insensitive to the change in extracellular Ca. This is easily understood:

1. Because transmembrane Ca conductivity is rather small when, at rest, the myocardial membrane potential is high.

2. Because, at rest, the pathways of ATP utilization presumably differ from those during activity with respect to Ca requirements.

II. Basic Mechanisms of Cardiodepression by Interference with Transmembrane Ca Supply

To lower cardiac tension development at a constant extracellular Ca concentration there are two principal ways which lead to a decrease in transmembrane Ca influx:

The first way consists of an abbreviation of membrane excitation, particularly by shortening the plateau of action potential. The result is a decrease in Ca supply to the contractile system due to restriction of the length of time of transmembrane Ca entry (and intracellular Ca release). In this case, Ca conductivity of the depolarized membrane and all other steps of excitation–contraction coupling may remain completely intact. Acetylcholine, for instance, exerts its negative inotropic action on frog hearts and mammalian atria merely by abbreviation of the action potentials (Figs. 14 and 15). This conclusion was further substantiated in a thorough study by ANTONI and ROTMANN (1968). Interestingly enough, contractile force can be selectively restored in the presence of acetylcholine by increasing the extracellular Ca concentration, whereas the shortening of action potential persists (Fig. 15). In contrast to acetylcholine, a great number of other compounds, which also abbreviate cardiac action potential, do this by producing more or less irreversible alterations of membrane function or cardiac metabolism. Thus shortening or loss of the plateau phase of the action potential is a rather commom phenomenon in myocardial fiber damage. Accordingly in all these cases a depression of systolic force ensues even if excitation–contraction coupling and the contractile system itself are not seriously affected. It should also be noted in this connection that the extreme decay of tension in a fibrillating heart is another example of severe contractile failure resulting from a situation in which the duration of the cardiac fiber action potentials is minimized.

The second way of interfering with the Ca supply to the excited myocardial fibers consists of a direct inhibition of the transmembrane Ca influx by blocking the so-called "slow channel". This produces excitation–contraction uncoupling because contractile force declines selectively whereas height and duration of the action potentials do not change appreciably. When excess Ca is administered, the block of transmembrane Ca conductivity may also be overcome.

Thus both the fibers with abbreviated action potentials as well as those with deficient excitation–contraction coupling behave similarly, in that contractile force recovers, at least in part, if the extracellular Ca concentration rises to supernormal values. From this it becomes obvious that a suitable differentiation of the mechanisms of action of negative inotropic agents requires the use of modern electrophysiological techniques such as recording of single fiber action potentials (with intracellular microelectrodes), registration of isometric tension development (with ultrasensitive mechano-electronic transducers) and, in addition, direct measurements of the transmembrane Ca conductivity (with the voltage clamp technique).

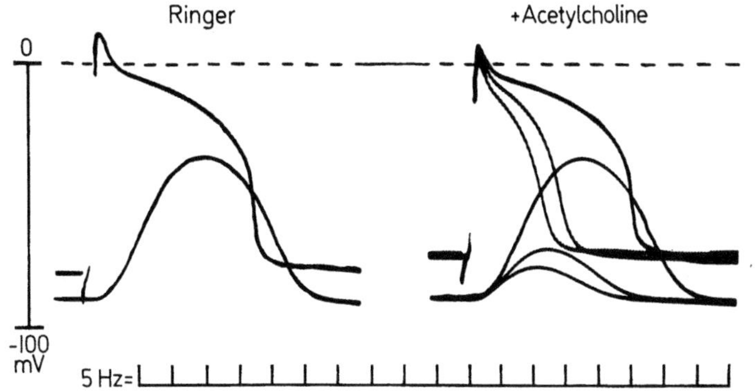

Fig. 14. Depression of the contractile force of a strip of frog ventricle by abbreviation of the action potential in an acetylcholine-containing Ringer's solution. Measurements of potentials and isometric tensions as in Fig. 9 (Fleckenstein, 1963a; Antoni and Rotmann, 1968)

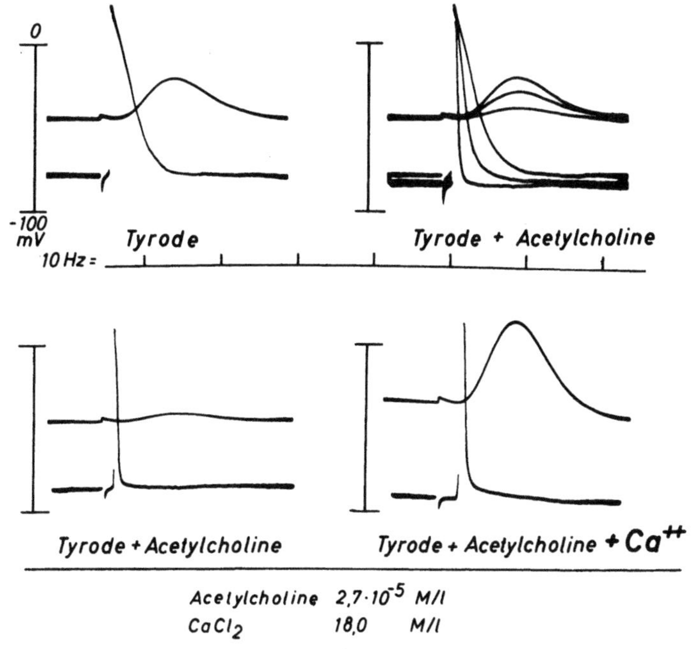

Fig. 15. Depression of the contractile force of isolated atrial tissue of a guinea pig by abbreviation of the action potential in an acetylcholine-containing Tyrode solution. Restitution of the strength of contraction by addition of excess Ca without an appreciable re-prolongation of action potential (Antoni and Fleckenstein; see Fleckenstein, 1963a)

III. Excitation-Contraction Uncoupling of Heart Muscle by Ca-Antagonistic Bivalent Ni, Co, and Mn Cations

Although cardiodepression produced by cobalt, nickel, or manganese ions is not exclusively due to excitation–contraction uncoupling, it may serve as an interesting example of direct interference with the activator Ca (Kaufmann and Fleckenstein, 1965). As shown in Fig. 16, a nearly complete loss of myocardial

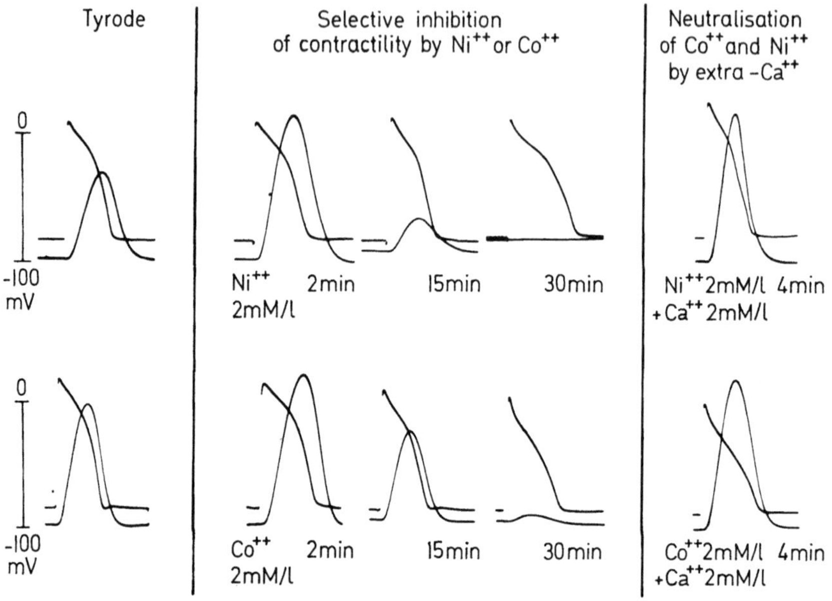

Fig. 16. Isolated guinea pig papillary muscles lose their contractility within 30 min after addition of 2 mM $NiCl_2$ or $CoCl_2$ to a normal Tyrode solution containing 1.8 mM Ca/l, whereas the single fiber action potentials persist. The effects of Co and Ni can be rapidly neutralized by an extra-dose of 2 mM $CaCl_2$/l, so that contractility recovers within 4 min. Rate of stimulation: 30 shocks/min. Temperature: 33° C. Methods as in Fig. 9 (KAUFMANN and FLECKENSTEIN, 1965)

contractility can be produced by Ni or Co without major changes in resting or action potential. Here, 2 mM/l $NiCl_2$ or $CoCl_2$ were added to an ordinary Tyrode solution (1.8 mM Ca/l), in which 2 isolated guinea pig papillary muscles were continuously stimulated with 30 shocks/min. Excitation–contraction uncoupling took place within 30 min. However, as soon as an extra dose of 2 mM $CaCl_2$/l was administered, after contractility had disappeared, the original strength of contraction returned to normal within 4 min. Ni, Co, and Mn ions inhibit the transmembrane Ca inward current through the slow channel as was shown by KOHLHARDT, BAUER, KRAUSE, and FLECKENSTEIN (1973) with the voltage clamp technique (Fig. 17). It is to be assumed that these bivalent cations compete with Ca for some common binding sites at the sarcolemma membrane or, more specifically, at the Ca transport system itself. Thus, with the help of excess Ca, the transmembrane Ca influx through the slow channel can be restored in the presence of Co or Ni.

Our publication on acute Co-induced cardiac failure in 1965 was followed, one year later, by clinical reports, in which a chronic form of Co-induced cardiac incompetence was described (MCDERMOTT, DELANEY, EGAN, and SULLIVAN, 1966; MORIN and DANIEL, 1967; MORIN, FOLEY, MARTINEAU, and ROUSSEL, 1967). This new disease occurred in heavy beer drinkers and resulted from the surprising fact that some Canadian breweries had added $CoCl_2$ to the beer to improve the foam; about 50 persons died before this dangerous procedure could be stopped. Unfortunately, treatment with Ca was not administered. Subsequent animal experiments have shown that chronic poisoning with $CoCl_2$ leads to an intracellular accumulation of Co in the hearts pari passu with a displacement of myocardial Ca

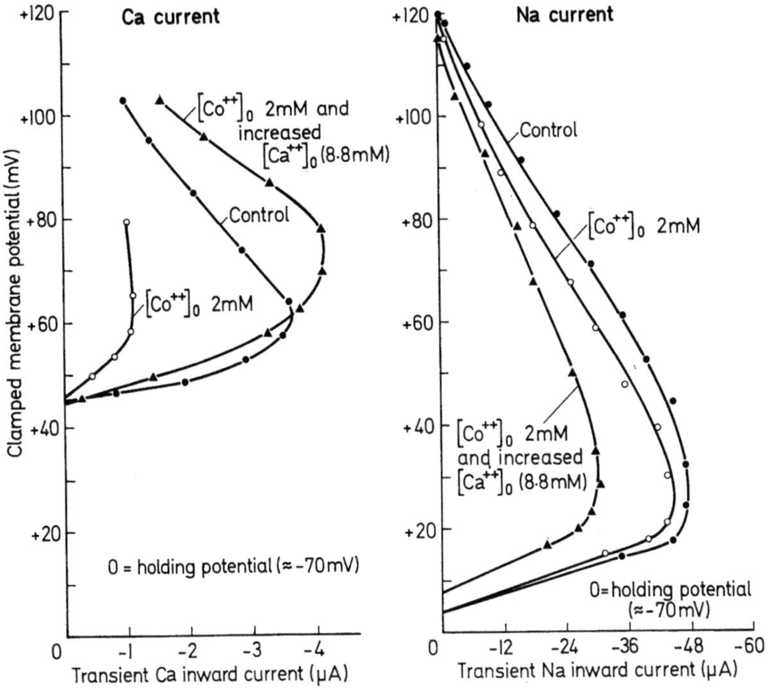

Fig. 17. Current–voltage relationships of both the slow Ca and the fast Na inward currents obtained on a trabecula from the right ventricle of a cat using the voltage clamp technique. The ordinate shows the clamped (depolarized) potential; 0 indicates the holding potential (approximately −70 mV). By addition of $CoCl_2$ (2 mM/l) to a normal Tyrode solution with 2.2 mM $CaCl_2$/l, the current–voltage relationship curve of the slow Ca inward current is shifted to lower values indicating a reduced transmembrane Ca conductivity. By increasing the extracellular Ca concentration up to 8.8 mM/l the effect of Co on the transmembrane Ca current is more than compensated. The influence of Co on the fast Na inward current is relatively weak. Additional Ca reduced the transmembrane Na conductivity even more (KOHLHARDT, BAUER, KRAUSE, and FLECKENSTEIN, 1973)

(SULLIVAN, PARKER, and CARSON, 1968; KNIERIEM and HERBERTZ, 1969; KASPEREK, SILLER, and KNIERIEM, 1969). However, it should be noted in this connection that chronic treatment with Co not only impairs excitation–contraction coupling but also produces severe myocardial damage. This applies particularly to function and ultrastructure of the mitochondria (RONA and CHAPPEL, 1971). With regard to certain inhibitory side effects on intracellular enzyme systems, which have nothing to do with excitation–contraction coupling, the etiology of cobalt-induced cardiac failure is considered to be multifactorial.

IV. Restriction of Myocardial Contractility by Organic Compounds with Ca-Antagonistic Side Effects

The first report on excitation–contraction uncoupling of heart muscle produced by Ca-antagonistic drugs (FLECKENSTEIN, 1964) was based on studies with certain sympathetic β-receptor blocking agents, barbituric acid derivatives and 2 new compounds, namely prenylamine (Segontin) and verapamil (Isoptin). When large doses of these drugs were administered in guinea pigs (open chest

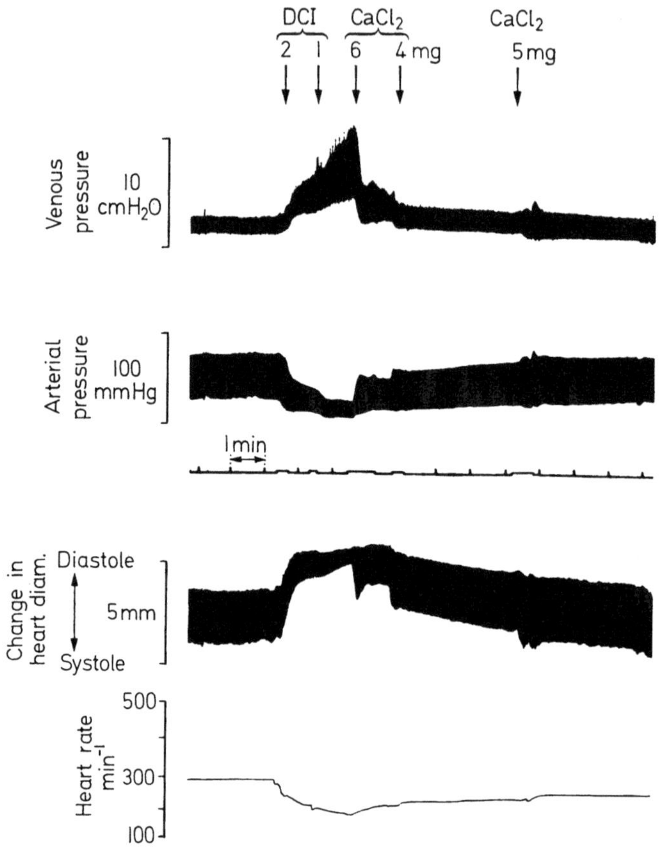

Fig. 18. Acute contractile failure of a guinea pig heart (open chest preparation with the peri cardium removed) after i.v. injection of 10 mg dichloroisoproterenol/kg body weight. Rapid restoration of contractility (contraction amplitude, heart diameter) and of the original arterial and venous blood pressures by $CaCl_2$. Throughout the 700 open chest experiments of this standard type, suitable Statham elements were used for the blood pressure registration in the left jugular vein (P 23 BB) and in the right carotid artery (P 23 Db) under nembutal-ether anesthesia. In many cases, acute ventricular dilation produced by Ca-antagonistic inhibitors of utilization of high-energy phosphates was accompanied by insufficiency of the tricuspidal valve leading to a positive venous pulsation (FLECKENSTEIN, 1964)

preparations) an acute loss of cardiac tone and contractility was produced, whereas the excitatory processes remained more or less unaffected. Hemodynamically, the behavior of the failing hearts was quite similar to cases of cardiac incompentence resulting from ischemia or anoxia. But the metabolic background proved to be totally different because, instead of the well-known high-energy phosphate exhaustion in anoxia, elevated levels of ATP and CP were found closely resembling those in Ca deficiency. Thus we concluded that high concentrations of these drugs suppress myocardial contractility by interfering with the Ca-dependent utilization of high-energy phosphates. Accordingly, the mechanical function of the hearts could be restored by i.v. injection of appropriate amounts of $CaCl_2$ (Figs. 18, 19, and 20).

Ca-antagonistic excitation–contraction uncoupling of heart muscle by sympathetic β-receptor blocking agents or barbituric acid derivatives is to be considered as a side effect which merely occurs in a supernormal concentration range.

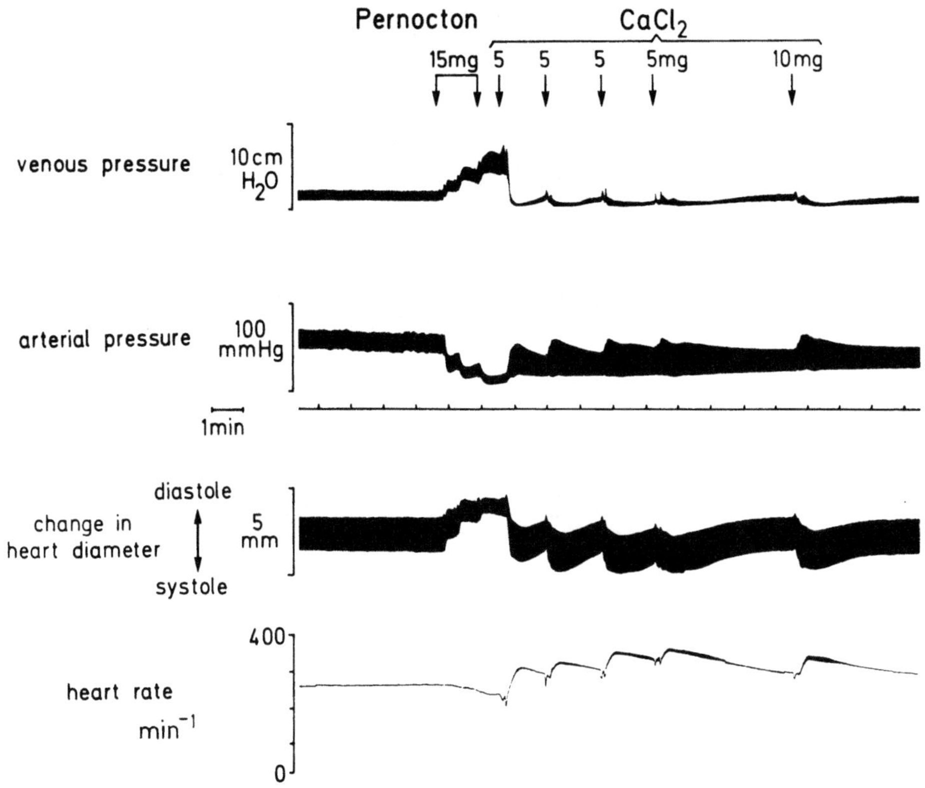

Fig. 19. Acute contractile failure of a guinea pig heart (open chest preparation with the pericardium removed) after i.v. injection of Pernocton (= butyl-bromallyl-barbituric acid). The total dose was 15 mg (≈ 45 mg/kg body weight). Rapid recovery of contractile cardiac function following i.v. administration of $CaCl_2$. Methods as in Fig. 18 (FLECKENSTEIN, 1965/66)

Table 4. Substances with Ca-antagonistic side effects on excitation-contraction coupling (FLECKENSTEIN, DÖRING, and KAMMERMEIER, 1967)

Substances	Effective doses for causing contractile failure of guinea pig hearts (mg/kg)	Effective[a] doses for blocking β-receptors in guinea pig hearts (mg/kg)
Propranolol (Inderal, Dociton)	1.5–6	0.3
Pronethalol (Alderlin, Nethalide)	3–5	0.5
Dichloroisoproterenol	6–25	1.5
Pernocton (= butyl-bromallyl-barbituric acid)	75	no effect
Luminal (= phenyl-ethyl-barbituric acid)	180	no effect
Nembutal (= ethyl-methyl-butyl-barbituric acid)	200	no effect
Somnifen (= diethyl-barbituric allyl-isopropyl-barbituric acid)	190	no effect

[a] The "effective" doses for blocking β-receptors indicate, arbitrarily, the amount of substance which completely inhibits the chronotropic action of 0.1 μg isoproterenol on guinea pig hearts (i.v. administration on open chest preparations).

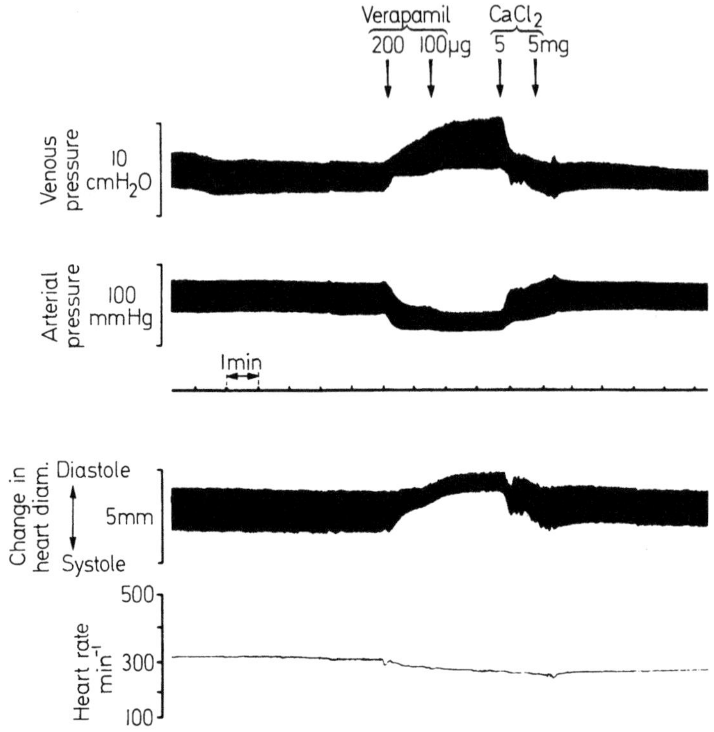

Fig. 20. Acute contractile failure of a guinea pig heart (open chest preparation with the pericardium removed) after i.v. injection of a total of 300 µg verapamil (≈ 0.9 mg/kg body weight). Rapid restoration of cardiac performance by $CaCl_2$. Methods as in Fig. 18 (FLECKENSTEIN, 1970/71a)

For instance, the effective doses of propranolol, pronethalol, or dichloroisoproterenol, which cause contractile failure of guinea pig hearts, are roughly 10 times greater than those needed for β-receptor blockade (Table 4). Similarly cardiodepression by barbiturates requires much higher doses than general anesthesia. Moreover, there is no quantitative correlation between the effective doses for excitation–contraction uncoupling and β-receptor blockade. This becomes evident from the fact that some highly potent β-receptor blocking agents such as pindolol (Visken, LB 46) and MJ 1999 are practically unable to produce contractile failure of the heart because they lack an appreciable Ca-antagonistic side effect. On the other hand, cardiac incompetence produced by propranolol, pronethalol, or dichloroisoproterenol is rapidly overcome by i.v. administration of $CaCl_2$ whereas the β-blockade persists. Furthermore, barbituric acid derivatives which do not possess any remarkable β-adrenolytic efficacy cause the same type of cardiac incompetence as the β-receptor blocking agents listed in Table 4. Hence the only common denominator of the strong cardiodepression (exceeding the mild negative-inotropic influence of a simple β-receptor blockade) is the Ca-antagonistic action of the drugs under examination. Thus the cardiac effects of large doses appear rather uniform. The characteristic features are as follows:

1. A drop of isometric peak tension or at least of the velocity of tension development in isolated heart muscle preparations. Accordingly, a reduction of stroke volume or systemic output occurs in heart–lung preparations or in the beating heart *in situ*.

2. An increase in heart diameter which is partly due to a reduction of the diastolic tonus.

3. A more or less selective inhibition of contractility without a major impairment of the intracellularly recorded action potentials. In other words this means excitation–contraction uncoupling.

4. A supranormal or, at least, normal high-energy phosphate content of the myocardium, even in the state of full contractile failure as a result of inhibition of high-energy phosphate utilization.

5. A decrease in oxygen demand per heart beat.

6. A rapid and complete reversal of all these typical symptoms by an extra dose of $CaCl_2$.

7. A quick recovery of the contractile function under the influence of Ca-synergistic promoters of excitation–contraction coupling such as β-adrenergic catecholamines and cardiac glycosides (these effects are discussed later; see Chapter D, VI).

It is interesting to note that in earlier studies on cardiac incompetence produced by barbiturates, some of the characteristics listed above had already been obersved but remained unexplained. This applies particularly:

a) To the selectivity of contractile depression by Pernocton or Somnifen at persisting action potentials (KRAYER and SCHÜTZ, 1932).

b) To the high myocardial ATP and CP contents at the climax of contractile failure (WOLLENBERGER, 1947; FAWAZ and HAWA, 1953; DÖRING and KAMMERMEIER, 1961).

c) To the easy restitution of contractile force by cardiac glycosides (KRAYER, 1931; SCHWIEGK, 1931) or adrenaline (KRAYER and SCHÜTZ, 1932).

It is obvious that Ca-antagonism provides a reasonable basis for the understanding of all these scattered experimental findings. Another achievement to be mentioned is that the number of negative inotropic agents with Ca-antagonistic side effects has rapidly grown during the last decade. Today more than 30 substances of this type are known: barbiturates, β-receptor blocking agents as well as other compounds, pharmacologically categorized as antifibrillatory drugs, local anesthetics etc.

V. Discovery of a New Group of Specific Ca-Antagonistic Inhibitors of Excitation-Contraction Coupling

Our main interest, however, has become more and more concentrated since 1964 on a new group of substances which, according to our observations, are capable of blocking excitation–contraction coupling "specifically". "Specificity" means that the Ca-antagonistic inhibitory action of these compounds on excitation–contraction coupling of heart (and smooth muscle) is so predominant that all other pharmacodynamic properties, at least in a reasonable dosage range, are more or less negligible. The most important drugs of this type are given in Table 5. The first compound of this list, prenylamine, was still relatively weak and of modest specificity. The following compounds, however, namely verapamil, D 600, and nifedipine (Bay a 1040, Adalat) are very powerful. The same is true for diltiazem, whereas fendiline closely resembles prenylamine. The inhibitory effects of these drugs on cardiac performance had been observed earlier by the following authors: LINDNER (1960) for prenylamine; HAAS and HÄRTFELDER (1962) for verapamil; HAAS and BUSCH (1967) for D 600; and VATER, KRONEBERG, HOFFMEISTER, KALLER, MENG, OBERDORF, PULS, SCHLOSSMANN, and STOEPEL (1972)

Table 5. Ca-antagonistic inhibitors of excitation-contraction coupling in mammalian myocardium and vascular smooth muscle

Prenylamine (Segontin)	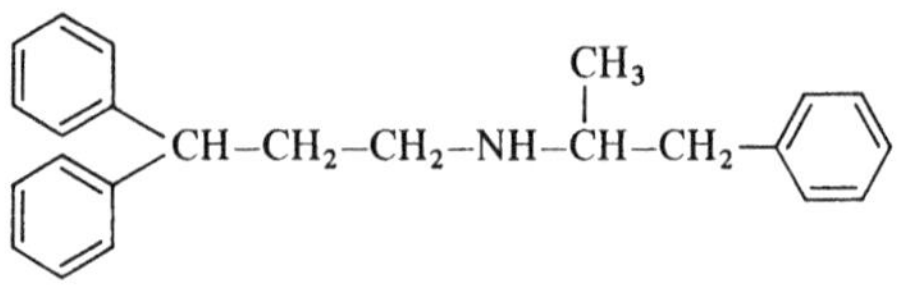
Fendiline (Sensit)	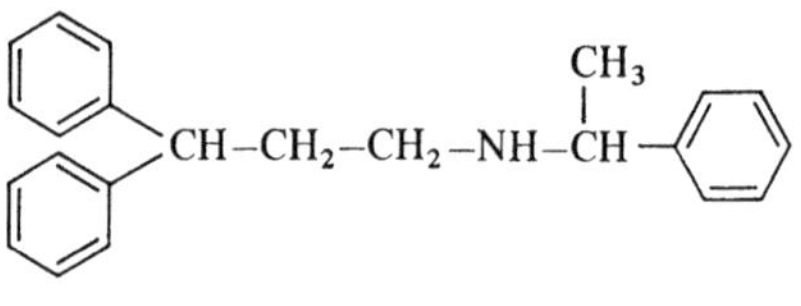
Verapamil (Isoptin)	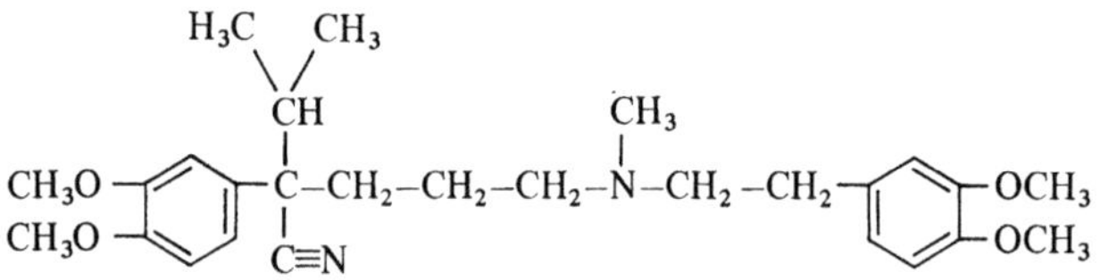
Compound D600	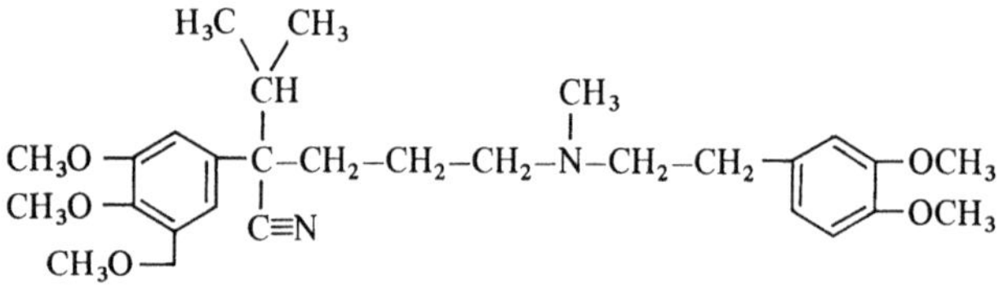
Nifedipine (Adalat, Bay a1040)	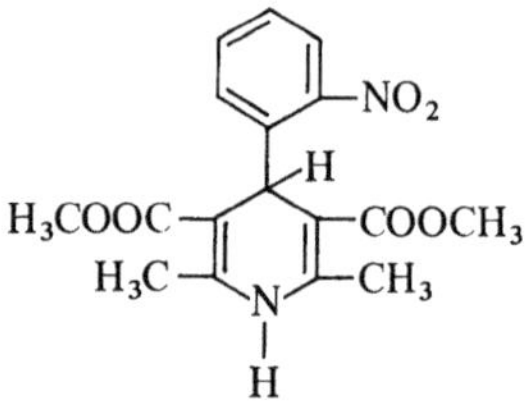
Diltiazeme (Herbesser)	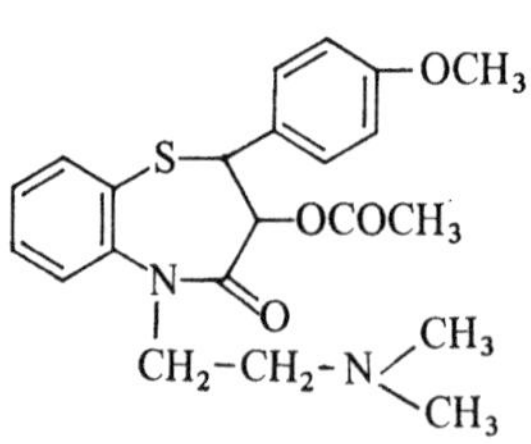

for nifedipine. But the mechanism of action remained unexplained until we found that all these drugs can produce a selective depression of myocardial contractility as in Ca-deficiency. For instance, verapamil, D 600, or nifedipine, in a concentration range as low as 0.1 to 1.0 mg/l Tyrode solution, blocked excitation–contraction coupling completely. D 600 and nifedipine are the most powerful agents (FLECKENSTEIN, TRITTHART, DÖRING, and BYON, 1972). Their Ca-antagonistic action:

1. Is several thousand times stronger than that of Co or Ni ions.
2. Does not cause structural damage of cardiac muscle or other tissues.
3. Is highly specific because, when injected into the intact animal, apparently no effects other than excitation–contraction uncoupling of heart muscle (and vascular smooth muscle[3]) are produced.
4. Is fully reversible upon administration of suitable amounts of $CaCl_2$.

All specific inhibitors of excitation–contraction coupling reduced the contractile response of the myocardium without a considerable change of the electric excitation process. Fig. 21 shows two experiments on cat papillary muscles in which an 80% loss of contractility was obtained by 400 µg of nifedipine/l, whereas the height and the shape of the single fiber action potentials practically did not change. On the right side of the figure contractility was restored by extra-calcium, as shown in the upper curve, or by isoproterenol as can be seen from the lower record. The experiment with verapamil in Fig. 22 is perhaps even more impressive since in this case contractility was completely abolished whereas, again, the action potentials persisted. In this experiment each molecule of verapamil antagonized approximately 200 Ca ions. The ratio will rise, in the case of nifedipine, up to a value as high as 1 to several thousand. With isoproterenol, in the lowest part of the figure, the original height of the mechanical responses returned to normal. Isoproterenol promotes the Ca influx so that the effect of verapamil is neutralized. The graphs in Fig. 23 represent a quantitative evaluation of such an experiment with verapamil. Obviously, resting potential as well as the action potential parameters, upstroke velocity, and height of the overshoot, which indicate the transmembrane Na influx, remain at a consistently high level, whereas the Ca-dependent

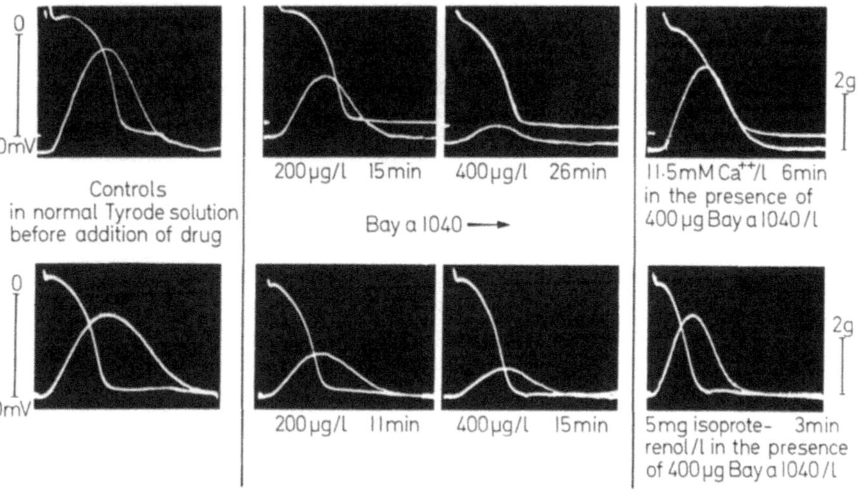

Fig. 21. Selective inhibition of contractile force of 2 cat papillary muscles by nifedipine (Bay a 1040). Restoration of contractility by additional Ca (upper experiment) or by isoproterenol (lower experiment). Single fiber action potentials and isometric contractions were measured using the same techniques as in Fig. 9 (FLECKENSTEIN, TRITTHART, DÖRING, and BYON, 1972)

[3] For excitation–contraction uncoupling of smooth muscle see: FLECKENSTEIN, GRÜN, TRITTHART, and BYON: Klin. Wschr. **49**, 32–41 (1971); GRÜN and FLECKENSTEIN: Arzneimittelforsch. (Drug Res.) **22**, 334–344 (1972); HAEUSLER: J. Pharmacol. a. exp. Therap. **180**, 672–682 (1972); PEIPER and SCHMIDT: Pflügers Arch. ges. Physiol. **337**, 107–117 (1972).

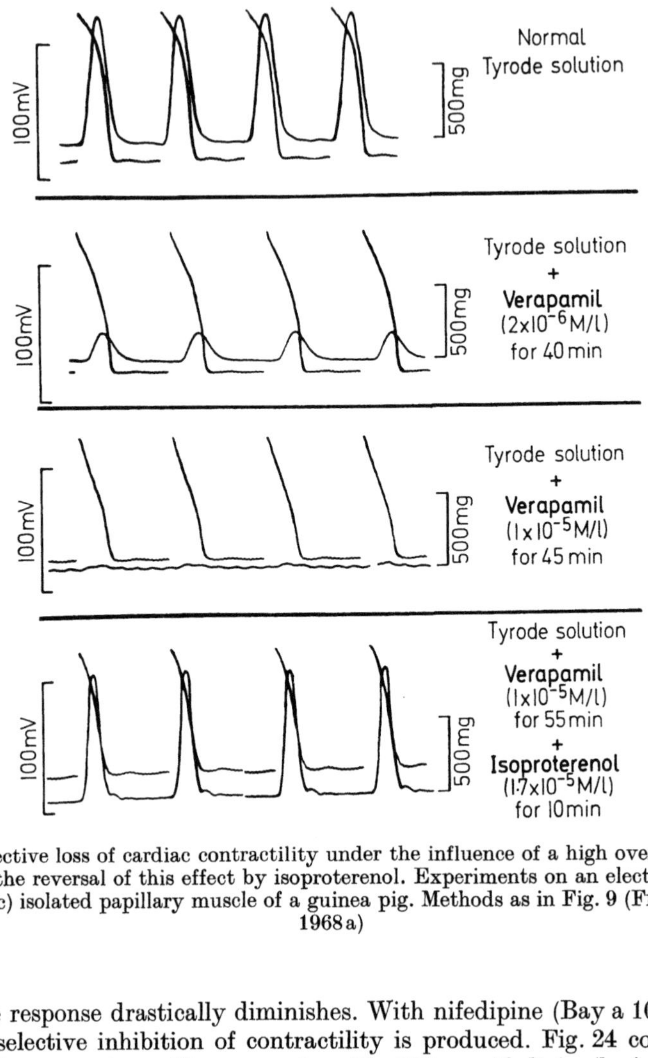

Fig. 22. Selective loss of cardiac contractility under the influence of a high overdose of verapamil, and the reversal of this effect by isoproterenol. Experiments on an electrically driven (2 shocks/sec) isolated papillary muscle of a guinea pig. Methods as in Fig. 9 (Fleckenstein, 1968a)

contractile response drastically diminishes. With nifedipine (Bay a 1040, Adalat) the same selective inhibition of contractility is produced. Fig. 24 contains data obtained from a cat papillary muscle with 100 μg nifedipine/l. Again resting potential, upstroke velocity, and duration of the plateau of the action potential persisted, whereas contractility declined.

In a further attempt to clarify the specific mechanism of action of these powerful drugs, separate measurements of the transmembrane Na and Ca currents were performed on ventricular trabeculae of cats with the use of a special voltage clamp technique by Kohlhardt, Bauer, Krause, and Fleckenstein (1972). The following results were obtained: verapamil and compound D 600 even in a dose as low as 0.5 to 2.0 mg/l produce a drastic reduction in the transmembrane Ca conductivity. In some experiments, D 600 blocked the Ca currents completely. This effect can be neutralized by addition of excess Ca to the bathing fluid even in the presence of the inhibitors. But in contrast to their strong inhibitory effect on the passive transmembrane Ca movements, verapamil and D 600 in corresponding concentrations do not block the fast Na current. The graphs in Fig. 25 demonstrate both the transmembrane Ca and Na currents—expressed in μA—on the abscissa, plotted against the clamped membrane potentials on the ordinate. As can be

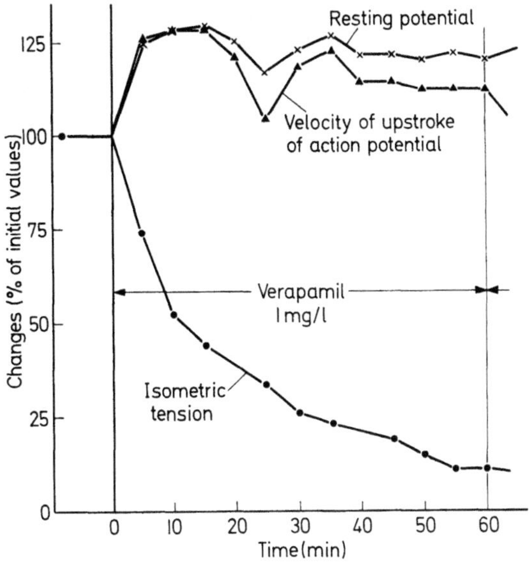

Fig. 23. Selective reduction of the Ca-dependent contractile force of a guinea pig papillary muscle to $^1/_{10}$ of normal by 1 mg/l verapamil within 60 min, whilst the upstroke velocity and the height of the overshoot of the cardiac action potential, which indicate the transmembrane Na influx, did not decrease. Continuous microelectrode recordings were taken from the same cardiac fiber for 90 min. The absolute values (100%) at the beginning of the experiment were as follows: Resting potential (−75 mV); upstroke velocity (130 V/sec); isometric peak tension (700 mg). Temperature 36° C. Frequency of stimulation 2/sec (FLECKENSTEIN, 1970/71a)

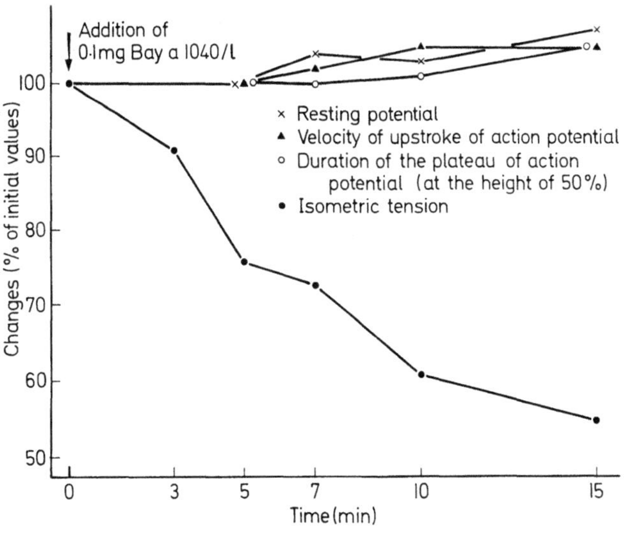

Fig. 24. Nifedipine (Bay a 1040): Selective inhibition of the contractile force of a cat papillary muscle without reduction of resting potential and without influence on velocity of rise, and duration of the plateau of action potential. Experimental procedure as in Fig. 23. × resting potential; ▲ velocity of upstroke of action potential; ○ duration of the plateau of action potential (at a height of 50%) (FLECKENSTEIN, TRITTHART, DÖRING, and BYON, 1972)

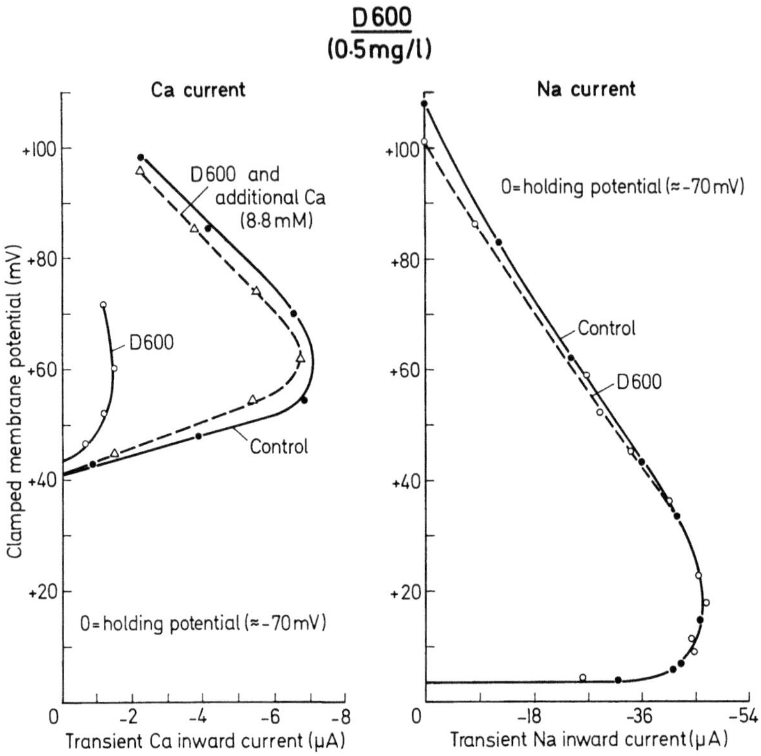

Fig. 25. Current–voltage relationship curves of the slow transmembrane Ca current and the fast Na current under the influence of D 600 (0.5 mg/l). Observations on an isolated trabecula from the right ventricle of a cat. By addition of D 600 to normal Tyrode solution containing 2.2 mM $CaCl_2$/l, the current–voltage relationship curve of the slow Ca inward current is shifted to very low values indicating a strong inhibition of the transmembrane Ca influx through the slow channel. By increasing the extracellular Ca concentration up to 8.8 mM/l, the effect of D 600 on the transmembrane Ca current is nearly neutralized. The influence of D 600 on the fast Na inward current is negligible. Temperature 32° C, pH 7.35 (KOHLHARDT, BAUER, KRAUSE, and FLECKENSTEIN, 1972)

seen from the left side of the figure the current–voltage relationship curve of the transmembrane Ca currents is shifted by D 600 to very low values. But as soon as the extracellular Ca concentration is increased from 2.2 up to 8.8 mM/l, by addition of excess Ca to the D 600-containing medium, the Ca currents almost returned to normal. The fast Na conductivity, on the other hand, is not altered by D 600, as shown on the right side of the figure. Here the current–voltage relationship curves of the fast Na inward currents are practically identical regardless of whether D 600 had been given or not. Quite similar results were obtained with verapamil (Fig. 26). Verapamil and D 600 differ in this respect from common local anesthetic compounds such as xylocaine (lidocaine) or procaine which interfere much more with the transmembrane Na conductivity than with the Ca conductivity. The selective depression of the Ca or the Na conductivity by specific inhibitors indicates that during excitation the influxes of Na and Ca are independent of each other. Therefore, in the mammalian myocardium the existence of two separate channels for Na and Ca has to be assumed.

As a functional consequence of this dual membrane transport system it is possible to change the contractile force by inotropic substances which act on the

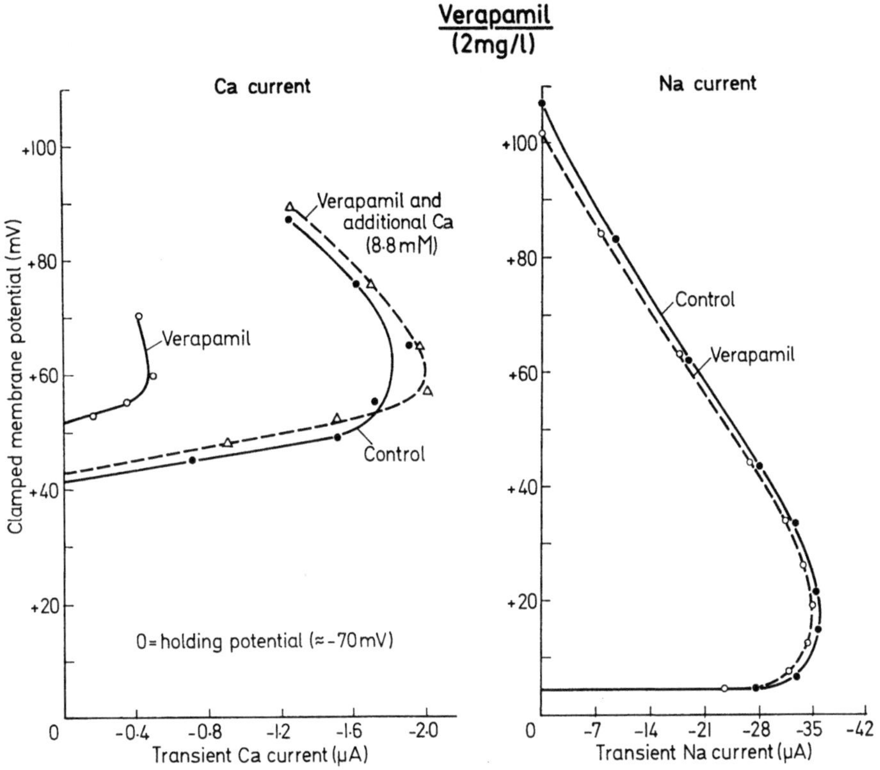

Fig. 26. Current–voltage relationship curves of the slow transmembrane Ca current and the fast Na current under the influence of verapamil (2 mg/l). With this dose the transmembrane Ca conductivity is reduced to a similar extent as with 0.5 mg/l D 600. There is again no significant change in the fast Na current. The measurements were carried out on a trabecula from the right ventricle of a cat. Experimental procedures as in the Fig. 17 and 25 (Kohlhardt, Bauer, Krause, and Fleckenstein, 1972)

Ca conductivity without a corresponding influence on Na-dependent excitation. This possibility of controlling contractile force by acting on the Ca channel is lost in skinned myocardial fibers which we have prepared by glycerin–water extraction or according to Winegrad's technique. In such skinned fibers the Ca-antagonistic compounds exert no inhibitory effect when contraction is directly induced by addition of ATP and Ca (Weder and Grün, 1973). This means that the inhibitors of the transmembrane Ca transport system, such as verapamil or D 600, lose their power if the Ca ions have free access to the contractile system where ATP is split. The same is true for the cobalt and nickel ions which also block primarily the transmembrane Ca inward movement, but have no comparable effect on the Ca-activated myofibrillar ATPase itself (Kohlhardt, Krause, Bauer, and Fleckenstein, 1973).

Despite these clear results, a number of other questions have not yet been fully answered. So the possibility is still not definitely excluded that Ca-antagonistic inhibitors of excitation–contraction coupling, apart from their well-established action on the "slow membrane channel", might also interfere in some way with intracellular Ca movements. Admittedly, in isolated mitochondria only excessive concentrations of verapamil were capable of reducing Ca uptake (Janke and Frey,

1972). Similarly, in isolated sarcoplasmic reticulum, all direct attempts of showing an inhibitory effect of negative inotropic doses of verapamil on accumulation, binding, or exchange of Ca have failed (NAYLER and SZETO, 1972; ENTMAN, ALLEN, BORNET, GILLETTE, WALLICK, and SCHWARTZ, 1972; WATANABE and BESCH, JR., 1974). The same is true for some model studies regarding the kinetics of the verapamil action which were carried out by means of an analog computer (HENNEKES, BAYER, and KAUFMANN, 1974). More sophisticated than helpful, such calculations on a presumed interaction of verapamil with intracellular Ca movements (between unidentified compartments) are no substitute for solid experimental data obtained on isolated organelles. Nevertheless, with respect to the growing number of Ca-antagonistic substances of widely different chemical structure, the lack of results using verapamil should not discourage further work in this field.

More promising, however, are some recent investigations about the particular action of verapamil on isolated cardiac sarcolemma membranes. Here a membrane-located Ca store was found by NAYLER and SZETO (1972) which could be depleted by verapamil. The reduced amount of Ca taken up per beat when verapamil is present may result from the effect the drug has on the Ca accumulating activity of these membrane-located sites. According to WILLIAMSON, WOODROW, and SCARPA (1973) there are two different types of Ca storage in cardiac sarcolemma membranes, one at low and another at high affinity Ca binding sites. Verapamil specifically inhibits low affinity Ca binding. These observations as well as other findings justify the assumption that the Ca ions which enter the excited myocardial fibers are derived from an intermediate pool of superficially bound membrane Ca. If this hypothesis is correct, then the principal action of verapamil would consist of imparing the Ca binding capacity or the refilling of this sarcolemma Ca store so that the availability of Ca to the "slow membrane channel" is restricted. However, further work is needed to establish this attractive theory.

VI. Neutralization of Ca-Antagonistic Compounds by β-Adrenergic Catecholamines and Cardiac Glycosides

Apart from Ca ions, cardiac glycosides and β-adrenergic catecholamines are also capable of restoring the utilization of high-energy phosphates in contraction so that the negative inotropic influence of Ca-antagonistic compounds is overcome. However, even these agents seem to act through the mediation of Ca. As early as 1917, O. LOEWI was the first to attribute the cardiac effects of digitalis glycosides to an interaction with Ca. But more than 40 years passed before LOEWI's hypothesis was further substantiated by THOMAS, JOLLEY, and GRECHMAN (1958) and by HOLLAND and his group (HOLLAND and SEKUL, 1959; SEKUL and HOLLAND, 1960; LÜLLMANN and HOLLAND, 1962; GERSMEYER and HOLLAND, 1963; and the review articles of KLAUS, 1964 and REPKE, 1964). This work established that ouabain causes an increased rate of ^{45}Ca uptake in frog hearts and in rabbit or rat atria. The influence on ^{45}Ca uptake was small but statistically significant during the positive inotropic action of ouabain, whereas the uptake rates rose sharply with the onset of ouabain-induced contractures. Accordingly, in our experiments on isolated rabbit atria, small inotropic effects of ouabain were accompanied by a slight decrease of the ratio CP/inorganic P, whereas a more obvious high-energy phosphate breakdown occurred in toxic concentrations. But there was no clear influence of ouabain on CP and inorganic P in the resting state of the myocardium or in a Ca-free medium. The experimental data suggest that

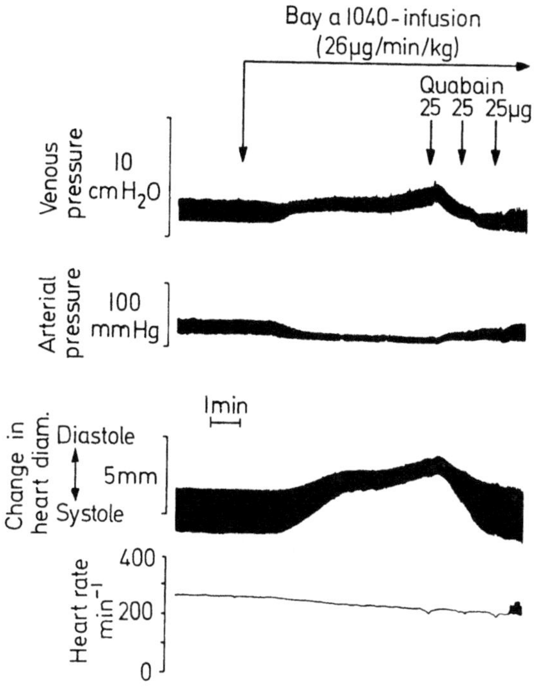

Fiig. 27. Acute contractile failure of a guinea pig heart (open chest preparation) produced by intravenous infusion of nifedipine (26 µg/min/kg). Recovery of cardiac function takes place within 3 to 4 min following intravenous injection of ouabain (FLECKENSTEIN, TRITTHART, DÖRING, and BYON, 1972)

cardiac glycosides facilitate the process of Ca entry (or Ca release from certain binding sites), by which the action potential gives rise to contractions. By this effect the cardiodepression produced by Ca-antagonistic drugs is easily abolished (Figs. 27 and 28).

Evidence has accumulated in recent years that the mechanism of action of positive inotropic catecholamines also consists of a potentiation of Ca-dependent excitation–contraction coupling (ANTONI, ENGSTFELD, and FLECKENSTEIN, 1960). For instance, sympathomimetic amines with β-receptor stimulating properties such as epinephrine or isoproterenol influence the transmembrane Ca conductivity exactly in the opposite sense as the Ca-antagonistic drugs, in that they potentiate the Ca influx through the excited myocardial fiber membranes (REUTER, 1965; JANKE and FLECKENSTEIN; see FLECKENSTEIN, 1970/71 a, b). The result of these opposite cardiac actions is simply that Ca-antagonistic compounds and β-adrenergic catecholamines neutralize each other. Among the sympathomimetic amines tested in this respect, isoproterenol was by far the most powerful Ca promoter. Therefore, in all cases of contractile cardiac failure due to inhibition of Ca-dependent utilization of high-energy phosphates, the biochemical and mechanical functions could be restored by suitable doses of isoproterenol with a minimum Ca requirement. Isoproterenol-induced recovery usually takes place within 10 to 20 sec. This applies not only to isolated preparations of cardiac tissue (Fig. 22) but also to hearts *in situ*. Fig. 29 shows, for example, the development of severe contractile failure of a guinea pig heart after i.v. administration of a total dose of about 1 mg verapamil/kg. There was an increase in central venous pressure and a decrease in

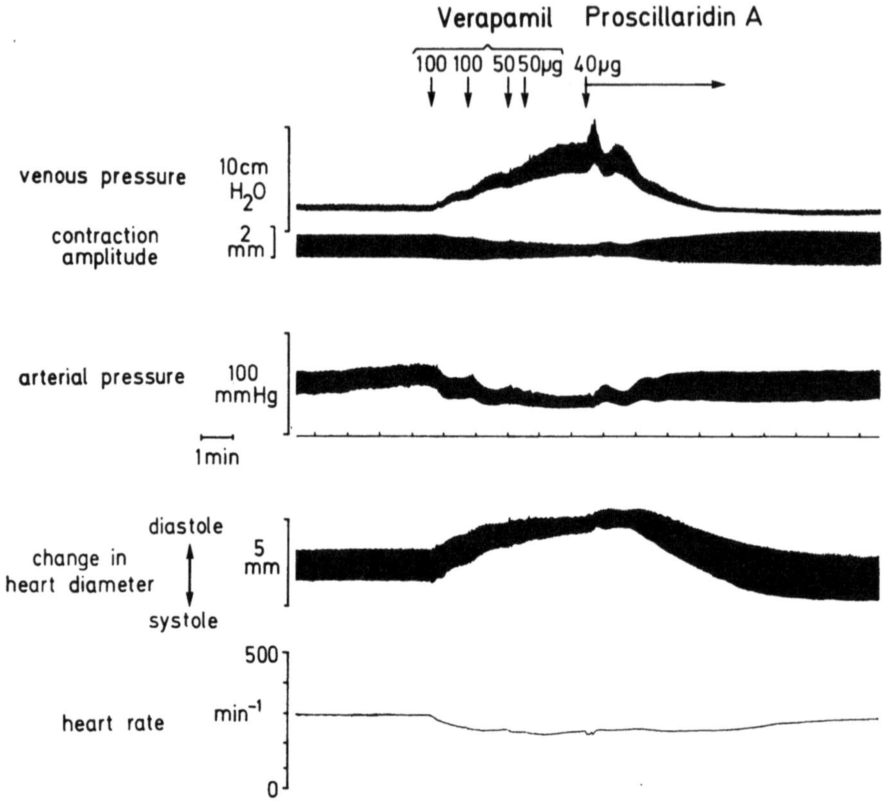

Fig. 28. Acute contractile failure of a guinea pig heart (open chest preparation) produced by a large i.v. overdose of verapamil (≈ 1 mg/kg). Following i.v. administration of 0.13 mg/kg proscillaridin A (Talusin) the cardiovascular effects of verapamil are completely neutralized within 5 min (DÖRING and KAMMERMEIER, unpublished, 1964)

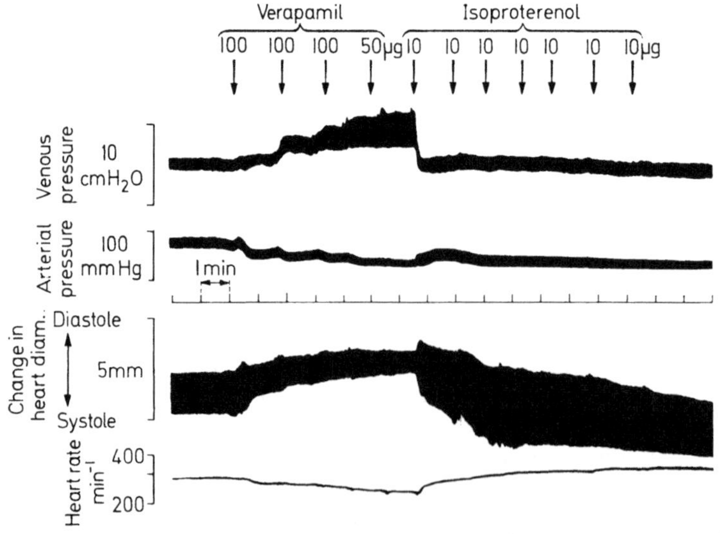

Fig. 29. Acute contractile failure of a guinea pig heart (open chest preparation) produced by a large overdose (1.2 mg/kg) of verapamil. After the first therapeutic dose of 10 µg isoproterenol (which corresponds to 35 µg/kg isoproterenol), contractility and venous blood pressure returned to normal within 20 to 30 sec (FLECKENSTEIN, 1964)

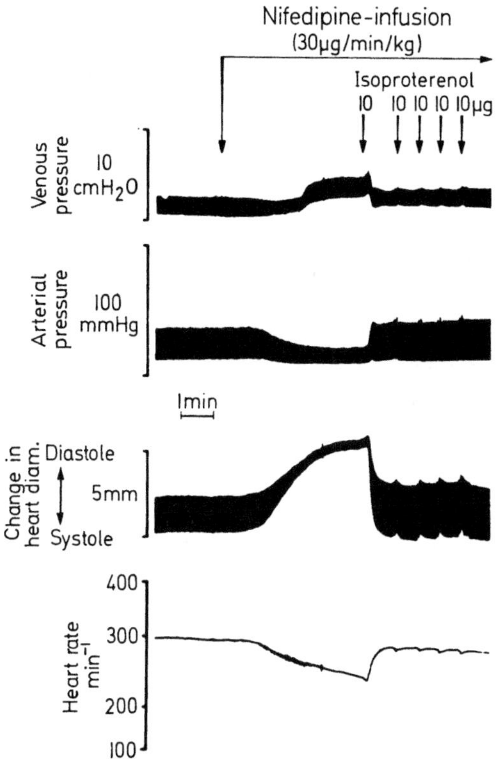

Fig. 30. Acute contractile failure of a guinea pig heart (open chest preparation) produced by i.v. infusion of nifedipine (30 µg/min/kg). The first therapeutic dose of 10 µg isoproterenol (≈ 30 µg/kg body weight) restores the contractile function of the heart almost completely within 20 to 30 sec (FLECKENSTEIN, TRITTHART, DÖRING, and BYON, 1972)

the aortic pressure, whilst the heart was more and more dilated and the contraction amplitude strongly reduced. But after the i.v. injection of a single dose of 10 µg isoproterenol, the contractile function of the heart quickly returned to normal within 20 sec. A similar experiment, using nifedipine instead of verapamil, is shown in Fig. 30. Further extensive studies on the mutual neutralization of verapamil and isoproterenol were carried out by NAYLER, MCINNES, SWANN, PRICE, CARSON, RACE, and LOWE (1968).

VII. Influence of Inhibitors and Promoters of Ca Action on Myocardial High-Energy Phosphate Consumption

Our experiments demonstrate that there are many inhibitors and promoters of the Ca action in excitation–contraction coupling. By this basic mechanism they can intensify or restrict the utilization of high-energy phosphates in the contractile machinery or even block it. Because less ATP is consumed by the Ca-deficient myocardium or under the influence of Ca-antagonistic inhibitors of excitation–contraction coupling, mechanical tension decreases while high-energy phosphates accumulate in the cardiac muscle. So the contractile failure produced by Ca-antagonistic drugs is generally accompanied by an elevated CP or ATP level and by a diminution in the orthophosphate fraction. This is true for the isolated myocardium as well as for hearts *in situ* after i.v. administration of Ca-antagonistic com-

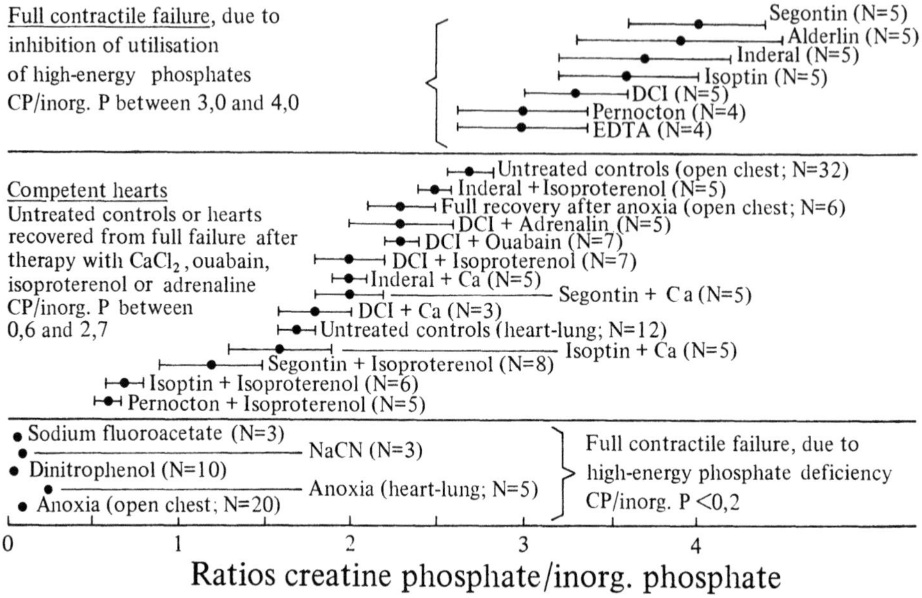

Fig. 31. Increase of the creatine phosphate/inorganic phosphate ratio (up to a value of 3–4) in the left ventricular myocardium of guinea pig hearts *in situ* during the contractile failure produced by Ca-antagonistic interference with excitation–contraction coupling. To cause this type of cardiac incompetence overdoses of verapamil (0.4 to 1.0 mg/kg) and prenylamine (6 to 12 mg/kg) were given i.v. to guinea pigs (open chest preparations). Moreover, several substances with Ca-antagonistic side effects such as propranolol (1.5 to 6 mg/kg), pronethalol (3 to 5 mg/kg), dichloroisoproterenol (6 to 25 mg/kg), and butyl-bromallyl barbituric acid (Somnifen, 75 mg/kg) were administered until severe contractile failure of the hearts developed. I.v. injection of EDTA (40 to 70 mg/kg), by simple chelation of Ca, had a similar effect. In all these cases the Ca-dependent high-energy phosphate consumption in the contractile system was restricted so that the CP content, in relation to inorganic P, rose. If, however, the high-energy phosphate utilization was restored by $CaCl_2$ (45 mg/kg), isoproterenol (150 µg/kg), epinephrine (300 µg/kg), or ouabain (150 to 300 µg/kg), the creatine phosphate/inorganic phosphate ratio rapidly fell to the normal range pari passu with the recovery of the contractile tension. For comparison, the graph also shows the very low ratios (0.1 to 0.2) found in the left ventricular myocardium under the influence of anoxia or metabolic poisons (10 mg/kg NaCN; 15 mg/kg sodium fluoroacetate; 30 mg/kg 2,4-dinitrophenol) when contractile failure developed due to a nearly complete high-energy phosphate exhaustion. The absolute concentrations of the acid-soluble phosphate compounds in 32 untreated control hearts *in situ* (expressed as µM/g blood-free tissue wet weight) were as follows: creatine phosphate 8.3 ($\pm$ 0.25 = SE of mean); inorganic phosphate 3.2 ($\pm$ 0.11), ATP 4.6 ($\pm$ 0.08), ADP 0.8 ($\pm$ 0.03), total acid-soluble phosphorus 1160 ($\pm$ 13) µg P/g. The corresponding control values for the left ventricular myocardium of 12 competent heart–lung preparations were: creatine phosphate 7.9 ($\pm$ 0.2), inorganic phosphate 4.4 ($\pm$ 0.05), ATP 4.6 ($\pm$ 0.2), ADP 0.8 ($\pm$ 0.03), total acid-soluble phosphorus 1145 ($\pm$ 21) µg P/g (FLECKENSTEIN, DÖRING, and KAMMERMEIER, 1966/67)

pounds (FLECKENSTEIN, KAMMERMEIER, DÖRING, and FREUND, 1967). We have carried out several hundred experiments on guinea pig hearts *in situ* (open chest preparations) in which the effects of large doses of a wide variety of specific and non-specific Ca-antagonistic drugs on heart diameter, contraction amplitude, cardiac frequency, and on arterial and venous blood pressure were investigated together with the changes in the high-energy phosphate content of the left ventricular myocardium. A summary of some of our biochemical results is given in Fig. 31. The graph shows that the creatine phosphate/inorganic phosphate ratio was consistently increased above normal (up to 3–4) when severe symptoms of heart incompetence appeared after i.v. administration of the Ca-antagonistic compounds. If, however, the high-energy phosphate consumption was restored by the administration of Ca or by therapeutic doses of sympathomimetic amines or cardiac glycosides, the myocardial creatine phosphate/inorganic phosphate ratio rapidly fell to the normal range of 0.6 to 2.7 simultaneously with the recovery of the contractile force. The graph also shows the extremely low figure of 0.1 to 0.2 in all cases of contractile failure resulting from high-energy phosphate deficiency. The present results also explain why the two types of cardiac incompetence widely differ with respect to their responses to therapeutic doses of $CaCl_2$, cardiac glycosides, or β-adrenergic catecholamines: In all cases of contractile failure due to a lack of ATP or CP the effect of this treatment is necessarily small, transient, or totally absent. In contrast, cardiac incompetence resulting from deficient high-energy phosphate utilization is greatly susceptible to this therapy and responds with full and long-lasting recovery of the mechanical function.

As to the significance of our results for human cardiology, it is interesting to note that the usual congestive heart failure resulting from chronic valvular disease has probably more in common with contractile failure due to deficient utilization of high-energy phosphates than with the cardiac disorders in anoxia or ischemia. This conclusion is mainly based on two observations, namely:

1. That the myocardial high-energy phosphate concentrations are not critically diminished in such incompetent human hearts. This also applies to experimental cardiac failure produced by coarctation of the aorta or pulmonary artery (FEINSTEIN, 1962; FOX, WIKLER, and REED, 1965; CHIDSEY, WEINBACH, POOL, and MORROW, 1966; POOL, SPANN, BUCCINO, SONNENBLICK, and BRAUNWALD, 1967; HEIN, FLECKENSTEIN, JANKE, ECKARDT, and LUDIN, 1972). Moreover, isolated mitochondria from such incompetent hearts showed no damage of oxidative phosphorylation so that the ATP supply seems to be unaltered (SOBEL, SPANN, POOL, SONNENBLICK, and BRAUNWALD, 1967).

2. That cardiac glycosides are particularly helpful in the treatment of congestive cardiac failure, whereas all agents which interfere with excitation–contraction coupling aggravate the disease as has been shown by many clinical case reports.

All these results disprove the classical concept of HARRISON (1935) and others who postulated a decisive role of hypoxia or deficient oxidative metabolism in the production of congestive cardiac failure in men. Therefore, we have suggested as an alternative hypothesis that, in hypertrophied heart muscle fibers, the enlargement in diameter, the relative increase in mass or thickness of myofibrils, or ultrastructural alterations in the transverse tubular system might possibly impair excitation–contraction coupling by reducing the availability of Ca (FLECKENSTEIN, 1965/66, 1968a). This could be simply due to an increase in the distance over which Ca has to move. In addition, the utilization of high-energy phosphates could also be decreased as a result of the catecholamine depletion which takes place when contractile failure develops (SPANN, CHIDSEY, POOL, and BRAUNWALD, 1965).

VIII. Drug-Induced Changes in Cardiac Oxygen Requirement

As already discussed in a preceding chapter (D, I) not only the utilization of ATP for tension development but also the consecutive rise in oxygen consumption of active cardiac muscle above resting level is necessarily Ca-dependent. Therefore,

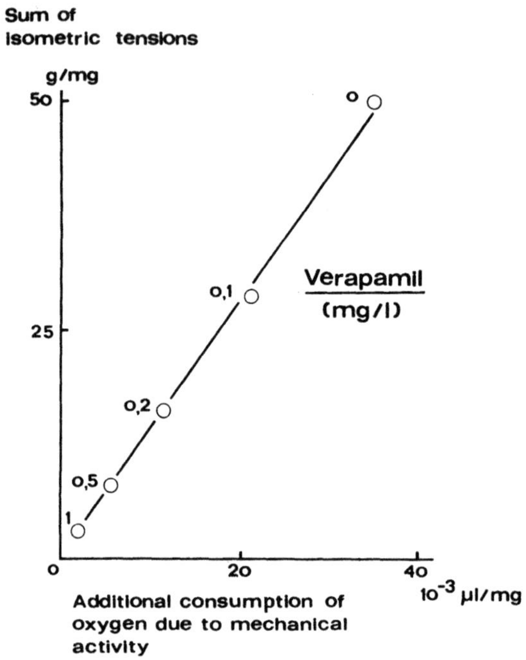

Fig. 32. Verapamil: Linear reduction of isometric tension and additional consumption of oxygen due to mechanical activity under the influence of increasing doses of the drug (0.1, 0.2, 0.5, and 1.0 mg/l) in Tyrode solution containing 2.0 mM Ca/l. The experiment was carried out on a rabbit papillary muscle (1.7 mg wet weight) which was incubated at rest in the different media each time for 20 min and then stimulated for 3 min at a frequency of 60 sec. Measurements of the rates of oxygen consumption with a platinum electrode and of mechanical tension with a mechano-electronic displacement transducer were made throughout the experiment at 30° C (BYON and FLECKENSTEIN, 1969; see FLECKENSTEIN, 1970/71b)

it is easily understood that Ca-antagonistic drugs, in reducing high-energy phosphate consumption in the contractile system, also lower cardiac oxygen requirement per heart beat. The decrease in cardiac oxygen demand strictly parallels that of contractile force. Fig. 32 demonstrates the proportional reduction of isometric tension and extra-consumption of oxygen under the influence of increasing doses of verapamil. It was interesting that in this case a 50% decrease of contractile force and extra-consumption of oxygen was produced by a dose as low as 0.1 mg verapamil/l. With a higher dose of 1 mg verapamil/l both tension and oxygen consumption dropped almost to the resting level since the persisting electric activity of the myocardial fibers influences the rate of respiration to a rather insignificant extent. The results of two other experiments of this type with the use of prenylamine and nifedipine are shown in Fig. 33 and 34. As can be seen from Fig. 34, only 0.01 mg nifedipine/l is required for an almost 50% inhibition of isometric tension and extra-oxygen consumption. By increasing the extracellular Ca concentration up to 16 mM/l, mechanical activity and oxygen consumption were rapidly restored to normal even if the contractile system had previously been almost paralyzed.

In contrast to the Ca sensitivity of extra-oxygen consumption during mechanical activity, the oxygen uptake of cardiac tissue preparations at rest does

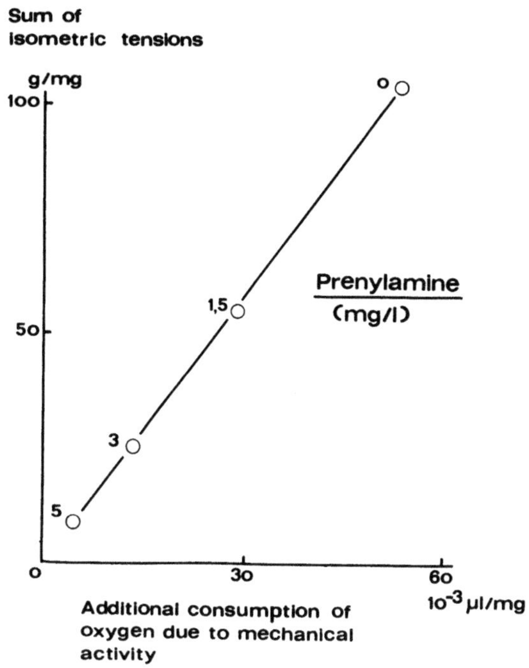

Fig. 33. Prenylamine: Linear reduction of isometric tension and additional consumption of oxygen due to mechanical activity under the influence of increasing doses of the drug (1.5, 3.0, and 5.0 mg/l) in Tyrode solution containing 2.0 mM Ca/l. The experiment was carried out on a rabbit papillary muscle (0.6 mg wet weight). Experimental procedure as in Fig. 32 (Byon and Fleckenstein, 1969; see Fleckenstein, 1970/71b)

not show any depression when the Ca-antagonistic inhibitors of excitation–contraction coupling are administered even in relatively big doses. So their oxygen-saving effect is only due to a restriction of the cardiac activity metabolism in which the Ca ions play the key-role, whereas all other ATP-consuming metabolic reactions which are not connected with mechanical activity are not affected by these drugs.

The new Ca-antagonistic inhibitors of excitation–contraction coupling deserve more than academic interest since in patients with a hyperkinetic heart function or in cases of angina pectoris and of other forms of coronary disease a certain restriction of the cardiac activity metabolism may be helpful in order to re-establish a suitable balance between a reduced coronary oxygen supply and the actual cardiac oxygen requirement. In this respect the Ca-antagonistic drugs exert the same beneficial influence on patients with angina pectoris as the adrenergic β-receptor blocking agents do. Needless to say that the relatively small doses of Ca-antagonistic drugs used in human therapy cannot produce more than a moderate reduction of tension development. Moreover, on the heart *in situ*, the negative inotropic effects of Ca-antagonistic drugs are limited by a reflex activation of the sympathetic system if there is an unproportionate fall of arterial blood pressure. In this situation the hearts are still responsive to sympathetic transmitter substances because the specific Ca-antagonistic drugs, in the therapeutic dosage range, do not possess any remarkable β-receptor blocking activity.

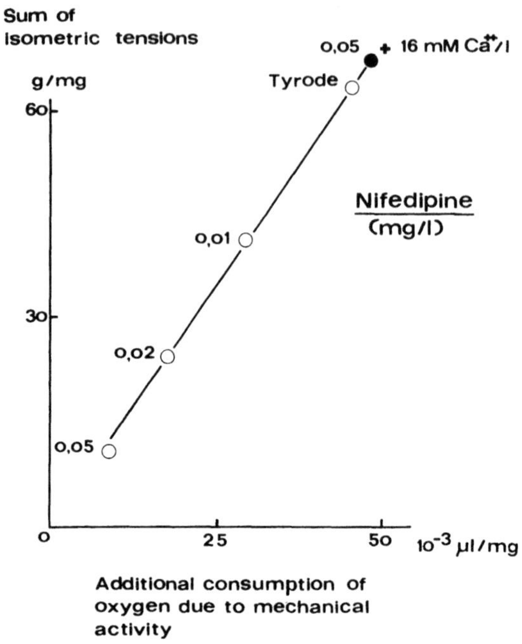

Fig. 34. Nifedipine: Linear reduction of isometric tension and additional consumption of oxygen due to mechanical activity under the influence of increasing doses of the drug (0.01 mg, 0.02 mg, and 0.05 mg/l) in Tyrode solution containing 2.0 mM Ca/l. With 0.05 mg/l tension, development and extra-consumption of oxygen were greatly depressed. This drug effect could be completely neutralized by increasing the extracellular Ca concentration up to 16 mM/l in the presence of 0.05 mg/l nifedipine. Experimental procedure as in the Figs. 32 and 33 (FLECKENSTEIN, TRITTHART, DÖRING, and BYON, 1972)

E. Myocardial High-Energy Phosphate Depletion and Structural Decay

I. The Fundamental Role of High-Energy Phosphates in Cardiac Resting Metabolism

The maintenance of structural integrity and the permanent regeneration of the myocardial tissue require a sufficient supply of ATP for many energy-consuming synthetic processes which continue whether the heart is active or not. Obviously the myocardial fiber, like every other living structure, is in a state of dynamic equilibrium between spontaneous degradation and opposite recovery reactions which operate at the expense of phosphate-bond energy. For instance, the rate of steady-state oxygen consumption of the quiescent mammalian myocardium amounts to approximately 0.01 to 0.02 ml O_2/g tissue/min at 37° C. At a P/O ratio of 3, these figures correspond to a quantity of 2.5 to 5 μM high-energy phosphate/g myocardial tissue/min which is metabolized under the conditions of cardiac arrest. With regard to the fact that the total high-energy phosphate content does not exceed 15 to 20 μM/g myocardial tissue, this rate of ATP consumption is surprisingly high: in the case of a total blockade of ATP synthesis, the high-energy phosphate stores would be completely exhausted within 4 to 8 min even in the absence of any mechanical activity. Due to glycolysis this critical state is certainly

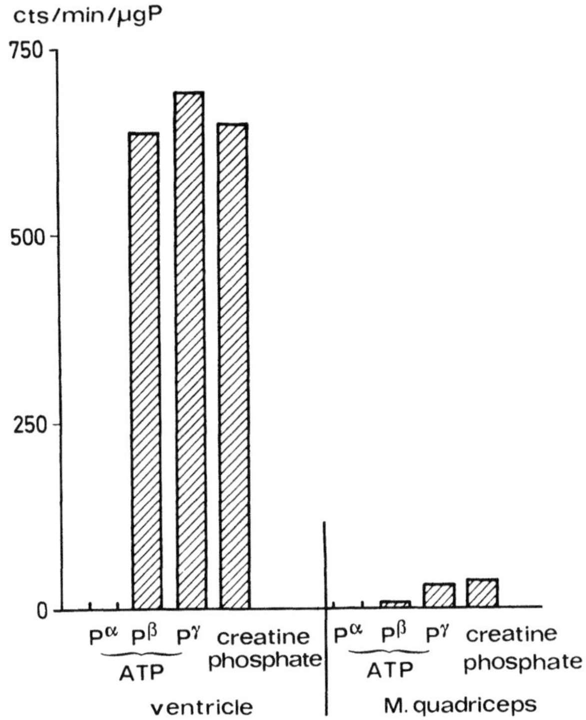

Fig. 35. Rate of ^{32}P-incorporation into ATP and creatine phosphate in cardiac and skeletal muscle of rats after i.v. injection of 0.2 mCi ^{32}P-labelled orthophosphate. The anesthetized animals were killed by immersion in liquid nitrogen 20 min after the ^{32}P-injection (FLECKENSTEIN and JANKE, 1959)

somewhat postponed in the anoxic or ischemic myocardium (Fig. 5). Nevertheless, as shown by BÜCHNER and ONISHI (1968) in oxygen-deprived rat hearts, the first signs of degradation of the mitochondrial and myofibrillar structures appear as early as within 5 to 10 min.

Interestingly enough, the resting oxygen requirement of cardiac muscle is much greater than that of skeletal muscle: According to the classical studies of CLARK and WHITE (1929) the respiration rates of quiescent tortoise and frog atria exceed those of resting skeletal muscles by a factor of 10–20. Approximately the same proportion was found in our own experiments on rats. Similarly, in cardiac muscle, the intracellular turnover rates of ATP and CP are considerable greater than in skeletal muscle (FLECKENSTEIN and JANKE, 1958, 1959; FLECKENSTEIN JANKE and GERLACH, 1959; FLECKENSTEIN, 1961, 1963). Fig. 35 shows experiments in which ^{32}P-labelled orthophosphate was i.v. administered to anesthetized rats, and the ^{32}P-uptake into the ventricular and skeletal ATP and CP fractions were measured. As can be easily seen there was, in the myocardium, a 10 to 20 times faster incorporation of radiophosphorus into CP and the different phosphate groups of ATP than in the M. quadriceps of the same animals. These figures reveal large differences in the rates of oxidative phosphorylation which are probably due to the fact that the myocardial fibers—in contrast to skeletal muscle—contain an exceedingly large number of mitochondria. The individual ^{32}P-uptake rates remain in the same order of magnitude whether cardiac and skeletal muscle preparations are stimulated or not; they are, however, largely influenced by changes

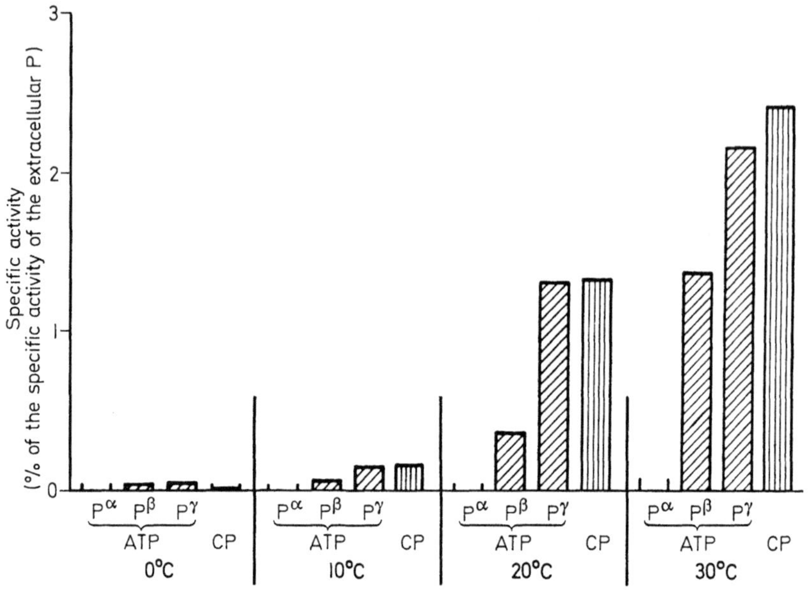

Fig. 36. Influence of temperature on the cardiac high-energy phosphate metabolism at rest: Quiescent rabbit auricles were exposed to a Tyrode solution containing 0.4 μM/ml orthophosphate of an activity of about 100 μCi/ml for 15 min at 0, 10, 20, and 30° C. Then the ^{32}P-uptake rates into CP and the 3 phosphate groups of ATP were determined. The specific activities measured are expressed as percent of the specific activity of the extracellular P (FLECKENSTEIN, JANKE, and GERLACH, 1959)

Table 6. Uptake of ^{18}O from $H_2{}^{18}O$ into the 3 phosphate groups of ATP according to their individual turnover rates at different temperatures (FLECKENSTEIN, JANKE, and MARMIER, 1965)

	Temp. (° C)	Total Uptake (atom ^{18}O per molecule)	Distribution: Adenosine·O-P^{α}(=O)(OH)—O	—P^{β}(=O)(OH)—O—	—P^{γ}(=O)(OH)—OH	Number of Exp.
M. rectus abdomin. (frog)	0	0.012	0	0	0.012 (100%)	5
	10	0.046	0	0	0.046 (100%)	8
	20	0.15	0	0.02 (13%)	0.13 (87%)	6
Isolated rabbit auricle	10	0.34	$>$0.01	0.06 (18%)	0.28 (82%)	5
	20	0.97	0.01 (1%)	0.13 (13%)	0.83 (86%)	5

in temperature. When, for instance, the temperature was lowered from 30 to 0° C the absolute concentrations of ATP and CP in quiescent rabbit auricles did not change, but the rate of ^{32}P-uptake into these high-energy phosphate fractions was reduced to approximately $^1/_{100}$ of the original value (Fig. 36). Because all "catabolic" reactions are considerably slower at low temperature, less ATP is split and resynthesized to cover the energy expenses for cellular regeneration of the resting auricular tissue. Thus, at low temperature, the oxygen requirement declines in parallel with the high-energy phosphate turnover.

Our results obtained with radioactive ^{32}P-labelled orthophosphate were accomplished by further turnover studies with ^{18}O-labelled water. This technique is based on the ^{18}O-uptake from $H_2{}^{18}O$ and allows estimations of the *absolute turnover rates* of the intracellular phosphate fractions (FLECKENSTEIN, GERLACH, JANKE, and MARMIER, 1959, 1960; FLECKENSTEIN, 1961, 1963b; FLECKENSTEIN and JANKE, 1964; FLECKENSTEIN, JANKE, and MARMIER, 1965; JANKE, MARMIER, and FLECKENSTEIN, 1965; JANKE, FLECKENSTEIN, MARMIER, and KOENIG, 1966). Measurements of ^{32}P-uptake only indicate *relative turnover rates* of the intracellular organophosphate fractions because the orthophosphate transfer from the extracellular space to the internal compartments is not only restricted by a low sarcolemma membrane permeability but also influenced by the height of the transmembrane orthophosphate gradient. In contrast, $H_2{}^{18}O$ permeates freely toward all intracellular sites where organophosphate compounds are hydrolytically split and resynthesized. Table 6 contains some data about the ^{18}O incorporation into the different phosphate groups of ATP, both in resting frog skeletal muscle and in quiescent rabbit auricles. As shown by these figures, two principal findings previously obtained with radiophosphorus, were confirmed with the more reliable ^{18}O-technique:

1. The resting ATP turnover is considerable and changes with a factor of about 3 at a temperature variation of 10° C.
2. At a given temperature, resting ATP turnover of cardiac muscle is many times faster than that of sceletal muscle. This applies to frogs as well as to mammals.

In conclusion it is to be stated that the great amount of metabolic energy required for basic maintenance reactions at 37° C renders the myocardial cells particularly sensitive to any interruption of high-energy phosphate supply whether this may be caused by simple oxygen lack or inhibitors of ATP synthesis. Therefore, as commonly known, the only possible way of protecting anoxic or ischemic hearts against rapid cellular disintegration consists of cooling in order to reduce their basic energy requirement.

II. Myocardial Fiber Damage Caused by Exhaustive High-Energy Phosphate Consumption due to Ca Overload

A negative myocardial energy balance is not only produced by an insufficient rate of ATP synthesis. Another important reason why the high-energy phosphates may be exhausted is an excessive ATP consumption due to mechanical hyperactivity. This applies particularly to β-adrenergic overstimulation of the heart. As regards the mechanism of action, in physiological doses, the sympathetic catecholamines increase the force of the beating heart by enhancing the utilization of high-energy phosphates in the contractile machinery. This effect is primarily due to an augmentation of the transmembrane Ca influx during excitation, so that the Ca-dependent myofibrillar ATPase, which transforms phosphate-bond energy into mechanical work, is more activated. With increasing doses of catecholamines, however, Ca uptake and high-energy phosphate breakdown may become so excessive that not enough ATP is left for the various synthetic processes which are involved in the regeneration of the living structures. In other words, overdoses of β-adrenergic catecholamines, leading to an abundant Ca influx, waste ATP

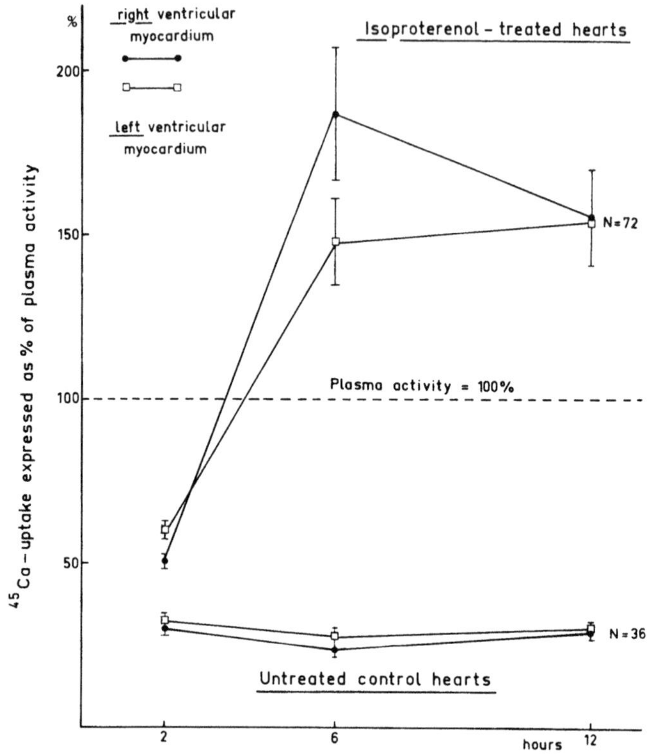

Fig. 37. Increase of the net radiocalcium uptake into the left and right ventricular myocardium of rats produced by the s.c. injection of 30 mg/kg isoproterenol. The ^{45}Ca uptake into 1 g of fresh cardiac tissue is expressed as a percentage of the corresponding ^{45}Ca activity in 1 ml of plasma during an observation period of 12 hr after i.p. administration of 10 μCi ^{45}Ca/kg body weight

which is necessary for the maintenance and survival of the myocardial cells, in useless mechanical reactions.

According to our observations on rat and guinea pig hearts, the high-energy phosphate breakdown becomes critical when the ATP concentration in the left or right ventricular myocardium is lowered by more than 50 to 60% and the corresponding CP concentration falls by more than 80%. A simple method of producing such a deleterious fall in ATP and CP is the subcutaneous injection of isoproterenol. Fig. 37 shows the tremendous increase of ^{45}Ca uptake in the rat heart *in situ* as a function of time under the influence of a high subcutaneous dose of this drug (30 mg/kg body weight). In the untreated control rat hearts, the ^{45}Ca incorporation is relatively small. Here, the radioactivity of 1 g of fresh cardiac tissue, for instance, never exceeds 30% of the radioactivity simultaneously measured in 1 ml of the blood plasma. But after administration of the isoproterenol, the net radiocalcium uptake into the myocardium was increased by a factor of 6 to 7 within a few hours. The simultaneous changes in the high-energy phosphate concentrations in the left ventricular myocardium of 90 rats during an observation period of 24 hrs following isoproterenol injection is shown in Fig. 38. Due to the excessive transmembrane Ca influx, a 50% loss of ATP and an 85% loss of creatine phosphate occurred within 2 hrs; but later, there was partial recovery. Nevertheless, disseminated myocardial fiber necroses developed in all cases. The

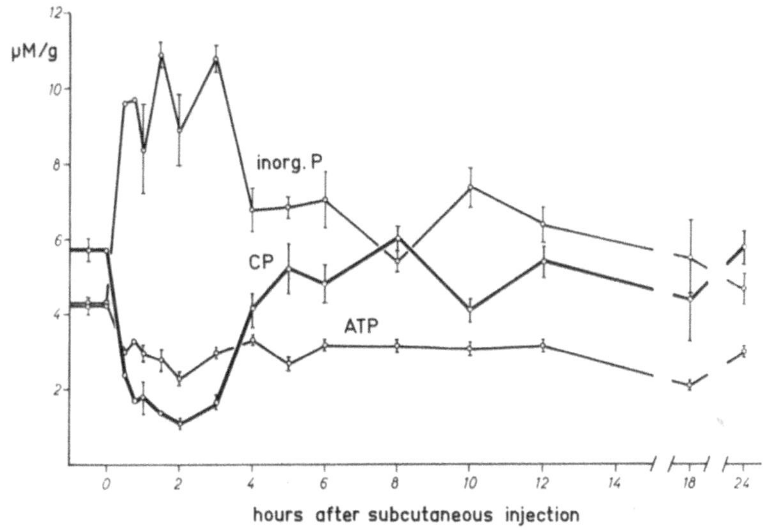

Fig. 38. Isoproterenol-induced changes in the concentrations of ATP, creatine phosphate, and orthophosphate in the left ventricular myocardium of 90 rat hearts after s.c. injection of 30 mg/kg isoproterenol during an observation period of 24 hr (from FLECKENSTEIN, DÖRING, and LEDER, 1969)

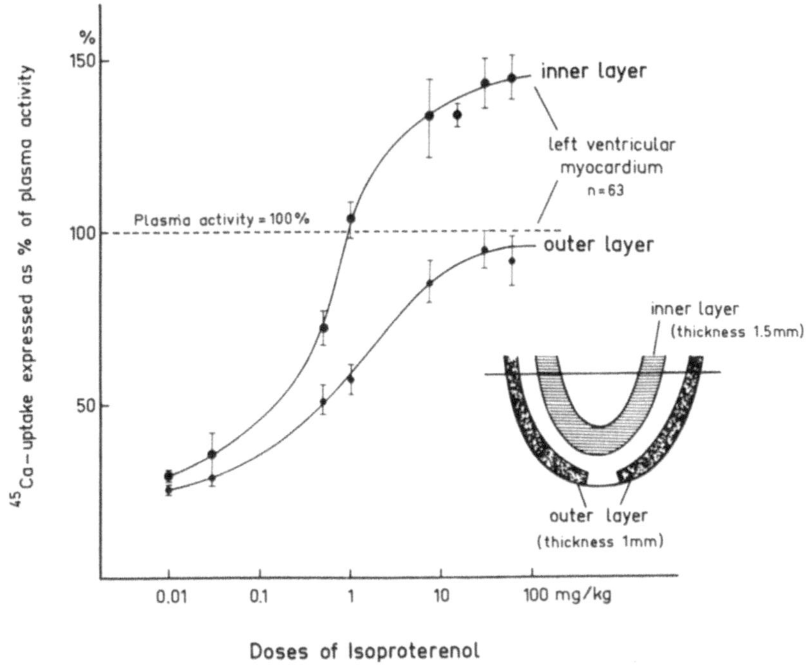

Fig. 39. Log dose-response curves of the isoproterenol-induced net ^{45}Ca uptake into the inner and outer layer of the left ventricular myocardium of rats (apical region). The measurements were carried out 6 hr after injection of different s.c. doses of isoproterenol and of 10 μCi ^{45}Ca/kg i.p. (FLECKENSTEIN, JANKE, DÖRING, and LEDER, 1974)

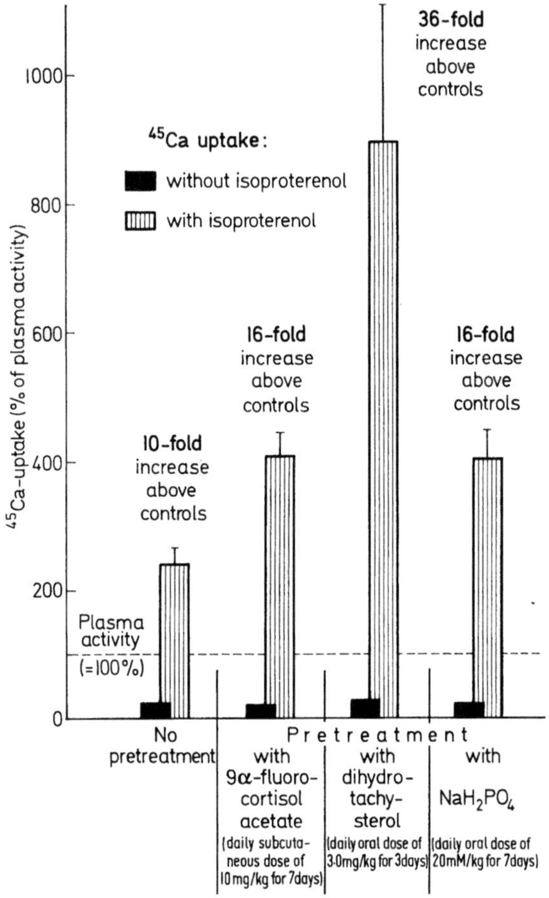

Fig. 40. Sensitization to the isoproterenol-induced radiocalcium uptake into the right ventricular myocardium of rats by pretreatment with 9 α-fluorocortisol acetate, dihydrotachysterol, or NaH_2PO_4. All measurements were carried out 6 hr after s.c. administration of isoproterenol (30 mg/kg)

size and density of the necrotic areas correspond to the intensity of uptake of labelled Ca into the different regions of the heart. Fig. 39 shows log dose response curves of the isoproterenol-induced net radiocalcium uptake into the inner and outer layers of the left ventricular myocardium of rats. Obviously the inner layer, where most of the necroses are localized, incorporates more labelled Ca than the subepicardial region. Accordingly, the high-energy phosphate breakdown was always more pronounced in the inner layer.

In their investigations regarding the factors that enhance myocardial necrotization, Selye (1960) and Bajusz (1963) discovered that rats can be sensitized for the production of cardiac necroses by pretreatment with certain corticosteroids, dihydrotachysterol, or monosodium phosphate. According to the observations of Rona, Chappel, and Kahn (1963), the same substances aggravate the cardiotoxicity of isoproterenol. Therefore, we have also examined how these sensitizing substances can influence the radiocalcium uptake. As shown in Fig. 40 the pretreatment with 9 α-fluoro-cortisol acetate, dihydrotachysterol, and NaH_2PO_4 apparently

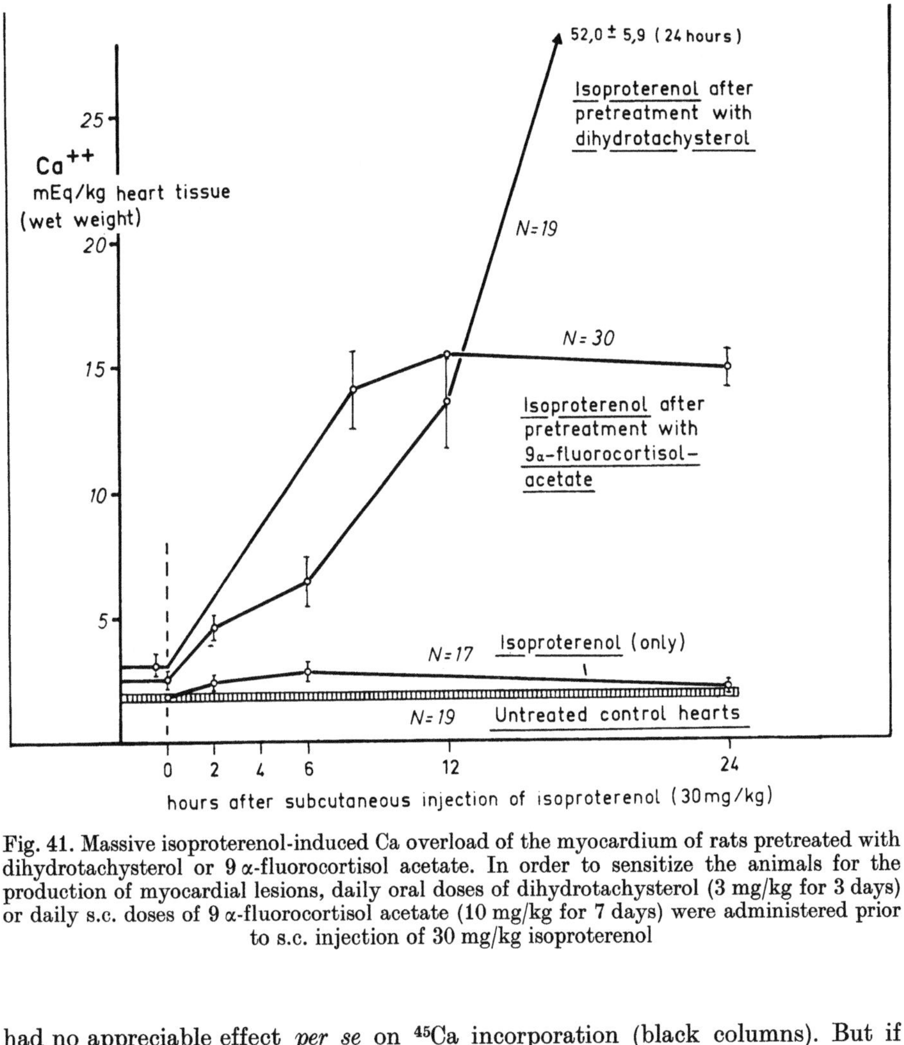

Fig. 41. Massive isoproterenol-induced Ca overload of the myocardium of rats pretreated with dihydrotachysterol or 9 α-fluorocortisol acetate. In order to sensitize the animals for the production of myocardial lesions, daily oral doses of dihydrotachysterol (3 mg/kg for 3 days) or daily s.c. doses of 9 α-fluorocortisol acetate (10 mg/kg for 7 days) were administered prior to s.c. injection of 30 mg/kg isoproterenol

had no appreciable effect *per se* on ^{45}Ca incorporation (black columns). But if isoproterenol was administered after pretreatment with these sensitizing agents, a tremendous increase in ^{45}Ca uptake occurred (striped columns). For instance, in the hearts of dihydrotachysterol-pretreated rats a radiocalcium accumulation was found 6 hrs after administration of isoproterenol which was 36 times greater than the normal control value. After sensitization by 9α-fluoro-cortisol-acetate or monosodium phosphate, the increase was 16-fold. Fig. 41 depicts the simultaneous changes in the myocardial Ca concentration expressed in mEq/kg wet weight. Again, the normal control value, amounting to about 2 mEq Ca/kg heart tissue, was not markedly influenced by pretreatment with the sensitizing agents. But as soon as isoproterenol was administered, the myocardial Ca concentration rose steeply. In the hearts of dihydrotachysterol-pretreated rats, a Ca accumulation up to 52 mEq/kg wet weight was found 24 hrs after the administration of isoproterenol. This concentration exceeds the normal control value of 2 mEq Ca/kg by a factor of 26. After sensitization by 9 α-fluoro-cortisol-acetate, the increase was 8-fold. Most of this Ca is concentrated in the mitochondria. But the mitochondria are badly damaged by this excessive Ca overload both morphologically and in relation to

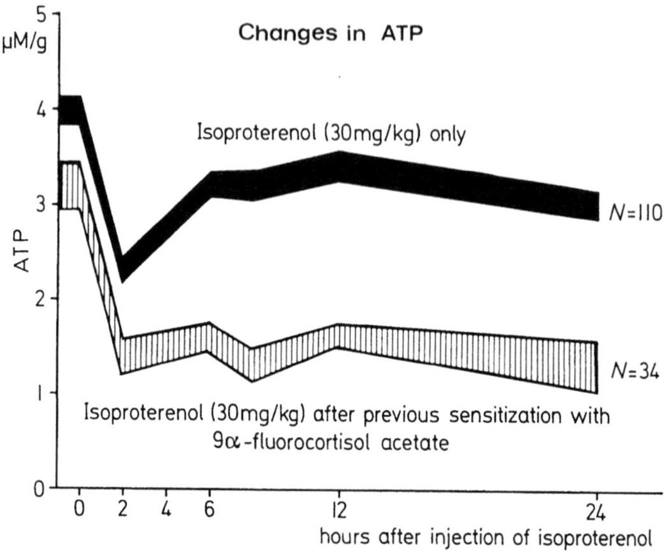

Fig. 42. Accentuation of the isoproterenol-induced fall in the ATP content of the left ventricular myocardium of rats by pretreatment with 9 α-fluorocortisol acetate. For the sensitization of the animals a daily dose of 10 mg/kg 9 α-fluorocortisol acetate was administered s.c. for 7 consecutive days (DÖRING and FLECKENSTEIN; see FLECKENSTEIN, 1970/71a, b)

their biochemical function, since they become swollen and their respiratory control and phosphorylation capacity is seen to deteriorate[4].

As to the concomitant changes in the high-energy phosphate fractions, it is not surprising that pretreatment with sensitizing agents leads to a further augmentation and prolongation of the isoproterenol-induced fall in the myocardial ATP and CP concentrations. As can be seen from Fig. 42, isoproterenol lowered the cardiac ATP level in the fluoro-cortisol-pretreated rats to less than 50% of the normal ATP content, with no sign of recovery. The simultaneous potentiation of the isoproterenol-induced CP breakdown is shown in Fig. 43. The magnitude of this myocardial high-energy phosphate deficiency is critical and could not be survived in many cases for more than a few hours after the isoproterenol administration. The hearts of such animals exhibited infarct-like confluent necrotic areas as described previously by RONA, CHAPPEL, BALAZS, and GAUDRY (1959); RONA, CHAPPEL, and KAHN (1963); and RONA, KAHN, and CHAPPEL (1963). It is obvious that the energetic state of the myocardium of isoproterenol-treated animals—especially after sensitization—is comparable to the metabolic situation of the heart muscle in anoxia and ischemia, or under the influence of metabolic poisons such as cyanide or 2,4-dinitrophenol, insofar as in all these cases, cardiac function and structural integrity cannot be maintained because the high-energy phosphate pool is exhausted. All these observations justify the statement that Ca overload leading

[4] Concerning the influence of Ca on cardiac mitochondria see SLATER, E. C. and CLELAND, K. W. [Biochem. J. **55**, 566–580 (1953)]. Similar Ca effects were observed on mitochondria from liver, see ROSSI, C. S. and LEHNINGER, A. L. [J. biol. Chem. **239**, 3971 (1964)], CARAFOLI, E. and ROSSI, S. C. [Europ. J. Biochem. **2**, 224 (1967)], AZZI, A. and AZZONE, G. F. [Biochem. biophys. Acta **113**, 438 (1966); COHN, D. V., BAWDON, R., NEWMAN, R. R., and HAMILTON, J. W., J. biol. Chem. **243**, 1089 (1968)], from kidney [COHN, D. V., BAWDON, R., and ELLER, G., J. biol. Chem. **242**, 1253 (1967)] and from suprarenal cortex [WHYSNER, J. A., PAULE, W. J., NELSON, D. H., and HARDING, B. W., Clin. Res. **14**, 180 (1966)].

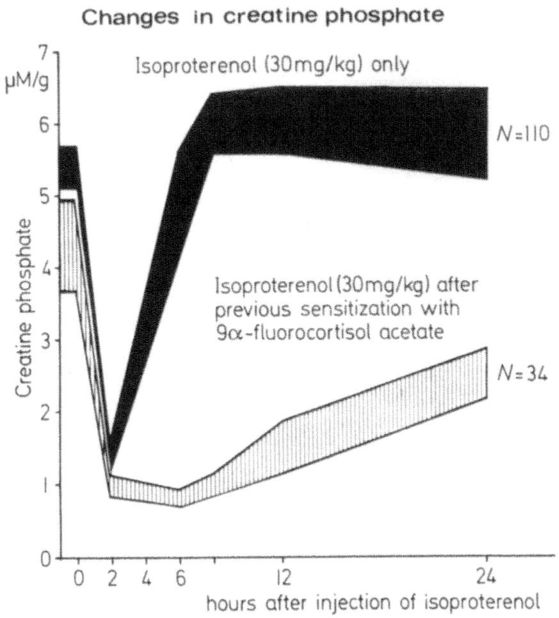

Fig. 43. Accentuation and prolongation of the isoproterenol-induced creatine phosphate (CP) deficiency by pretreatment with 9 α-fluorocortisol acetate. The determinations of the CP content were carried out on the same specimens of cardiac tissue as the ATP analysis in Fig. 42 (DÖRING and FLECKENSTEIN; see FLECKENSTEIN, 1970/71a, b)

to high-energy phosphate deficiency is a determinant factor in the production of non-coronarogenic myocardial lesions (FLECKENSTEIN, 1968, 1969, 1970/71a, b; FLECKENSTEIN, DÖRING, and LEDER, 1969; JANKE, FLECKENSTEIN, and JÄDICKE, 1970; FLECKENSTEIN, JANKE, DÖRING, and PACHINGER, 1973; FLECKENSTEIN, JANKE, DÖRING, and LEDER, 1971, 1974).

III. Prevention by Ca-Antagonistic Drugs of Cardiac ATP-Wasting and Necrotization

If the Ca concept concerning the etiology of isoproterenol-induced cardiac necroses is correct, it is to be expected that any substance or procedure that inhibits the transmembrane Ca influx into the excited myocardial fibers will protect the isoproterenol-treated hearts against the deleterious breakdown of ATP and creatine phosphate and, as a result of this, against structural damage. We have proved these conclusions with the help of specific Ca-antagonistic compounds, namely verapamil, D 600, and prenylamine, which reduce the Ca conductivity of mammalian cardiac fiber membranes. By this action the Ca-antagonistic compounds can neutralize even the effects of overdoses of sympathomimetic catecholamines on the Ca channel, without influencing the sympathetic β-receptors. Fig. 44 shows the log dose-response curves of isoproterenol-induced radiocalcium uptake into the right ventricular myocardium of rats. The measurements were made 6 hrs after subcutaneous injection of different amounts of isoproterenol. The rise in ^{45}Ca uptake above the control level begins with a dose as small as 0.1 mg/kg and

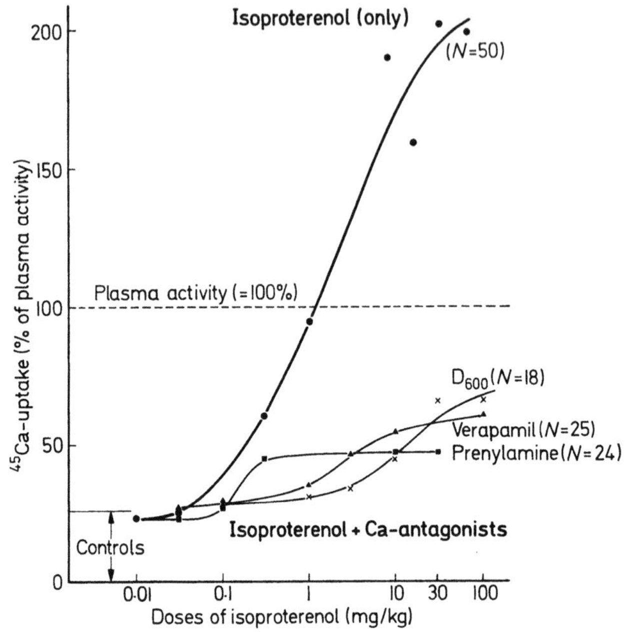

Fig. 44. Prevention of excessive isoproterenol-induced uptake of labelled Ca into the right ventricular myocardium of rats by three Ca-antagonistic compounds: Log dose-response curves of the isoproterenol-induced radiocalcium incorporation obtained with or without simultaneous administration of D 600 (10 mg/kg), verapamil (17 mg/kg) or prenylamine (250 mg/kg). All measurements were made 6 hr after s.c. injection of the drugs (JANKE and FLECKENSTEIN; see FLECKENSTEIN, 1970/71 a, b)

proceeds steeply to a maximum that is beyond the high dose of 30 mg/kg. Obviously, the Ca-antagonistic compounds, verapamil, D 600, or prenylamine, inhibit the isoproterenol-induced radiocalcium uptake by a rather impressive degree, if they are injected simultaneously with the isoproterenol. Small doses of isoproterenol are completely neutralized, whilst the effects of higher doses are greatly diminished. By this action, the Ca-antagonistic compounds also prevent the Ca-induced high-energy phosphate exhaustion. Therefore, the same doses of D 600, verapamil, or prenylamine that inhibit the cardiac ^{45}Ca uptake are also fully effective in preventing the isoproterenol-induced breakdown of the ATP and CP fractions in the left ventricular myocardium of rats (Fig. 46). Moreover, together with the stabilization of the high-energy phosphate content of the myocardium, the hearts are also protected by the Ca-antagonistic compounds against isoproterenol-induced tissue damage (Fig. 45). This prophylactic effect could be demonstrated by histological methods (hematoxylin–eosin stain, fuchsinophilic reaction, v. Kossa's stain for the detection of Ca precipitates) as well as by enzyme tests. The fuchsinophilic reaction is particularly suitable for a most impressive illustration of the cardioprotective action of verapamil (Fig. 49).

In their studies dealing with the factors that prevent myocardial necrotization, SELYE, BAJUSZ and RONA, among others, noted the usefulness of K and Mg salts; but the mechanism of action remained unknown. Our present results show, however, that KCl and $MgCl_2$ also exhibit surprisingly strong Ca-antagonistic potencies. Nevertheless, the site of action of K and Mg ions as physiological Ca-antagonists seems to differ from that of verapamil and D 600, since the K and Mg

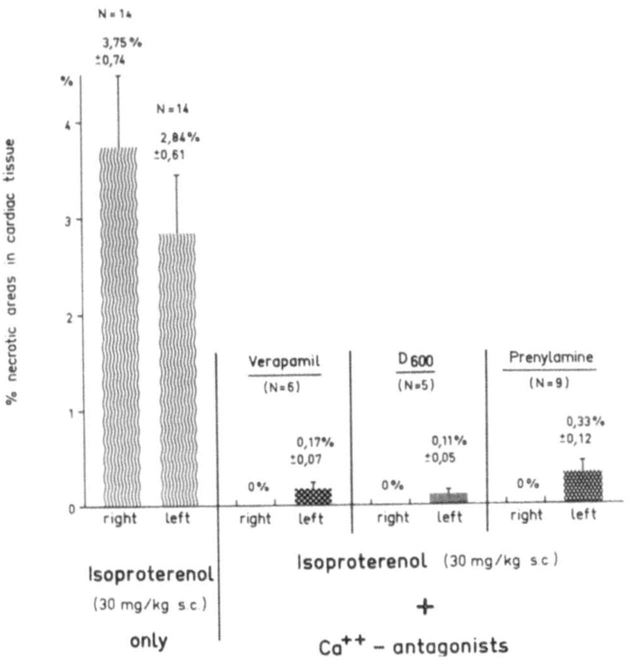

Fig. 45. Proportion of necrotic myocardial tissue 6 hr after isoproterenol with or without prophylactic administration of Ca-antagonistic compounds. Evaluation was carried out with the use of the Zeiss integration plate No. 1 on the right and left ventricular myocardium of rats (FLECKENSTEIN, JANKE, DÖRING, and LEDER, 1974)

ions do not block the transmembrane Ca influx; this was shown in our laboratory by KOHLHARDT, using direct measurements with the voltage-clamp technique (unpublished observations, 1970). Presumably, the K and Mg ions only restrict the intracellular Ca accumulation acting on intracellular structures in a competitive way. As can be seen from Fig. 47, a single oral dose of 10 mM KCl or $MgCl_2$ per kg body weight can enormously depress the log dose-response curve of the isoproterenol-induced ^{45}Ca uptake into the left ventricular myocardium of rats. Prophylactic treatment with oral doses of KCl or $MgCl_2$ was also effective against myocardial Ca overload, high-energy phosphate breakdown, and cardiac necrotization, in rats sensitized by corticosteroids, dihydrotachysterol, or NaH_2PO_4. Conversely, cardiac lesions can be produced or, at least, aggravated by a K- or Mg-deficient diet.

We have recently found that hydrogen ions are also able to antagonize isoproterenol-induced ^{45}Ca uptake into the ventricular myocardium (FLECKENSTEIN, JANKE, DÖRING, and LEDER, 1974). Similar results obtained on isolated guinea pig atria were reported by MORGENSTERN, NOAK, and KÖHLER (1972). Accordingly, in our experiments on rat hearts *in situ*, acidification by oral doses of NH_4Cl or CO_2 respiration (Fig. 48) restricted the radiocalcium incorporation considerably, whereas alkalization by oral doses of $NaHCO_3$ led to a potentiation of the isoproterenol effects. This was true of the incorporation of labelled Ca, as well as of the high-energy phosphate breakdown and the subsequent production of myocardial lesions. The preventive effectiveness of NH_4Cl in isoproterenol-induced myo-

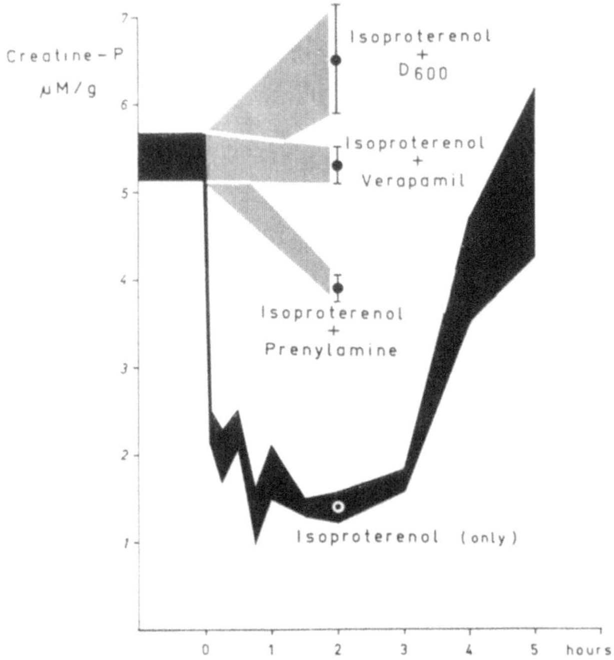

Fig. 46. Inhibition of the isoproterenol-induced creatine phosphate breakdown in the left ventricular myocardium of rats by three Ca-antagonistic compounds. The drugs were applied simultaneously by single s.c. injections at separate sites. The following doses were administered: isoproterenol (30 mg/kg), verapamil (50 mg/kg), compound D 600 (20 mg/kg), prenylamine (250 mg/kg) (FLECKENSTEIN, DÖRING, and LEDER, 1969)

cardial injury was also observed by LEHR, CHAU, and KAPLAN (1972), but these authors suggested that the beneficial effect of NH_4Cl is primarily based upon removal of Na. As to the mechanism of action, H ions compete with Ca for at least two sites: One is at the membrane or, possibly, at the transmembrane Ca channel, whilst the second is at the myofibrillar ATPase itself, as shown by SCHÄDLER, RÜEGG, and others (SCHÄDLER, 1967).

Extracellular Ca concentration is another important factor which determines the isoproterenol-induced uptake of labelled Ca into the heart, and consequently the number and size of necroses. Thus, a simple reduction in the plasma Ca concentration of rats to about 50% of normal by means of calcitonin (Table 7) serves to lower the cardiotoxic effects of isoproterenol considerably (FLECKENSTEIN, PACHINGER, LEDER, HEIN, and JANKE, 1972). Similarly, URBANEK, VASKU, BED-

---

Fig. 47. Prevention of excessive isoproterenol-induced ^{45}Ca uptake into the inner layer of the left ventricular myocardium of rats by a single oral standard dose of KCl (10 mM/kg) or $MgCl_2$ (10 mM/kg). The log dose-response curves were obtained 6 hr after s.c. injection of different amounts of isoproterenol, with and without KCl or $MgCl_2$ (JANKE and FLECKENSTEIN; see FLECKENSTEIN, 1970/71a, b)

Fig. 48. Restriction of the isoproterenol-induced net ^{45}Ca uptake into the myocardium of rats by CO_2 respiration (10% CO_2, 40% O_2, 50% N_2). The measurements were carried out 6 hr after i.p. ^{45}Ca injection. The isoproterenol was administered s.c. at the same time as ^{45}Ca

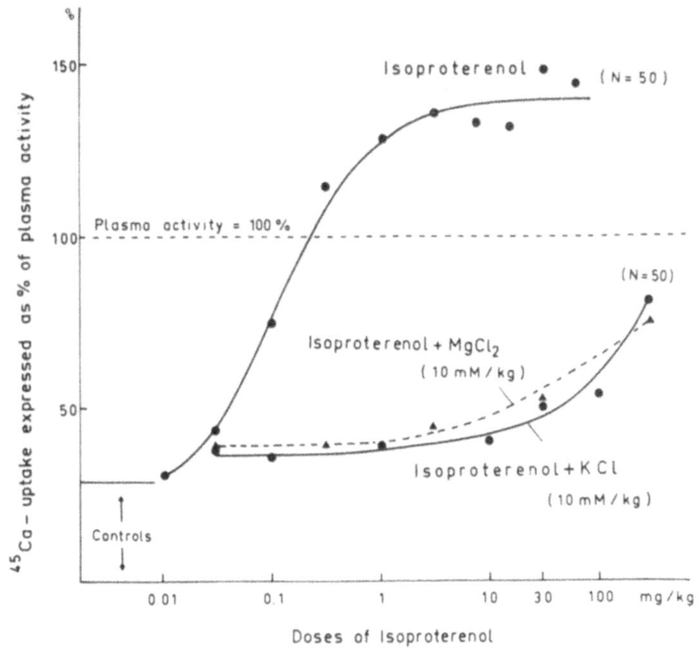
%
150
100
50
^{45}Ca - uptake expressed as % of plasma activity
Isoproterenol
(N = 50)
Plasma activity = 100 %
(N = 50)
Isoproterenol + MgCl$_2$
(10 mM / kg)
Isoproterenol + KCl
(10 mM / kg)
Controls
0.01
0.1
1
10
30
100
mg/kg
Doses of Isoproterenol

Fig. 47

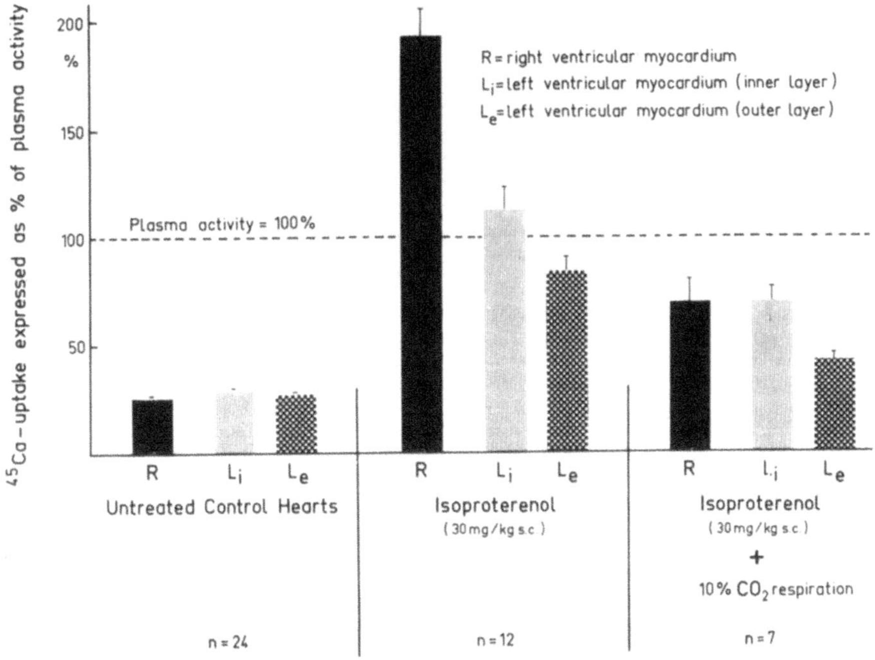
200
%
150
100
50
^{45}Ca - uptake expressed as % of plasma activity
R = right ventricular myocardium
L$_i$ = left ventricular myocardium (inner layer)
L$_e$ = left ventricular myocardium (outer layer)
Plasma activity = 100%
R
L$_i$
L$_e$
Untreated Control Hearts
Isoproterenol
(30 mg/kg s.c.)
Isoproterenol
(30 mg/kg s.c.)
+
10% CO$_2$ respiration
n = 24
n = 12
n = 7

Fig. 48

a
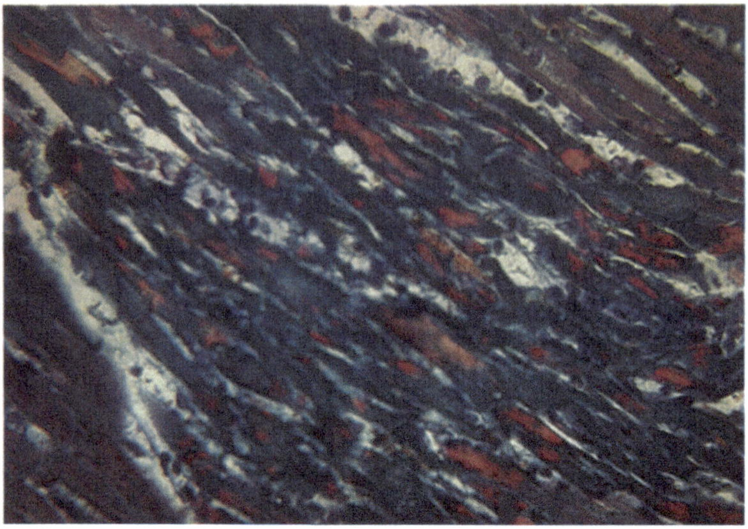

b
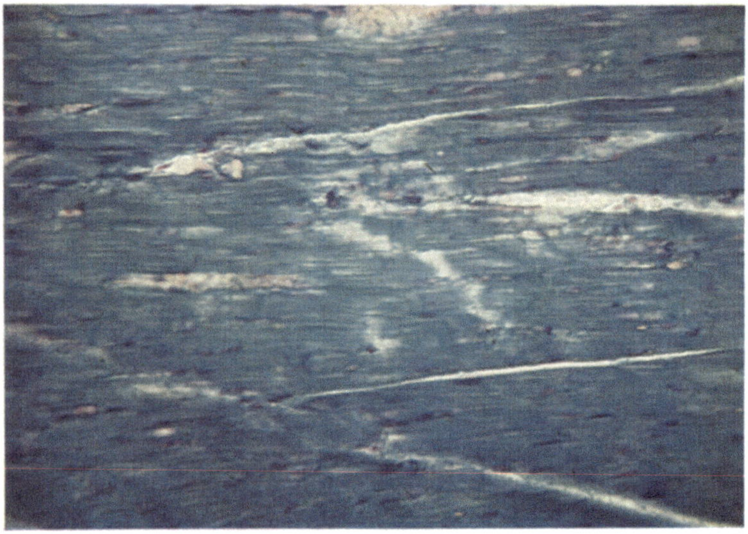

Fig. 49a and b. *Fuchsinophilic reaction:* Demonstration of the cardioprotective action of verapamil. (a) Disseminated structural lesions in the right ventricular myocardium of a rat 24 hrs after s.c. administration of 30 mg/kg isoproterenol only. Necrotic and prenecrotic fibres are visualized by their positive fuchsinophilic reaction (red or pink colour), whereas normal myocardial tissue appears blue (O. Leder, unpublished, 1969). (b) Prevention of isoproterenol-induced myocardial necrotization by simultaneous administration of verapamil. Right ventricular myocardium of a rat 24 hrs after s.c. injection of 30 mg/kg isoproterenol *and* 50 mg/kg verapamil at different sites. The absence of red-colored necrotic tissue is obvious. The pink-colored material in the cross-sectioned capillaries merely consists of erythrocytes (O. Leder, unpublished, 1969)

narik, and Urbankova (1969) observed a prophylactic effect of EDTA against necroses in corticosteroid-cardiomyopathic rats which was also related to the inhibition of Ca overload. The cardioprotective influence of calcitonin (or EDTA) seems to be, at least in part, the reverse of the sensitization to necroses by di-

Table 7. Plasma Ca concentration in rats

	$mEq\ Ca^{++}/l$
Untreated control rats	4.77 ($\pm$0.09)
After pretreatment with *dihydrotachysterol* (daily oral dose of 3.0 mg/kg for 3 days)	7.13 ($\pm$0.23)
After *Calcitonin* injection (6 hrs after 2×40 units/kg s.c.)	2.30 ($\pm$0.10)

hydrotachysterol, since dihydrotachysterol by increasing the plasma Ca concentration, obviously acts in the opposite direction.

The results indicate that the myocardial Ca uptake is not only influenced by drugs acting on the transmembrane Ca conductivity but also by factors which change the ionic composition of the extracellular fluid. Thus, it is obvious that the intracellular Ca incorporation, with all its consequences, is largely modified by the extracellular cation ratio as schematically shown in Table 8: If Mg, K, or H ions

Table 8. Basic influence of changing cation ratios on the production or prevention of myocardial necrotization

Ca / Mg, K, H	Ca / Mg, K, H,	Ca / Mg, K, H
Prevention of necroses	Normal cationic balance	Production of necroses

predominate myocardial Ca overload and necrotization can be prevented. But if, on the other hand, the extracellular Mg, K, or H ion concentrations are too low, Ca uptake and necrotization are facilitated.

References

ALLELA, A.: Steuerung der Coronardurchblutung. In: Probleme der Coronardurchblutung. Bad Oeynhausener Gespräche, Bd. II. Berlin-Göttingen-Heidelberg: Springer 1958.

ANTONI, H., ROTMANN, M.: The negative inotropic mechanism of acetylcholine in the isolated frog's myocardium. Pflügers Arch. ges. Physiol. **300**, 67–86 (1968).

ANTONI, H., ENGSTFELD, G., FLECKENSTEIN, A.: Inotrope Effekte von ATP und Adrenalin am hypodynamen Froschmyokard nach elektro-mechanischer Entkoppelung durch Ca^{++}-Entzug. Pflügers Arch. ges. Physiol. **272**, 91–106 (1960).

BAJUSZ, E.: Conditioning factors for cardiac necroses. Basel-New York: Karger-Verlag 1963.

BARCROFT, J.: Die Atmungsfunktion des Blutes, Bd. I. Berlin: Springer 1927.

BENSON, E. S., EVANS, G. T., HALLAWAY, B. E., PHIBBS, C., FREIER, E. P.: Myocardial creatine phosphate and nucleotides in anoxic cardiac arrest and recovery. Amer. J. Physiol. **201**, 687–693 (1961).

BRETSCHNEIDER, H. J.: Über den Mechanismus der hypoxischen Coronarerweiterung. In: „Probleme der Coronardurchblutung", Bad Oeynhausener Gespräche, Bd. II. Berlin-Göttingen-Heidelberg: Springer 1958.

BÜCHNER, F., IIJIMA, S., BÜCHNER, F.: Die allgemeine Pathologie des Blutkreislaufs. In: Handbuch Allgem. Pathologie, vol. 5, part I, p. 820 (1961).
BÜCHNER, F., ONISHI, S.: Der Herzmuskel bei akuter Koronarinsuffizienz im elektronenmikroskopischen Bild. München: Urban u. Schwarzenberg 1968.
BYON, K. Y., FLECKENSTEIN, A.: Parallele Beeinflussung von isometrischer Spannungsentwicklung und O_2-Verbrauch isolierter Papillarmuskeln unter dem Einfluß von Ca^{++}-Ionen, Adrenalin, Isoproterenol und organischen Ca^{++}-Antagonisten (Iproveratril, D 600, Prenylamin). Pflügers Arch. ges. Physiol. **312**, R 8/9 (1969).
CHIDSEY, C. A., WEINBACH, E. C., POOL, P. E., MORROW, A. C.: Biochemical studies of energy production in the failing human heart. J. clin. Invest. **45**, 40–50 (1966).
CLARK, A. J., WHITE, A. C.: The oxygen consumption of the auricles of the frog and of the tortoise. J. Physiol. **68**, 406–432 (1929).
COPER, H., HERKEN, H., SENFT, G.: Der Gehalt des Herzmuskels an Adenosintriphosphorsäure bei experimentellen Ödemen. Arch. exp. Path. Pharmakol. **233**, 192–200 (1958).
DÖRING, H. J., KAMMERMEIER, H.: Das Verhalten der energiereichen Phosphor-Verbindungen des Myokards bei unterschiedlichen Belastungsformen sowie bei verschiedenen Arten experimenteller Insuffizienz am Herz-Lungen-Präparat. Verh. dtsch. Ges. Kreisl.-Forsch. **27**, 227–232 (1961).
DÖRING, H. J., KAMMERMEIER, H.: Änderungen des Herzquerdurchmessers unter dem Einfluß von Sauerstoffmangel, Stoffwechsel-Inhibitoren und erregungshemmenden Substanzen. In: Kreislaufmessungen. Vorträge des 4. Freiburger Colloquiums über Kreislaufmessungen vom 4.—6. April 1963 (A. FLECKENSTEIN, ed.), p. 45—56. München-Gräfelfing: Werk Verlag Dr. E. Banaschewski 1963.
DÖRING, H. J., KAMMERMEIER, H., BYON, Y. K.: Changes of cardiac tonus and high-energy phosphate concentrations of the heart due to anoxia or metabolic inhibitors. XXII Internat. Congress of Physiol. Sciences in Leiden, 10.–17. Sept. 1962. Excerpta Medica, Internat. Congr. Ser. 48.
EBASHI, S., ENDO, M.: Calcium ions and muscle contraction. Progr. Biophys. Molec. Biol. 18, 123–183 (1968).
EBASHI, S., LIPMANN, F.: Adenosine triphosphate-linked concentration of calcium ions in a particulate fraction of rabbit muscle. J. Cell. Biol. **14**, 389–400 (1962).
EGGLETON, P., EGGLETON, G. P.: The physiological significance of "phosphagen". J. Physiol. **63**, 155–161 (1927).
ENTMAN, M. L., ALLEN, J. C., BORNET, E. P., GILLETTE, P. C., WALLICK, E. T., SCHWARTZ, A.: Mechanisms of calcium accumulation and transport in cardiac relaxing system (sarcoplasmic reticulum membranes): Effects of verapamil, D 600, X537A and A23187. J. Molec. Cell. Cardiology **4**, 681–687 (1972).
FANBURG, B., FINKEL, R. M., MARTONOSI, A.: The role of calcium in the mechanism of relaxation of cardiac muscle. J. biol. Chem. **239**, 2298–2306 (1964).
FAWAZ, G., HAWA, E. S.: Phosphocreatine content of mammalian cardiac muscle. Proc. Soc. exp. Biol. (N.Y.) **84**, 277–280 (1953).
FAWAZ, G., HAWA, E. S., TUTUNJI, B.: The effect of dinitrophenol, hypoxaemia and ischaemia on the phosphorus compounds of the dog heart. Brit. J. Pharmacol. **12**, 270–272 (1957).
FEINSTEIN, M.: Effects of experimental congestive heart failure, ouabain, and asphyxia on the high-energy phosphate and creatine content of the guinea pig heart. Circulat. Res. **10**, 333–346 (1962).
FLECKENSTEIN, A.: Enzymregulation im Herzstoffwechsel. In: Enzymatische Regulationen in der Klinik. Proc. 6. Internat. Congress of Internal Med., Basel 1960 (A. GIGON and H. LUDWIG, eds.), p. 37–51. Basel-Stuttgart: Benno Schwabe 1960.
FLECKENSTEIN, A.: Aktuelle Probleme der Muskelphysiologie und ihre Analyse mit Isotopen. In Handbuch: Künstliche radioaktive Isotope in Physiologie, Diagnostik und Therapie (H. SCHWIEGK und F. TURBA, eds.), 2nd ed., p. 179–228. Berlin-Göttingen-Heidelberg: Springer 1961.
FLECKENSTEIN, A.: Metabolic aspects of the excitation-contraction coupling. In: The cellular functions of membrane transport. Symposium of the Society of General Physiologists in Woods Hole, Mass., Sept. 4–7 (J. F. HOFFMANN, ed.), p. 71–93. Prentice-Hall, Englewood Cliffs, N.J. (USA) 1963a.
FLECKENSTEIN, A.: Physiologie und Pathophysiologie des Myokard-Stoffwechsels im Zusammenspiel mit den bioelektrischen und mechanischen Fundamentalprozessen. In: Das Herz des Menschen (W. BARGMANN und W. DOERR, eds.), p. 355–411. Stuttgart: Georg Thieme 1963b.
FLECKENSTEIN, A.: Die Bedeutung der energiereichen Phosphate für Kontraktilität und Tonus des Myokards. 70th Congress, Verh. dtsch. Ges. inn. Med., 81–99 (1964).
FLECKENSTEIN, A.: Myokardstoffwechsel und Insuffizienz. In: Kreislaufmessungen. Vorträge

des 5. Freiburger Colloquiums über Kreislaufmessungen vom 1.–3. April 1965 (H. REINDELL und H. KLEPZIG, eds.), p. 36–55. München-Gäfelfing: Werk-Verlag Dr. E. Banaschewski 1966.

FLECKENSTEIN, A.: Stoffwechselprobleme bei der Myokard-Insuffizienz. Verh. dtsch. Ges. Pathologie, 51. Tagung in Göttingen vom 25.–29. April 1967, p. 15–29. Stuttgart: Gustav Fischer 1967.

FLECKENSTEIN, A.: Experimentelle Pathologie der akuten und chronischen Herzinsuffizienz. Verh. dtsch. Ges. Kreisl-Forsch. **34**, 15–34 (1968a).

FLECKENSTEIN, A.: Myokardstoffwechsel und Nekrose. In: VI Symposium der Dtsch, Gesellsch. f. Fortschritte auf d. Gebiet der Inneren Medizin über „Herzinfarkt und Schock", 8. Nov. 1968 in Freiburg (L. HEILMEYER und H.-J. HOLTMEIER, eds.), p. 94–109. Stuttgart: Georg Thieme 1968b.

FLECKENSTEIN, A.: Pathophysiologische Kausalfaktoren bei Myokardnekrose und Infarkt. Wien. Z. inn. Med. **52**, 133–143 (1971).

FLECKENSTEIN, A.: Specific inhibitors and promoters of calcium action in the excitation-contraction coupling of heart muscle and their role in the prevention or production of myocardial lesions. In: Calcium and the Heart (P. HARRIS and L. OPIE, eds.), p. 135–188. London-New York: Academic Press 1970/71a.

FLECKENSTEIN, A.: Neuere Ergebnisse zur Physiologie, Pharmakologie und Pathologie der elektromechanischen Koppelungsprozesse im Warmblütermyokard. In: Vorträge der Erlanger Physiologentagung 1970 (W. D. KEIDEL und K.-H. PLATTIG, eds.), p. 13–52. Berlin-Heidelberg-New York: Springer 1970/71b.

FLECKENSTEIN, A.: Drug-induced changes in cardiac energy. In: The Myocardium. Advanc. Cardiol., vol. 12, p. 183–197. Basel: Karger 1974.

FLECKENSTEIN, A., DÖRING, H. J., KAMMERMEIER, H.: Experimental heart failure due to inhibition of utilisation of high-energy phosphates. Internat. Symposium on the Coronary Circulation and Energetics of the Myocardium, in Milan 1966, p. 220–236. Basel-New York: Karger 1967.

FLECKENSTEIN, A., DÖRING, H. J., KAMMERMEIER, H.: Myokardstoffwechsel und Insuffizienz. Ärztl. Forschung **21**, 1–14 (1967).

FLECKENSTEIN, A., DÖRING, H. J., KAMMERMEIER, H.: Einfluß von Beta-Receptorenblockern und verwandten Substanzen auf Erregung, Kontraktion und Energiestoffwechsel der Myokardfaser. Klin. Wschr. **46**, 343–351 (1968).

FLECKENSTEIN, A., DÖRING, H. J., KAMMERMEIER, H.: Beziehung zwischen den Spiegeln an energiereichem Phosphat und verschiedenen Insuffizienzformen. In: Herzinsuffizienz, Pathophysiologie und Klinik. Internat. Symposium 2.–5. Nov. 1967 in Hinterzarten (H. REINDELL, J. KEUL und E. DOLL, eds.), p. 216–226. Stuttgart: Georg Thieme 1968a.

FLECKENSTEIN, A., DÖRING, H. J., LEDER, O.: The significance of high-energy phosphate exhaustion in the etiology of isoproterenol-induced cardiac necrosis and its prevention by iproveratril, compound D 600 or prenylamine. In: Symposium International on Drugs and Metabolism of Myocardium and Striated Muscle (M. LAMARCHE and R. ROYER, eds.), p. 11–12. Nancy 1969.

FLECKENSTEIN, A., GERLACH, E., JANKE, J., MARMIER, P.: Die Bestimmung des Turnovers von ATP, Kreatinphosphat und Orthophosphat in lebenden Muskeln mittels H_2O^{18} und anschließender Aktivierung durch Protonen-Beschuß. Naturwissenschaften **46**, 365–367 (1959).

FLECKENSTEIN, A., GERLACH, E., JANKE, J., MARMIER, P.: Die Inkorporation von markiertem Sauerstoff aus Wasser in die ATP-, Kreatinphosphat- und Orthophosphat-Fraktion intakter Muskeln bei Ruhe, tetanischer Reizung und Erholung. Neue Wege der intracellulären Turnover-Messung mit Hilfe von H_2O^{18} und anschließender Aktivierung der O^{18}-haltigen Phosphat-Fraktionen durch Protonen-Beschuß. Pflügers Arch. ges. Physiol. **271**, 75–104 (1960).

FLECKENSTEIN, A., JANKE, J.: The turnover rates of labile compounds in skeletal and heart muscle during activity and rest. An investigation with the use of radiophosphorus and paper chromatography. In: Radioisotopes in Scientific Research, **4**, 60–73 (Proc. 1st UNESCO Int. Conf., Paris 1957). London-New York-Paris: Pergamon Press 1958.

FLECKENSTEIN, A., JANKE, J.: The metabolism of organophosphates in cardiac tissue as studied with radiophosphorus and paper chromatography. Proc. 2nd International Conf., Geneva, Sept. 1958 on United Nations Peaceful Uses of Atomic Energy, p. 39–44. London-New York-Paris-Los Angeles: Pergamon Press 1959.

FLECKENSTEIN, A., JANKE, J.: L'application biologique de l'analyse d'activation de l'oxygène 18. In: L'analyse par radioactivation et ses applications aux sciences biologiques. 3e Colloque International de Biologie de Saclay en Sept. 1963, p. 267–285. Imprimerie des Presses Universitaires de France, Vendôme 1964.

FLECKENSTEIN, A., JANKE, J., DÖRING, H. J., LEDER, O.: Die intracelluläre Überladung mit

Kalzium als entscheidender Kausalfaktor bei der Entstehung nicht-coronarogener Myokard-Nekrosen. Verh. dtsch. Ges. Kreisl.-Forsch. **37**, 345–353 (1971).

FLECKENSTEIN, A., JANKE, J., DÖRING, H. J., LEDER, O.: Myocardial fiber necrosis due to intracellular Ca overload—a new principle in cardiac pathophysiology. In: Myocardial biology, recent advances in studies on cardiac structure and metabolism, vol. 4, p. 563–579. Baltimore-London-Tokyo: University Park Press 1974.

FLECKENSTEIN, A., JANKE, J., DÖRING, H. J., PACHINGER, O.: Ca overload as the determinant factor in the production of catecholamine-induced myocardial lesions. In: Cardiomyopathies, recent advances in studies on cardiac structure and metabolism, vol. 2, p. 455–466. Baltimore-London-Tokyo: University Park Press 1973.

FLECKENSTEIN, A., JANKE, J., GERLACH, E.: Über den tatsächlichen Gehalt des Rattenherzens an Adeninnucleotiden. Naunyn-Schmiedebergs Arch. exp. Path. Pharmak. **235**, 243–246 (1959).

FLECKENSTEIN, A., JANKE, J., GERLACH, E.: Konzentration und Turnover der energiereichen Phosphate des Herzens nach Studien mit Papierchromatographie und Radiophosphor. Klin. Wschr. **37**, 451–459 (1959a).

FLECKENSTEIN, A., JANKE, J., MARMIER, P.: Biological application of the activation analysis of O^{18}. In: Isotopes in Experimental Pharmacology (L. J. ROTH, ed.), p. 33–45. The University of Chicago Press 1965.

FLECKENSTEIN, A., KAMMERMEIER, H., DÖRING, H. J., FREUND, H. J.: Zum Wirkungsmechanismus neuartiger Koronardilatatoren mit gleichzeitig Sauerstoff-einsparenden Myokard-Effekten, Prenylamin und Iproveratril. Z. Kreisl.-Forsch. **56**, 716–744, 839–853 (1967).

FLECKENSTEIN, A., PACHINGER, O., LEDER, O., HEIN, B., JANKE, J.: Verhütung Isoproterenol-induzierter Myocard-Nekrosen durch Senkung des Plasma-Calcium-Spiegels mittels Calcitonin. Pflügers Arch. **332**, R 40 (1972).

FLECKENSTEIN, A., SCHWOERER, W.: Die Bedeutung der Ca-Ionen für die Spaltung von energiereichem Phosphat während verschiedener reversibler Kontrakturen und irreversibler Starre-Verkürzungen des Frosch-Rectus. Pflügers Arch. ges. Physiol. **274**, 8–9 (1961).

FLECKENSTEIN, A., SCHWOERER, W., JANKE, J.: Parallele Beeinflussung der mechanischen Spannungsentwicklung und der Spaltung von energiereichem Phosphat bei der Kaliumkontraktur des Froschrectus in Lösungen mit variiertem K^+- und Ca^{++}-Gehalt. Pflügers Arch. ges. Physiol. **273**, 483–498 (1961).

FLECKENSTEIN, A., TRITTHART, H., DÖRING, H. J., BYON, Y. K.: Bay a 1040 — ein hochaktiver Ca^{++}-antagonistischer Inhibitor der elektro-mechanischen Koppelungsprozesse im Warmblüter-Myokard. Arzneimittel-Forsch. **22**, 22–33 (1972).

FOX, A. C., WIKLER, N. S., REED, G. E.: High energy phosphate compounds in the myocardium during experimental congestive heart failure: purine and pyrimidine nucleotides, creatine, and creatine phosphate in normal and in failing hearts. J. clin. Invest. **44**, 202–218 (1965).

FÜHNER, H., STARLING, E. H.: Experiments on the pulmonary circulation. J. Physiol. **47**, 286–304 (1913).

GERLACH, E., DEUTICKE, B., DREISBACH, R. H.: Der Nucleotid-Abbau im Herzmuskel bei Sauerstoffmangel und seine mögliche Bedeutung für die Coronardurchblutung. Naturwissenschaften **50**, 228–229 (1963).

GERSMEYER, G., HOLLAND, W. C.: Influence of ouabain on contractile force, resting tension, Ca^{45} entry and tissue Ca content in rat atria. Circulat. Res. **12**, 620–622 (1963).

GORLIN, R., LEWIS, B. M.: Circulatory adjustments to hypoxia in dogs. J. appl. Physiol. **7**, 180–185 (1954).

GREMELS, H., STARLING, E. H.: On the influence of hydrogen ion concentration and of anoxaemia upon the heart volume. J. Physiol. **61**, 297–304 (1926).

HAAS, H., BUSCH, E.: Vergleichende Untersuchungen der Wirkung von α-Isopropyl-α-(N-methyl-N-homoveratryl)-γ-aminopropyl)-3,4-dimethoxy-phenyl-acetonitril, seiner Derivate sowie einiger anderer Coronardilatatoren und β-Receptor-affiner Substanzen. Arzneimittel-Forsch. **17**, 257–271 (1967).

HAAS, H., HÄRTFELDER, G.: α-Isopropyl-α-(-N-methyl-homoveratryl)-γ-aminopropyl)-3,4-dimethoxy-phenylacetonitril, eine Substanz mit coronargefäßerweiternden Eigenschaften. Arzneimittel-Forsch. **12**, 549–558 (1962).

HASSELBACH, W., MAKINOSE, F.: Die Ca^{++}-Pumpe der Erschlaffungsgrana des Muskels und ihre Abhängigkeit von der ATP-Spaltung. Biochem. Z. **333**, 518–528 (1961).

HASSELBACH, W., WEBER, H. H.: Die intrazelluläre Regulation der Muskelaktivität. Naturwissenschaften **52**, 121–128 (1965).

HEIN, B., FLECKENSTEIN, A., JANKE, J., ECKARDT, K., LUDIN, H. J.: Einschränkung der Isoproterenol-induzierten ^{45}Ca-Netto-Aufnahme und der Utilisation von energiereichem

Phosphat am hypertrophierten Rattenmyocard. Verh. Dtsch. Ges. Kreislaufforsch. **38**, 196–201 (1972).

HENNEKES, R., BAYER, R., KAUFMANN, R.: The influence of verapamil on steady state and dynamic strength-interval relationship in mammalian cardiac muscle. Pflügers Arch. Suppl. vol. **347**, R 1 (1974).

HOLLAND, W. C., SEKUL, A.: Effect of ouabain on Ca^{45} and Cl^{36} exchange in isolated rabbit atria. Amer. J. Physiol. **197**, 757–760 (1959).

ISSELHARD, W.: Das Verhalten des Energiestoffwechsels im Warmblüterherz bei künstlichem Herzstillstand. Pflügers Arch. ges. Physiol. **271**, 347–360 (1960).

JANKE, J., FLECKENSTEIN, A., JAEDICKE, W.: Hemmung der Isoproterenol-induzierten $^{45}Ca^{++}$-Netto-Aufnahme in das Ventrikelmyokard durch Ca^{++}-antagonistische Hemmstoffe der elektro-mechanischen Koppelung (Isoptin = Verapamil, Iproveratril und Substanz D 600. Pflügers Arch. **316**, R 10 (1970).

JANKE, J., FLECKENSTEIN, A., MARMIER, P., KOENIG, L.: Steigerung der absoluten ATP-Umsetzungsrate in der isolierten Skelettmuskulatur unter dem Einfluß von 2,4-Dinitrophenol. Turnover-Studien mit P^{32}-markiertem Orthophosphat und H_2O^{18}. Pflügers Arch. ges. Physiol. **287**, 9–28 (1966).

JANKE, J., FREY, M.: Unpublished observation (1972).

JANKE, J., MARMIER, P., FLECKENSTEIN, A.: Die Bestimmung der absoluten Umsetzungsraten von ATP, Kreatinphosphat und Orthophosphat in der ruhenden Skelettmuskulatur mit Hilfe von H_2O^{18} als Tracer. Pflügers Arch. ges. Physiol. **282**, 119–134 (1965).

JARISCH, A., WASTL, H.: Observations on the effect of anoxaemia upon heart and circulation. J. Physiol. **61**, 583–592 (1926).

KAMMERMEIER, H.: Verhalten von Adenin-Nukleotiden und Kreatinphosphat im Herzmuskel bei funktioneller Erholung nach länger dauernder Asphyxie. In: Herzstillstand, Herzstilllegung und Wiederbelebung des Herzens. Verh. dtsch. Ges. Kreisl.-Forsch. **30**, 206–211 (1964).

KASPEREK, K., SILLER, V., KNIERIEM, H. J.: Neutronenaktivierungsanalytische Bestimmung von Kobalt und Calcium bei der experimentellen Herzinsuffizienz durch Kobalt-chlorid. Z. ges. exp. Med. **150**, 316–324 (1969).

KATZ, A. M.: Contractile proteins of the heart. Physiol. Rev. **50**, 63–158 (1970).

KAUFMANN, R., FLECKENSTEIN, A.: Ca^{++}-kompetitive elektro-mechanische Entkoppelung durch Ni^{++}- und Co^{++}-Ionen am Warmblütermyokard. Pflügers Arch. ges. Physiol. **282**, 290–297 (1965).

KLAUS, W.: Neuere Aspekte über den Wirkungsmechanismus der Herzglykoside. Z. naturwiss.-med. Grundl.-Forsch. **2**, 43–117 (1964).

KNIERIEM, H. J., HERBERTZ, G.: Elektronenmikroskopische Befunde sowie photometrische und aktivierungsanalytische Ergebnisse bei experimenteller Herzinsuffizienz durch Kobaltchlorid. Virchows Arch. Abt. B **2**, 32–46 (1969).

KOHLHARDT, M., BAUER, B., KRAUSE, H., FLECKENSTEIN, A.: Differentiation of the transmembrane Na and Ca channel in mammalian cardiac fibres by the use of specific inhibitors. Pflügers Arch. **335**, 309–322 (1972).

KOHLHARDT, M., BAUER, B., KRAUSE, H., FLECKENSTEIN, A.: Selective inhibition of the transmembrane Ca conductivity of mammalian myocardial fibres by Ni, Co and Mn ions. Pflügers Arch. **338**, 115–123 (1973).

KRAYER, O.: Versuche am insuffizienten Herzen. Naunyn-Schmiedebergs Arch. exp. Path. Pharmak. **162**, 1–28 (1931).

KRAYER, O., SCHÜTZ, E.: Mechanische Leistung und einphasisches Elektrogramm am Herz-Lungen-Präparat des Hundes. Z. Biol. **92**, 453–461 (1932).

LAMPRECHT, W., MICHAL, G., NÄGLE, S.: Der Stoffwechsel des hypoxischen und anoxischen Herzmuskels. Klin. Wschr. **39**, 358–364 (1961).

LEHR, D., CHAU, R., KAPLAN, J.: Prevention of experimental myocardial necrosis by electrolyte solutions. In: Myocardiology, recent advances in studies on cardiac structure and metabolism, vol. 1, p. 684–698. Baltimore-London-Tokyo: University Park Press 1972.

LE PAGE, G. A.: Biological energy transformations during shock as shown by tissue analysis. Amer. J. Physiol. **146**, 267–281 (1946).

LINDNER, E.: Phenyl-propyl-diphenyl-propyl-amin, eine neue Substanz mit coronargefäßerweiternder Wirkung. Arzneimittel-Forsch. **10**, 569–573 (1960).

LOEWI, O.: Über den Zusammenhang zwischen Digitalis- und Calciumwirkung. Naunyn-Schmiedebergs Arch. exp. Path. Pharmakol. **82**, 131–158 (1917).

LOEWY, A., MAYER, E.: Über experimentell erzeugte akute Herzerweiterungen beim Menschen. Klin. Wschr. **5**, 1213–1216 (1926).

LÜLLMANN, H., HOLLAND, W. C.: Influence of ouabain on an exchangeable calcium fraction, contractile force, and resting tension of guinea-pig atria. J. Pharmacol. exp. Therap. **137**, 186–192 (1962).

MATHISON, G. C.: The action of asphyxia upon the spinal animal. J. Physiol. **41**, 416–449 (1910).
MCDERMOTT, P. H., DELANEY, R. L., EGAN, J. D., SULLIVAN, J. F.: Myocardosis and cardiac failure in men. J. Amer. med. Ass. **198**, 253–256 (1966).
MERCKER, H.: Zur Frage der Herzinsuffizienz im Sauerstoffmangel. Luftfahrtmed. 8, 217–223 (1943).
MICHAL, G., NAEGLE, S., DANFORTH, W. H., BALLARD, F. B.: BING, R. J.: Metabolic changes in heart muscle during anoxia. Amer. J. Physiol. **197**, 1147–1151 (1959).
MOMMAERTS, W. F. H. M.: Muscular contraction, a topic in molecular physiology. Interscience Publishers New York 1950.
MOMMAERTS, W. F. H. M.: Phosphate metabolism in the activity of skeletal and cardiac muscle. In: MCELROY and GLASS, Phosphorus metabolism, vol. I, p. 551. Baltimore: The Johns Hopkins Press 1951.
MORGENSTERN, M., NOACK, E., KÖHLER, E.: The effects of isoprenaline and tyramine on the ^{45}calcium uptake, the total calcium content and the contraction force of isolated guinea-pig atria in dependence on different extracellular hydrogen ion concentrations. Naunyn-Schmiedebergs Arch. Pharmak. **274**, 125–137 (1972).
MORIN, Y., DANIEL, P.: Quebec beer-drinkers' cardiomyopathy: etiological considerations. Canad. med. Ass. J. **97**, 926–928 (1967).
MORIN, Y. L., FOLEY, A. R., MARTINEAU, G., ROUSSEL, J.: Quebec beer-drinkers' cardiomyopathy: forty-eight cases. Canad. med. Ass. J. **97**, 881–883 (1967).
NÄGLE, S., HOCKERTS, TH., BÖGELMANN, G.: Die Beeinflussung des Kreatinphosphokinase-Gleichgewichts durch pH-Abfall im Herzmuskel unter ischämischen Bedingungen. Klin. Wschr. **42**, 780–784 (1964).
NAYLER, W. G., MCINNES, I., SWANN, J. B., PRICE, J. M., CARSON, V., RACE, D., LOWE, T. E.: Some effects of iproveratril (Isoptin) on the cardiovascular system. J. Pharmacol. exp. Therap. **161**, 247–260 (1968).
NAYLER, W. G., SZETO, J.: Effect of verapamil on contractility, oxygen utilization and calcium exchangeability in mammalian heart muscle. Cardiovasc. Res. **6**, 120–128 (1972).
OPITZ, E., SCHNEIDER, M.: Über die Sauerstoffversorgung des Gehirns und den Mechanismus von Mangelwirkungen. Ergebn. Physiol. **46**, 126–260 (1950).
POOL, P. E., SPANN, J. F., BUCCINO, R. A., SONNENBLICK, E. H., BRAUNWALD, E.: Myocardial high energy phosphate stores in cardiac hypertrophy and heart failure. Circulat. Res. **21**, 365–373 (1967).
REPKE, K.: Über den biochemischen Wirkungsmodus von Digitalis. Klin. Wschr. **42**, 157–165 (1964).
REUTER, H.: Über die Wirkung von Adrenalin auf den cellulären Ca-Umsatz des Meerschweinchenvorhofs. Naunyn-Schmiedebergs Arch. exp. Path. Pharmak. **251**, 401–412 (1965).
RONA, G., CHAPPEL, C. I.: Pathogenesis and pathology of cobalt cardiomyopathy. In: Cardiomyopathies, recent advances in studies on cardiac structure and metabolism, vol. 2, p. 407–422. Baltimore-London-Tokyo: University Park Press 1973.
RONA, G., CHAPPEL, C. I., BALAZS, T., GAUDRY, R.: An infarct-like myocardial lesion and other toxic manifestations produced by isoproterenol in the rat. A.M.A. Arch. Path. **67**, 443–455 (1959).
RONA, G., CHAPPEL, C. I., KAHN, D. S.: The significance of factors modifying the development of isoproterenol-induced myocardial necrosis. Amer. Heart J. **66**, 389–395 (1963).
RONA, G., KAHN, D. S., CHAPPEL, C. I.: Studies on infarct-like myocardial necrosis produced by isoproterenol: a review. Rev. Canad. Biol. **22**, 241–255 (1963).
RUSHMER, R. F.: Cardiovascular dynamics, p. 183. Philadelphia-London: W. B. Saunders 1961.
SCHÄDLER, M.: Proportionale Aktivierung von ATPase-Aktivität und Kontraktionsspannung durch Calciumionen in isolierten kontraktilen Strukturen verschiedener Muskelarten. Pflügers Arch. ges. Physiol. **296**, 70–90 (1967).
SCHILDBERG, F. W., FLECKENSTEIN, A.: Die Bedeutung der extracellulären Calciumkonzentration für die Spaltung von energiereichem Phosphat in ruhendem und tätigem Myokardgewebe. Pflügers Arch. ges. Physiol. **283**, 137–150 (1965).
SCHMITZ, H.: Vorkommen und Bedeutung von freien Nucleotiden in Zellen und Geweben. 11. Coll. Ges. Physiol. Chem., p. 1–25. Berlin-Göttingen-Heidelberg: Springer 1961.
SCHWIEGK, H.: Kreislaufwirkung eines Glykosides aus Digitalis lanata. Naunyn Schmiedebergs Arch. exp. Path. Pharmak. **162**, 56–69 (1931).
SEIDEL, J. C., GERGELY, J.: Studies on myofibrillar adenosine triphosphatase with calcium-free adenosine triphosphate. J. biol. Chem. **238**, 3648–3653 (1963).
SEKUL, A., HOLLAND, W. C.: Effects of ouabain on Ca^{45} entry in quiescent and electrically driven rabbit atria. Amer. J. Physiol. **199**, 457–459 (1960).

SELYE, H.: Elektrolyte, Streß und Herznekrose. Basel: Benno Schwabe 1960.

SOBEL, B. E., SPANN, J. F., POOL, P. E., SONNENBLICK, E. H., BRAUNWALD, E.: Normal oxidative phosphorylation in mitochondria from the failing heart. Circulat. Res. **21**, 355–363 (1967).

SPANN, J. F., CHIDSEY, C. A., POOL, P. E., BRAUNWALD, E.: Mechanism of norepinephrine depletion in experimental heart failure produced by aortic constriction in the guinea pig. Circulat. Res. **17**, 312–321 (1965).

STRUGHOLD, H.: A cinematographic study of systolic and diastolic heart size with special reference to the effects of anoxemia. Amer. J. Physiol. **94**, 641–655 (1930).

SULLIVAN, J., PARKER, M., CARSON, S. B.: Tissue cobald content in "beer drinkers" myocardiopathy. J. Lab. clin. Med. **71**, 893–896 (1968).

SZEKERES, L., SCHEIN, M.: Cell metabolism of overloaded mammalian heart in situ. Cardiologia **34**, 19–27 (1959).

TAKEUCHI, K.: The relation between the size of the heart and the oxygen content of the arterial blood. J. Physiol. **60**, 208–214 (1925).

THOMAS, L. J., JOLLEY, W. B., GRECHMAN, R.: Effect of potassium lack and ouabain on calcium^{45} uptake in frog's heart. Fed. Proc. **17**, 162 (1958) [see THOMAS, L. J.: Ouabain contracture of frog heart: Ca^{45} movements and effect of EDTA. Amer. J. Physiol. **199**, 146–150 (1960)].

THORN, W., HEIMANN, J., MÜLDENER, B., ISSELHARD, W., GERCKEN, G.: Herzstoffwechsel in Abhängigkeit von Versuchsanordnung, Gewebsgewinnung und anoxischer Belastung. Pflügers Arch. ges. Physiol. **269**, 214–231 (1959).

URBANEK, E., VASKU, J., BEDNARIK, B., URBANKOVA, H.: Influence of Na_2-EDTA upon development of experimental cardiomyopathies. Proceedings of the Second Annual Meeting of the International Study Group for Research in Cardiac Metabolism, Istituto Lombardo, Fondazione Baselli, p. 242–249 (1969).

VATER, W., KRONEBERG, G., HOFFMEISTER, F., KALLER, H., MENG, K., OBERDORF, A., PULS, W., SCHLOSSMANN, K., STOEPEL, K.: Zur Pharmakologie von 4-(2′-Nitrophenyl)-2,6-dimethyl-1,4-dihydropyridin-3,5-dicarbonsäuredimethylester (Nifedipine), Bay a 1040). Arzneimittel-Forsch. **22**, 1–14 (1972).

WATANABE, A. M., BESCH, H. R., JR.: Subcellular myocardial effects of verapamil and D 600: comparison with propranolol. J. Pharmacol. exp. Therap. **191**, 241–251 (1974).

WEBER, A., HERZ, R.: The binding of calcium to actomyosin systems in relation to their biological activity. J. biol. Chem. **238**, 599–605 (1963).

WEBER, A., WINICUR, S.: The role of calcium in the superprecipitation of actomyosin. J. biol. Chem. **236**, 3198–3202 (1961).

WEDER, U., GRÜN, G.: Ca^{++}-antagonistische elektro-mechanische Entkoppelung der glatten Gefäßmuskulatur als Wirkungsprinzip vasodilatatorischer Nitroverbindungen. Naunyn-Schmiedebergs Arch. Pharmacol. Suppl. vol. **277**, R 88 (1973).

WILLIAMSON, J. R., WOODROW, M. L., SCARPA, A.: Calcium binding to cardiac sarcolemma. In: Recent Advances in Studies on Cardiac Structure and Metabolism, vol. 5, p. 61–71. Baltimore-London-Tokyo: University Park Press 1975.

WINEGRAD, S.: Studies of cardiac muscle with a high permeability to calcium produced by treatment with ethylenediamine-tetraacetic acid. J. gen. Physiol. **58**, 71–93 (1971).

WOLLENBERGER, A.: On the energy-rich phosphate supply of the failing heart. Amer. J. Physiol. **150**, 733–745 (1947).

ZONDEK, H.: Herzbefunde bei Leuchtgasvergifteten. Ein Beitrag zur Lehre von der Organdisposition des Herzens. Dtsch. Med. Wschr. **45**, 678–680 (1919).

Experimental Models of Hemorrhagic Shock*

R. CARLSON and M. H. WEIL

I. Introduction

Prior to the landmark experiments of WIGGERS and his colleagues (WIGGERS, 1917; WERLE et al., 1942; WIGGERS, 1942; WIGGERS and WERLE, 1942; WIGGERS et al., 1946; WIGGERS, 1950), a standardized method for the production of hemorrhagic shock did not exist, and the pathophysiology of this form of shock in man or the experimental animal was poorly understood. The modern era of research in this field of shock can therefore be traced to the innovative studies by WIGGERS and other farsighted investigators of his generation (FINE and SELIGMAN, 1943; FINE and SELIGMAN, 1945; FRANK et al., 1945).

In designing his experiments WIGGERS defined several goals. He initially sought to develop a method for standardizing the production of hypovolemic shock and to determine criteria for identifying and quantitating perfusion failure. The method could then be used to provide data which would lead to a more complete understanding of the syndrome. The technique would also serve as a basis for developing more effective therapy of the clinical equivalent of this form of shock. In large measure the results of those early experiments achieved these goals. Since his studies new techniques as well as further insight into the mechanisms which lead to shock have evolved. However, the goals outlined by Doctor WIGGERS more than 40 years ago remain applicable for the investigator today.

The purpose of this chapter is to briefly review the procedures utilized to induce hypovolemic shock in the laboratory and the pathophysiology of this syndrome, with special reference to variabilities resulting from the choice of experimental technique.

II. Definition of Problem

Hypovolemic shock may be defined as perfusion failure due to a critical reduction in blood volume. Cardiac output and the supply of oxygen and other nutrients are lowered. The multisystem failure which emerges can be directly traced to a reduction in nutritive blood flow. Oxidative metabolism is curtailed and anerobic pathways are utilized to supply energy requirements. However, this leads to the production and accumulation of lactic acid and other acid metabolites, which include inorganic phosphates derived from the breakdown of nucleotides. Progressive metabolic acidosis and acidemia in themselves alter cardiovascular function. The animal initially responds with compensatory cir-

* From the Shock Research Unit and the Department of Medicine, University of Southern California School of Medicine, the Los Angeles County/USC Medical Center, and the Center for the Critically Ill, Hollywood Presbyterian Medical Center, Los Angeles, California.

culatory adjustments; subsequently, the responses are decompensatory, terminating in death.

Within the past few years it has become possible to reliably measure the severity of perfusion failure by analysis of the concentration of lactic acid in blood. Stemming in part from studies originating in our own Unit (BRODER and WEIL, 1964; WEIL and AFIFI, 1970), the onset of perfusion failure may be correlated with a sharp increase in blood lactate. The severity of the shock state may then be monitored by sequential determinations of this metabolite.

A. Techniques for the Production of Hemorrhagic Shock

I. Pressure-Resistance Model

Several techniques may be selected to induce hemorrhagic shock in the laboratory. However, all methods involve bleeding controlled either by reducing arterial pressure or by the removal of specified volumes of blood. The first method is often termed the pressure or resistance model. The technique developed by WIGGERS is an example of this type, although several modifications have been developed since the initial description by WIGGERS (FRANK et al., 1945; LAMSON and DETURK, 1945; LANSING and STEVENSON, 1957; SELKURT and ROTHE, 1961; BUTCHER and BRAITBERG, 1969; KIM et al., 1969; MONAFO et al., 1969; MACDONALD et al., 1975).

The essential feature of this model is the removal of blood to induce a predetermined level of arterial hypotension. The animal is bled rapidly through an arterial catheter into a glass or plastic reservoir containing an anticoagulant. Bleeding continues until the mean arterial pressure is between 35 and 50 mm Hg. Maximum bleedout occurs within two hours and is approximately 50 ml of blood per kilogram of body weight. This represents a hemorrhage of nearly two-thirds of the total blood volume. Subsequently, additional aliquots of blood are removed or reinfused to maintain the arterial pressure at the preselected level. The height of the reservoir bottle may be adjusted or pressure may be applied to the bottle (LAMSON and DETURK, 1945) to achieve the desired hydrostatic pressure. If the system is hydrostatically controlled in such a manner, the arterial catheter can be opened and arterial pressure will equilibrate with the pressure in the reservoir. This method for bleeding the conscious dog is well established. With this technique both bleeding and subsequent reinfusion can be automatically controlled by the arterial pressure level. As the period of hypotension is lengthened, usually beyond 90 min, the animal's arterial pressure declines to less than the reservoir pressure and blood is spontaneously reinfused. This is known as the uptake phenomenon (FRANK et al., 1945; GREEN, 1961; HOLLENBERG and NICKERSON, 1970; ROTHE, 1970; NAGLER and LEVENSON, 1974). Criteria of the severity of the insult include the uptake of a specified percentage of shed blood or the duration of hypotension. If the interval of hypotension is prolonged, or a significant percentage of blood spontaneously reinfuses, survival of the animal is unlikely even if the remainder of the shed blood is reinfused. This phenomenon has led to use of the term "irreversible" shock (FRANK et al., 1945).

The pressure model creates an artificial situation by partially ablating the compensatory vasoconstriction by the vasculature, yet the volumes of blood removed are predictable as is the severity of insult as judged by ultimate survival. The method is easily standardized and constitutes the most frequently used technique. However, this technique is not directly comparable to the insult which follows acute blood loss in patients and constitutes the clinical syndrome of hemorrhagic shock.

II. Volume Model

The second method for the experimental production of hemorrhagic shock involves the removal of a specified volume of blood. A percentage of the measured or estimated blood volume of the animal is selected (SELKURT and ROTHE, 1961; MARKS et al., 1967; BROBMANN et al., 1970, 1971; SPITZER and SPITZER, 1972; NELSON and SWAN, 1974; ZWEIFACH, 1974). At least one-third of the blood volume must be removed to induce perfusion failure, and considerably greater volumes must be removed if the hemorrhage is to be lethal.

Several techniques may be selected. Small aliquots may be removed in stepwise fashion, a single rapid hemorrhage may be performed, or the animal may be subjected to a slow, continuous hemorrhage. The duration of ischemia and the subsequent reinfusion of blood are other variables which must be controlled. Stepwise bleeding in the rat has been reported by our group (WHIGHAM and WEIL, 1966). Some methods do not include the reinfusion of blood, allowing the investigator to study the pathophysiologic responses of the organism without the complicating factors induced by reinfusion.

If stepwise bleeding is selected, this technique allows the study of the compensatory mechanisms called into action by the animal, and in large measure duplicates the condition seen clinically. However, this method may be less predictable. Individual differences in cardiac output and peripheral resistance may alter the response to hemorrhage. In addition, the post-hemorrhage residual blood volume of the animal may vary, after bleeding a fixed percentage of the total blood volume, due to the duration of hemorrhage and the compensatory mechanisms to restore blood volume. The slow, continuous hemorrhage may more closely mimic the clinical state but has the additional disadvantage that the experiments are unduly prolonged.

Another variation is the single rapid bleed of a fixed volume (ZWEIFACH, 1974). This allows the investigator to study compensatory mechanisms, often without reinfusion. Using this technique less hemorrhage volume is required to produce a lethal insult than if blood is removed more slowly. Another variation is the rapid removal of a fixed percentage of blood volume, usually 40%, followed by a slower rate of bleeding.

B. Pathophysiology of Hemorrhagic Shock

Hemorrhage induced by either the pressure or volume method leads to characteristic pathophysiologic responses common to both methods. As blood volume decreases resistance (precapillary) and capacitance (postcapillary) vessels constrict. The former serves as a compensatory mechanism which supports perfusion in the face of a reduced blood volume and cardiac output (SELKURT and ROTHE, 1961; CHIEN, 1967; BROBMANN et al., 1971). The coronary and cerebral circulations do not participate in this general vasoconstrictive response, but perfusion of less critical regions, and particularly skin and muscle, may be drastically reduced. Venoconstriction augments the return of blood to the heart. Early in the course of hemorrhage the ratio of precapillary to postcapillary resistance increases (MELLANDER and LEWIS, 1963; HOLLENBERG and NICKERSON, 1970; BROBMANN et al., 1971). This results in a decrease in the hydrostatic pressure within the capillary bed. The balance of hydrostatic and oncotic forces described by the Starling equation then favors a movement of protein-poor fluid from the interstitium into the vascular space. This process is termed transcapillary refill. The fluid entering the circulation from the interstitium partially restores the vascular volume, but produces a decrease in the hematocrit and plasma oncotic pressure. This process may be monitored by sequential determinations of hematocrit and plasma protein concentration. Oncotic pressure may be calculated from the protein concentration or measured directly with a transducer-membrane system. A decline in oncotic pressure following hemorrhage has been documented by us (unpublished). Viscosity of blood is also reduced, which favorably affects small vessel blood flow even though the calculated peripheral vascular resistance is greatly increased. Transcapillary refill begins shortly after the initiation of hemorrhage and may persist for hours. The process slows and ceases as the balance of hydrostatic and oncotic forces achieve a new equilibrium. At this point plasma volume has been partially restored. A major source of fluid for transcapillary refill originates from the splanchnic bed. Full restitution of the blood volume and restoration of the plasma oncotic pressure usually require a longer interval, typically in excess of 24 hrs. The lymphatics participate in this secondary response and facilitate restoration of both fluid volume and protein content. Although new protein is rapidly synthesized and enters the circulation, recent studies suggest that it is the mobilization of preformed protein stored in the interstitium which accounts for the major source of protein entering the circulation within the first 24 hrs after hemorrhage (MARKS et al., 1967; PIRKLE and GANN, 1975). The adrenal corticosteroids play an important role in the mobilization of this protein. In addition to the fluid shifts between the interstitium and the vascular space, the intracellular volume supplies a portion of the fluid reserve which restores blood volume after hemorrhage.

In addition to the pre- and postcapillary resistance changes during hypovolemia, capillary compliance, microcirculatory blood flow and the permeability of the microvasculature also determine the balance of fluid movement. The pre- and postcapillary resistance changes are mediated by the sympathetic nervous system, the local release of neurotransmitters, the concentration of circulating catecholamines and other vasoactive substances, and by the effects of local metabolites (GREEN, 1916; MELLANDER and LEWIS, 1963; HADDY et al., 1965; CHIEN, 1967; BROBMANN et al., 1970; HOLLENBERG et al., 1970; GLENN and LEFER, 1971; NAGLER and LEVENSON, 1974; ZWEIFACH, 1974). Although levels of angiotensin and other vasoconstrictors in the blood increase with hemorrhage, peripheral resistance changes during hemorrhagic shock are temporally related to serum catecholamine levels (MCNEILL et al., 1970; JAKSCHIK et al., 1974). In late shock, local tissue metabolites exert a pronounced vasodilating effect with subsequent decompensation. However, the administration of alphalytic and beta-minetic catecholamines may improve tissue perfusion and improve survival if instituted prior to irreversible decompensation (JACOB et al., 1956; GREEN, 1961; MELLANDER and LEWIS, 1963; FINE, 1965; CHIEN, 1967; BROBMANN et al., 1970; HOLLENBERG and NICKERSON, 1970; BROBMANN et al., 1971; WHIGHAM et al., 1973).

When the ischemic episode is prolonged, the vasoconstrictor response of the precapillary resistance vessels is less pronounced. After three to four hours, vasomotion is severely disturbed and the microvasculature responds in a more passive manner to changes in arterial pressure. At this time the balance of pre- and postcapillary resistance favors an increase in hydrostatic pressure within the capillary bed. This process creates a situation in which fluid is lost from the circulation to the interstitium; a reversal of transcapillary refill (Wiggers et al., 1946; Mellander and Lewis, 1963; Gillett and Halmagyi, 1966; Rothe, 1970; Cook et al., 1971; Chien et al., 1973). In studies using the pressure method of hemorrhage, this late decline in blood volume is heralded by an increase in hematocrit and oncotic pressure, as well as the phenomenon of uptake (Hollenberg and Nickerson, 1970; Hollenberg et al., 1970; Rothe, 1970; Chien et al., 1973; Zweifach, 1974). As more blood is spontaneously reinfused during the uptake interval, more fluid is lost from the vascular space. Thus, uptake signals a major decompensatory phase of the syndrome and often correlates with the ultimate death of the animal. However, hemoconcentration is not commonly observed in the clinical setting.

Sludging of flow, increases in viscosity, and the accumulation of local metabolites of themselves hamper the exchange of nutrients and metabolites within the microcirculation. The progressive decline in venous return and cardiac output, and the variable effects of anoxia, together with the effect of circulating as well as local toxins, explain terminal deterioration with myocardial and peripheral vascular decompensation (Green, 1961; Kim et al., 1969; Glenn and Lefer, 1971; Nagler and Levenson, 1974; Nelson and Swan, 1974; Zweifach, 1974; MacDonald et al., 1975).

C. Technical Considerations

I. Anesthesia

In experiments of hemorrhagic shock which utilize general anesthesia, this condition complicates the interpretation of results. Unanesthetized animals have a stronger cardiovascular and respiratory response to the stress and tolerate a greater loss of blood. In addition, most of the general anesthetic agents have profound direct effects on the nervous and cardiovascular systems. Therefore, if possible, general anesthesia should be avoided. If surgical procedures are required for the study, these should be completed several days in advance of the acute experiment. Local anesthesia should be used for placement of catheters. These experiments are best conducted on the conscious animal (Priano et al., 1969).

II. Sterile Technique

Under ideal conditions all experiments should be performed with surgical aseptic precautions. As a minimum, clean if not sterile procedures must be used. Special precautions should be observed to insure that the blood is not exposed to contaminated catheters or equipment. If the experiment is prolonged, or involves significant surgical manipulation, sterile technique should be observed.

III. Blood Trauma and Microembolization

In addition to the potential exposure of blood to microorganisms, with any procedure in which the shed blood is held in a reservoir, the exposure of that fluid to air, glass or other container surface may induce deleterious effects upon reinfusion. The plasma proteins, and particularly the clotting factors, as well as the formed elements, may be damaged by surface contact or trauma in handling. Heparin or a citrate solution is usually added to the reservoir to prevent clotting. Some investigators also maintain the shed blood at 37° prior to reinfusion. The blood may be returned to the animal by way of the arterial catheter, in which case the systemic vascular bed acts as a primary filter for the particulate matter which may have formed. The blood can be infused by increasing the pressure in the reservoir bottle and opening the arterial catheter, by manual infusion using a syringe, or with the aid of an infusion pump. The latter technique assures a constant rate of infusion and results in less trauma to the blood. The blood may also be returned to the animal by way of a venous catheter. If this method is selected, it is desirable to monitor central venous pressure, pulmonary artery wedge (occluded) pressure or left ventricular end-diastolic pressure to avoid inducing cardiac decompensation. Recently, blood ultrafiltration systems have become widely available. These devices remove particulate matter as small as 20 μ in diameter and are therefore helpful in minimizing the exogenous microembolization which occurs with massive transfusions. If the blood is reinfused into a vein, the use of these filtering systems helps prevent the accumulation and subsequent deleterious effects of particulate matter in the pulmonary circulation (Jenevein and Weiss, 1964; Connell and Swank, 1971; Connell et al., 1975).

IV. Species

The choice of an experimental animal is an important consideration. Investigators are likely to select an animal species which is readily available, inexpensive, free of disease, uniform in size, sex and genetic strain, and in which the physiologic responses to the insult duplicate those observed in man. Although virtually all domesticated animals and several exotic species have been utilized, the rat, subhuman primate, and the dog are most often selected. Investigators are well advised to confirm and compare the results of studies in at least two species (Selkurt and Rothe, 1961; Zweifach, 1961).

The rat offers the advantage of uniformity of size and strain (Jacob et al., 1956; Whigham and Weil, 1966; Butcher and Braitberg, 1969; Monafo et al., 1969; Whigham et al., 1973; Nagler and Levenson, 1974). The rat by virtue of its size and ease of handling permits the study of several animals simultaneously. For this reason this species is well suited to studies of survival and the evaluation of experimental therapy. However, because of its size, the amount of blood which may be removed must be carefully controlled. It is usually necessary to prepare donor animals for replacement of blood utilized for laboratory procedures.

The subhuman primates are excellent subjects in that their responses often correlate well with the clinical condition. However, availability and cost are major considerations limiting their more widespread use.

The dog has been the subject for more hemorrhage experiments than any other animal. However, the exaggerated hemodynamic responses of the hepatosplanchnic viscera must be taken into consideration when interpreting canine studies.

The spleen of the dog is a reservoir of blood containing a high red cell mass (Guntheroth and Mullins, 1963; Brooksby and Donald, 1972; Chien et al., 1973). When the animal is subjected to stress the spleen contracts, augmenting the circulating blood volume and producing a marked rise in hematocrit. This may complicate studies in which the investigator wishes to examine the early interval after hemorrhage. Some investigators therefore perform splenectomies on their subjects prior to hemorrhage. However, in dogs with an intact spleen, a larger bleeding volume is tolerated. There is less transcapillary refill and a greater peripheral vascular resistance and blood viscosity are observed in animals with an intact spleen (Chien et al., 1973).

The splanchnic viscera predominate in the canine response. During hemorrhage the liver becomes engorged because of sphincteric constriction of small hepatic veins. Bloody diarrhea is a common finding after reinfusion of shed blood following prolonged hemorrhagic shock (Crowell and Nelson, 1975). This phenomenon is related to both splanchnic ischemia and portal venous congestion. Marked increases in the hydrostatic pressure of the portal circulation and alterations in visceral capillary permeability following severe ischemia have been documented (Wiggers et al., 1946; Selkurt and Rothe, 1961; Fine, 1965; Cook et al., 1971).

D. Summary and Conclusions

Although the animal model provides understanding of the clinical condition of hemorrhagic shock without jeapordizing human life, it is important to recognize that any experimental method designed to produce shock represents an artificial situation. The investigator induces hypotension or removes a measured volume of blood. In contrast, once hypovolemia is recognized clinically, treatment is instituted. The clinician can rarely quantitate the volume of blood lost by his patient or the duration of hemorrhage. Even with the more general availability of radioisotopic techniques for the measurement of blood volume, results of these studies are not immediately available to the clinician and compensatory responses by the patient or volume repletion prior to measurement may make interpretation more difficult. Therefore, although experimental models of hypovolemic shock may did not duplicate the clinical picture, they allow the study of the natural evolution of the process and provide a basis for evaluating methods by which circulatory failure and tissue injury may be reversed.

The research program of the Shock Research Unit and the Center for the Critically Ill have been supported by United States Public Health Service Research Grant HL-05570 from the National Heart, Lung, and Blood Institute, GM-16462 from the National Institute of General Medical Sciences, RO1 HS 01474 from Health Resources Administration, and the Parker B. Francis Foundation of Kansas City, Missouri.

References

Brobmann, G. F., Ulano, H. B., Moore, G., Meyer, P., Brecher, G. A., Jacobson, E. D.: Effect of acute hemorrhage on arterial and venous resistance. Amer. J. Physiol. **220**, 12–15 (1971).

Brobmann, G. F., Underwood, L. D., McCoy, J., Price, W. E., Jacobson, E. D.: Early regional vascular responses to hemorrhage and reinfusion in dogs. Surg. Gynec. Obstet. **131**, 409–416 (1970).

Broder, G., Weil, M. H.: Excess lactate: An index of reversibility of shock in human patients. Science **143**, 1457–1459 (1964).

Brooksby, G. A., Donald, D. E.: Release of blood from the splanchnic circulation in dogs. Circulat. Res. **31**, 105–118 (1972).

Butcher, H. R., Braitberg, A.: Hemorrhagic shock in rats. Arch. Surg. **98**, 685–693 (1969).

Chien, S.: Role of the sympathetic nervous system in hemorrhage. Physiol. Rev. **47**, 214–288 (1967).

Chien, S., Dellenback, R. J., Usami, S., Burton, D. A., Gustavson, P. F., Magazinovic, V.: Blood volume, hemodynamic, and metabolic changes in hemorrhagic shock in normal and splenectomized dogs. Amer. J. Physiol. **225**, 866–879 (1973).

Connell, R. S., Swank, R. L.: Pulmonary fine structure after hemorrhagic shock and transfusion of ageing blood. In: Microcirculatory approaches to current therapeutic problems. Symposia. 6th Europ. Conf. Microcirculation, Aalborg 1970, p. 49–58. Basel: Karger 1971.
Connell, R. S., Swank, R. L., McWebb, M. C.: The development of pulmonary ultrastructural lesions during hemorrhagic shock. J. Trauma **15**, 116–128 (1975).
Cook, B. H., Wilson, E. R., Jr., Taylor, A. E.: Intestinal fluid loss in hemorrhagic shock. Amer. J. Physiol. **221**, 1494–1498 (1971).
Crowell, J. W., Nelson, K. M.: Mechanisms of bloody diarrhea in shock. Circ. Shock **2**, 21–28 (1975).
Fell, C.: Plasma loss in dogs in irreversible hemorrhagic shock. Amer. J. Physiol. **211**, 885–889 (1966).
Fine, J.: Shock and peripheral circulatory insufficiency In: Handbook of physiology, sect. 2, Circulation, vol. III (eds. W. F. Hamilton and P. Dow), p. 2037–2069. Washington, D.C.: Amer. Physiol. Soc. 1965.
Fine, J., Seligman, A. M.: Traumatic shock: An experimental study including evidence against the capillary leakage hypothesis. Ann. Surg. **118**, 238–243 (1943).
Fine, J., Seligman, A. M.: Traumatic shock. VII. A study of the problem of the "lost plasma" in hemorrhagic, tourniquet and burn shock by the use of radioactive iodoplasma protein. J. clin. Invest. **23**, 720–730 (1945).
Frank, H. A., Seligman, A. M., Fine, J.: Traumatic shock. X. The treatment of hemorrhagic shock irreversible to replacement of blood volume deficiency. J. clin. Invest. **24**, 435–443 (1945).
Gillett, D. J., Halmagyi, D. F. J.: Blood volume in reversible and irreversible posthemorrhagic shock in sheep. J. Surg. Res. **6**, 259–261 (1966).
Glenn, T. M., Lefer, A. M.: Significance of splanchnic proteases in the production of a toxic factor in hemorrhagic shock. Circulat. Res. **29**, 338–343 (1971).
Green, H. D.: Physiology of peripheral circulation in shock. Fed. Proc. **20**, 61–68 (1961).
Guntheroth, W. G., Mullins, G. L.: Liver and spleen as venous reservoirs. Amer. J. Physiol. **204**, 35–41 (1963).
Haddy, F. J., Scott, J. B., Molnar, J. I.: Mechanism of volume replacement and vascular constriction following hemorrhage. Amer. J. Physiol. **208**, 169–181 (1965).
Hollenberg, N. K., Nickerson, M.: Changes in pre- and postcapillary resistance in pathogenesis of hemorrhagic shock. Amer. J. Physiol. **219**, 1483–1489 (1970).
Hollenberg, N. K., Waters, J. R., Toews, M. R., Davies, R. O. Nickerson, M.: Nature of cardiovascular decompensation during hemorrhagic hypotension. Amer. J. Physiol. **219**, 1476–1482 (1970).
Jacob, S., Friedman, E. W., Levenson, S., Glotzer, P., Frank, H. A., Fine, J.: Antiadrenergic and antihistaminic therapy in hemorrhagic shock in dog and rat. Amer. J. Physiol. **186**, 79–83 (1956).
Jakschik, B. A., Marshall, G. B., Kourik, J. L., Needleman, P.: Profile of circulating vasoactive substances in hemorrhagic shock and their pharmacologic manipulation. J. clin. Invest. **54**, 842–852 (1974).
Jenevein, E. P., Weiss, D. L.: Platelet microemboli associated with massive blood transfusions. Amer. J. Path. **45**, 313–326 (1964).
Kim, S. I., Desai, J. M., Shoemaker, W. C.: Sequence of cardiorespiratory alterations after gradual prolonged hemorrhage in conscious dogs. Amer. J. Physiol. **216**, 1044–1050 (1969).
Lamson, P. D., DeTurk, W. E.: Studies on shock induced by hemorrhage. XI. A method for the accurate control of blood pressure. J. Pharmacol. exp. Ther. **83**, 250–252 (1945).
Lansing, A. M., Stevenson, J. A. F.: The standardization of stress in the production of hemorrhagic shock. Canad. J. Biochem. **35**, 1085–1092 (1957).
Lansing, A. M., Stevenson, J. A. F.: Mechanism of action of norepinephrine in hemorrhagic shock. Amer. J. Physiol. **193**, 289–293 (1958).
MacDonald, J. A. E., Milligan, G. F., Mellon, A., Ledingham, I. McA.: Ventricular function in experimental hemorrhagic shock. Surg. Gynec. Obstet. **140**, 572–581 (1975).
Marks, L. J., King, D. W., McCarthy, H. F.: Physiological role of cortisone in the plasma volume response to hemorrhage. Surgery **61**, 422–426 (1967).
McNeill, J. R., Stark, R. D., Greenway, C. V.: Intestinal vasoconstriction after hemorrhage: Roles of vasopressin and angiotensin. Amer. J. Physiol. **219**, 1342–1347 (1970).
Mellander, S., Lewis, D. H.: Effect of hemorrhagic shock on the reactivity of resistance and capacitance vessels and on capillary transfer in cat skeletal muscle. Circulat. Res. **13**, 105–118 (1963).
Monafo, W. W., Wachtel, T. L., Deitz, F.: Bioassay of hemorrhagic shock in rats. Arch. Surg. **98**, 275–280 (1969).

NAGLER, A. L., LEVENSON, S. M.: The nature of the toxic material in the blood of rats subjected to irreversible hemorrhagic shock. Circ. Shock **1**, 251–258 (1974).
NELSON, A. W., SWAN, H.: Hemorrhage: Responses determining survival. Circ. Shock **1**, 273–285 (1974).
PIRKLE, J. C., GANN, D. S.: Restitution of blood volume after hemorrhage: Mathematical description. Amer. J. Physiol. **228**, 821–827 (1975).
PRIANO, L. L., TRABER, D., WILSON, R. D.: Barbiturate anesthesia: An abnormal physiologic situation. J. Pharmacol. exp. Ther. **165**, 126–130 (1969).
ROTHE, C. F.: Heart failure and fluid loss in hemorrhagic shock. Fed. Proc. **29**, 1854–1860 (1970).
SELKURT, E.E.: Status of investigative aspects of hemorrhagic shock. Fed. Proc. **29**, 1832–1835 (1970).
SELKURT, E. E., ROTHE, C. F.: Critical analysis of experimental hemorrhagic shock models. Fed. Proc. **20**, 30–48 (1961).
SPITZER, J. J., SPITZER, J. A.: Myocardial metabolism in dogs during hemorrhagic shock. Amer. J. Physiol. **222**, 101–105 (1972).
SWINGLE, W. W., PFIFFNER, J. J., VARS, H. M., PARKINS, W. M.: The effect of hemorrhage on the normal and adrenalectomized dog. Amer. J. Physiol. **107**, 259–264 (1934).
WEIL, M. H., AFIFI, A. A.: Experimental and clinical studies on lactate and pyruvate as indicators of severity of acute circulatory failure (shock). Circulation **44**, 989–994 (1970).
WEIL, M. H., WHIGHAM, H.: Corticosteroids for reversal of hemorrhagic shock in rats. Amer. J. Physiol. **209**, 815–818 (1965).
WERLE, J. M., COSBY, R. S., WIGGERS, C. J.: Observations on hemorrhagic hypotension and hemorrhagic shock. Amer. J. Physiol. **136**, 401–420 (1942).
WHIGHAM, H., WEIL, M. H.: A model for the study of hemorrhagic shock in the rat: Development of the method. J. appl. Physiol. **21**, 1860–1863 (1966).
WHIGHAM, H., WEIL, M. H., SHUBIN, H.: Effects of isoproterenol during hemorrhagic shock in the rat. J. Pharmacol. exp. Ther. **186**, 355–365 (1973).
WIGGERS, C. J.: The initial and progressive stages of circulatory failure in abdominal shock. Amer. J. Physiol. **45**, 485–490 (1917).
WIGGERS, C. J.: The present status of the shock problem. Physiol. Rev. **22**, 74–102 (1942).
WIGGERS, C. J.: Physiology of shock. New York: New York Commonwealth Fund 1950.
WIGGERS, C. J., OPDYKE, D. F., JOHNSON, J. R.: Portal pressure gradients under experimental conditions, including hemorrhagic shock. Amer. J. Physiol. **146**, 192–206 (1946).
WIGGERS, C. J., WERLE, J. M.: Cardiac and peripheral resistance factors as determinants of circulatory failure in hemorrhagic shock. Amer. J. Physiol. **136**, 421–432 (1942).
ZWEIFACH, B. W.: Aspects of comparative physiology of laboratory animals relative to the problem of experimental shock. Fed. Proc. **20**, 18–27 (1961).
ZWEIFACH, B. W.: Mechanisms of blood flow and fluid exchange in microvessels: Hemorrhagic hypotension model. Anesthesiology **42**, 157–168 (1974).

Some Experimental Shock Models: Traumatic Shock, Catecholamine Shock, Burn Shock and Other Shock Forms

H. D. Schmidt

Numerous models are available for the investigation of problems relating to shock in animal experimentation. Before a particular model is selected the investigator should be clear in his own mind about his expectations of the model and the pronouncements reached by its application and use. There are various requirements which a model might be expected to meet, depending on the problem being investigated. Some of these are listed below.

1. The experimental model should be similar to the clinical situation. In this case experimental shock should as far as possible correspond to the resp. form of shock in the human patient. The extent to which this demand is met varies widely in various shock models. Only an approximation to the clinical situation is possible, however, even in the most favorable cases. In addition, many patients affected by shock are already ill prior to going into a state of shock and suffer from organic insufficiencies, whereas animal experients are almost without exception performed on healthy animals. This fact must be borne in mind when conclusions reached as the result of the animal experimentation are applied to the human organism.

2. The means of eliciting the state of shock must be unequivocally defined. This means that the method of precipitating the state of shock must be qualitatively as well as quantitatively defined as precisely as possible. The manner in which this clearly defined intervention impairs the homeostasis of the organism should also be extensively known. In noradrenaline shock, e.g., these two demands are met to a large extent. The infused dosage or, still better, the catecholamine level in the plasma can be exactly determined and the pharmacological action of noradrenaline is wellknown.

In the case of drum shock, in contrast, the precipitating factor cannot be precisely defined (unless the number and speed of revolutions is thought to constitute an acceptable definition), and nor are the mechanisms by which this treatment causes the state of shock sufficiently clear. The necessity for this demand to be met increases in proportion as the wish to investigate basic pathophysiological laws in the shock tests intensifies. In most cases it is thus difficult to reconcile it with the demand for similarity to the clinical situation.

3. The shock model must be easily put into practice and easily standardized. This requirement is met to a large extent in, for example, hemorrhagic shock, which is probably the reason for the widespread use of this model. Reliable therapeutic investigations are only possible when the severity of the intervention leading to the state of shock is comparable in the individual animals.

4. It must be possible to abolish the primary cause of shock. In many shock models the intervention that elicits the shock cannot be reversed, but continues to act on the organism until death occurs (e.g. endotoxin shock, burn shock, cardiogenic shock). In such models, in the late stages of shock it is no longer possible to recognize which pathophysiological changes are due to the continued effect of the primary cause of the shock and which should be regarded as secondary effects of the shock itself. In addition, in some cases (e.g. septic shock) the factor that originally causes the shock can change without this being noted. Thus, when the consequences of shock only are being investigated, it must be possible after some time to abolish the shock producing factor.

In the case of shock induced by oxygen deficiency, for example, this can easily be achieved by switching over to room air (see below).

The most commonly used experimental models for shock are described briefly below. As cardiogenic and septic shock are described in detail elsewhere in this volume, they are not included here. The list given is by no means complete. But anyone carrying out shock experiments would be well advised to give preference to the models that have already been extensively examined in other laboratories and for which a standard course has been devised; only then will comparison of his results with those of other authors be valid. The general term *Traumatic shock* includes widely varying forms of shock. In this group, shock is induced by direct destruction of tissues, by ischemia of the tissues, or by hypoxia and anoxia of the tissues. Hemorrhagic shock and catecholamine shock can thus also be classified as traumatic shock. A typical model for traumatic shock, however, is the tourniquet shock.

A. Tourniquet Shock

In this form of shock the blood flow to one or more extremities is interrupted for a defined length of time. When the ligation is released a state of shock sets in.

Interruption of blood flow can be achieved in various ways. In dog, the hair is removed from the hind legs and a piece of thick rubber tubing is wrapped round each hind leg as high up and as tightly possible. Complete occlusion of the artery in the leg is obtained with greater certainty with the aid of flexible synthetic-coated steel wire tightened with conventional wire tighteners [57]. When the arteries in both hind legs are occluded for 5 h, the 48-h mortality is almost 100%, the average length of survival being 7–8 h [42, 57, 77]. Tourniquet shock also occurs when both legs are tightly wrapped with rubber tubing from ankle to groin. If this compression is released after 6 h the mortality is more than 90% and the average length of survival is 14 h [30]. When rats and mice are used the hind legs are tied round with a rubber band or linen thread as high up as possible [70]. This can also be done with rubber rings that have first been mounted on a metal pipe through which the extremity is pulled. Threads placed through the rubber rings are then used to pull the rings from the pipe and they are fixed as high up as possible on the upper tigh. The ligatures are secured with sutures to prevent them from slipping on the conical thighs. The hair should be moved from the animals' legs before application of the tourniquets.

In one method developed specifically for use with small animals, the animals are placed in metal cylinders; the hind legs protrude through openings in the sides. A second cylinder is slipped over the first, with conical recesses corresponding to the openings. In this way, both hind limbs can be crushed quite simply [25].

When the blood flow to both hind limbs is interrupted for 4–5 h in rats or mice, the mortality is 90–100%; the length of survival can be 2–5 h or even more [34, 41, 63, 70, 78]. If the ligatures are left in place for only 2.5 h, rather more than 50% of the animals die within 24 h [38].

All these mortality data relate, of course, to tests performed at room temperature. If the limbs are cooled during or before ligation the tolerance is higher [68, 74]. If the legs are encased in tight plaster immediately after release of the tourniquet death is not prevented, but it is delayed [40].

In the induction of tourniquet shock it is important to make sure that the ligatures really do occlude the blood flow to the extremities completely; if this is so the extremities quickly become cold and pale, without the development of clear-cut edema. It is advisable to test the adequacy of the tourniquets by giving an injection of a dye or of a radioactive indicator; the indicator should not pass into the vasculature of the ligated legs.

In tourniquet shock the state of shock does not set in until the ligatures are removed. The blood pressure first falls abruptly and then rises slightly, remaining at the plateau reached at this point—usually 50–70 mm Hg—for up to several hours [10, 11]. The final fall in blood pressure is usually rather sudden and rapid.

Experimental tourniquet shock is easy to induce and a good degree of standardization is possible. It corresponds quite closely to the crush syndrome seen in clinical practice. The mortality can be varied by changing the duration of occlusion or the amount of tissue affected (e.g. by tying off a different number of extremities). As this experimental model meets most of the requirements that can be asked of experimental shock models, tourniquet shock seems to be particularly well suited to the investigation of traumatic shock [73].

B. Shock Induced by Occlusion of the Superior Mesenteric Artery (SMA Shock)

Shock induced by occlusion of the superior mesenteric artery (SMA shock) is basically a variant of tourniquet shock. The abdomen is opened under sterile conditions and the intestinal artery is occluded; this occlusion is maintained for several hours. The state of shock again sets in as soon as the blood flow is restored. The artery can also be reached from the retroperitoneal approach, avoiding opening of the peritoneum [33]. The artery can be occluded with an atraumatic artery clamp or with a ligature. Reopening of the artery is particularly simple if a glass rod is tied into the ligature; this can be pulled out on a thread while the abdomen remains closed [37, 39].

The size of the intestinal area that becomes ischemic after occlusion of the artery is dependent on the size of the supply area of the occluded artery and on the standard of collateral supply available. The course of the experiment can therefore vary widely after reopening of the occluded artery. In dog, the mortality (48-h limit) after occlusion of the superior mesenteric artery for 3 h is about 50%; after ligation for 4 h it is 80%, and when the occlusion is maintained for 5 h the mortality averages 90% [51]. In rabbit the mortality is 50–90% even when the artery is occluded for only 1–1.5 h. The mortality is similar in rat after the same duration of occlusion [5,, 45].

The main reason for the onset of the state of shock after opening of the mesenteric occlusion is the loss of fluid in the damaged area of the intestine. Endotoxemia seems to be of no great significance [17, 54].

The method of induction of SMA shock can be varied by the additional occlusion of further intestinal vessels; this of course lowers the tolerance [28, 48, 69]. Again, it is important to make quite sure that the artery is completely occluded. This is usually easily recognized by the paleness of the intestinal segment affected and the absence of arterial pulsations. It is also necessary to test whether reopening of the artery really leads to a release of the blood flow. The blood flow has been released if the pulsations resume and the intestine becomes pink.

On the whole, SMA shock is assessed in a similar way to tourniquet shock. The main disadvantage of this model is the necessity for surgery, which is an additional trauma. The trauma can be kept slight by means of a careful technique and/or retroperitoneal exposure of the mesenteric artery. SMA shock has a clinical counterpart in intestinal infarction. In addition, an area of tissue is directly affected in this model, which plays an important part in other forms of shock such as hemorrhagic shock and endotoxin shock, especially in dog.

C. Drum Shock

In this model, small mammals, usually rats, mice, or guinea-pigs, are placed in a drum approximately 40 cm in diameter and 17.5 cm deep. Their paws are tied and they are not anesthetized. Two ledges about 5 cm wide are fixed at the edge of the drum opposite to each other. As the drum turns the animals are taken up on these ledges and then fall onto the edge of the drum once or twice per revolution [16]. The animals obviously become unconscious the first time they fall, as they do not show any pain reaction. Drum shock was first reported by NOBEL and COLLIP in 1942 [55]. The speed of revolution of the drum is generally 40–45 revolutions per minute. The mortality is dependent on the total number of revolutions. After 300 revolutions the 12-h mortality is about 10–15%, after 500–600 revolution it is 75–80% [16, 18], and after 1000 revolutions it is practically 100% [56].

The requirement for unequivocal definition of the event causing shock is not met with this model, for the extent and localization of the tissue injuries are largely a matter of chance and cannot be stated quantitatively. In addition, only a very general qualitative description of the intervention is possible. Intra-abdominal injuries seem to play an important part. When the mortality is calculated, animals that die in the drum while it is revolving or within 20 min after being taken out must not be included in the calculation. Animals found at autopsy to have suffered severe intestinal hemorrhage, intracranial hemorrhage, or broken limbs are also excluded from the calculation [4].

The advantage of this model is that it is very easily set up and a large number of traumatic shock experiments can be performed in small animals within a short time and with relatively low expenditure. In therapeutic tests, several treatment and control groups can be exposed to drum shock simultaneously, which allows optimum comparability. In addition, the numbers necessary for statistical significance of the results are very quickly reached in this way. It must be noted, however, that the posttraumatic course can vary very widely with a low number of revolutions. Better reproducibility can be attained only with more severe trauma [62].

D. Shock Induced by Direct Destruction of Tissue

Experimental shock research began with direct trauma to the tissues [8, 14]. An enormous number of different techniques were used. One method proved to be relatively practicable. The extremities of an animal—usually a dog or a cat—are struck with a soft hammer. In dog, after 100 blows on each hind limb (in animals weighing about 20 kg) the blood pressure and cardiac output fall continuously and the animals die within 3–6 h. If only one extremity is processed irreversible shock occurs only in some of the animals [8, 59, 67, 75, 76]. The muscles in the upper and lower leg are traumatized without breaking the bones. It is easy to elicit shock by direct destruction of the tissues in this way. This model contrasts with drum shock in that the extent and site of the tissue destruction can be stated fairly accurately, and with tourniquet in that the state of shock is the direct result of tissue damage and not elicited by ischemia of the tissues. The shock in this model is more like the form of shock observed in clinical practice. In contrast to the situation in tourniquet shock, in this model the state of shock sets in immediately after administration of the blows with the hammer, so that it is not necessary to wait for 3–5 h with ligatures in place. The difficulty with this model is that it is difficult to reproduce the severity of the trauma inflicted satisfactorily in the different animals [32]. Two different experimenters achieve trauma of different grades of severity when they administer the same number of blows and "apply the same force". If the severity selected is thus that not all the animals die, the posttraumatic course varies very widely and the survival rate found in any series cannot normally be duplicated [32].

E. Catecholamine Shock

A typical state of shock can be elicited by the administration of an intravenous infusion of a catecholamine such as noradrenaline over several hours. The vasoconstriction induced leads to hypoxia in the areas affected, which leads in turn to irreversible and ultimately fatal changes if the infusion is continued over a sufficiently long period. In hemorrhagic shock and endotoxin shock the excessive vasoconstriction caused by endogenously released catecholamines is a significant feature in the pathogenesis. In one way, catecholamine shock is therefore related to these two other forms of shock. When the infusion is begun, the blood pressure initially rises steeply, the level reached corresponding to the dose/time. It can reach levels of up to 300 mm Hg [2, 29]. Even when the infusion is continued, the blood pressure then falls again slowly. If the infusion is discontinued after 3–4 h the blood pressure first falls abruptly and then slowly diminishes until the animal dies. The mortality depends on the duration of the infusion and on the dose infused. When 1.5 μg/kg·min is given over 3 h, practically all the dogs survive [31]. Irreversible shock is elicited in a high proportion of the animals when 2 μg/kg·min is given over 4 h]79[. After the infusion of 3μg/kg·min over more than 3 h the 48-hour mortality is almost 100% in dogs [19, 31]. Catecholamine infusions regularly cause a distinct rise in the hematocrit [31, 44, 53], which is a point of difference between catecholamine shock and hemorrhagic shock, though otherwise there are many similarities in the pathophysiology of these two forms of shock, despite the very different blood-pressure levels. If adrenaline is given in the infusion instead of noradrenaline the course of the shock reaction and the mortality are about the same, providing the same doses are used [31].

In one modification of catecholamine shock, the blood pressure is kept constant instead of the speed of infusion. The selected dose is such that the blood pressure first rises by a certain amount (e.g. 60 mm Hg) and is then maintained at the new level by continuously increasing the speed of the infusion [26]. The course of the shock reaction is practically the same as that caused by an infusion of the catecholamine at constant speed.

Catecholamine shock is extremely easy to elicit, and a good degree of standardization is possible [24]. The primary cause of the state of shock is well defined. The requirement of similarity to the clinical situation is not met with this model, however, as catecholamine shock does not occur spontaneously in man in the form described. The mortality can be deliberately varied in catecholamine shock by changing the dose infused or the duration of the infusion. It is advisable, however, to give reasonably low doses of noradrenaline (about 2–3 μg/kg·min) over a fairly long period, to avoid unphysiologically high pressures that could have a direct deleterious effect on the heart [26, 53]. The shock-inducing process can be abolished completely within a very short time by discontinuation of the infusion. It is, of course, also possible to continue the infusion until a fatal outcome is reached [2].

The simplicity of the method, the possibility of unequivocal definition, and the easy management combine to make catecholamine shock well suited to the examination of basic questions relating to shock.

F. Burn Shock

In experimental burn shock the state of shock is elicited by either burning or scalding, and it is therefore more correct to refer to it as shock by high temperature. The expression 'burn shock' has gained general acceptance, however, and will therefore be used in this article. Burn shock also occurs in man after burns and scalds, so that there is a very close similarity between the experimental model and the clinical situation.

In principle, burn shock is easily elicited in animal experimentation. It is very difficult, however, to attain satisfactory standardization and reproducibility with this model and a series of requirements must be met before these can be adequate:

1. Exactly corresponding areas of the body and the same proportion of the body surface must be affected in each animal.
2. The depth of the burn wound must be practically uniform all over the burnt area.
3. The boundary between burnt and nonburnt areas must be as sharp as possible.
4. The duration of action of the heat must be exactly definable.
5. The effective temperature must remain constant throughout the application.

In addition, the thermal damage should affect only the skin, and as far as possible deeper tissues and organs should be left unaffected.

Experimental burn shock is more often elicited by scalding, as this is easier than burning. Small animals such as mice and rats are almost always used. The simplest experimental method involves shaving the animals from the tail to the axilla and then immersing them up to the axilla in water at 70–100°C for a few seconds [15, 35, 36, 47, 50]. If the animals are not shaved it is advisable to add, a wetting agent to the water [35]. The survival rate depends on the area affected, the temperature of the water, and the duration of immersion. If two-thirds of the body surface is scalded for 5–6 sec with water at 70°C, 73–100% of the animals die within 24 h [47, 50]. If only one hind leg is scalded, in contrast, water at 95°C must be allowed to take effect for 15 sec for 24-hour mortality of 82% and 48-hour mortality of 100% [47]. If rats are immersed up to the neck in water at 75°C for 15 sec the 48-hour mortality is 87% [36]. Shock has also been elicited by scalding in dog [21, 52, 58], pig [46], and monkey [23].

One drawback always encountered with this simple method is that the extent of the scalded area cannot be accurately stated. It is also very difficult to decide in advance on a certain region to be scalded and to keep to the same area in all the animals. It is possible to circumvent this difficulty with small animals by applying adhesive dressings to them, with a hole corresponding in size to the area the experimenter wishes to be scalded situated over the back [6]. This also allows quite clear differentiation between the burnt and nonburnt areas of skin. When large animals are used this can be achieved by the use of several layers of crepe bandage that leave only the area to be scalded exposed. This area can be measured and expressed as a proportion of the total body surface area. Appropriate formulas have been published for the calculation of total body surface area for small rodents [7, 43], dogs [18], and pigs [46]. Scalding of the skin with water at 90°C for 20 sec results in third-degree lesions. In rat the mortality is 100% when more than 40% of the total body surface is scalded in this way, and 50% when about 30% of the body surface is scalded under these conditions [6]. The results are similar in dog: when an average of 43% of the body surface is immersed in water at 100°C for 10 sec all the animals die [21].

Most of the experimental studies on burn shock reported in the literature have been based on scalding. The cases of burn shock seen in clinical practice, however, are generally caused by the direct action of dry heat. Experimental burning is even more difficult to standardize than experimental scalding, however. Dry heat of 60–250°C is usually used for the burns. Metal stamps made of iron, copper, and other metals are used for this purpose; they are first heated to the required temperature by means of a heating element such as is used in an electric iron [12, 72], or by immersion in water at a thermostatically controlled temperature [9], or simply in an oil bath [60]. The hot metal is then pressed onto the shaven skin for 12–20 sec. Several of these brands can be made next to each other. The application pressure is usually supplied by the weight of the metal stamp. A constant temperature can only be maintained ,however, if heating of the stamp is continued while the burn is inflicted. In rabbit, when 30% of the body surface area is burnt with an iron at 250°C for 15 sec all the animals die within 24 h [12].

Direct burning with flames is probably best achieved by the ignition of powdered magnesium. The brief flash, lasts only 0.7 sec, and temperatures of over 1000°C are generated. When the shaven skin of monkeys is about 10 cm away from the powdered magnesium and third-degree burns are inflicted in this way over 25% of the body surface, all the animals die after an average of 24 h [22, 23].

Another method involves exposing animals to the thermal energy from irradiation lamps (750 W) with parabolic reflectors [13, 27]. The irradiation energy at the focal point can certainly be accurately recorded, but the declining intensity out to the sides cannot be defined as the parts of the body being irradiated are not plane surfaces. The edge of the burnt area is indistinct.

A burn model for use in mouse has recently been described, which allows the infliction of burns and scalds under controlled conditions and also comparison of the two [71]. An area of skin up to 5×2 cm in size is shaved and raised away from the animals back, remaining attached along the two long sides. A Pyrex glass spatula is inserted into the resulting tunnel. The animal is lifted by the glass spatula, and the prepared skin, which is also stretched by the lifting, is pressed at constant pressure against an electrically heated stamp fitted with a thermostat, so that burning results. For scalding, the skin is prepared in the same way and the prepared area is pressed against a cover plate with a rectangular opening. Steam or hot water is directed onto the skin exposed within the opening, from a vaporizing head with numerous tiny openings. When shock is elicited by scalding the area treated has to be twice the size of the area exposed to dry heat for the same mortality to result if the duration of exposure to heat is the same in both cases [22, 71]. This shock model largely fulfils the requirements expected of experimental burn shock.

G. Shock Induced by Acute Anemia

In this experimental shock model severe anemia is induced without changing the total blood volume [61, 64, 65]. The anemic state is then maintained for several hours, as nearly as possible at the same level of severity. The method has been described in detail elsewhere [65]: 2.5 ml blood/min·kg is taken from each animal, and a plasma substitute at body temperature is infused simultaneously at the same speed until the hemoglobin value has fallen to 20–25% of the normal value. The blood taken is immediately and carefully centrifuged, and the plasma obtained is used together with the plasma substitute for dilution of the circulating blood. Thus all animals get back all the plasma initially taken away. Small infusions must be given at frequent intervals over the next few hours to keep the hemoglobin value constant. Care must be taken not to let the blood pressure fall below 90 mm Hg, to avoid adding hypotonia to the anemic state. When the anemia has been maintained for about 4 h, all erythrocytes are suspended in 100–200 ml Ringer's solution and reinfused at a speed of 1.25 ml/min·kg. If such a severe anemia is maintained in dogs for 4 h by means of dilution of the blood with dextran or gelatin solution, only about 20–30% of the animals survive for over 48 h. The advantage of this form of shock over hemorrhagic shock is that the blood volume remains constant, the cardiac output is not diminished but tends to rise and there is no centralization of the circulation, which would entail hemostasis with all its consequences. It must be admitted that the technique is quite elaborate and costly. No corresponding form of shock is encountered in clinical practice.

A combination of hypotonia and anemia can occur during the treatment of hypovolemia with plasma substitutes, however, which could cause a state of shock. Shock induced by anemia is best suited to the examination of basic questions relating to shock.

H. Shock Induced by Respiratory Oxygen Deficiency

In this model the animals spontaneously breathe a mixture of gases that is deficient in oxygen or are respirated with a mixture of this type for a predetermined time after muscle relaxation [1, 3, 65].

When the mixture used for spontaneous respiration is 6.5–10.5 ml O_2 per 100 ml N_2 and this is provided for 6.5 h or until respiratory arrest occurs, the 48-hour mortality is 46%. When the animals are artificially respirated for an average of 2.5 h with resting minute volume and an oxygen concentration of 9.5–15.0 ml per 100 ml in the breathing mixture, the average mortality is 54% [1, 65]. It is relatively easy to induce shock by means of oxygen deficiency, and standardization is also comparatively simple with this model. The procedure is clearly defined. The cause of shock can be abolished at any time by switching over to ordinary air in the respiration apparatus. The mortality can be influenced by variation of the duration of hypoxia and the composition of the oxygen-deficient mixture. This model is also best suited to the investigation of basic and theoretical questions relating to shock, as it has no close counterpart in clinical practice; a similar state of shock is sometimes observed in human patients in the presence of severe impairment of oxygen diffusion (e.g. hyaline membranes, pulmonary contusion, etc.).

I. Conclusion

The severity of the state of shock can be varied in almost all shock models by changes in the severity of the intervention used to elicit the shock. Death of the experimental animals despite abolition of the primary cause of shock is the only sure criterion of irreversible shock. It is usual to assess any animals still alive after 48 h as surviving. If reversible shock is elicited the animals survive.

In investigations based on experimental shock models, the severity of the state of shock induced should generally be such that irreversible shock occurs in a high proportion of the animals. This is particularly important in therapeutic studies, in which the mortality should be 70–90% in the control group if possible; it is only under these circumstances that any therapeutic effect is clearly recognizable. If all the control animals die it is possible that the severity of the intervention is such that even an effective therapeutic treatment could not improve the survival rate.

The information given in the literature on mortality and thus on the severity of the shock elicited can only be taken as a rough guide. Every experimenter concerned with shock experiments must test for himself how severe a state of shock he obtains with a standardized procedure in *his* laboratory animals and under the conditions in *his* laboratory. In all shock experiments it is therefore necessary to observe the subsequent fate of the animals and to determine the survival rate. The length of survival is quite an unsatisfactory criterion. If the survival rate is determined a condition cannot be defined as a state of shock without in fact being so. For example, if only one lower leg is tied off in an animal, tourniquet shock cannot develop. Even if this ligature is left in place for many hours there will be no direct fatal consequences when it is removed. Ligation of the main trunk of the left coronary artery at its root almost always leads to acute cardiac insufficiency with a critical fall in blood pressure and cardiac output. But this condition would also be incorrectly described as a state of shock. If the ligature is removed promptly full recovery is generally possible within a short time.

We believe that "shock is a state of tissue hypoxidosis that leads to irreversible and ultimately fatal changes if it persists sufficiently long" [3, 65, 66]. Thus the intervention eliciting the shock reaction leads to irreversible damage that results in the death of the total organism, even long after the stimulus causing the initial damage has ceased to be directly effective. If the original intervention results directly in death, as in the case of ligation of the main trunk of the coronary artery, there is no state of shock.

If basic rules of the type discussed in this paper are observed, and tests are carried out with as well-standardized models as possible, experimental shock research can make a substantial contribution to the solution of pathophysiological and therapeutic problems relating to shock.

References

1. ACKERN, K. VAN, MEHMEL, H., SCHMIDT, H. D., SCHMIER, J.: Schock durch gesteuerten Sauerstoffmangel. Z. ärztl. Forsch. **10**, 309–315 (1971).
2. ACKERN, K. VAN, BRÜCKNER, U. B., HAKIMI, B., LEINBERGER, H., SCHMIER, J.: Tödlicher Schock durch Nor-Adrenalin-Infusion im Tierexperiment. Langenbecks Arch. Chir. **336**, 115–123 (1974).
3. ACKERN, K. VAN, MEHMEL, H., SCHMIDT, H. D., SCHMIER, J.: Sauerstoffschuld und Acidose im Schock durch gesteuerte Hypoxämie. Langenbecks Arch. Chir. **331**, 131–147 (1972).
4. ALTURA, B. M., HSU, R., MAZZIA, V. D. B., HERSHEY, S. G.: Influence of vasopressors on survival after traumatic intestinal ischemia and endotoxin shock in rats. Proc. Soc. exp. Biol. **119**, 389 (1965).
5. ALTURA, B. M., HERSHEY, S. G., MAZZIA, V. D. B.: Microcirculatory approach to vasopressor therapy in intestinal ischemic (SMA) shock. Amer. J. Surg. **111**, 186–192 (1966).
6. ARTURSON, G.: The infliction and healing of a large standard burn in rats. Acta path. microbiol. scandinav. **61**, 353–364 (1964).
7. BHATT, R. M., PATEL, B., SHETTY, V.: Effect of high and low protein diets on post burn hepatic enzyme changes in experimental animals. In: Research in burns. Eds.: MATTER, P., BARCELAY, T. L., KONICKOWA, Z. Berne: Huber 1970, p. 557–560.
8. BLALOCK, A.: Experimental shock: the cause of the low blood pressure produced by muscle injury. Arch. Surg. **20**, 959–996 (1930).
9. BROOKS, J. W., ROBINETT, P., LARGEN, T. L., EVANS, I. E.: A standard contact burn. Method of production and observations of the blood picture following its production in dogs. Surg. Gynec. Obst. **93**, 543–554 (1951).
10. BRÜCKNER, U. B., HERRMANN, H., SCHMIER, J., STENGER, E., ULMER, H. E.: Hämodynamische Veränderungen im Tourniquet-Schock des Hundes. Z. Kreislaufforsch. **60**, 740–751 (1971).
11. BRÜCKNER, U. B., OPHERK, D., SCHMIER, J., TREUMER, H., SCHWARZ, G.: Kreislaufdynamik und Kontraktilität des Herzens im Tourniquet-Schock des Hundes bei Hemmung der Blutgerinnung und der Xanthinoxydase. Z. Kreislaufforsch. **61**, 161–178 (1972).
12. BURRI, C., ALLGÖWER, M.: Die Wirksamkeit zweier Plasmaexpander im experimentellen Verbrennungs-Schock. Schw. med. Wschr. **94**, 816–819 (1964).
13. CALDWELL, F. T., OSTERHOLM, J. H., LOWER, N. D., HOYER, C. A.: Metabolic response to thermal trauma of normal and thyroprivic rats at three environmental temperatures. Ann. Surg. **150**, 976–988 (1959).
14. CANNON, W. B., BAYLISS, W. M.: Note on muscle injury in relation to shock. Report of Shock Committee, Medical Research Committee No. **26**, 19–23 (1919).
15. MCCARTHY, M. D., MCCARTHY, M. D.: Coombs' (Antiglobulin) reaction in severely-burned rats. Ann. Surg. **157**, 446–452 (1963).
16. CHAMBERS, R., ZWEIFACH, B. W., LOWENSTEIN, B. E.: Circulatory reactions of rats traumatized in the Noble-Collip drum. Amer. J. Physiol. **139**, 123–128 (1943).
17. CHU-JENG CHIU, M. D., SCOTT, H. J., GURD, F. N.: Volume deficit versus toxic absorption: A study of canine shock after mesenteric arterial occlusion. Ann. Surg. **175**, 479–488 (1972).
18. COWGILL, G. R., DRABKIN, D. L.: Determination of a formula for the surface area of the dog together with a consideration of formulae available for other species. Amer. J. Physiol. **81**, 36–61 (1927).
19. DRUCKER, W. R., KINGSBURY, B., POWERS, A., O'REILLEY, M.: Metabolic changes in lethal shock produced by norepinephrine. J. lab. clin. Med. **60**, 871 (1962).
20. EIGLER, F. W., STOCK, W., HÖFER, I.: Wirkung eines Proteinaseinhibitors auf das Tourniquet-Syndrom der Ratte, Z. ges. exp. Med. **151**, 55–63 (1969).
21. ELROD, P. D., MCCLEERY, R. S., BALL, C. O. T.: An experimental study of the effect of heparin on survival time following lethals burns. Surg. Gynec. Obstet. **92**, 35–42 (1951).
22. FOX, C. L., LASKER, S. E., WINFIELD, J. M.: Relative lack of efficacy of fluid therapy. Comparison of flash burns and scalds in monkeys. Amer. J. Surg. **99**, 690–693 (1960).

23. Fox, C. L., Lasker, S. E.: Fluid and electrolyte alterations in burned monkeys. Ann. New York Acad. Sci. **150**, 611–617 (1968).
24. Freeman, N. E., Freedman, H., Miller, C. C.: The production of shock by the prolonged continuous injection of adrenalin in unanesthetised dogs. Amer. J. Physiol. **131**, 545–553 (1941).
25. Friedmann, J. J.: Alterations in tissue blood volume induced by tourniquet application. Amer. J. Physiol. **198**, 886–890 (1960).
26. Gilbert, R. P., Hohf, R.: Hemodynamic basis of norepinephrine shock. Proc. Soc. exp. Biol. **116**, 43–46 (1964).
27. Gilmore, J. P., Handford,, S. W.: Hemodynamic response of the dog to thermal radiation. J. Appl. Physiol. **8**, 393–398 (1956).
28. Glenn, T. M., Lefer, A. M.: Role of lysosomes in the pathogenesis of splanchnic ischemia shock in cats. Circul. Res. **27**, 783–797 (1970).
29. Gomez, H. J., Yard, A. C.: Cardiac and vascular changes in acute tolerance to norepinephrine infusions. J. Pharmacol. exp. Therap. **164**, 270–279 (1968).
30. Green, H. D., Dworkin, R. M., Antos, R. J., Bergeron, G. A.: Ischemic compression shock with an analysis of local fluid loss. Amer. J. Physiol. **142**, 494–507 (1944).
31. Grega, G. J., Haddy, F. J.: Forelimb transcapillary fluid fluxes and vascular resistances in catecholamine shock. Amer. J. Physiol. **220**, 1448–1462 (1971).
32. Gregersen, M. I.: Shock. Ann. Rev. Physiol. **8**, 335–354 (1946).
33. Gruber, U. F.: Intestinale Faktoren im Schock: Darmtoxine. Langenbecks Arch. klin. Chir. **319**, 909–925 (1967).
34. Hamolsky, M. W., Gierlach, Z. S., Jensen, H.: Uptake and conversion of radioactive iodine (I^{131}) by thyroid gland *in vivo* and *vitro* in tourniquet shock in rats. Amer. J. Physiol. **164**, 35–43 (1951).
35. Harkins, H. N., Long, C. N. H.: Metabolic changes in shock after burns. Amer. J. Physiol. **144**, 661–668 (1945).
36. Hazan, S. J., Treadwell, C. R.: Saline and methionine-saline effects on survival rate of rats receiving standardized burn shock. Proc. Soc. exp. Biol. **68**, 684–686 (1948).
37. Hershey, S. G., Baez, S., Rovenstine, E. A.: Intestinal ischemia shock in normal and Dibenzyline-protected dogs. Amer. J. Physiol. **200**, 1239–1244 (1961).
38. Ingle, D. J.: The survival of non-adrenalectomized rats in shock with and without adrenal cortical hormone treatment. Amer. J. Physiol. **139**, 460–463 (1943).
39. Janoff, A., Nagler, A. L., Baez, S., Zweifach, B. W.: Pathogenesis of experimental shock. III. A lethal factor in the blood of rabbits following occlusion of the superior mesenteric artery. J. exp. Med. **114**, 205–216 (1961).
40. Koletsky, S. G., Gustafson, G. E.: Effect of plaster on tourniquet shock. Proc. Soc. exp. Biol. **75**, 776–778 (1950).
41. Koletsky, S. G., Gustafson, G. E.: Tourniquet shock in rats. Reversibility in the terminal phase. Amer. J. Physiol. **178**, 229–232 (1954).
42. Kovach, A. G. B., Takacs, L.: Responsiveness of the vegetative nervous system in shock. Acta physiol. hung. **8**, 91–101 (1952).
43. Lee, M. O.: Determination of the surface area of the white rat with its application. Amer. J. Physiol. **89**, 24–33 (1929).
44. Lillehei, R. C., Longerbeam, J. K., Block, J. H., Manax, W. G.: The nature of experimental irreversible shock with its clinical application. In: Shock. Ed. Hershey, S. G. London: Churchill 1964.
45. Lin, M. K., Zweifach, B. W.: Effects of preptreatment with antibiotics on survival following mesenteric arterial occlusion in rats. Proc. Soc. exp. Biol. **108**, 27 (1961).
46. Lyon, J. L., Emery, A. J., Jr., Davis, T. P., Pearse, H. E.: The relationship of thermal induced hemoglobinanemia to volume of skin burn. Surgery **40**, 234–246 (1956).
47. Markley, J., Smallman, E., Evans, G., McDaniel, E.: Mortality of germ free and conventional mice after thermal trauma. Amer. J. Physiol. **209**, 365–370 (1965).
48. Mavor, G. E., Lyall, A. D., Chrystal, K. M. R., Proctor, D. M.: Observation of experimental occlusion of the superior mesenteric artery. Brit. J. Surg. **50**, 536–541 (1963).
49. Mehmel, H., Ackern, K. van, Schmidt, H. D., Schmier, J.: Schock durch gesteuerte Hypoxämie. Pflügers Arch. **291**, R 34 (1966).
50. Millican, R. C., Tabor, H., Rosenthal, S. M.: Traumatic shock in mice. Comparison of survival rates following therapy. Amer. J. Physiol. **170**, 179–186 (1952).
51. Milliken, J., Nahor, A., Fine, J.: A study of the factors involved in the development of peripheral vascular collapse following release of the occluded superior mesenteric artery. Brit. J. Surg. **52**, 699–704 (1965).
52. Moncrieff, J. A.: Effects of various fluid regimens and pharmacologic agents on the circulatory hemodynamics of the immediate postburn period. Ann. Surg. **164**, 723–750 (1966).

53. Moss, A. J., Vittands, J., Schenk, E. A.: Cardiovascular effects of sustained norepinephrine infusion. I. Hemodynamics. Circulat. Res. **18**, 596–604 (1966).
54. Murli, Manohar, Tyagi, R. P. S.: Experimental intestinal shock in dogs. Amer. J. Physiol. **225**, 887–892 (1973).
55. Noble, R. L., Collip, I. B.: A quantitative method for the production of experimental traumatic shock without hemorrhage in unanaesthetized animals. Quart. J. exp. Physiol. **31**, 187–199 (1942).
56. Noble, R. L.: The development of resistance by rats and guinea pigs to amounts of trauma usually fatal. Amer. J. Physiol. **138**, 346–351 (1943).
57. Opherk, D.: Kreislaufdynamik und Kontraktilität im Tourniquet-Schock des Hundes bei Hemmung der Blutgerinnung, der Proteinasen und der Xanthinoxidase. Thesis, Heidelberg 1970.
58. Raker, J. W., Rovit, R. L.: Acute red blood cell destruction following severe thermal trauma in dogs: based on use of radioactive chromate tagged red blood cells. Surg. Gynec. Obstet. **98**, 169–176 (1954).
59. Remington, J. W., Hamilton, W. F., Caddell, H. M., Boyd, G. H., Jr., Wheeler, N. C., Pickering, R. W.: Vasoconstriction as a precipitating factor in traumatic shock in the dog. Amer. J. Physiol. **161**, 125–132 (1950).
60. Renner, K.: Der Einfluß der Defektgröße auf die Heilung unter dem Schorf. Verbrennungsexperimente an der Schweinehaut. Strahlentherapie **132**, 33–39 (1967).
61. Rentrop, P., Schmidt, H. D., Schmier, J.: Shock resulting from hemodilution, the dependence of tolerance of the blood fluid substitute. Bibliog. haemat. **33**, 254–260 (1969).
62. Rittmann, W. W., Gruber, U. F.: Der traumatische Schock. Z. prakt. Anästh. **2**, 65–71 (1969).
63. Rosenthal, S. M., Tabor, H., Little, R. D.: The local nature of acquired resistance to trauma. Amer. J. Physiol. **143**, 402–406 (1945).
64. Schmidt, H. D., Schmier, J.: Schock durch akute Verminderung der Sauerstofftransportkapazität des Blutes. Pflügers Arch. ges. Physiol. **291**, 34 (1966).
65. Schmidt, H. D.: Experimenteller Nachweis der entscheidenden Bedeutung der Gewebshypoxidose im Schock. Thesis, Heidelberg 1969.
66. Schmidt, H. D.: Definition des Begriffes „Schock". In: H. Lutz: „Schock". Munich-Berlin-Vienna: Urban & Schwarzenberg (in press).
67. Schönian, R., Ackern, K. von, Brückner, U. B., Deuster, J. E., Füchte, I., Schmier, J.: Pulmonary artery resistance and myocardial contractility in canine traumatic shock. Proc. Intern. Union Physiol. Science **9**, 501 (1971 (XXV Internat. Congress, Munich).
68. Schwiegk, H.: Kreislaufveränderungen nach Esmarchscher Blutleere. Klin. Wschr. **22**, 477–481 (1943).
69. Selkurt, E. E.: Intestinal ischemic shock and the protective role of the liver. Amer. J. Physiol. **197**, 281–285 (1959).
70. Shipley, E. G., Meyer, R. K., McShan, W. H.: Shock produced by the application of tourniquets to the hind limbs of rats. Proc. Soc. exp. Biol. **60**, 340–344 (1945).
71. Städtler, K., Allgöwer, M., Cueni, L. B., Schönenberger, G. A.: Pathophysiologische Untersuchungen an einem Verbrennungsmodel der Maus. Res. exp. Med. **158**, 23–33 (1972).
72. Stenberg, T.: Studies of the liver function in experimental burns. I. A standardized back burn procedure for the rabbit and observations on blood volume and some blood components after a 10% burn. Acta chir. scand. **123**, 159–170 (1962).
73. Stoner, H. B.: Critical analysis of traumatic shock models. Fed. Proc. **20**, 38–48 (1961).
74. Stoner, H. B.: Studies on the mechanism of shock. The effect of previous exposure to cold. Brit. J. exp. Path. **46**, 278–291 (1965).
75. Swank, R. L., Seaman, G. V. F., Hissen, W., Lino, L.: Physicochemical changes in blood induced by trauma. Surg. Gynec. Obstet. **123**, 251–259 (1966).
76. Swank, R. L., Hissen, W., Bergentz, S. E.: 5-Hydroxytryptamine and aggregation of blood elements after trauma. Surg. Gynec. Obstet. **119**, 779–784 (1964).
77. Swingle, W. W., Remington, J. W.: An experimental study of the tourniquet as a method for inducing circulatory failure in the dog. Amer. J. Physiol. **138**, 156–165 (1942).
78. Van der Meer, C., Valkenburg, P. W., Ariens, A. T., Benthem, R. M. J. van: Cause of death in tourniquet shock in rats. Amer. J. Physiol. **210**, 513–525 (1966).
79. Yard, A. C., Nickerson, M.: Shock produced in dogs by infusion of norepinephrine. Fed. Proc. **15**, 502 (1956).
80. Zweifach, B. W., Metz, D. B., Shorr, E.: Participation of VEM and VDM mechanism in drum shock and in development of resistance to drum trauma. Amer. J. Physiol. **164**, 91–104 (1951).

Microcirculatory Disturbances Induced by Generalized Intravascular Coagulation

G. MÜLLER-BERGHAUS[1] and H.-G. LASCH

With 38 Figures

A. Introduction

The primary function of the circulation of the blood consists in transporting the substances necessary for the maintenance of the metabolic activity of the tissue cells. The circulation is itself dependent on a functioning cardiovascular system in the macrocirculation and, equally important, in the microcirculation. Substances are exchanged between the tissue cells and the blood in the microcirculation, so that any impairment of the microcirculation can also influence the macrocirculation. In the same way, changes in the cardiovascular system of the macrocirculation will also have repercussions on the microcirculation. Figure 1 illustrates the dependence of the microcirculation both on the metabolic processes in the peripheral blood vessels and on the macrocirculation.

According to present ideas about the peripheral blood vessels, the microcirculation can be thought of as a functional entity with three compartments, namely vessel content, vessel wall and tissue. This chapter deals mainly with substances and cells that are contained in the vessels and exert some influence on the vessel wall and tissue. The changes that are sometimes observed in these substances and cells are described variously as sludge, skimming, stasis, change in viscosity, vasoconstriction, vasodilatation and impaired permeability. The coagulation system is involved in these disorders in the peripheral blood vessels, since the vessel wall, the bloodstream and the coagulation system are all interdependent (Fig. 1). Disorders in the microcirculation can cause activation of intravascular coagulation, which sometimes persists to the point where coagulation factors and thrombocytes are used up (consumption of substrate), which in turn can result in the occurrence of microclots in the peripheral blood vessels.

This chapter summarizes the methodological data and the pathophysiologic factors concerned, together with their connections with the occurrence of generalized intravascular coagulation and disseminated development of microclots. The volume of literature on this subject makes it impossible to give a wider or more detailed account of the angles from which experimental investigations have been tackled. Particular stress is laid on the pathophysiologic connections, to enable even an inexperienced experimenter to think or work his way into this sometimes difficult area.

---

[1] Author's experiments described in this article were supported by the Deutsche Forschungsgemeinschaft, Bad Godesberg.

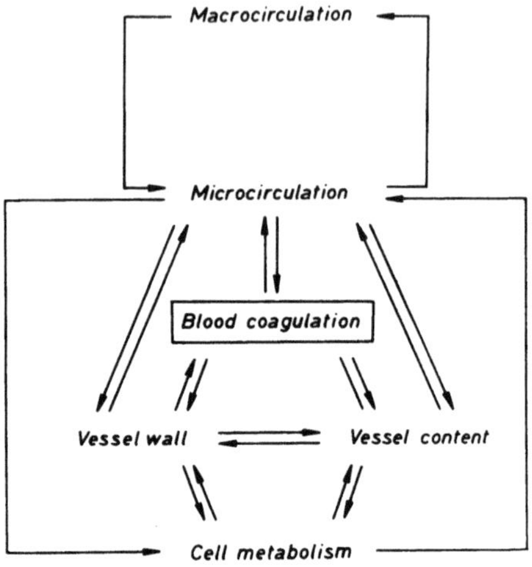

Fig. 1. Dependence of microcirculation on macrocirculation as well as vessel wall and vessel content

B. Historical Notes

The earliest observations bearing on impairments of the microcirculation in relation to coagulation of the blood are concerned with the description of microclots in various pathologic states and animal investigations. LANDOIS (1875) observed microclots in numerous capillaries following the injection of heterologous blood. KLEBS (1876) described hyaline clots in small vessels in a patient who had died of the sequelae of burning. After the injection of tissue fluid, WOOLDRIDGE (1886) found clot formation and, even more interesting, massive hemorrhage. This publication is the first to establish the coexistence of intravascular coagulation and an hemorrhagic diathesis. In 1888, ROUX and YERSIN described abnormal coagulation of the blood following intravenous injection of live diphtheria bacilli to rabbit. Multiple hemorrhages were found in kidneys, lungs and adrenals. WELTI (1889) reported microclots after skin burns in the rabbit. In 1891, WELCH and FLEXNER injected live diphtheria bacilli and subsequently observed hyaline substances occluding the lumina of the glomerular capillaries. These descriptions of the effects seen after the administration of bacteria, such as changes in blood coagulation, the occurrence of microclots (hyaline material) and hemorrhages, are the earliest observations on the effects of bacterial products on blood coagulation and on its consequences; these effects are now referred to as consumption coagulopathy (LASCH et al., 1961a) or disseminated intravascular coagulation (SCHNEIDER, 1951; MCKAY, 1964; HARDAWAY, 1966).

KUSAMA (1913) and SANARELLI (1924) developed the model in which bacterial products are intravenously given in two sublethal doses. The experimental model is now known as the Sanarelli-Shwartzman phenomenon (SSP) or the generalized Shwartzman reaction (GSR). In 1923 and 1924, SANARELLI reported that small amounts of cholera virus, E. coli or typhoid toxin administered in two doses 24 hrs or 48 hrs apart led to death of the animals and an hemorrhagic diathesis, neither of which was observed after a single injection of the agent. KUSAMA (1913) is credited with being the first to indicate the pathogenetically significant finding of extensive microclots with this experimental model. According to KUSAMA'S reports, microclots occurred with particular frequency in the capillaries of lungs, liver and spleen.

It was not until 1927 that SHWARTZMAN and HANGER, working independently of one another, reported a local cutaneous reaction at the site of injection when an *intracutaneous* injection of B. typhosus filtrate was followed 24 hrs later by an intravenous injection of the same material. After intracutaneous injection of endotoxin alone there was no hemorrhagic necrosis. It was APITZ, who in 1935 referred to the appearance of a hemorrhagic necrosis after endotoxin by intracutaneous injection and by intravenous injection 24 hrs later as the *local* Shwartzman reaction. The *generalized* Shwartzman reaction, in contrast, is elicited by two intravenous injections of endotoxin administered 24 hrs apart.

C. Terms and Definitions

I. Intravascular Coagulation

Both clinicians and pathologists generally use the term intravascular coagulation to describe thrombotic processes in the vessel areas of artery and vein. In this context, coagulation means the transformation of fibrinogen to fibrin, which makes up a part of the thrombus that adheres to the vessel wall. In contrast to the formation of microclots, the thrombotic process can be seen with the naked eye on the walls of veins and arteries, while microclots can be detected only by histological examination. This macroscopically visible thrombosis is a localized process, so that it can be described as *local intravascular coagulation*. The coagulation situation is usually normal in the rest of the vascular system, even when an increased tendency to coagulation (hypercoagulability) favors the development of macrothrombosis.

II. Generalized or Disseminated Intravascular Coagulation

When intravascular coagulation is activated in *many* vessel areas, the phenomenon is referred to as disseminated intravascular coagulation or generalized intravascular coagulation; it is often not easy to decide in any particular case whether activation of the intravascular coagulation starts at various points, and has varying preferences for some vascular areas, or whether it begins in all vascular areas (MÜLLER-BERGHAUS, 1971). In this text, preference will be given to the term generalized intravascular coagulation from this point onwards.

III. Consumption Coagulopathy

Either generalized or disseminated activation of the coagulation system will lead to the consumption of plasmatic coagulation factors and also to both numerical and functional changes in the platelets. The term consumption coagulopathy was suggested by LASCH et al. (1961a) to characterize the dynamic process of the activation of intravascular coagulation with consumption of the coagulation components.

Definition: Consumption coagulopathy is defined as an acquired coagulation defect, the main principle in its pathogenesis being increased elimination (increased elimination rate) of plasmatic coagulation factors and platelets due to a *generalized* intravascular coagulation process.

An increased turnover of coagulation factors does not exclusively describe the process in question (LASCH et al., 1971), as the increased turnover of coagulation factors is not necessarily identical with an increased elimination rate (fractional catabolic rate). In this text, generalized intravascular coagulation and consumption coagulopathy are used as synonyms.

IV. Dynamics of Generalized Intravascular Coagulation

McKAY and MÜLLER-BERGHAUS (1967) described the dynamics of generalized intravascular coagulation as follows: Generalized intravascular coagulation (consumption coagulopathy) begins when some procoagulant material or activity enters the circulating blood; it progresses to the stage of free thrombin activity within the circulation, with the formation of fibrin monomers and the occurrence of thrombin-induced platelet aggregation; it is associated with activation of the fibrinolytic system, which leads to the formation of fibrin-split and/or fibrinogen-split products; and it is not complete until the coagulation system, the fibrinolytic system and the hemodynamics have returned to normal. Generalized intravascular coagulation is sometimes accompanied by occlusion of arterioles, capillaries and venules of various organs by fibrin-rich microclots, but this is not a mandatory feature. Impairment of specific organ functions and shock may develop only as secondary phenomena.

V. Generalized Shwartzman Reaction

Definition: The generalized Shwartzman reaction may be defined as occlusion of the glomerular capillaries with fibrin-rich microclots persisting sufficiently long to produce renal cortical necroses (McKAY, 1963).

The term generalized Shwartzman reaction is applied only if microclots occur in the kidneys, as there is obviously a particular mechanism behind the formation of fibrin-rich microclots in the kidneys (McKAY, 1973; MÜLLER-BERGHAUS, 1969). Furthermore, it should be pointed out that the terms generalized Shwartzman reaction and generalized (= disseminated) intravascular coagulation (= consumption coagulopathy) should really not be used as synonyms, as the term generalized intravascular coagulation represents a wider concept, and the generalized Shwartzman reaction is one of many forms of generalized intravascular coagulation.

D. Generalized Intravascular Coagulation

I. Methods of Induction

1. Endotoxin

a) Chemistry and Demonstration of Endotoxin

Endotoxins (or lipopolysaccharides) are components mainly of gram-negative bacteria and are found adjacent to the outer layer of the bacterial cell. They are macromolecules consisting of approximately 70% polysaccharides, 20% lipid moiety, and 10% polypeptides (for references see NOWOTNY, 1966, 1971). The decisive role in the biological activity of an endotoxin is ascribed to the lipid moiety of the endotoxin molecule or to "lipid A" in the terminology of WESTPHAL and LÜDERITZ (1954). A so-called endotoxoid is obtained by way of chemical changes in the endotoxin molecule. Endotoxoid is still capable of evoking a nonspecific resistance to bacteria but it has lost many of its biological properties (NOWOTNY, 1963; URBASCHEK and NOWOTNY, 1968; URBASCHEK et al., 1968).

Endotoxin can specifically be estimated in small amounts by means of the Limulus test (LEVIN and BANG, 1964; LEVIN et al., 1970). It has not yet been recognized with certainty, however, whether coagulation derivatives that arise during an intravascular coagulation process might possibly have a nonspecific effect on the result of the limulus test. Other methods of estimation are based on the biological effect of the endotoxin concerned (for references see NOWOTNY, 1971; URBASCHEK et al., 1975).

b) Single Injection of Endotoxin

A single intravenous injection of endotoxin initiates the activation of intravascular coagulation (APITZ, 1934, 1935a; BRUNSON et al., 1955a; McKAY and SHAPIRO, 1958; KRECKE, 1964; LERNER et al., 1968a; PHILLIPS et al., 1968; THEISS and BELLER, 1973). Endotoxin preparations (lipopolysaccharides) from various strains of bacteria can be used, e.g. E. coli, Shigella flexneri, S. marcescens, and Salmonella abortus equi (THOMAS and GOOD, 1951; KRECKE, 1964). It has also become apparent that endotoxin isolated according to different methods does not vary in its effect on the activation of intravascular coagulation. Endotoxin can be obtained either by BOIVIN's trichloroacetic acid method (1933) or by the modification of PALMER and GERLOUGH's (1940) phenol water method used by WESTPHAL et al. (1952). As a rule, between 50 and 500 μg endotoxin/kg body weight is given by the intravenous route, depending on how active the endotoxin used is.

The dose of endotoxin actually used should be selected so as to allow the animal to survive the injection by 10 to 48 hrs and not die within a few hours after receiving it. The dose given must be potent enough to cause detectable microclots in the lungs, liver, and spleen of even nonpregnant animals.

c) Two Injections of Endotoxin

Two intravenous injections of bacterial endotoxin administered approximately 24 hrs apart produce the generalized Shwartzman reaction in 50 to 100% of the animals depending on the activity of the endotoxin. The interval between the two injections of endotoxin can vary from 6 to 72 hrs, but the optimum reaction is obtained with an interval of 16 to 28 hrs (for references see KRECKE, 1964; SELYE, 1966). The most usual procedure is to give two injections of the same dose of endotoxin (e.g. 2×50 μg endotoxin derived from E. coli) 24 hrs apart. It is also possible, however, to give a lower dose in the first injection, and a correspondingly higher one in the second (e.g. 0.5 μg/kg in the first and 500 μg/kg in the second injection) (KRECKE, 1964). In the model of the generalized Shwartzman reaction the first injection of endotoxin is generally referred to as the *preparatory* injection and the second as the *provoking* injection. After the first injection eosinophilic material is found, which can occlude some capillary lumina in lungs, liver and spleen. The renal capillaries generally remain unobtrusive. If no second injection of endotoxin is given the animals survive. If, however, a second intravenous injection is given about 24 hrs later, about 50 to 100% of the animals fall into a protracted state of shock, develop a hemorrhagic diathesis, and if they survive, die of the sequelae of complete anuria. Histologic examination again reveals eosinophilic material, but in much larger quantities, in lungs, liver and spleen of these animals. The occlusion of the renal glomerular capillaries by eosinophilic material is particularly striking, however. This occlusion results in necrosis of the renal tubules and, if the animals survive long enough, bilateral symmetrical renal cortical necrosis, which is easily visible even to the naked eye. Diagnosis of the generalized Shwartzman reaction is only justified if these renal changes appear (see Chapter C.).

d) Continuous Infusion of Endotoxin

A generalized Shwartzman reaction with fibrin-rich microclots in the renal glomerular capillaries and development of bilateral renal cortical necrosis can be produced by means of a continuous intravenous infusion of 10 to 50 μg endotoxin per kg of body weight per hour for 10 to 14 hrs (BELLER and GRAEFF, 1967; GRAEFF and BELLER, 1968; SCHOENDORF et al., 1971; GLASER, 1973; MÜLLER-BERGHAUS and LOHMANN, 1974). The results of pathoanatomical investigations (p. 452) as well as coagulation studies (p.443) are similar to those obtained after the second provoking injection of endotoxin (see c). The infusion of endotoxin only leads to the generalized Shwartzman reaction when the endotoxin is dissolved in isotonic saline solution, and not when it is dissolved in dextrose (THEISS and BELLER, 1973).

e) Single Injection of Endotoxin into the Pregnant Animal

Induction of the generalized Shwartzman reaction in the pregnant rabbit and the pregnant rat by means of a single injection of endotoxin has been described by APITZ (1935), TAKEDA and TSUCHIYA (1953), MCKAY et al. (1960), KALEY et al. (1962), WONG (1962) and RODRÍGUEZ-ERDMANN (1964b). The results of the coagulation analyses and the patho-anatomical findings appear to be similar to those seen in the case of the classical generalized Shwartzman reaction (RODRÍGUEZ-ERDMANN, 1964b; MÜLLER-BERGHAUS et al., 1967a; PHILLIPS et al., 1968; OBST et al., 1971), although MCKAY et al. (1960) have described a different pattern of distribution for the microclots.

f) Single Injection of Endotoxin into Animals with Reduced Phagocytic Function of the Reticulo-endothelial System

Phagocytosis of the reticulo-endothelial system (RES) is considerably reduced after an injection of Thorotrast (3 ml/kg) (BEESON, 1947a; CREMER and WATSON, 1957). If a single dose of endotoxin is given immediately after or 24 hrs after the injection of Thorotrast, changes such as are observed in the classical generalized Shwartzman reaction are found in the results both of coagulation analysis and of patho-anatomical examination (GOOD and THOMAS, 1952; LEE, 1962; LEVIN and CLUFF, 1965a; LEVIN and BECK, 1966; MÜLLER-BERGHAUS and SCHNEBERGER, 1971). There are other substances besides Thorotrast that have the necessary properties to prepare the organism for the generalized Shwartzman reaction by limiting phagocytosis of the RES, so that a single injection of endotoxin is sufficient to produce the reaction. These substances include trypan blue, colloidal iron, India ink (GOOD and THOMAS, 1952; THOMAS and SMITH, 1954) and denaturated albumin (LEE, 1962). LEE's findings (1962) also suggest that epsilon-aminocaproic acid (EACA) which is generally used as an antifibrinolytic agent, also limits the phagocytic function of the RES. According to this, it is possible to produce the generalized Shwartzman reaction by means of a single injection of endotoxin and epsilon-aminocaproic acid (LEE, 1962; PHILLIPS et al., 1968).

The hyperlipoproteinemia observed by MÜLLER-BERGHAUS et al. (1964) and HIRSCH et al. (1964) after the injection of endotoxin may contribute to the development of the generalized Shwartzman reaction by way of a reduction in the phagocytic function of the RES, as HUTH et al. (1967) were able to produce changes in the coagulation system such as are typically found in the generalized Shwartzman reaction by infusing an oil-in-water emulsion (2 g fat/kg body weight over 2 hrs) and giving a single injection of endotoxin.

g) Single Injection of Endotoxin in the Presence of Inhibited Fibrinolysis

LEE (1962) succeeded in producing the generalized Shwartzman reaction with a single injection of endotoxin if he administered epsilon-aminocaproic acid (EACA) with this injection (cf. Section I.f.). Fibrinolysis can be blocked in the rabbit if EACA is given in a dosageof 0.2 to 0.5 g/kg and hr. LEE (1962) interpreted the effect of EACA in the production of the generalized Shwartzman reaction as an influence on the phagocytic function of the RES. Investigations performed by MARGARETTEN et al. (1967) and GRAEFF et al. (1968) leave the significance of the inhibition of fibrinolysis in the formation of microclots in no doubt.

h) Single Injection of Endotoxin after Stimulation of the Alpha-Adrenergic Receptor Sites

If rabbits receive a single injection of endotoxin, followed by an infusion of norepinephrine over the next four hours (1.25 μg/kg and hr), microclots such as are typical of the generalized Shwartzman reaction are found in the glomerular capillaries of the kidney (McKAY and MÜLLER-BERGHAUS, 1968; McKAY et al., 1969). The effect of norepinephrine is attributed to localization or precipitation of soluble fibrin monomer complexes in the kidneys (MÜLLER-BERGHAUS and HOCKE, 1972, 1973; MÜLLER-BERGHAUS and MANN, 1973).

i) Single Injection of Endotoxin after Administration of Glucocorticoids

Another modification of the generalized Shwartzman reaction is seen in the experimental set-up described by THOMAS and GOOD (1951, 1952a). If rabbits are treated for four days with 25 mg cortisone per day, the generalized Shwartzman reaction is produced by a single injection of endotoxin given on the fourth day after the beginning of cortisone medication. This has been confirmed by various experimenters (McKAY and MERRIAM, 1960; LERNER et al., 1968b; LATOUR et al., 1971). Triamcinolone can be used instead of cortisone, but mineralocorticoids do not prepare the organism for the generalized Shwartzman reaction (LATOUR et al., 1971). The effect of glucocorticoids is attributed to a reduction in the phagocytic function of the RES (THOMAS and GOOD, 1951, 1952a) or to intensified sensitivity of the microcirculation to catecholamines (LATOUR et al., 1971).

2. Antigen-Antibody Reaction

Intravenous injection or infusion of an antigen to a rabbit that has been sensitized to it produces generalized intravascular coagulation; it is not known for certain whether the intravascular coagulation is initiated by the anaphylactic circulatory reaction of the circulation or by the generated immune complexes. According to studies by LAMBERT and SALMON (1966), SALMON et al. (1968, 1971), ovalbumin given by intravenous injection is sufficient to produce generalized intravascular coagulation and the generalized Shwartzman reaction in rabbits immunized against this antigen. The carefully documented studies of LEE (1963) show that rabbits immunized against bovine serum albumin do not develop the generalized Shwartzman reaction after an intravenous infusion of the same antigen (50 mg bovine serum albumin infused over 15 min). This observation of LEE's has been confirmed by various groups (MÜLLER-BERGHAUS and MUELLER-ECKHARDT, 1970; MUELLER-ECKHARDT and MÜLLER-BERGHAUS, 1971; EVENSEN et al., 1972). It can, however, safely be assumed that the induction of an immune reaction *in vivo* activates the intravascular coagulation process (LAMBERT and SALMON, 1966; BLOMBÄCK et al., 1967; MUELLER-ECKHARDT and MÜLLER-BERGHAUS, 1971; WARDLE, 1973). If the immunized rabbits receive Thorotrast before the provoking injection of antigen, however, bilateral renal cortical necrosis develops in addition (LEE, 1963).

In the immunized rabbit, the injection of antigen for the induction of intravascular coagulation can be replaced by the administration of a soluble antigen-antibody complex produced *in vitro*. The generalized Shwartzman reaction can also be produced by a single injection of a leukocyte antiserum followed after five minutes by a single injection of endotoxin (MARGARETTEN and MCKAY, 1969a). In the same way, an injection of bovine serum albumin to immunized animals combined with a single injection of endotoxin can also elicit the generalized Shwartzman reaction (MARGARETTEN and MCKAY, 1969a). Injection of an antiplatelet serum also causes activation of intravascular coagulation in the rabbit (LEVIN and CLUFF, 1965a; LEVIN and BECK, 1966; EVENSEN and FOLLING ELGJO, 1972). The generalized Shwartzman reaction only occurs, however, when Thorotrast (3 ml/kg) is administered to the animals by the intravenous route before administration of the antiplatelet serum (LEVIN and BECK, 1966). In rabbits immunized against bovine serum albumin the generalized Shwartzman reaction can also be produced if EACA and noradrenaline are given by continuous infusion in addition to the antigen given for the activation of intravascular coagulation (MÜLLER-BERGHAUS and MUELLER-ECKHARDT, 1970; MUELLER-ECKHARDT and MÜLLER-BERGHAUS, 1971). In Masugi nephritis, which is induced by a single injection of an antiserum to renal tissue, i.e. by heterologous nephrotropic antibodies (for references see ROTHER, 1965; ROTHER and TILL, 1974), activation of intravascular coagulation also occurs, with particularly pronouced fibrin-rich microclots in the renal glomerular capillaries (VASSALLI and MCCLUSKEY, 1964; ROTHER et al., 1967). In this case, however, it is probably a local clotting process within the vascular system of the kidney that is involved, rather than a generalized intravascular coagulation process. Thus it may be that the pathogenetic mechanism that leads to the generalized Shwartzman reaction has no part in Masugi nephritis.

3. Thromboplastin and Thrombin

Generalized intravascular coagulation can be induced in any mammal after the administration of thromboplastin or thrombin. It is important that homologous thromboplastin be used in each case, as there are species specificities for thromboplastin. Slow infusion of thromboplastin causes generalized intravascular coagulation to the point of complete incoagulability of the blood and afibrinogenemia (RATNOFF and CONLEY, 1951; SCHNEIDER, 1947, 1951, 1969; PENICK et al., 1958; VASSALLI et al., 1963; IZAK and GALEWSKY, 1966; RAPAPORT et al., 1966; NORDSTRØM and ZETTERQVIST, 1969; SLAASTAD et al., 1974; MORIAU et al., 1974). In such cases, thromboplastin activates the coagulation system by way of activation of Factor X in the presence of Factor VII as accelerator (NEMERSON and SPAET, 1964; for further references see NEMERSON and PITLICK, 1972). Thromboplastin for the induction of generalized intravascular coagulation can be obtained from brain, lung or placenta, all of which are rich in this procoagulant.

Intravascular coagulation can also be initiated by the infusion of thrombin instead of thromboplastin, and thrombin by infusion allows more accurate regulation of the speed at which the generalized intravascular coagulation process takes place. The model for induction of generalized intravascular coagulation and the generalized Shwartzman reaction by means of slow intravenous infusion of thrombin goes back to JÜRGENS and STUDER (1948). Their experiments have been repeated with different species with identical results (QUICK et al., 1959; HARDAWAY, 1961; LEE, 1962; VASSALLI et al., 1963; KOWALSKI et al., 1965; GIROLAMI et al., 1966a; COLLINS et al., 1968; WHITAKER and MCKAY, 1969; BUSCH and SALDEEN, 1973; MÜLLER-BERGHAUS et al., 1974).

4. Snake Venoms

Generalized intravascular coagulation can be produced by the administration of snake venoms or purified fractions of snake venoms. Varying types of reaction within the coagulation system are observed, depending on the mechanism of action of the snake venom concerned. Thus the injection of ancrod, the procoagulant fraction of the venom of Agkistrodon rhodostoma, of reptilase, the procoagulant fraction taken from Bothrops atrox, or of the procoagulant fraction of the venom of Crotalus adamanteus (WEISS et al., 1969) produces defibrination, which comes about because of a direct effect of the snake venom on the fibrinogen molecule. Coagulation factors other than fibrinogen are not affected by ancrod or reptilase (REGOECZI et al., 1966; MARSTEN et al., 1966; KWAAN and BARLOW, 1971; EGBERG et al., 1971; MÜLLER-BERGHAUS and HOCKE, 1973). After injection of the venom of the sand rattle snake (Echis carinata), the activation of intravascular coagulation observed is due to a primary effect of the snake venom on the factors of the prothrombin complex (ZIMMERMANN et al., 1971).

Russel's viper venom activates coagulation Factor X. Activation of intravascular coagulation has been described after intravenous injection of this snake venom (LEANDOER and NILÉHN, 1969). A similar effect of the venom of Echis colorata on factor X is known. Afibrinogenemia occurs if the venom is administered to an animal (DE VRIES et al., 1965).

Other snake venoms with specific mechanisms of action on the coagulation system are known, but ancrod and reptilase are used for preference in experimental and clinical research.

5. Viruses

In animal experiments various viruses can be used to activate intravascular coagulation. Thus, generalized intravascular coagulation occurs in the experimental Aleutian mink disease, in acute hog cholera and in fowl plague of chickens (MCKAY et al., 1967b; GAGEL et al., 1970; HEENE et al., 1971). It is not known how viruses trigger an intravascular coagulation process

6. Nonbiological Substances

a) Liquoid

Liquoid is a synthetic acid polymer (sodium polyanethol sulfonate) that is generally used *in vitro* as an anticomplementary agent in blood cultures. HAUSMAN and DREYFUS (1953) observed the formation of hyaline microclots in the renal glomerular capillaries and the development of multiple hemorrhages in various organs after intravenous injection of Liquoid into rabbits. Generalized intravascular coagulation and the generalized Shwartzman reaction can regularly be induced with a single intravenous injection of 5 to 15 mg Liquoid/kg body weight (BOHLE et al., 1959; RODRÍGUEZ-ERDMANN et al., 1960; EVENSEN et al., 1967; MÜLLER-BERGHAUS and LASCH, 1970, 1971).

b) Carrageenin

Carrageenin is a vegetable extract prepared from red algae and used in industry. In rats and in rabbits the injection or infusion of carrageenin causes generalized intravascular coagulation (SELYE, 1965, 1966; HUTH et al., 1966; SCHIMPF et al., 1969).

c) Ellagic Acid

Substances which act on contact factors of blood coagulation, such as ellagic acid, are particularly interesting in the study of a controlled activation of coagulation. Infusion of ellagic acid alone activates the Hageman factor (clotting factor XII) but does not cause any generalized intravascular coagulation (BOTTI and RATNOFF, 1964; GIROLAMI et al., 1966b). The activation of intravascular coagulation as well as the generalized Shwartzman reaction can be induced if in addition to ellagic acid EACA and norepinephrine are infused into animals (MCKAY and MÜLLER-BERGHAUS, 1968; MCKAY et al., 1969).

d) Colchicine

Intravenous injection of colchicine into the pregnant golden hamster or the pregnant rat elicits the generalized Shwartzman reaction (GALTON, 1963, 1966; MÜLLER-BERGHAUS and OBST, 1972). Intravascular coagulation can also be activated by colchicine in the nonpregnant rat (MÜLLER-BERGHAUS and OBST, 1972). The mechanism of the activation of intravascular coagulation following the administration of colchicine is not known.

e) Galactosamine

D-galactosamine induces experimental hepatitis in various species (KEPPLER et al., 1968; REUTTER et al., 1968). When galactosamine and EACA are administered to rabbits,, generalized intravascular coagulation and the generalized Shwartzman reaction develop (MÜLLER-BERGHAUS and REUTER, 1972; MAHN et al., 1974).

7. Impaired Perfusion of the Circulatory Periphery—Shock

Paragraphs 1–6 deal with substances by means of which activation of intravascular coagulation can be obtained. In view of the delicate connections linking vessel content, vessel wall, and circulation of the blood in the periphery of the circulation, it is understandable that a primary influence on the circulation will also affect the homeostasis of blood coagulation. All forms of circulatory shock resulting from a slowing-down of the bloodstream will lead to activation of the coagulation process if the circulatory shock is sufficiently intense and lasts long enough. The best model for induction of generalized intravascular coagulation by way of inadequate capillary perfusion is hemorrhagic shock (CROWELL and READ, 1955; LASCH et al., 1957, 1961 b; HARDAWAY et al., 1962; ENCKE et al., 1969; NEUHOF et al., 1973; for further references see HARDAWAY, 1966). In other forms of shock, intravascular coagulation is activated by pathogenetically important factors in addition to alterations caused by circulatory changes. In septic shock, endotoxin is an additional activator involved in the initiation of the intravascular coagulation process, in traumatic shock thromboplastin, and in anaphylactic shock the antigen-antibody reaction. It is possible that in every form of circulatory shock endotoxin enters the circulation in fairly large quantities and persists for some time, and provokes the changes described under the heading of endotoxin-induced shock (FINE et al., 1959a; RAVIN et al., 1960; GANS and MATSUMOTO, 1974).

8. Production of the Generalized Shwartzman Reaction by Means of Substances with Defined Mechanisms of Action

The generalized Shwartzman reaction can be produced with great regularity with endotoxin, but the polyvalence of endotoxin makes it extraordinarily difficult to explain the pathogenesis of the generalized Shwartzman reaction. For this reason there have been attempts to simulate individual mechanisms that are triggered by endotoxin and appear to be significant in the pathogenesis.

a) Activation of Intravascular Coagulation

One of the main effects of endotoxin in the generalized Shwartzman reaction is the activation of intravascular coagulation. The appropriate model is the infusion of small amounts of thrombin or thromboplastin. When thromboplastin or thrombin are given by continuous infusion over several hours no microclots are generally observed to persist for any significant length of time in either rabbit or rat. It is important in this situation that the speed of the infusion of thrombin or thromboplastin be slow, to avoid acute obstruction of the pulmonary circulation with substantial fibrin clots and death of the animal. The fibrinogen level should fall by 50–70% of the initial value in a period of approximately 2 hrs. When these conditions are observed and the animals sacrificed immediately after discontinuation of the thrombin infusion, i.e. 2 to 4 hrs after it is begun, microclots are found in lungs, liver, spleen, and kidneys. If the animals are allowed to survive for a longer period of time, however, microclots are no longer demonstrable in the kidneys 24 hrs later, which indicates pronounced local fibrinolysis in the kidneys (MARGARETTEN et al., 1964; BELLER et al., 1967; GRAEFF et al., 1968; LIPINSKI et al., 1968; BERGSTEIN and MICHAEL, 1973a).

Tissue thromboplastin can be used instead of thrombin in all models for the production of a synthetic generalized Shwartzman reaction. Apart from the varying activity of the thromboplastins used and the difficulty of inferring the *in vivo* effect of any thromboplastin from its activity *in vitro*, species specificity must also be mentioned. It is best to infuse rabbit thromboplastin when rabbits are used, and thromboplastin obtained from rat organs when the experimental animals are rats. The thromboplastin should be given over 1 to 4 hrs, and it is best to dose the amount of thromboplastin so that the fibrinogen level falls to 50–30% of the initial value.

b) Inhibition of Fibrinolysis

The administration of an inhibitor of the fibrinolytic system in addition to the infusion of thrombin or thromboplastin makes it possible to protect the microclots formed from fibrinolysis, so that they can still be found by histological examination 24 hrs after the infusion of thrombin or thromboplastin is begun.

c) Pregnancy

If thrombin is infused into pregnant rats, microclots generate in the renal glomerular capillaries and are not lysed over the next 24 hrs, so that they cause renal cortical necrosis .When the same amount of thrombin is infused into non-pregnant rats microclots are also found, but they will be lysed within a short time following spontaneous activation of the fibrinolytic system (MARGARETTEN et al., 1964).

d) Thorotrast

Thorotrast can be used instead of substances that inhibit activation of the fibrinolytic system to prepare the organism for the generalized Shwartzman reaction. The mechanism of action of this substance is attributed to its influence on the phagocytic function of the RES, to the inhibition of fibrinolysis, and to its protein-precipitating properties (see Chapter F. III. 2. and F. V.). If 3 ml Thorotrast/kg body weight are injected into a rabbit, a subsequent infusion of thrombin elicits the generalized Shwartzman reaction (LEE, 1962).

e) Synthetic Generalized Shwartzman Reaction

On the basis of the idea that intravascular coagulation might be initiated in some pathologic states by activation of contact factors of blood coagulation, ellagic acid was infused into rabbits in order to activate Factor XII. In comparison to thrombin or thromboplastin, ellagic acid produces only a weak activation of intravascular coagulation, so that neither BOTTI and RATNOFF (1964) nor GIROLAMI et al. (1966b) observed any microclots after infusions of ellagic acid, even if injections of Thorotrast were given in addition. When, however, continuous intravenous infusions of norepinephrine to stimulate the alpha-receptor sites in the kidney (see Section D.I.1.h) and EACA to inhibit fibrinolysis (see Sections D.I.1.g and D.I.8.b) were given in addition to ellagic acid, occlusion of the peripheral blood vessels with microclots was observed in both rabbit and monkey (MCKAY and MÜLLER-BERGHAUS, 1968; MCKAY et al., 1969). In this experimental set-up ellagic acid can be replaced by sodium stearate in order to activate contact factors of blood coagulation (MÜLLER-BERGHAUS, 1969). With these experimental models it is possible to elicit the generalized Shwartzman reaction by means of substances with defined mechanisms of action. Only the combination of activation of the contact phase of blood coagulation and infusion of EACA and norepinephrine led to the synthetic generalized Shwartzman reaction.

II. Results

1. Hematologic Investigations

a) Endotoxin

A pronounced fall in leukocyte and platelet counts is observed both after the first injection of endotoxin and after the second (SANARELLI, 1924; STETSON, 1951; McKAY and SHAPIRO, 1958; SHIMAMOTO et al., 1958a; KLEINMAIER et al., 1959; DAVIS, 1960; LASCH et al., 1960). It is obvious that endotoxin has a direct action on these blood cells, for lowering of platelet and leukocyte counts is observed even one minute after endotoxin injection (DAVIS et al., 1960, 1961). By 24 hrs after the first injection the leukocyte count has risen again to the initial value, and generally reached about twice the initial figure (Fig. 2). In contrast to leukocyte counts, platelet counts do not rise before the second injection of endotoxin. Leukocyte and platelet counts fall immediately after the second injection as they do after the first (Fig. 2).

Not only a fall in platelet counts, but also qualitative changes are observed in these cells after injections of endotoxin. LASCH et al. (1960) described a lowering of the activity of platelet factor 3 in the platelets of rabbits that had been injected with endotoxin, while HOROWITZ et al. (1962) noted a transitory rise in the activity of platelet factor 3 in the platelet-poor plasma after endotoxin injection. Investigations by WEBER et al. (1963) showed that the platelet-dependent retraction is impaired after the injection of endotoxin, and in addition the platelets have lost ATP and ADP and other nucleotides.

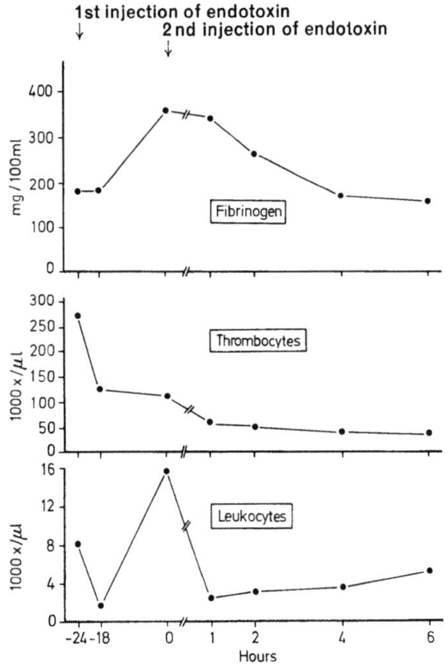

Fig. 2. Changes in mean fibrinogen levels and leukocyte as well as platelet counts after two i.v. injections of endotoxin into rabbits 24 hrs apart. Each curve represents 10 animal experiments

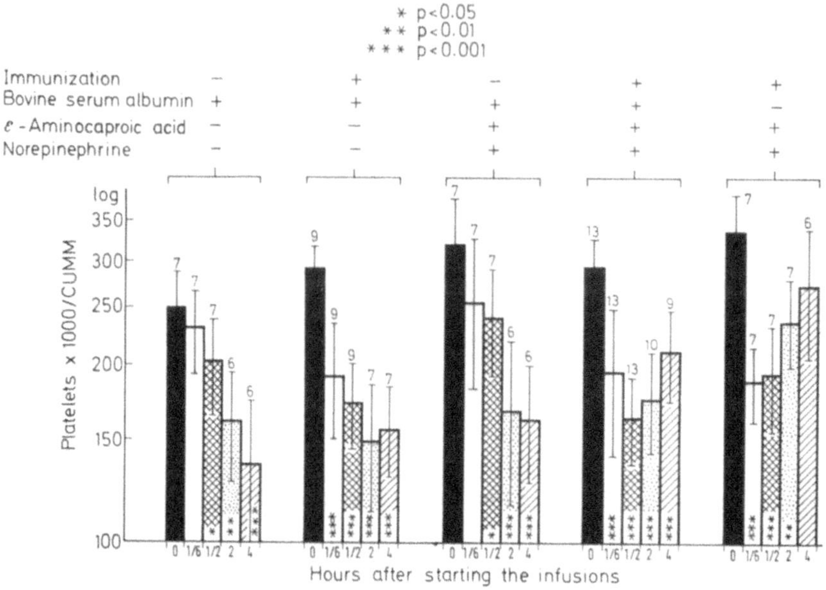

Fig. 3. Decrease in mean platelet counts after administration of bovine serum albumin, EACA and/or norepinephrine to immunized and nonimmunized rabbits. Standard deviation, number of animals, and the levels of significance are given. (From Mueller-Eckhardt, C. and Müller-Berghaus, G., 1971)

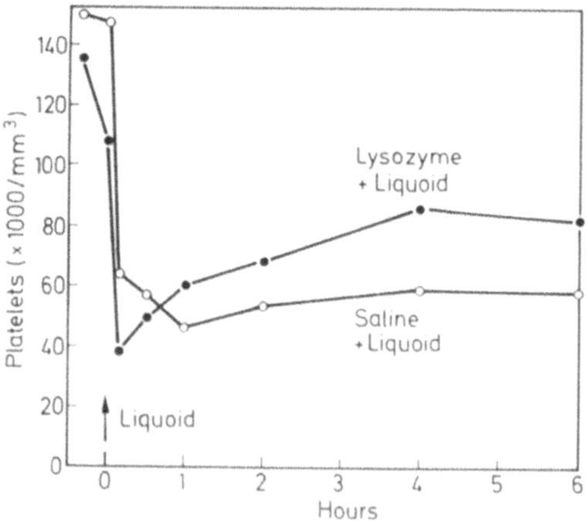

Fig. 4. Changes in platelet counts after injection of Liquoid into rabbits treated with lysozyme or saline (control). Lysozyme treatment does not prevent decrease in platelet counts, although it prevented the occurrence of the generalized Shwartzman reaction. (From Müller-Berghaus, G. and Lasch, H. G., 1970)

Apart from a lowering of the hematocrit value due to frequent blood sampling, erythrocyte counts do not seem to undergo any decisive change during the experiment. There is, however, a rise in the free plasma hemoglobin level after the second injection of endotoxin, a finding that correlates with the formation of fibrin-rich microlots. BELLER and THEISS (1973) interpret the presence of free plasma hemoglobin as a sign of the formation of microclots.

b) Procoagulant Substances Other than Endotoxin

A fall in platelet counts is also observed in models for the induction of intravascular coagulation in which endotoxin is not involved, e.g. in the case of an antigen-antibody reaction (Fig. 3), after infusion of thromboplastin or thrombin, after the administration of snake venoms, in experimental viral infections, after administration of Liquoid (Fig. 4), carrageenin, ellagic acid, colchicine or galactosamine, and in shock (for references see the section on methods of induction).

2. Coagulation Studies

a) Endotoxin

Changes in the plasmatic coagulation system are observed both after the first injection of endotoxin and after the second; these changes are of the same type in both cases but vary substantially in intensity (Fig. 5). In the rabbit, the first injection of endotoxin is followed by a minimal fall in the fibrinogen level, which then rises over the next 24 hrs by an average of 50% varying from animal to animal (Fig. 2) (MCKAY and SHAPIRO, 1958; LERNER et al., 1968a). After the second provoking injection there is a definite fall in the plasma concentration of fibrinogen, which reaches its minimum value 6 hrs after the injection and then gradually rises. Investigations with ^{131}I-labelled fibrinogen have shown that the synthis is countered by increased catabolism after the second than after the first thesis of fibrinogen is intensified after both injections of endotoxin, but that injection (LERNER et al., 1968a). The fall in the fibrinogen level is much more marked in the rat than in the rabbit (PHILLIPS et al., 1968; THEISS and BELLER, 1973). However, a single injection of endotoxin does not induce the generalized Shwartzman reaction in the rat unless additional mechanisms such as inhibition of fibrinolysis and/or localization mechanisms are triggered.

As the fibrinogen concentration falls, soluble fibrinogen derivatives occur in the blood (THOMAS et al., 1955b; SHAINOFF and PAGE, 1960, 1962; LIPINSKI

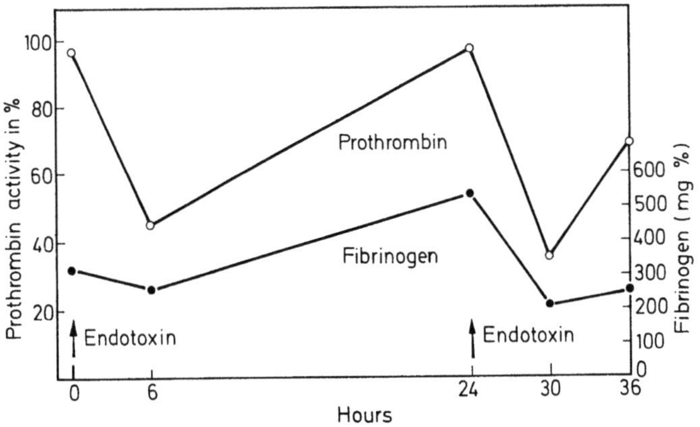

Fig. 5. Changes in prothrombin activities and fibrinogen levels after each of 2 i.v. injections of endotoxin into rabbits. The response to the second injection of endotoxin is much more pronounced than to the first injection. (From MÜLLER-BERGHAUS, G., 1969)

Table 1. Incidence of positive ethanol gelation tests (expressed as number of positive results over total number of rabbits studied) after single i.v. injection of endotoxin into rabbits (From MÜLLER-BERGHAUS, G. and HOCKE, M., 1973)

Treatment	Before endotoxin	After endotoxin injection			
		1 hr	2 hr	4 hr	6 hr
Endotoxin	0/9	4/9	9/9	9/9	8/9

et al., 1968; MÜLLER-BERGHAUS and HOCKE, 1973; VON HUGO et al., 1975). One feature of this stage is that the ethanol gelation test (Table 1) (MÜLLER-BERGHAUS and HOCKE, 1973) and the protamine sulfate test (LIPINSKI et al., 1968) are positive, a sign that circulating soluble fibrin monomer complexes are present. Another feature is that there is an increased amount of fibrinolytic split products (FDP) in the serum after the injection of endotoxin (FONG and GOOD, 1971). The fibrinolytic split products can be estimated either with the staphylococcal clumping test (HAWIGER et al., 1970) or with the tanned red cell hemagglutination inhibition immunoassay (MERSKEY et al., 1969). Soluble fibrin monomer complexes are estimated with the ethanol gelation test (GODAL and ABILDGAARD, 1966), the protamine sulfate test (NIEWIAROWSKI and GUREWICH, 1971), or gel chromatography to separate the high-molecular-weight fibrinogen derivatives from the fibrinogen molecule (GRAEFF and VON HUGO, 1972).

After the first injection of endotoxin and after the second there is a fall in prothrombin activity and also in the activities of Factors V, VII, IX, X, XII, and XIII (Fig. 6) (McKAY and SHAPIRO, 1958; KLEINMAIER et al., 1959; ALEXANDER et al., 1962; MÜLLER-BERGHAUS and LASCH, 1963; LERNER et al., 1968b; HEENE, 1969; MÜLLER-BERGHAUS and SCHNEBERGER, 1971). The changes observed in screening tests are in keeping with the findings obtained in specific tests for individual factor activities. Thus the thromboplastin time according to Quick, the partial thromboplastin time, the whole blood coagulation time ac-

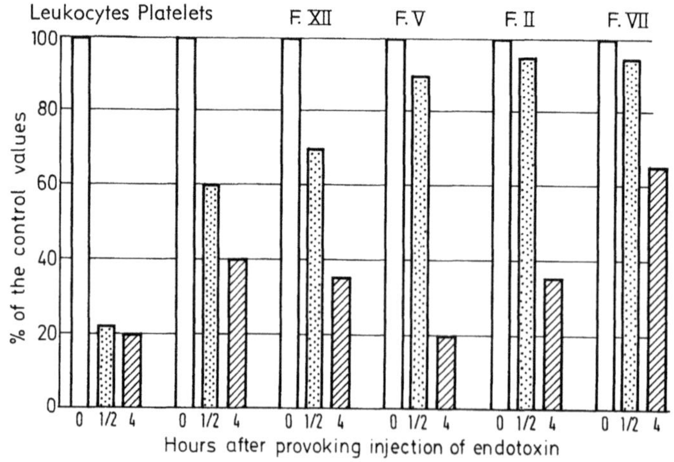

Fig. 6. Changes in leukocyte as well as in platelet counts, Hageman factor (Factor XII), Factor V, prothrombin (Factor II), and Factor VII activities $^1/_2$ and 4 hrs after second provoking injection of endotoxin into rabbits. (From MÜLLER-BERGHAUS, G., 1969)

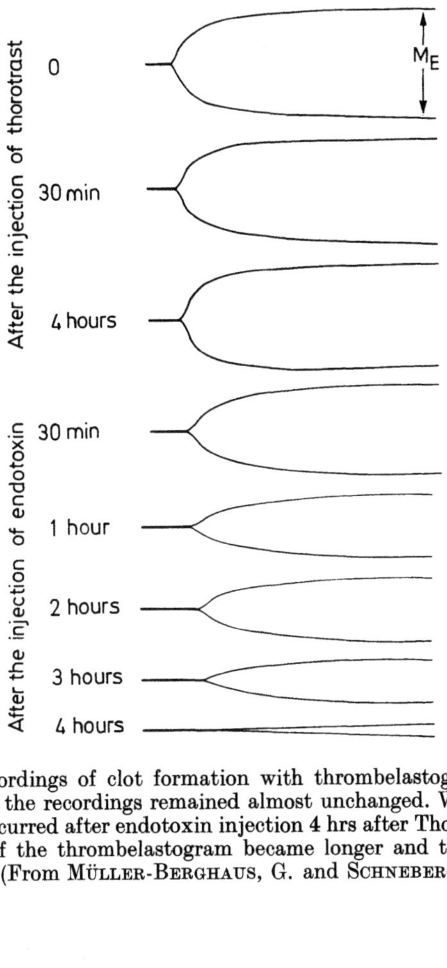

Fig. 7. Continuous recordings of clot formation with thrombelastogram. After Thorotrast injection into a rabbit, the recordings remained almost unchanged. When generalized intravascular coagulation occurred after endotoxin injection 4 hrs after Thorotrast administration, the coagulation time of the thrombelastogram became longer and the maximal amplitude M_E narrower. (From MÜLLER-BERGHAUS, G. and SCHNEBERGER, R., 1971)

cording to Lee and White, the r-time of the thrombelastogram (Fig. 7), and the thrombin time are lengthened. The maximal amplitude of the thrombelastogram is reduced after the injection of endotoxin (Fig. 8). As the activities of individual coagulation factors fall there is also a reduction in the inhibitors of the coagulation system, such as antithrombin III and antithrombokinase (LASCH etal., 1961c; SCHIMPF and CIBELIUS, 1964). Similar changes to those observed in the coagulation system after the injection of endotoxin have also been noted after endotoxin by infusion (Fig. 9–14) (BELLER and GRAEFF, 1967; GRAEFF and BELLER, 1968; GRAEFF et al., 1968; BELLER et al., 1969; SCHOENDORF et al., 1971; GLASER, 1973; MÜLLER-BERGHAUS and LOHMANN, 1974).

Changes in the fibrinolytic system are observed at the same time as those in the coagulation system. After the injection of endotoxin there is a fall in the plasminogen level (PHILLIPS et al., 1968) and a rise in fibrinolytic activity in the plasma (LIPINSKI et al., 1968). Changes in the fibrinolytic system are also recorded after infusion of endotoxin, and are interpreted as activation of this enzymatic system with subsequent consumption of the plasma proteins concerned (GRAEFF et al., 1968).

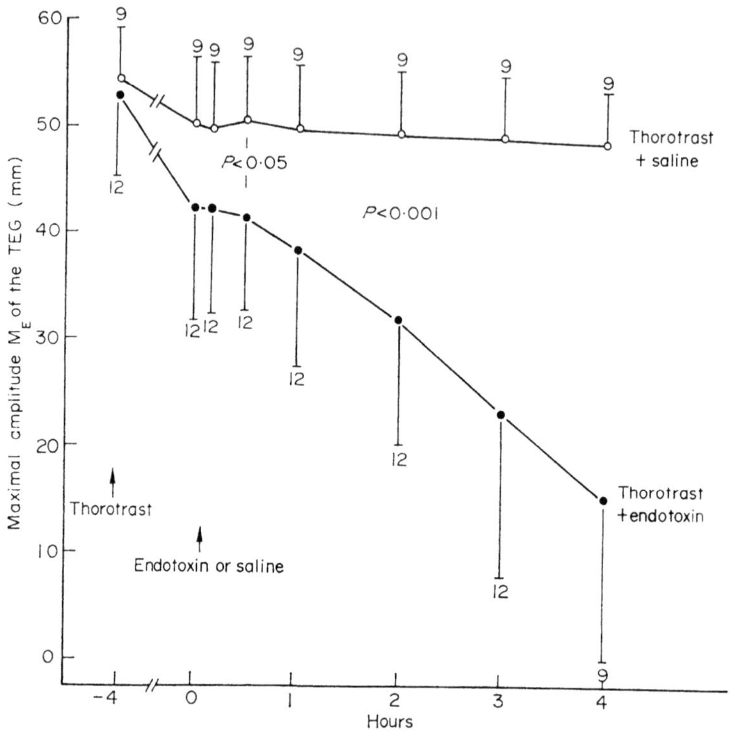

Fig. 8. The maximal amplitude M_E of the thrombelastogram after injections of Thorotrast and saline (control) or Thorotrast and endotoxin for induction of generalized intravascular coagulation. Mean values, standard deviations (drawn only from one side of the plotted points), and number of animals are indicated. Rabbits injected with Thorotrast (3 ml/kg) and endotoxin (20 μg) developed fibrin-rich microclots in glomerular capillaries. (From Müller-Berghaus, G. and Schneberger, R., 1971)

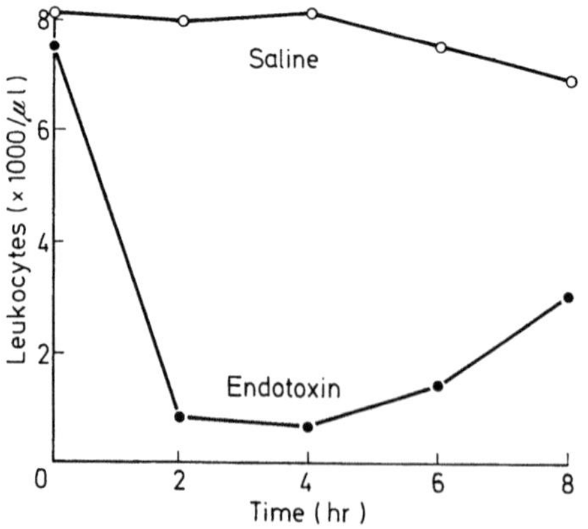

Fig. 9. Changes in mean leukocyte counts during continuous 8-hr infusion of endotoxin or saline into rabbits. Curves represent 10 animal experiments each. (Data from Müller-Berghaus, G. and Lohmann, E., 1974)

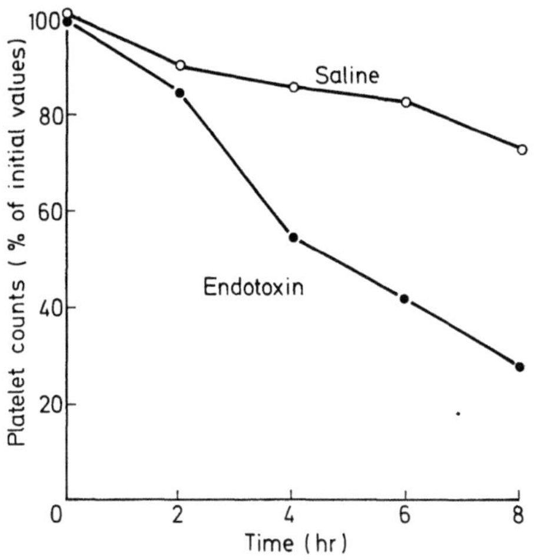

Fig. 10. Changes in mean platelet counts during continuous 8-hr infusion of endotoxin or saline into rabbits. The curves represent 10 animal experiments each. (Data from MÜLLER-BERGHAUS, G. and LOHMANN, E., 1974)

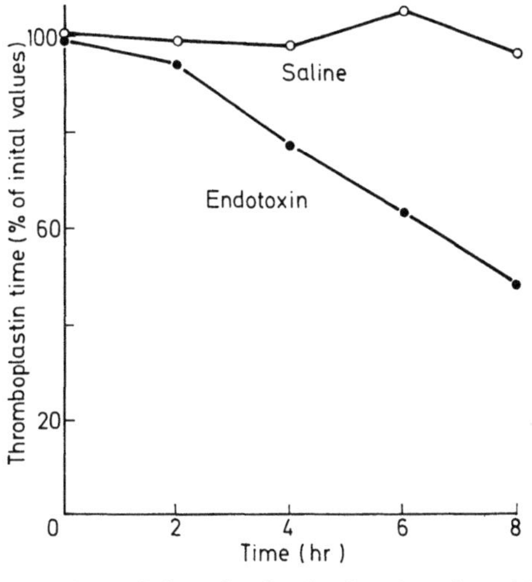

Fig. 11. Changes in mean values of thromboplastin time (prothrombin time activity) during continuous 8-hr infusion of endotoxin or saline into rabbits. The curve "endotoxin" represents 9 animal experiments, the curve "saline" 10 animal experiments. (Data from MÜLLER-BERGHAUS, G. and LOHMANN, E., 1974)

b) Procoagulant Substances Other than Endotoxin

A fall in plasma factors I, II, V, VII, VIII, IX, X, XI, and XII is also seen in models for the induction of generalized intravascular coagulation in which endotoxin is not involved for example in the case of the antigen-antibody reaction, after infusion of thromboplastin or thrombin, after the administration of snake venoms, in experimental viral infections, after the administration of

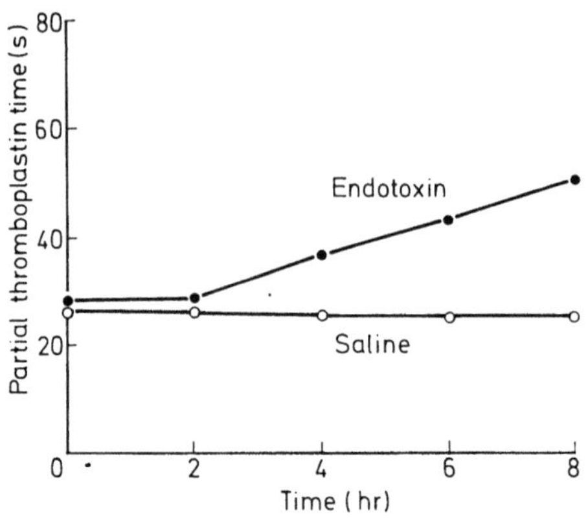

Fig. 12. Changes in mean values of partial thromboplastin time during continuous 8-hr infusion of endotoxin or saline into rabbits. Curves represent 10 animal experiments each. (Data from MÜLLER-BERGHAUS, G. and LOHMANN, E., 1974)

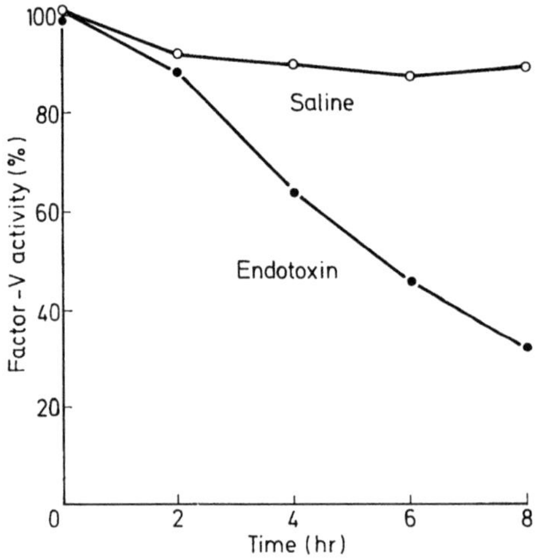

Fig. 13. Changes in mean Factor V activities during continuous 8-hr infusion of endotoxin or saline into rabbits. The curves represent 10 animal experiments each. (Data from MÜLLER-BERGHAUS, G. and LOHMANN, E., 1974)

Liquoid (Fig. 15), carrageenin, ellagic acid, colchicine, and galactosamine (Fig. 16), and in shock (for references see section on methods of induction).

3. Measurements of Circulatory Parameters

Continuous measurement of various circulatory parameters, including oxygen consumption, in the generalized Shwartzman reaction has been described by NEUHOF et al. (1970, 1973), who themselves devised a new method for studying these parameters (Fig. 17). This test procedure of continuous recording of oxygen consumption in relation to other circulatory parameters revealed a rise in the pressure in the right ventricle and in the pulmonary artery 15 to 20 min after

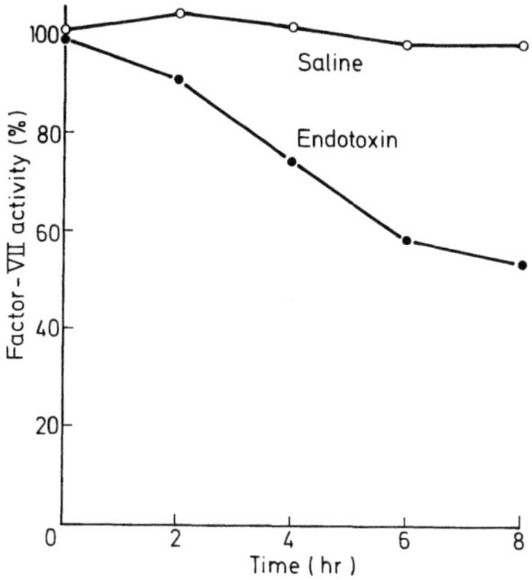

Fig. 14. Changes in mean Factor VII activities during continuous 8-hr infusion of endotoxin or saline into rabbits. The curves represent 10 animal experiments each. (Data from MÜLLER-BERGHAUS, G. and LOHMANN, E., 1974)

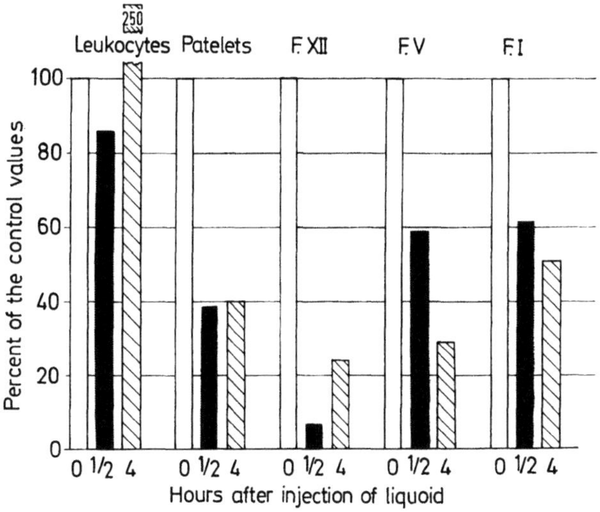

Fig. 15. Changes in mean leukocyte as well as platelet counts, Hageman factor (Factor XII), Factor V, and fibrinogen (Factor I) activities $^1/_2$ and 4 hrs after a single i.v. injection of Liquoid (10 mg/kg) into rabbits. (From MÜLLER-BERGHAUS, G., 1969)

the first injection of endotoxin (100 µg/kg body weight), due to an acute increase in the resistance in the pulmonary circulation (NEUHOF et al., 1970). There is no primary connection between this acute increase in resistance and the occlusion of the pulmonary peripheral blood vessels with platelets which aggregate after the injection of endotoxin. A similar rise in resistance is observed after an injection of endotoxin even in animals with low platelets counts (NEUHOF and KAUFMANN, 1968).

After the administration of endotoxin a marked reduction in the oxygen consumption of the total organism is recorded in the first phase (NEUHOF, 1975)

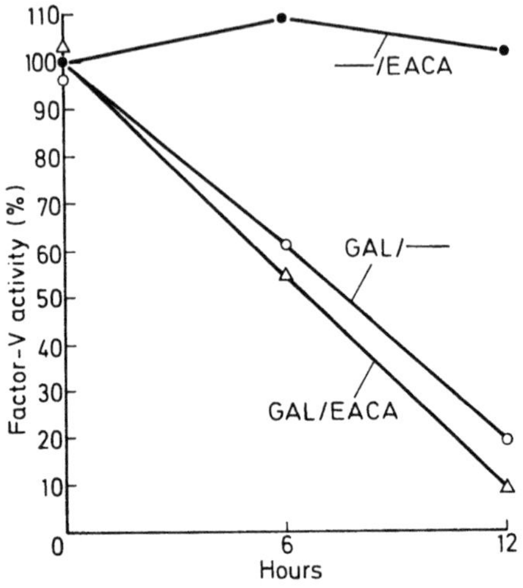

Fig. 16. Experimental hepatitis induced by galactosamine (GAL). Decrease in mean Factor V activities after infusion of galactosamine and saline, galactosamine and EACA, or saline and EACA into rabbits. Values are means of 10 rabbit experiments each. Rabbits infused with galactosamine developed generalized intravascular coagulation and in part the generalized Shwartzman reaction. (From Müller-Berghaus, G., and Reuter, C., 1972)

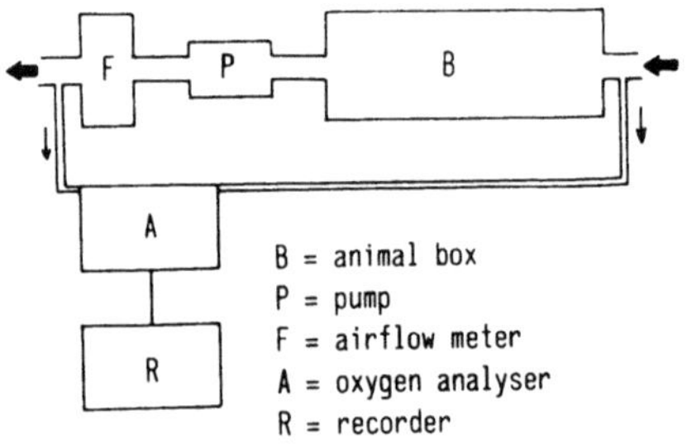

Fig. 17. Block diagram showing the various subunits for continuous registration of the body's total oxygen uptake. (From Neuhof, H. et al., 1970)

(Fig. 18). The main reason for the reduced oxygen consumption is the reduction in cardiac output. Later in the experiment the reduced oxygen supply to the tissues is followed by metabolic acidosis. Very soon (2 to 4 min) after the injection of endotoxin, a transient circulatory reaction is recorded in the form of reduced arterial pressure and raised systolic pressure in the right ventricle (Neuhof et al., 1970; Neuhof, 1975); this finding is attributable to the release of vasoactive substances (for references see Urbaschek, 1971). These circulatory changes are paralleled by the fall in the platelet count immediately after the injection of endotoxin. The changes in the circulatory parameters in the early phase of the reaction (15 to 30 min after an intravenous injection of endotoxin) arise independently of the coagulation system, as is seen from the fact that they cannot be affected by heparin treatment of the animals (Neuhof, 1975). The extent of the circulatory changes can certainly be substantially influenced in the late phase (2 to 4 hrs after administration of endotoxin), however (Neuhof, 1975). This

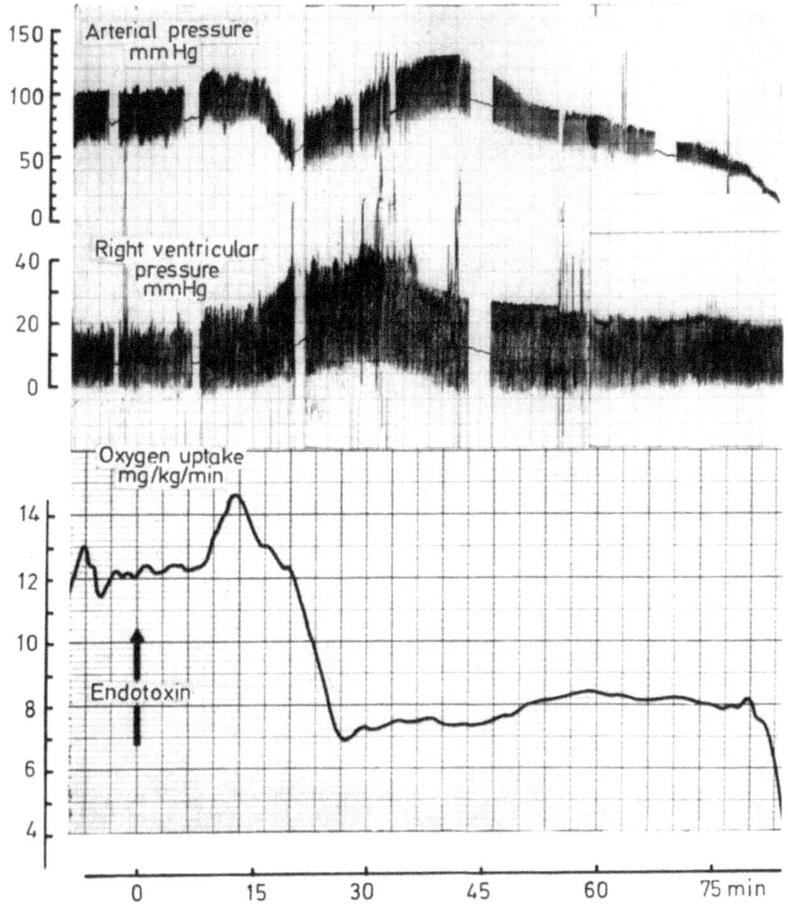

Fig. 18. Changes in arterial blood pressure, right ventricular pressure, and oxygen uptake in an unanesthetized rabbit after a single i.v. injection of endotoxin (*E. coli*, 100 μg/kg). (From NEUHOF, H., 1975)

is borne out by the findings of MARGARETTEN et al. (1967), which indicate that heparin medication prevents death in rats following the injection of a dose of endotoxin that would otherwise be lethal.

Figure 19 shows the temporal course of the hemodynamic changes correlated with the effect of fibrinolytic therapy. The circulatory changes are less pronounced after a second intravenous injection of endotoxin than after the first. If the animals die within the first 24 hrs after the second injection of endotoxin, circulatory changes such as are normally seen in animals in endotoxin-induced shock or hemorrhagic shock are observed (NEUHOF et al., 1973). The worsening of the circulatory situation after the second injection of endotoxin is conditioned partly by the intravascular coagulation process, as is borne out by the rise in arterial blood pressure and in the oxygen consumption of the total organism after treatment of the animals with streptokinase (NEUHOF et al., 1970). HARDAWAY (1966) has collected further literature on the connections between circulatory changes and coagulation of the blood.

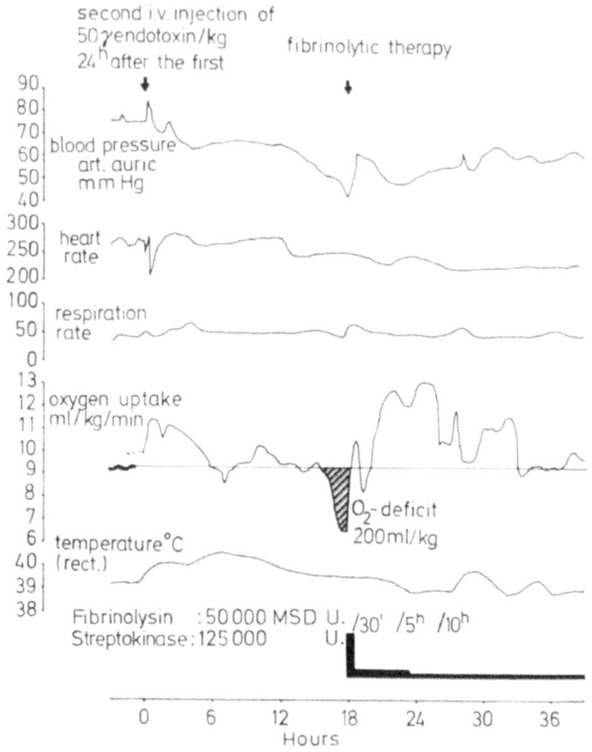

Fig. 19. Changes in blood pressure, heart rate, respiration rate, oxygen uptake, and rectal temperature after the second injection of endotoxin into an unanesthetized rabbit. Increasing oxygen debt becomes reversible and circulatory conditions normalize after starting fibrinolytic therapy. (From NEUHOF, H. et al., 1970)

4. Patho-anatomical Findings

Twenty four hrs after a single sublethal dose of endotoxin it is usual to find enlargement of the spleen,and multiple petechial hemorrhages in the liver. Fibrin-rich deposits on the surface of the liver are also occasionally found at this point. Histologic examination of the organs 24 hrs after a single injection of endotoxin reveals fibrin-rich microclots, varying in extent, in lungs, liver, and spleen (BRUNSON et al., 1955a; for references see McKAY, 1964; KRECKE, 1964). The intensity of the changes detectable by patho-anatomical examination depends on the amount of endotoxin administered. It is exceptional for microclots to be demonstrable in the kidneys after a single injection of endotoxin. If a sublethal dose of endotoxin is given and the animals are sacrificed 24 hrs later, microclots are never found in the kidneys. On this point there is a fundamental difference between the changes after the first injection of endotoxin and those after the second.

If the animals are sacrificed one hour after a single injection of endotoxin, platelet and leukocyte aggregates are found in the small vessels of the lungs and sometimes also of the liver. Fibrin-rich microclots have been reported to occur in lungs, liver, and particularly spleen 3 to 4 hrs after a single injection of endotoxin (McKAY, 1964).

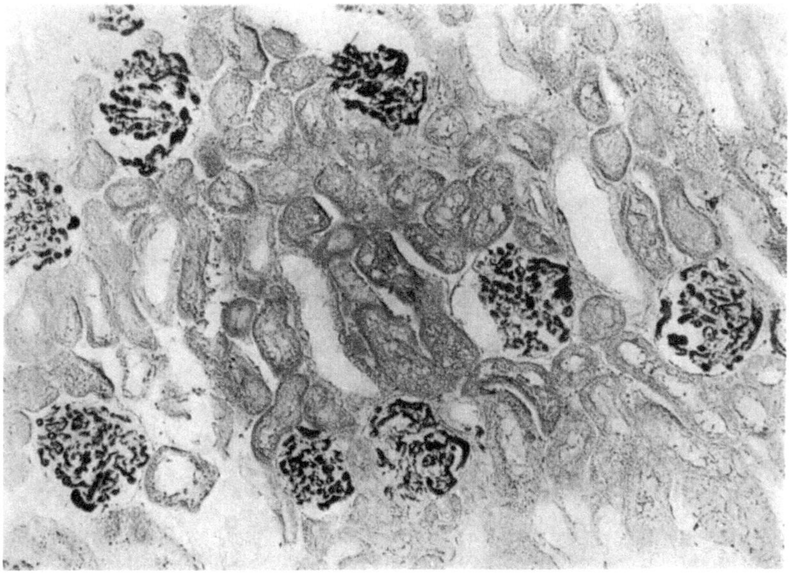

Fig. 20. Kidney section of a rabbit injected with 2 i.v. doses of endotoxin (*S. enteritidis*, 2 × 100 μg) 24 hrs apart and sacrificed 6 hrs after second injection of endotoxin. All renal glomerular capillaries are occluded by fibrin-rich microclots. Histochemistry, ×100

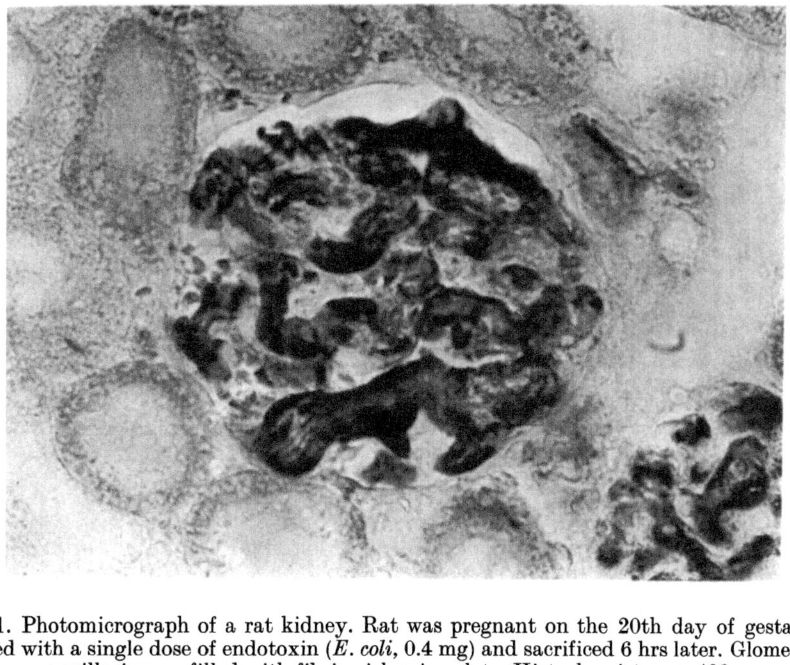

Fig. 21. Photomicrograph of a rat kidney. Rat was pregnant on the 20th day of gestation, injected with a single dose of endotoxin (*E. coli*, 0.4 mg) and sacrificed 6 hrs later. Glomerular capillaries are filled with fibrin-rich microclots. Histochemistry, ×400

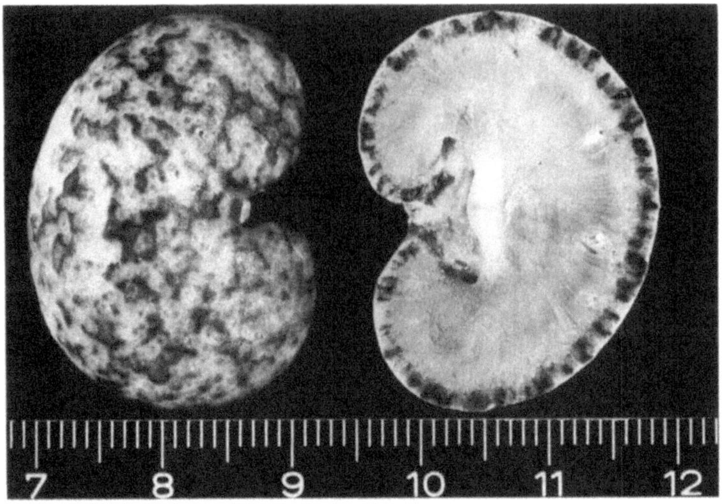

Fig. 22. Bilateral renal cortical necroses of a rabbit kidney typical of the generalized Shwartzman reaction. Rabbit was injected with 2 doses of endotoxin (*E. coli*, 2×100 µg) and sacrificed 24 hrs after second dose

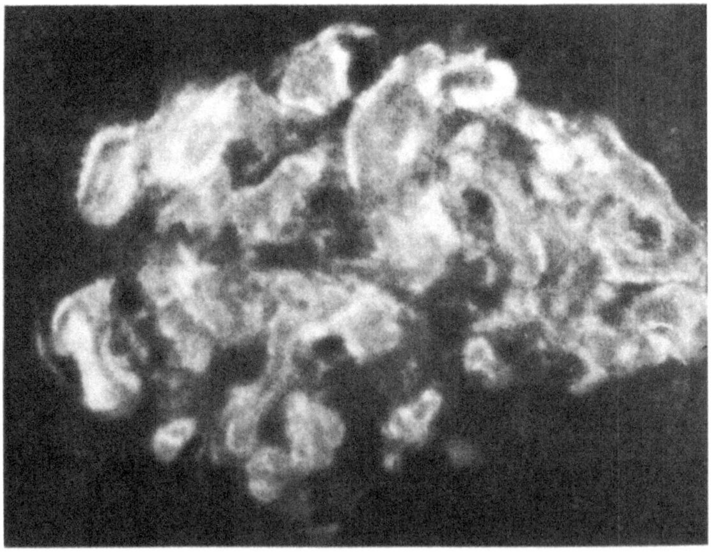

Fig. 23. Photomicrograph of a rabbit kidney. Rabbit was injected with ancrod, endotoxin, and heparin. Section was stained with fluorescent anti-rabbit fibrinogen antiserum. Magnification $\times 400$. (From MÜLLER-BERGHAUS, G. et al., 1972c)

If a second intravenous injection of endotoxin follows 24 hrs after the first, microclots are again found in lungs, liver, and spleen, but in much greater quantities (BRUNSON et al., 1955b). In the liver the intravascular microclots are found mainly in the interlobular capillaries and the central veins. In the spleen, the fibrin-rich substance appears to have a part-trabecular, part-reticular distribu-

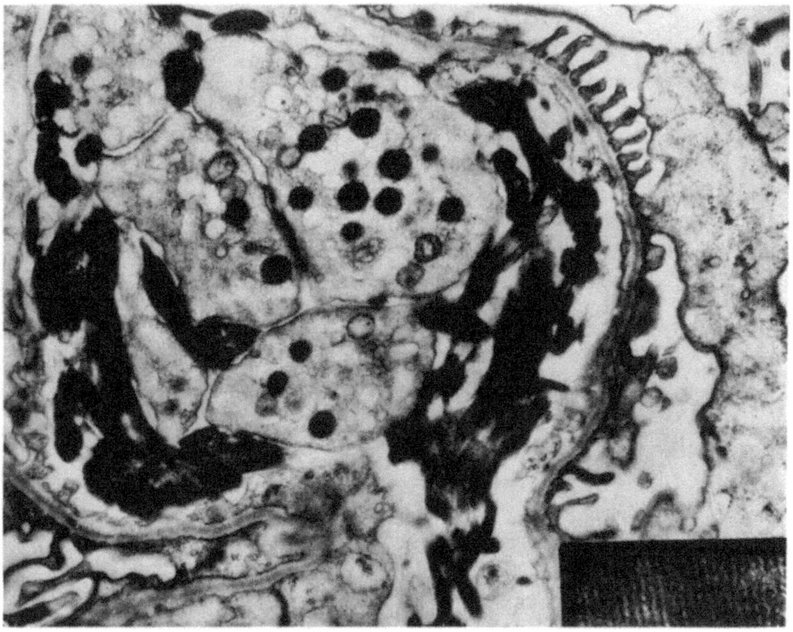

Fig. 24. Higher magnification of microclot in glomerular capillary with several platelets exhibiting partial degranulation. Magnification ×17600. *Inset* represents the periodicity of fibrin-like material (215 mμ). Magnification ×38850. (From McKAY, D. G. et al., 1969)

tion, and it is demonstrable both in the red pulpa and in the follicles (BOHLE et al., 1958; McKAY, 1964). A particularly striking feature is noted in the kidneys; in 60 to 100% of the animals fibrin-rich microclots are found in the glomerular capillaries of the kidneys 3 to 4 hrs after the provoking dose of endotoxin (Fig. 20 and 21). The occurrence of microclots in the kidneys is considered to be a typical finding in the generalized Shwartzman reaction (McKAY, 1963, 1964). If no microclots are detected in the glomerular capillaries of the kidneys 6 hrs after the second injection it is not to be expected that they will occur later. For this reason many experimenters sacrifice the animals as little as 4 or 6 hrs after the second provoking injection of endotoxin, as the histologic picture at this stage allows a definite diagnosis.

If the animals are allowed to survive after the second injection of endotoxin, macroscopically visible bilateral renal cortical necrosis is found 24 or 48 hrs later (Fig. 22). Disseminated necroses are often found as little as 6 to 8 hrs after the injection of endotoxin by means of histologic examination. In addition to kidneys, liver, spleen, and lungs, microclots are detected in the heart, adrenal glands and plexus chorioideus (BOHLE et al., 1958; for references see KRECKE, 1964).

Microscopic examination of the so-called fibrin-rich microclots reveals some homogeneous and some granulated or clumpy, eosinophilic, and PAS-positive substance that colors bright red with Goldner's trichrome stain (BOHLE et al., 1959; KRECKE, 1964) or blue with phosphotungstic acid (McKAY, 1964). Immunofluorescence microscopy with an antifibrinogen or antifibrin antiserum shows that the microclots contain a substance that can be derived from fibrinogen

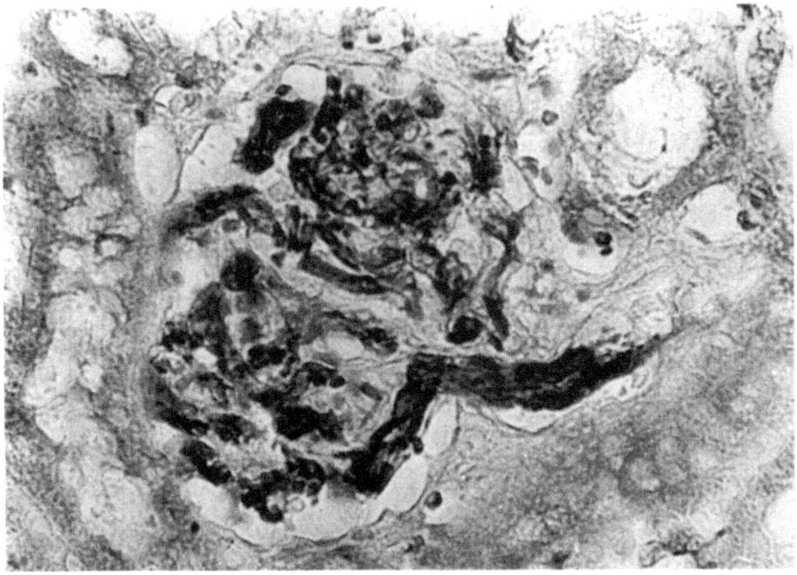

Fig. 25. Kidney section of a rabbit injected with single dose of Liquoid (10 mg/kg) and sacrificed 6 hrs thereafter. Many glomerular capillaries and afferent glomerular arteriole are occluded by fibrin-rich microclots. Histochemistry, ×400. (From MÜLLER-BERGHAUS, G., and LASCH, H. G., 1970)

(McKAY et al., 1959a) (Fig. 23). The antisera do not allow any distinction between fibrinogen and fibrinogen derivatives.

Electron microscope examination of the microclots reveals that they consist of leukocytes, platelets, a fibrinogen derivative, and neutral fats (BOHLE et al., 1959; McKAY et al., 1969). Some platelets are intact and some have lost their specific granula. In the same way, damaged erythrocytes are found, which may correspond to the fragmented red cells in the circulation (BRAIN et al., 1967). BOHLE et al. (1959) observed cross-striations by electron microscopy such as are considered typical of fibrin. According to the studies by BOHLE et al. (1959), this fibrin-like substance has an axial periodicity with an average period of 172 Å, whereas McKAY et al. (1966) measured 202 Å for the cross-striations of the fibrin strands after administration of endotoxin to rats. McKAY et al. (1969) observed a fibrin-like substance in the glomerular capillaries of the kidneys in rabbits after infusion of ellagic acid, EACA, and norepinephrine; the periodicity they recorded was 215 Å (Fig. 24). Whether this substance with the cross-striation detectable by electron microscopy is polymerized fibrin cannot clearly be answered at the moment. More recent investigations have cast a shadow on the unequivocal nature of the statement that the cross-striated substance is fibrin, as NIEWIAROWSKI et al. (1970), and STEWART and NIEWIAROWSKI (1971) have also been able to point out cross-striation of about 200 Å in aggregated fibrinogen. Similar electron microscope findings are obtained with precipitates of soluble fibrin monomer complexes (HORN et al., 1969).

It is certain that the microclots consist of some substance derived from fibrinogen. It has still not been decided, however, whether this is polymerized fibrin, precipitated fibrinogen, or aggregates of precipitated or polymerized fibrin monomer complexes. MÜLLER-BERGHAUS et al. (1973b) were able to produce

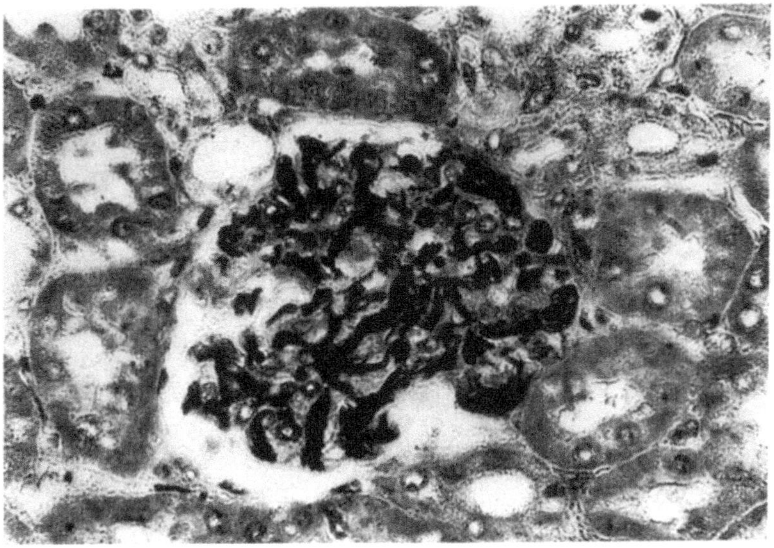

Fig. 26. Photomicrograph of monkey kidney. Monkey was infused with ellagic acid, EACA. and norepinephrine, and sacrificed 4 hrs after having started the infusions. Glomerular capillaries are filled with fibrin-rich microclots indicative of generalized Shwartzman reaction. Phosphotungstic acid hematoxylin, ×400. (From McKay, D. G. et al., 1969)

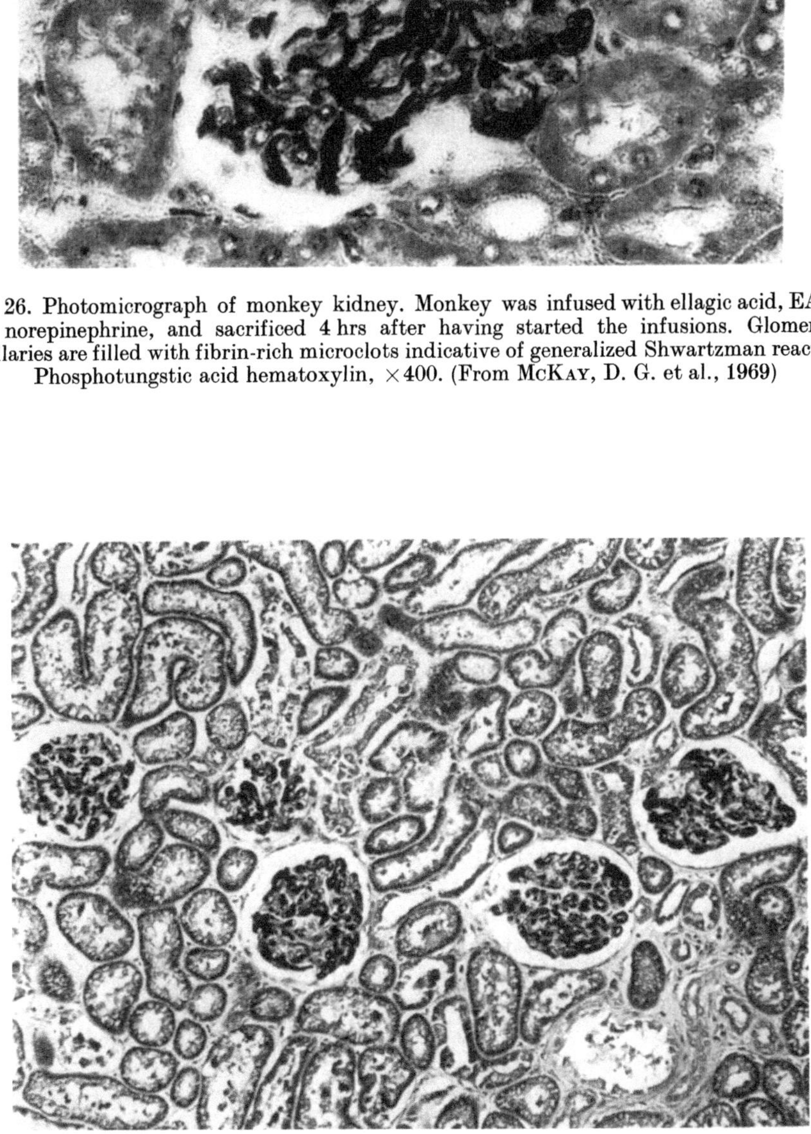

Fig. 27. Experimental hepatitis induced in a rabbit by i.v. administration of galactosamine and EACA. Renal glomerular capillaries are occluded with fibrin-rich microclots. Masson-Goldner, ×100. (Courtesy of Professor Uwe Bleyl, Heidelberg)

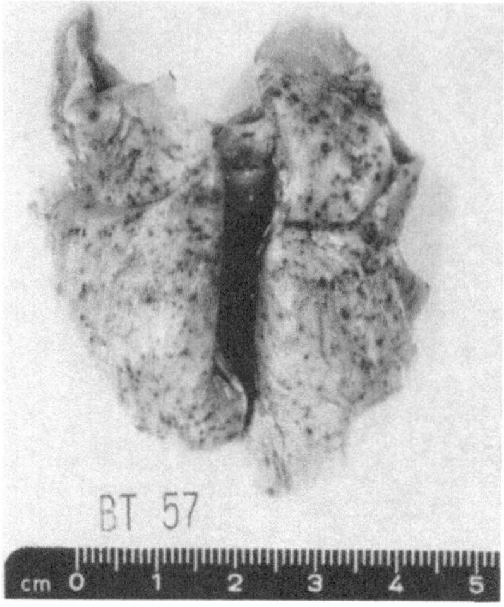

a

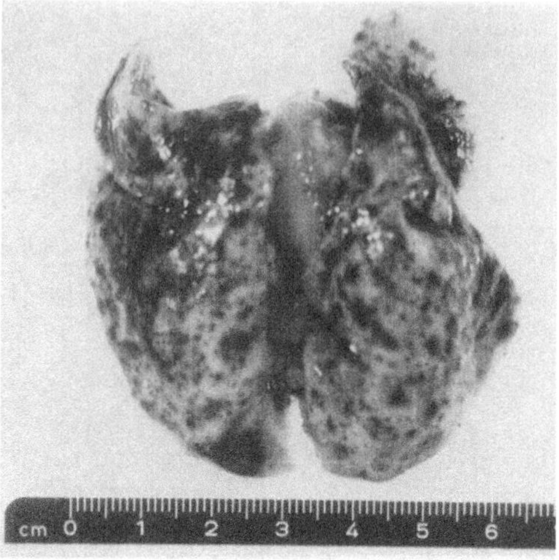

b

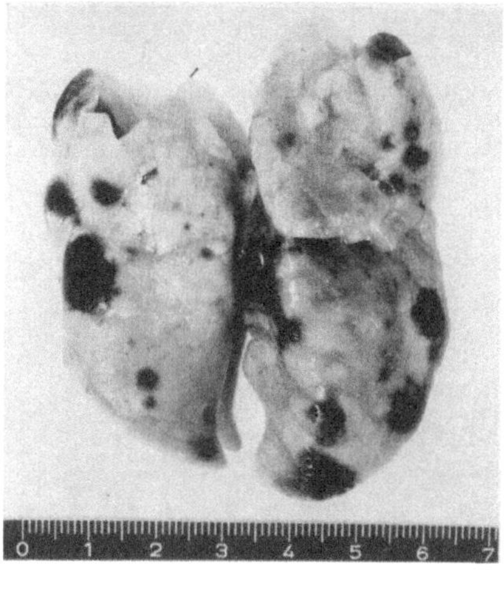

c

Fig. 28a—c. Hemorrhages of different sizes and intensities in lungs of rabbits after administration of galactosamine (a), Liquoid (b), and endotoxin (c)

microclots in the kidneys by means of an infusion of purified fibrin monomer even when the blood of the animals had been rendered incoagulable by heparinization. The experiment indicates that under *in vivo* conditions fibrin monomer complexes can form microclots. The same authors were able to precipitate circulating soluble fibrin monomer complexes in the kidneys even in animals with blocked coagulation systems; these microclots were not distinguishable under the light microscope from those observed in the generalized Shwartzman reaction (MÜLLER-BERGHAUS and HOCKE, 1972, 1973; MÜLLER-BERGHAUS and MANN, 1973). These investigations confirm that microclots may consist of entirely different fibrinogen derivatives.

The same kind of macroscopic and microscopic changes are observed after *infusion* of endotoxin as after *injection* of endotoxin (BELLER and GRAEFF, 1967; GRAEFF and BELLER, 1968; SCHOENDORF et al., 1971; GLASER, 1973; MÜLLER-BERGHAUS and LOHMANN, 1974). In rabbits, microclots are generally found six hours after an infusion of endotoxin is begun.

The staining qualities of the microclots and the electron microscope characteristics of cells and fibrinogen derivatives within the clots are identical in all models for the production of the generalized Shwartzman reaction, i.e. in the generalized Shwartzman reaction following an antigen-antibody reaction (LEE, 1963; MUELLER-ECKHARDT and MÜLLER-BERGHAUS, 1971; EVENSEN et al., 1963), after the infusion of thromboplastin or thrombin (VASSALLI et al., 1963; COLLINS et al., 1968; WHITAKER and MCKAY, 1969; BLEYL et al., 1969c, 1969d), after the administration of snake venom (KWAAN and BARLOW, 1971; MÜLLER-BERGHAUS et al., 1972c), in experimental viral infections (HOFFMANN et al., 1971), after administration of Liquoid (Fig. 25) (BOHLE et al., 1959; EVENSEN et al., 1967; MÜLLER-BERGHAUS and LASCH, 1970, 1971; SKJØRTEN and EVENSEN, 1972), carrageenin (SELYE, 1965, 1966), ellagic acid (Fig. 26) (MCKAY et al., 1969), colchicine (GALTON, 1963, 1966; MÜLLER-BERGHAUS and OBST, 1972) and galactosamine (Fig. 27) (MÜLLER-BERGHAUS and REUTER, 1972) and in shock (HARDAWAY, 1966; SANDRITTER and LASCH, 1967).

Histologic examination reveals pronounced hemorrhages in addition to fibrin-rich microclots in the peripheral blood vessels. Thus, extravasation of erythrocytes are observed in kidneys, liver, and, particularly, lungs (Fig. 28) and also in the adrenal glands, thymus, and intestine (MCKAY, 1964; KRECKE, 1964; HARDAWAY, 1966). The hemorrhages result from occlusion of arterioles, capillaries and venules, decreased coagulation factor activities, and increased fibrinolysis. Hemorrhage into the pericardium or hemorrhagic pulmonary edema can cause the death of the experimental animals.

BOHLE et al. (1959) and ALLARDYCE and GROVES (1969) have described the presence of neutral fats in the microclots in addition to blood cells and fibrinogen derivatives. These histological findings correspond to changes in the lipid metabolism after administration of endotoxin as it is expressed in hyperlipoproteinemia (MÜLLER-BERGHAUS et al., 1964; HIRSCH et al., 1964; HUTH and KARLICZEK, 1968; OBST et al., 1971).

5. Impairment of Organ Function

Dependent on the organ affected by the formation of capillary microclots, impairment of function can be expected in kidneys, liver, lungs, adrenal glands, brain, spleen, intestine, pancreas and heart. In animal experiments the functional impairment is investigated only in exceptional cases, while in patients functional disorders are familiar consequence of generalized intravascular coagulation (PFAU et al., 1960; MCKAY, 1964; HARDAWAY, 1966; LASCH and HEENE, 1967; LASCH et al., 1967, 1971; BLEYL et al., 1969a, 1969b; BLEYL and HÖPKER, 1970; KUHN and GRAEFF, 1970; MITTERMAYER et al., 1970; GRAEFF et al., 1971; NEUHOF et al., 1975).

Investigations of Renal Function

Changes in renal function are readily described in the generalized Shwartzman reaction following infusion of endotoxin. With the occurrence of microclots in the renal glomerular capillaries there is a reduction in the volume of urine excreted, which is followed in some cases by polyuric renal failure (GRAEFF et al., 1968; GLASER et al., 1971; GLASER, 1973; WARDLE, 1974). After transitory polyuria, the animals develop anuria, and the osmolal and free water clearance falls almost to zero (GRAEFF et al., 1968). The excretion of urokinase and the tissue plasminogen activator content of the kidney falls in proportion as the microclots are formed (GRAEFF et al., 1968). If the animals do survive for any length of time, renal cortical necrosis results, understandably, in anuria, with all the signs and symptoms associated with this condition.

During the infusion of endotoxin the animals develop metabolic acidosis (GRAEFF et al., 1968; GLASER, 1973), which is paralleled by a continuous increase in the arterio-venous oxygen difference. The decreasing oxygen consumption of the total organism allows the conclusion that the cardiac output begins to fall from the beginning of the experiment onwards (GLASER, 1973).

Lung function tests after infusions of endotoxin do not reveal any pronounced disorders (GLASER, 1973). The hemoglobin values also remain within normal limits, so that any reduction of the oxygen transport capacity can be excluded. In contrast to the findings after injections of endotoxin, no rapid fall in the arterial blood pressure is observed after continuous infusion of endotoxin; nor does the central venous pressure rise, according to GLASER's investigations (1973). In the experimental model in which endotoxin is given by continuous infusion, the arterial blood pressure may remain in the normal range until immediately before the animals die, while the oxygen consumption of the total organism and the central venous pH value fall throughout the infusion, so that one can only assume that damage to the peripheral blood vessels is developing progressively but can be compensated to such an extent that it is not reflected in the arterial blood pressure.

E. Prevention of Generalized Intravascular Coagulation and of the Generalized Shwartzman Reaction

Advancing knowledge of the pathogenesis of the generalized Shwartzman reaction has led to the use of agents with various modes of action to prevent generalized activation of intravascular coagulation and of the generalized Shwartzman reaction. It has proved possible to prevent both generalized intravascular coagulation and the generalized Shwartzman reaction with all substances with an inhibitory effect on the coagulation process. If substances such as endotoxin, which affect the coagulation system by way of mediators, are used for the activation of generalized intravascular coagulation, activation of the coagulation system can be prevented simply by manipulation of the mediator. As the generalized Shwartzman reaction is defined as generalized intravascular coagulation with the formation of microclots in the kidney, this reaction can also be prevented by means of substances that are responsible for the formation of microclots and their persistence (inhibition of fibrinolysis). Finally, the generalized Shwartzman reaction can be prevented by means of substances that lyse any microclots that have already formed.

I. Interference with the Activation of Intravascular Coagulation

1. Antithrombins

If heparin is administered in high doses (750 U/kg and hr) before or up to a maximum of 2 hrs after the second, provoking injection of endotoxin, generalized intravascular coagulation and the formation of microclots can completely be prevented (GOOD and THOMAS, 1953; CORRIGAN, 1970). Heparin is the antithrombin that is used most frequently for the prevention of generalized intravascular coagulation. Hirudin has been used only for the prevention of the local Shwartzman reaction (HAUSTEIN and MARKWARDT, 1965).

Table 2. Incidence of renal glomeralar microclots in phenprocoumon-pretreated and untreated rabbits. Generalized intravascular coagulation and generalized Shwartzman reaction (GSR) were induced with Thorotrast (3 ml/kg) and endotoxin (20 μg) or with Liquoid (10 mg/kg). (Data from MÜLLER-BERGHAUS, G., and LASCH, H. G., 1971; MÜLLER-BERGHAUS, G., and SCHNEBERGER, R., 1971)

Materials injected for induction of GSR	Untreated rabbits		Phenprocoumon-pretreated rabbits	
	No. of rabbits	Incidence of glomerular microclots[a]	No. of rabbits	Incidence of glomerular microclots[a]
Thorotrast and endotoxin	20	12/20	13	0/13
Liquoid	21	13/21	21	0/21

[a] Expressed as number of positive results over total number of rabbits studied.

Heparin also prevents the formation of microclots after the administration of endotoxin by infusion (GLASER, 1973) and of Liquoid (THOMAS et al., 1955a) or amniotic fluid (HARDAWAY and McKAY, 1959) by injection, and after an antigen-antibody reaction (LEE, 1963). The generalized Shwartzman reaction does not develop even in the pregnant rat when heparin is administered (MARGARETTEN et al., 1967). The generalized intravascular coagulation usually observed in experimental galactosamine-induced hepatitis can also be prevented by means of heparin. Liver damage and death of the animals are not affected by the anticoagulation (REUTER and MÜLLER-BERGHAUS, 1973; MAHN et al., 1974). Heparin cannot prevent the occurrence of glomerular microclots or bilateral renal cortical necrosis after the injection of staphylococcal toxin (NAKAI and MARGARETTEN, 1963).

2. Vitamin K Antagonists

It is possible to reduce the prothrombin time to less than 5% of the normal value in rabbits by the administration of several doses of a vitamin K antagonist. Sodium warfarin is used for this purpose in rabbits in a dosage of 90 to 700 mg (EVENSEN et al., 1967; LERNER et al., 1968b) and also phenprocoumon in a dosage of 60 to 80 mg (MÜLLER-BERGHAUS and SCHNEBERGER, 1971), administered over 4 to 5 days. In the resulting hypoprothrombinemic phase, generalized intravascular coagulation and the generalized Shwartzman reaction do not occur after two injections of endotoxin or after one injection each of cortisone and endotoxin or Thorotrast and endotoxin (Table 2) (SHAPIRO and McKAY, 1958; LERNER et al., 1968b; MÜLLER-BERGHAUS and SCHNEBERGER, 1971). In the same way, vitamin-K antagonists can prevent the Liquoid-induced generalized Shwartzman reaction (Table 2) (EVENSEN et al., 1967; MÜLLER-BERGHAUS and LASCH, 1971).

3. Hypofibrinogenemia

When hypofibrinogenemia is induced by means of several injections of ancrod, the procoagulant fraction of the venom of Agkistrodon rhodostoma, given over a fairly long period, the administration of Thorotrast and endotoxin does not result in the generalized Shwartzman reaction (BELL et al., 1972).

Table 3. Incidence of renal glomerular microclots in lysozyme-treated and untreated control rabbits. Generalized intravascular coagulation and generalized Shwartzman reaction (GSR) were induced with Thorotrast (3 ml/kg) and endotoxin (20 μg) or with Liquoid (10 mg/kg). (Data from MÜLLER-BERGHAUS, G., and LASCH, H. G., 1970; MÜLLER-BERGHAUS, G., and SCHNEBERGER, R., 1971)

Materials injected for induction of GSR	Control rabbits		Lysozyme-treated rabbits	
	No. of rabbits	Incidence of glomerular microclots[a]	No. of rabbits	Incidence of glomerular microclots[a]
Thorotrast and endotoxin	20	12/20	14	9/14
Liquoid	20	19/20	10	0/10

[a] Expressed as the number of positive results over the total number of rabbits studied.

4. Inhibition of Activation of the Hageman Factor

Lysozyme prevents activation of the Hageman factor induced by substances which initiate blood coagulation by contact-active agents (NOSSEL et al., 1968). A continuous infusion of lysozyme can prevent the generalized Shwartzman reaction after an injection of Liquoid (MÜLLER-BERGHAUS and LASCH, 1970), but has no effect on the generalized Shwartzman reaction produced by Thorotrast and endotoxin (Table 3) (MÜLLER-BERGHAUS and SCHNEBERGER, 1971). It is important to give lysozyme in a dosage calculated to increase the partial thromboplastin time from its initial value of approximately 30 sec to over 80 sec.

Administration of the proteinase inhibitor aprotinin can prevent the occurrence of the generalized Shwartzman reaction after Liquoid (MÜLLER-BERGHAUS et al., 1972a). In this model, aprotinin inhibits activation of Hageman factor (GIROLAMI et al., 1971, 1973). In addition, aprotinin inhibits the effect of thromboplastin on the activation of intravascular coagulation (NORDSTRØM, 1970; NORDSTRØM and ZETTERQVIST, 1969). Aprotinin has no effect, however, on the activation of intravascular coagulation and the generalized Shwartzman reaction after endotoxin by injection (MÜLLER-BERGHAUS et al., 1972b) or by infusion (GLASER, 1973).

5. Cytostatics

Pretreatment of animals with nitrogen mustard can prevent the generalized Shwartzman reaction normally evoked by two injections of endotoxin or by administration of cortisone and endotoxin or Thorotrast and endotoxin (THOMAS and GOOD, 1952b; LERNER et al., 1968b; HORN and COLLINS, 1968a; NIEMETZ and FANI, 1971; MÜLLER-BERGHAUS and ECKHARDT, 1975). In this experimental set-up, nitrogen mustard is given in a dosage of 1.75 mg/kg body weight four days prior to the second respectively provoking injection of endotoxin. Complete prevention of the generalized Shwartzman reaction is achieved only if granulocyte counts have fallen to values of less than 50/μl before the provoking or second injection of endotoxin. The platelet count plays no part in this (SMITH et al., 1968). In animals treated with nitrogen mustard, endotoxin injection is not followed by the activation of generalized intravascular coagulation, but the fall in platelet counts is not prevented (Fig. 29) (MÜLLER-BERGHAUS and ECKHARDT, 1975).

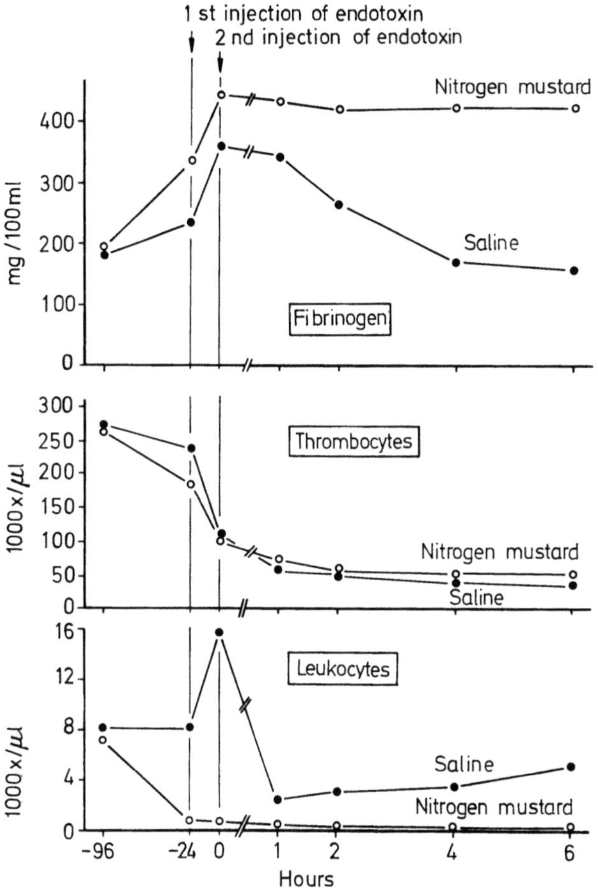

Fig. 29. Changes in mean leukocyte and platelet counts as well as fibrinogen levels after 2 i.v. injections of endotoxin (2×150 μg) into nitrogen mustard- or saline-pretreated rabbits. Before first injection of endotoxin, mean fibrinogen concentration of nitrogen mustard-treated rabbits was significantly higher than mean value of control animals. Each curve represents 10 animal experiments. Nitrogen mustard–pretreated rabbits did not show generalized intravascular coagulation although platelet counts decreased after endotoxin administration. (Data from MÜLLER-BERGHAUS, G. and ECKHARDT, T., 1975)

Nitrogen mustard cannot prevent the activation of generalized intravascular coagulation following Liquoid (THOMAS et al., 1955b; SKJØRTEN and EVENSEN, 1972).

Busulphan given by intraperitoneal injection or by mouth (2 doses of 25 mg/kg, 3 days apart) can produce thrombocytopenia and granulocytopenia in rabbits (EVENSEN et al., 1968; ECKHARDT and MÜLLER-BERGHAUS, 1975). Activation of intravascular coagulation by an antigen-antibody reaction (EVENSEN et al., 1972) can be prevented by busulphan pretreatment in dependence on platelet counts, but the generalized Shwartzman reaction occurs after the administration of Liquoid even in animals with very low platelet counts (EVENSEN and JEREMIC, 1968).

Table 4. Incidence of renal glomerular microclots in dibenzyline- or dibenamine-pretreated pregnant rats. Generalized Shwartzman reaction (GSR) was induced by single i.v. injection of endotoxin into pregnant rats (From MÜLLER-BERGHAUS, G., and MCKAY, D. G., 1967)

Material injected for induction of GSR	Untreated rats		Dibenamine- or Dibenzyline-pretreated rats	
	No. of rats	Incidence of glomerular microclots*	No. of rats	Incidence of glomerular microclots*
Endotoxin	39	25/39	39	5/39

* Expressed as number of positive results over total number of rats studied.

Neither nitrogen mustard nor busulphan prevent the precipitation of soluble fibrin after the injection of endotoxin (ECKHARDT and MÜLLER-BERGHAUS, 1974, 1975; MÜLLER-BERGHAUS and ECKHARDT, 1975).

6. Inhibitors of Platelet Aggregation

LATOUR (1974) reports prevention of the generalized Shwartzman reaction after two injections of endotoxin by means of pretreatment of the animals with acetylsalicylic acid, a powerful inhibitor of platelet aggregation. Prevention could only be achieved, if acetylsalicylic acid was administered before the first injection of endotoxin. SLABBER et al. (1972), however, did not find that pretreatment of animals with acetylsalicylic acid prevented the occurrence of fibrin deposits in the renal glomerular capillaries following infusion of endotoxin. The treatment of rabbits with pyrimido-pyrimidines certainly prevents the platelet count from falling during the infusion of endotoxin, but the generalized Shwartzman reaction still occurs in the same way (SLABBER et al., 1972).

7. Antibiotics

Production of the generalized Shwartzman reaction by two injections of endotoxin can be prevented by an intravenous injection of polymyxin B (5.0 mg) or colistin methate (5.0 mg) given at the same time as the second injection of endotoxin (CORRIGAN and BELL, 1971). It seems that both substances prevent the generalized Shwartzman reaction by way of their endotoxin-neutralizing properties (RIFKIND and HILL, 1967), as gentamicin, which has no neutralizing properties vis-à-vis endotoxin, cannot prevent the generalized Shwartzman reaction. Polymyxin B also regularly suppresses the activation of intravascular coagulation and the leukopenia and thrombocytopenia generally observed after endotoxin (CORRIGAN and BELL, 1971).

In the pregnant rat, the generalized Shwartzman reaction produced by feeding a diet rich in oxidized lipids can be prevented by giving resorbable and nonresorbable antibiotics by mouth (MCKAY and WONG, 1962). It is possible that the resorption of endotoxin from the gastrointestinal tract plays some part in this model, as is assumed to be the case in the generalized Shwartzman reaction following two injections of Thorotrast (FINE et al., 1959b).

II. Interference with the Additional Mechanisms of Microclot Formation

1. Alpha-Adrenergic Blocking Agents

Occurrence of the generalized Shwartzman reaction after endotoxin injection into the pregnant rat can be prevented by pretreatment of the animals with the alpha-receptor blocking agents dibenamine or dibenzyline (Table 4) (MÜLLER-BERGHAUS and MCKAY, 1967; MÜLLER-BERGHAUS et al., 1967a). Dibenzyline does not, however, suppress the activation of intravascular coagulation in this model (MÜLLER-BERGHAUS et al., 1967a). In the same way, dibenzyline can reduce the occurrence of microclots in the renal glomerular capillaries after the administration of cortisone and endotoxin (LATOUR et al., 1971).

The sympatholytic agent hexamethonium (5 mg/kg, 30 min before the second injection of endotoxin) also prevents the occurrence of microclots after two injections of endotoxin in much the same way as dibenzyline does (NASU et al., 1971).

2. Glucocorticoids

Various glucocorticoids (hydrocortisone, dexamethasone, triamcinolone) make it possible to reduce the frequency of microclots in the renal glomerular capillaries after two injections of endotoxin (LATOUR et al., 1972). For this purpose hydrocortisone (20 mg/kg), dexamethasone (1 mg/kg) or triamcinolone (5 mg/kg) is administered two hours before the second injection of endotoxin. It is also possible to prevent the generation of the generalized Shwartzman reaction that usually follows a single injection of endotoxin in the pregnant rat (LATOUR et al., 1972). DOCA and ACTH have no inhibitory effect on the occurrence of the generalized Shwartzman reaction.

3. Fibrinolysis Activators

The occurrence of the generalized Shwartzman reaction after two injections of endotoxin can be prevented by the administration of streptokinase, which activates the fibrinolytic enzyme system (CONDIE et al., 1957; KLIMAN and MCKAY, 1958). It is important that streptokinase treatment is begun not more than four hours, and preferably two hours, after the second injection of endotoxin. Treatment with an activator of fibrinolysis, however, does not prevent the occurrence of generalized intravascular coagulation (LASCH et al., 1962). Activation of the fibrinolytic enzyme system in the presence of generalized intravascular coagulation considerably intensifies the tendency to hemorrhage (MCKAY et al., 1959b).

The irreversible state of shock can be made reversible if animals are treated with a fibrinolytic activator (CROWELL and SMITH, 1956; LASCH et al., 1961b; HARDAWAY and BURNS, 1963; ENCKE et al., 1966, 1969).

F. Pathophysiology

Thrombosis and hemorrhage are generally considered as diametrically opposed phenomena, both of which are dysfunctions of the physiologic coagulation equilibrium. Impaired coagulation of the blood in the form of a hemorrhagic diathesis can, however, also be the paradoxical result of generalized or localized intravascular coagulation. SELYE (1966) proposed the term "thrombohemorrhagic phenomenon" to describe this process of intravascular coagulation with subsequent hemorrhagic diathesis. The breakdown of the hemostatic potential during the course of this phenomenon is caused by consumption of the coagulation factors and platelets; for this reason LASCH et al. (1961a, 1967) have termed the phenomenon "consumption coagulopathy".

Generalized intravascular coagulation (= consumption coagulopathy) is a syndrome in which the physiologic equilibrium between procoagulant and anticoagulant factors and the clearance of intermediate and end products of coagulation are disturbed. Even when the trigger mechanisms of intravascular coagulation are different, there is a general process of a chain reaction behind generalized intravascular coagulation. McKAY (1964), therefore, describes consumption coagulopathy as "disseminated intravascular coagulation" representing "an intermediary mechanism of disease". McKAY (1964) and HARDAWAY (1966) prefer the term "disseminated intravascular coagulation", which was coined by SCHNEIDER (1951).

I. Connections with Pathophysiology in Man

Although generalized or local intravascular coagulation can be set in motion by very different trigger mechanisms, the following etiologic factors can be distinguished leading to this specific form of microcirculatory impairment (Table 5):

Table 5. Etiologic factors of generalized intravascular coagulation. (From MÜLLER-BERGHAUS, G., 1969)

1. Bacterial endotoxin
2. Particulate or colloidal substances
3. Antigen-antibody complexes
4. Hypocirculation
5. Tissue thromboplastin
6. Proteolytic enzymes

1. Bacterial Endotoxin

Bacterial endotoxins can produce generalized intravascular coagulation such as is observed in purpura fulminans, chorioamnionitis, or septicemia (for references see McKAY, 1964; HJORT and RAPAPORT, 1965; SELYE, 1966; HARDAWAY, 1966; LASCH et al., 1966, 1967, 1969, 1971; McKAY and MÜLLER-BERGHAUS, 1967; ZANDER, 1968; KUHN and GRAEFF, 1970; McKAY, 1973; MINNA et al., 1974).

2. Particulate or Colloidal Substances

Particulate substances such as occur in amniotic fluid embolism can initiate generalized intravascular coagulation. Injection of the particulate portion of the amniotic fluid (STEINER and LUSHBAUGH, 1941) or of fat particles makes it possible to activate intravascular coagulation (BRUNSON et al., 1955c; McKAY, 1964; CONNOR et al., 1966; HUTH et al., 1967; MÜLLER-BERGHAUS, 1969; McKAY et al., 1969).

3. Antigen-Antibody Complexes

Antigen-antibody reactions regularly precipitate generalized intravascular coagulation, e.g. when incompatible blood is given by transfusion (HARDAWAY et al., 1956; McKay, 1964; Hardaway, 1966; Mueller-Eckhardt et al., 1969). In animal experiments, generalized intravascular coagulation can be produced in immunized animals after injection of antigen or infusion of immune complexes (see Section D.I.2.).

4. Hypocirculation

Shock, whether hemorrhagic, burn-induced or cardiogenic shock, is particularly likely to produce activation of intravascular coagulation in cases where the peripheral circulation of the blood has been substantially restricted for any length of time. In different animal species, various forms of shock have been induced, and activation of intravascular coagulation has regularly been recorded in each form (for references see McKay, 1964; Hardaway, 1966; Sandritter and Lasch, 1967; Lasch and Heene, 1970).

5. Tissue Thromboplastin

When organs that are rich in tissue thromboplastin are damaged, this procoagulant can enter the circulation and thus produce generalized intravascular coagulation. The same is known to be true of thromboplastin-rich tumor cells (for references see McKay, 1964; Penick and Roberts, 1964; Hardaway, 1966; Selye, 1966; Merskey et al., 1967; Schneider, 1969; Hilgard et al., 1973; Minna et al., 1974). In animal experiments the administration of tissue thromboplastin by infusion regularly produces generalized intravascular coagulation (see Section D.I.3.).

Generalized intravascular coagulation has been observed in viral infections such as measles, Rocky Mountain spotted fever, childhood diarrhea, and smallpox (for references see McKay, 1964, 1969; McKay and Margaretten, 1967; Dennis and Conrad, 1968). Certain viral infections seen in animal experiments, such as Aleutian mink disease (McKay et al., 1967b), fowl plapue of chickens (Gagel et al., 1970), acute hog cholera (Heene et al., 1971), and yellow fever (Dennis et al., 1969) are typically accompanied by generalized intravascular coagulation.

6. Proteolytic Enzymes

Proteolytic enzymes can cause generalized intravascular coagulation through their direct action on coagulation factors. Hemorrhagic diathesis has been known to result from generalized intravascular coagulation following snake bites (for references see Reid et al., 1963; McKay, 1964; Weiss et al., 1969). Injection of these snake venoms allows simulation of the hemorrhagic diathesis as a result of generalized intravascular coagulation in animal experiments (see Section D.I.4.).

The multiplicity of etiologic factors and wide variety of illnesses explains why each disease process connected with generalized intravascular coagulation has its own individual clinical picture and patho-anatomical correlate. There is a general principle behind the process of generalized intravascular coagulation, which does not always come out fully in clinical signs or in the results of diagnostic investigations, due to quantitative differences.

Even a description of the dynamic processes involved in generalized intravascular coagulation (= consumption coagulopathy) (see Section C) indicates the complexity of the mechanisms responsible for the variations in the course of generalized intravascular coagulation. We shall now give an account of the

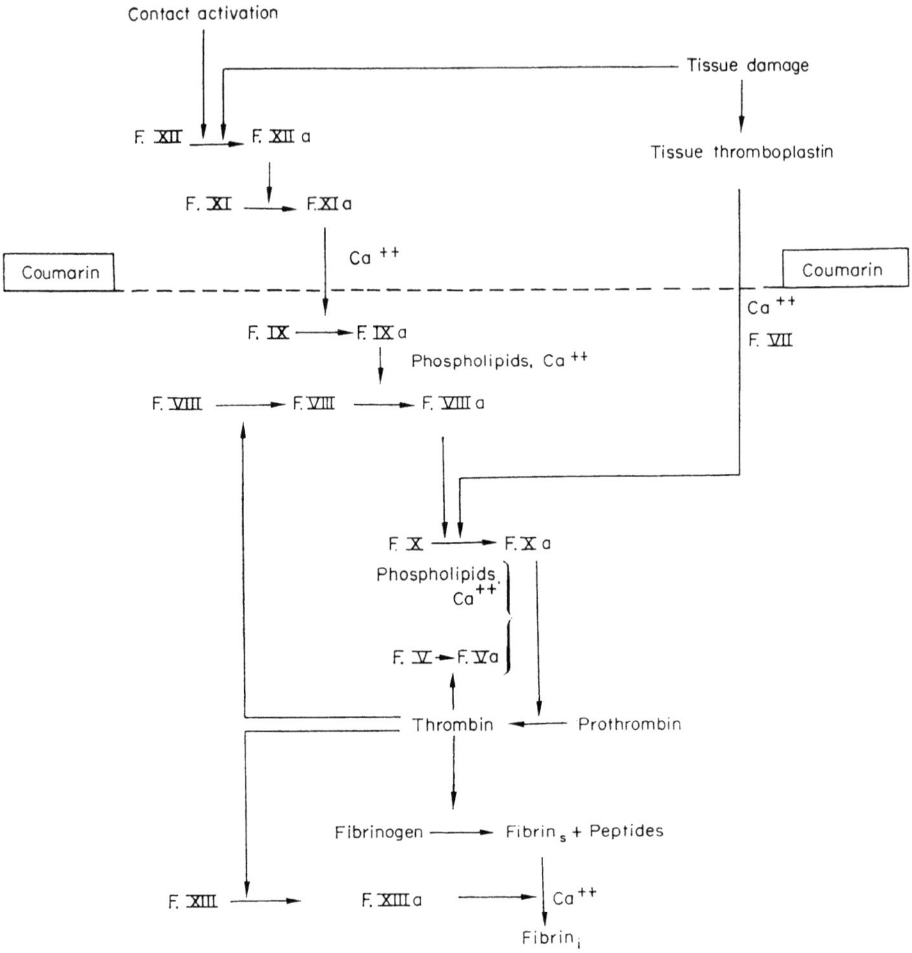

Fig. 30. Cascade of the blood coagulation system according to MACFARLANE (1964). Modification: Connection between intrinsic and extrinsic systems and interruption of the cascade by coumarin are indicated. Plasma coagulation factors are represented by Roman numerals; *a* indicates active form. (From MÜLLER-BERGHAUS, G., and SCHNEBERGER, R., 1971)

pathophysiologic mechanisms involved in an attempt to explain the varying courses of generalized intravascular coagulation, the varying intensity of the reactions, and its secondary consequences.

II. Coagulation System

1. Contact Factors of Blood Coagulation (Plasma Factors XII and XI)

According to the concept that activation of the coagulation system occurs in the form of a cascade, Hageman factor is the first factor to be activated in the intrinsic system of blood coagulation (Fig. 30). Recent studies by WALSH (1972) indicate the particular significance of plasma Factor XI for the initiation of coagulation in the intrinsic system (Fig. 31).

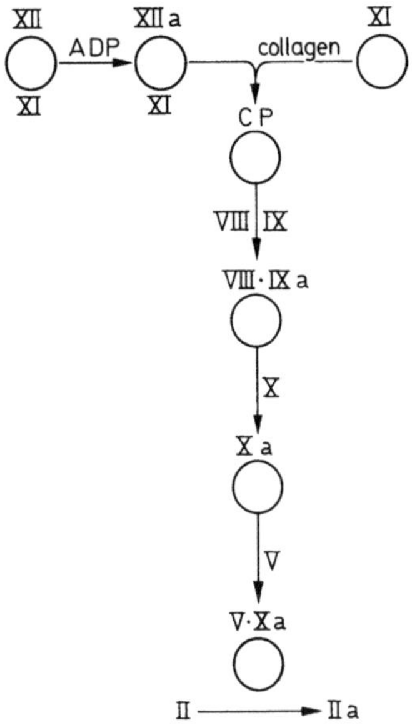

Fig. 31. Two postulated alternative pathways involving platelets in initiation of intrinsic coagulation according to WALSH (1972). Plasma coagulation factors are represented by Roman numerals; *a* indicates active form; CP (contact product) represents combined activities of activated Factors XII and XI. Open circles represent the platelet on the surface of which the activation of coagulation is thought to take place

RODRÍGUEZ-ERDMANN (1964c) observed a fall in the level of Hageman factor activity after endotoxin, and assumed from his studies that direct activation of Hageman factor triggers the coagulation process after endotoxin injection. This has not been confirmed, however; LERNER et al. (1968b) observed decreased Hageman factor activity after the injection of endotoxin into rabbits even if the animals had previously been treated with the vitamin K antagonist warfarin. A fall in the Hageman factor activity similar to that seen in the controls should have been observed in warfarin-pretreated animals even when endotoxin acted directly on Hageman factor, as vitamin K antagonists do not affect the first phase of the intrinsic pathway of the coagulation system (Fig. 30). In studies by LERNER et al. (1968b), the generalized Shwartzman reaction was induced by a single injection of endotoxin into animals pretreated with cortisone. MÜLLER-BERGHAUS and SCHNEBERGER (1971) obtained the same results: they produced the generalized Shwartzman reaction by injecting Thorotrast and endotoxin (Fig. 32). Furthermore, MÜLLER-BERGHAUS and SCHNEBERGER (1971) also showed that lysozyme, a substance that prevents activation of Hageman factor, does not suppress the endotoxin-induced generalized Shwartzman reaction (see Table 3). Thus, both experiments exclude the possibility that endotoxin is the direct activator of the Hageman factor. Studies by SHEN et al. (1973) support the assumption that endotoxin does not activate intravascular coagulation by way of the intrinsic system. SHEN et al. (1973) were able to produce the Shwartzman reaction induced by cortisone and endotoxin even in animals in which the activity of Factor VIII had been reduced to values below 10% of the norm by a Factor VIII antiserum. The experiments conducted by GAYNOR (1973) also exclude the possibility that damage to the vessel wall and release of collagen might activate

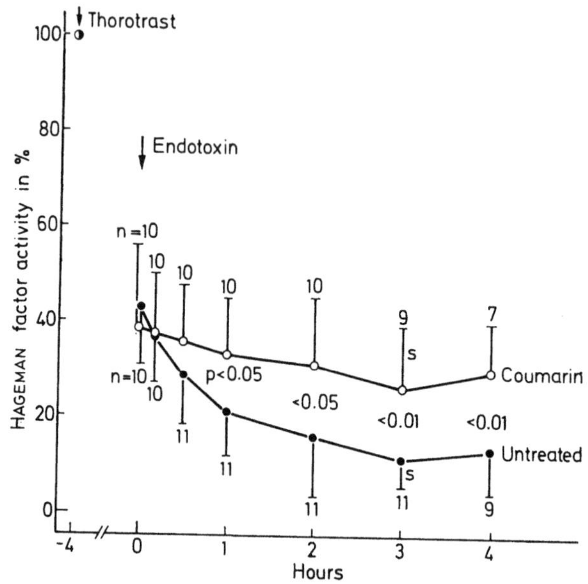

Fig. 32. Effect of coumarin pretreatment on Hageman factor activity after injections of Thorotrast (3 ml/kg) and endotoxin (20 μg). Coumarin pretreatment did not influence the decrease in Hageman factor activity after Thorotrast injection, but prevented its drop after endotoxin injection in the same way as it prevented the occurrence of generalized intravascular coagulation. Circles represent mean values, vertical lines refer to standard deviations drawn only from one side of the plotted points. The numbers at the end of the vertical lines indicate the number of animals at those points. (From MÜLLER-BERGHAUS, G., and SCHNEBERGER, R,. 1971)

Hageman factor, and thus in turn intravascular coagulation, as anticoagulation with warfarin prevents the in decrease Hageman factor activity but does not prevent endothelial injury.

In rabbits, a definite fall in Hageman factor activity is observed after the administration of endotoxin (LERNER et al., 1968b; MÜLLER-BERGHAUS and SCHNEBERGER, 1971). It is also possible to induce generalized intravascular coagulation with occurrence of microclots in the glomerular capillaries of the kidney by intravenously injecting Liquoid, a synthetic acidic polymer. This also produces a fall in Hageman factor activity (MÜLLER-BERGHAUS and LASCH, 1970, 1971). If rabbits are pretreated with lysozyme in this model, the Liquoid-induced generalized Shwartzman reaction is prevented (see Table 3) (MÜLLER-BERGHAUS and LASCH, 1970). Aprotinin, a proteinase inhibitor with inhibitory effects on the contact factors (GIROLAMI et al., 1971, 1973) has also been shown to prevent or reduce the appearance of the generalized Shwartzman reaction after Liquoid (MÜLLER-BERGHAUS et al., 1972a). In keeping with this, Hageman factor activity falls after injection of Liquoid even in animals pretreated with phenprocoumon to prevent the generalized Shwartzman reaction (MÜLLER-BERGHAUS and LASCH, 1971) (Fig. 33). These findings make it possible to distinguish between the trigger mechanism of generalized intravascular coagulation after injection of Liquoid from that following endotoxin injection.

While in various experimental models activation of Hageman factor had been demonstrated, this did not allow the conclusion that activation of Hageman

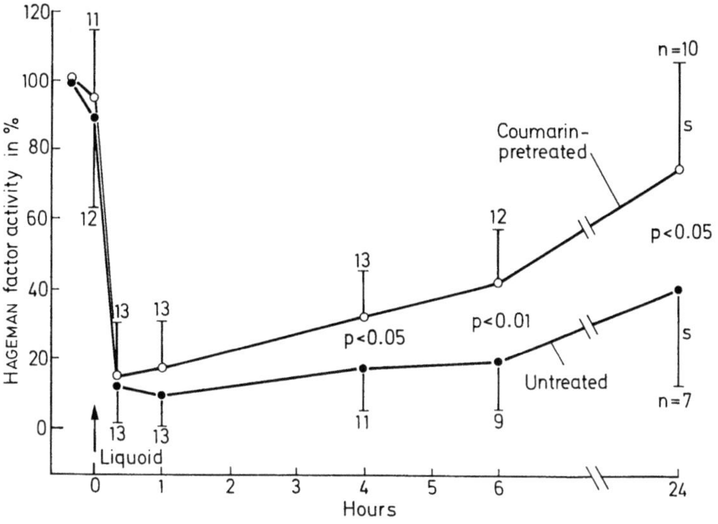

Fig. 33. Changes in Hageman factor activities after i.v. injection of Liquoid (10 mg/kg) into untreated and phenprocoumon (coumarin)-pretreated rabbits. Coumarin pretreatment did not prevent decrease in Hageman factor activities, although it prevented occurrence of generalized intravascular coagulation and generalized Shwartzman reaction after Liquoid injection. Circles represent mean values, vertical lines refer to standard deviations drawn only from one side of the plotted points. Numbers at the end of the vertical lines indicate number of animals at those points. (From MÜLLER-BERGHAUS, G., and LASCH, H.-G., 1971)

factor leads to generalized intravascular coagulation; since BOTTI and RATNOFF (1964) did not observe intravascular coagulation after injecting ellagic acid, which activates Hageman factor *in vitro*. Studies by McKAY and MÜLLER-BERGHAUS (1968) and McKAY et al. (1969) showed that after activation of Hageman factor by intravenous infusion of ellagic acid, generalized intravascular coagulation with fibrin-rich microclots in the glomerular capillaries of the kidney is observed only if the animals in addition receive EACA in order to inhibit fibrinolysis and norepinephrine for localizing microclots into the glomerular capillaries. The results of the studies are identical in rabbits and rhesus monkeys.

According to investigations performed by McKAY et al. (1970), stimulation of the alpha-adrenergic receptors with epinephrine leads to activation of Hageman factor. However, these experiments do not reveal any causal relationship between stimulation of the alpha-receptors and the activation of Hageman factor, as a disturbance of the microcirculation with occurrence of intravascular coagulation could initiate activation of Hageman factor as a secondary result. More recent studies allow the assumption that Hageman factor is activated by some hitherto unexplained feedback mechanism in every form of generalized intravascular coagulation, including that following infusion of thrombin (MÜLLER-BERGHAUS et al., 1974). Studies by McKAY et al. (1971 a) have shown beyond all doubt that activation of Hageman factor leads to generalized intravascular coagulation with microclot formation in the peripheral blood vessels. These investigators infused purified Hageman factor together with norepinephrine into pregnant rats, and thus produced the generalized Shwartzman reaction. In this model, pregnancy, with its tendency of low local fibrinolytic activity in the kidney

(MARGARETTEN et al., 1964; for references see p. 483), appears to take the place of EACA as used in the model described by McKAY and MÜLLER-BERGHAUS (1968).

2. Erythrocytes

In contrast to uninjured erythrocytes, hemolyzed erythrocytes show some coagulant activity (for references see SURGENOR, 1974). Washed and lysed erythrocytes have a weak thromboplastic activity *in vitro* (QUICK et al., 1954). *In vivo* studies have led to varying conclusions, however, mainly because mechanical hemolysis has been equated with immunologically mediated hemolysis. The secondary hemolysis that generally occurs in the presence of intravascular coagulation with microclot formation presents another complication (BRAIN et al., 1967; BRAIN, 1972; BELLER and THEISS, 1973). Hemolysis is usually observed during the infusion of tissue thromboplastin, endotoxin, or Liquoid (KRECKE, 1964; BRAIN et al., 1967; BRAIN and HOURIHANE, 1967; BENNETT et al., 1968; EVENSEN and JEREMIC, 1970; SLAASTAD and JEREMIC, 1973); this is probably due to the mechanical destruction of the erythrocytes during fibrin formation (KRECKE, 1964; BRAIN et al., 1967).

Hemolysate produced *in vitro* has an activity similar to that of platelet factor 3 (QUICK et al., 1954). In addition, an activity against the contact factors of the coagulation system can be ascribed to the membranes of the lysed erythrocytes (QUICK et al., 1954). A third activity of hemolyzed blood is inhibition of the activation of prothrombin (WALTHER, 1956), which has been confirmed by TRIANTAPHYLLOPOULOS (1971) and can be attributed to the presence of free hemoglobin. In this event, hemoglobin inhibits the activation of the contact factors of blood coagulation (TRIANTAPHYLLOPOULOS, 1971).

a) Mechanically Induced Hemolysis

Results obtained with the infusion of hemolyzed blood or components of hemolyzed blood allow an unequivocal assessment of the significance of hemolysis. The infusion of hemoglobin solutions that are free of cell stroma and lipid components has no effect on intravascular coagulation or kidney function tests; neither are there any toxic effects on liver or lungs (RABINER et al., 1967; BIRNDORF and LOPAS, 1970; RELIHAN and LITWIN, 1972). A wide variety of experimenters have failed to observe any activation of intravascular coagulation when autologous or homologous hemolyzed blood is given to dogs or rabbits by slow infusion (LANGDELL and HEDGPETH, 1959; JACOBI et al., 1971; HOCKE et al., 1973). It makes no difference whether the cells are hemolyzed by freezing and thawing of the blood or by ultrasonic treatment. Even the infusion of distilled water does not produce any signs of intravascular coagulation in rabbits (SLAASTAD and EIKA, 1973).

RABINER and FRIEDMAN (1968), working with dogs, as well as BIRNDORF et al. (1971), working with monkeys, obtained completely different results, as the authors mentioned above. RABINER and FRIEDMAN (1968) injected a large amount (10 ml/kg) of autologous hemolyzed blood within one minute, and observed changes in the coagulation system such as are typical of generalized intravascular coagulation. Pretreatment of the animals with carbon particles to block the reticulo-endothelial system led to a further intensification of generalized intravascular coagulation. In a similar way, BIRNDORF et al. (1971) induced generalized intravascular coagulation and renal failure by infusing ultrasonically treated autologous erythrocytes. It is important in this connection that the infusion of the erythrocyte stroma or ultrasonically treated erythrocytes respectively was given within the very short time of 5 min. This infusion of ultrasonically treated erythrocyte suspension raised the plasma hemoglobin concentration from 13 mg/100 ml to 2,200 mg/100 ml. Only under these extreme conditions, which led to circulatory shock and insome cases to death immediately after transfusion, was it possible to measure changes in the coagulation system such as are typically seen in generalized intravascular coagulation. Furthermore, in an account of the studies by BIRNDORF et al. (1971) and those of RABINER and FRIEDMAN (1968) it must be borne in mind that the animals were fully anesthetized, which would itself accelerate intravascular coagulation. Intravascular hemolysis obviously activates intravascular coagulation only when a shock syndrome develops at the same time. Shock is known to activate intravascular coagulation (HARDAWAY, 1966).

On the assumption that intravascular coagulation with formation of microclots in the peripheral blood vessels only comes about when the fibrinolytic system is inhibited and the alpha-adrenergic system stimulated at the same time as intravascular coagulation is activated (MÜLLER-BERGHAUS and MCKAY, 1968; MÜLLER-BERGHAUS, 1969), autologous blood hemolyzed by freezing and thawing was infused into rabbits in a concentration of 1 g hemoglobin equivalent/kg body weight over two hours. Under these experimental conditions the plasma hemoglobin level rose to 1,200 mg/100 ml (HOCKE et al., 1973). Even the additional infusion of EACA to inhibit activiation of fibrinolysis and norepinephrine to localize microclots in the peripheral blood vessels was not followed by the generation of microclots in small blood vessels (HOCKE et al., 1973; MÜLLER-BERGHAUS et al., 1973a). Obviously mechanically induced hemolysis cannot initiate generalized intravascular coagulation unless the cell stroma is administered in such large amounts that circulatory reactions follow and coagulation is activated by these reactions; this is known to happen in states of shock (HARDAWAY, 1966).

b) Immunologically Induced Hemolysis

Hemolysis induced by transfusions of incompatible blood or blood components should be distinguished from hemolysis induced by mechanical means. Generalized intravascular coagulation with the formation of microclots is described regularly in various species of animal after transfusion of incompatible blood or components of blood (LANDOIS, 1875; MCKAY et al., 1955; HARDAWAY et al., 1956; LANGDELL and HEDGPETH, 1959; SAMET and BOWMAN, 1961; LOPAS and BIRNDORF, 1971). JANZARIK et al. (1971) were also able to produce massive hemolysis and generalized intravascular coagulation in rabbits by means of injections of anti-rabbit erythrocyte serum. All these immunologically induced forms of hemolysis differ from those elicited by mechanical means in the development of massive intravascular coagulation. It must be considered very probable that the immune reaction by itself leads to activation of intravascular coagulation (see Section D.I.2.). In a comparative trial based on the model described by MCKAY and MÜLLER-BERGHAUS (1968) and MÜLLER-BERGHAUS (1969), the procoagulant activities compared were released by an intravascular immune reaction or by a mechanically induced hemolysis. Generalized intravascular coagulation with the generation of microclots in small blood vessels was produced only in the case of the immune reaction (MÜLLER-BERGHAUS and MUELLER-ECKHARDT, 1970; MUELLER-ECKHARDT and MÜLLER-BERGHAUS, 1971), while the hemolysis induced by mechanical means led to neither generalized intravascular coagulation nor the formation of microclots despite an identical experimental set-up (HOCKE et al., 1973).

c) Secondary Hemolysis after Formation of Microclots

A third connection between hemolysis and generalized intravascular coagulation consists in the occurrence of hemolysis after experimentally induced generalized intravascular coagulation with formation of microclots. Hemolysis, which according to BRAIN et al. (1962) as well as BULL and BRAIN (1968) is conditioned by intravascular formation of fibrin, is regularly observed after the infusion of tissue thromboplastin, endotoxin or Liquoid (BRAIN et al., 1967; BRAIN and HOURIHANE, 1967; BENNETT et al., 1968; EVENSEN and JEREMIC, 1970; SLAASTAD and JEREMIC, 1973; BELLER and THEISS, 1973). Fragmentocytes (schistocytes) are thought to result from the distortion and fragmentation of erythrocytes on the fibrin strands (BULL and BRAIN, 1968; BULL and KUHN, 1970).

3. Platelets

Incubation of platelet-rich rabbit plasma with endotoxin, the substance most frequently used in the study of generalized intravascular coagulation, results in platelet aggregation and the release of serotonin and platelet factor 3 into the surrounding medium (DES PREZ et al., 1961; HOROWITZ et al., 1962). Although extensive investigations of the effects of endotoxin on platelets are available, the chain of reactions culminating in the release of serotonin and platelet factor 3 is not known (for references see DES PREZ and MARNEY, 1971). Complement factors are involved in the reaction between platelets and endotoxin as well as calcium ions (GEWURZ et al., 1968; SANDBERG et al., 1975; for references see MERGENHAGEN et al., 1969). The release of serotonin (5-hydroxytryptamine), epinephrine, histamine, and adenosine nucleotides observed after the interaction of endotoxin and platelets can also be initiated by thrombin (for references see ARDLIE and HAN, 1974), by the contact of platelets with collagen (BOUNAMEAUX, 1961; ZUCKER and BORRELLI, 1962; for further references see VERMYLEN et al., 1970), epinephrine (O'BRIEN, 1964), by serotonin (MITCHELL and SHARP, 1964), by vasopressin (HASLAM and ROSSON, 1972), by large molecules (LÜSCHER et al., 1973), by antigen-antibody complexes (DAVEY and LÜSCHER, 1968; for references see PFUELLER and LÜSCHER, 1972), and, most importantly, by ADP (HELLEM, 1960; GAARDNER et al., 1961).

a) Activation of Intravascular Coagulation

Even though there is no doubt of the significance of platelets in the acceleration of blood clotting *in vitro*, the significance of platelets in the initiation of intravascular coagulation has not yet been unequivocally explained. When endotoxin is given by intravenous injection it becomes fixed on the surface of platelets, and also on that of leukocytes, within minutes (HERRING et al., 1963; BRAUDE et al., 1955). As little as 15 to 30 sec after the intravenous injection of endotoxin a fall in platelet counts and the release of serotonin into the plasma are observed (SHIMAMOTO et al., 1958a; DAVIS et al., 1960, 1961). The fall in platelet counts after endotoxin injection cannot be prevented by treating the animals with high doses of heparin, even if the activation of intravascular coagulation is suppressed (CORRIGAN, 1970).

Thrombocytopenia is a familiar observation after intravenous injection of endotoxin (Fig. 34) (STETSON, 1951; MCKAY and SHAPIRO, 1958; SHIMAMOTO et al., 1958a; KLEINMAIER, 1959). In addition, damage to the platelets becomes manifest *in vivo*, as the platelets that remain in the circulation have lost the major part of their content like platelets which have passed a release reaction

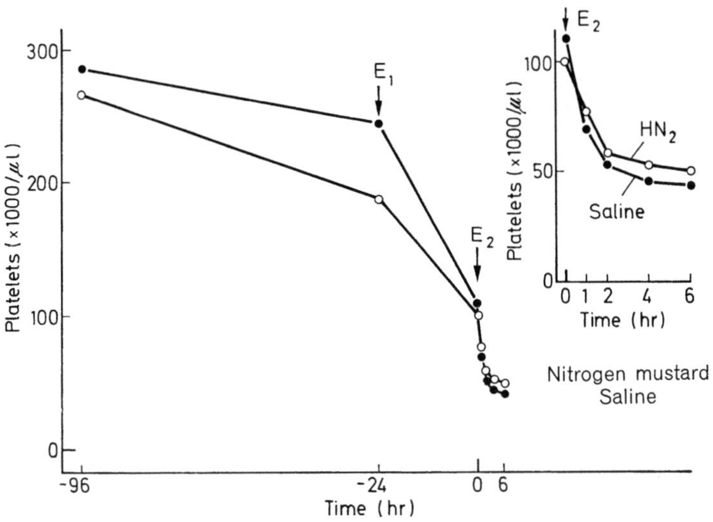

Fig. 34. Changes in mean platelet counts after 2 i.v. injections of endotoxin (E_1, E_2; 2× 150 μg) into nitrogen mustard (HN_2)- or saline-pretreated rabbits. *Inset:* higher magnification illustrates changes after second dose of endotoxin. Each curve represents 10 animal experiments. Curves after second endotoxin injection do not differ significantly from each other. The drop in platelet counts after endotoxin injections is independent of activation of intravascular coagulation, since nitrogen mustard-pretreated rabbits did not show generalized intravascular coagulation after endotoxin administration. (From MÜLLER-BERGHAUS, G., and ECKHARDT, T., 1975)

(LASCH et al., 1960; WEBER et al., 1963). Platelet factor 3 activity can be detected in the plasma after the administration of endotoxin by injection (HOROWITZ et al., 1962).

The platelet factor 3 activity released from platelets after the administration of endotoxin, and also after infusion of thrombin or thromboplastin, represents the most powerful procoagulant activity of the platelets. It was, therefore, felt that the infusion of platelet factor 3 would yield some insight into the role of this factor in the activation of intravascular coagulation. However, the infusion of purified platelet factor 3 or of phospholipid mixtures with a similar composition to platelet factor 3 did not produce intravascular coagulation with microclot formation in either rats or monkeys (MÜLLER-BERGHAUS et al., 1967b; MCKAY et al., 1969). In these studies the amount of platelet factor 3 activity injected into each animal was equivalent to 260 or 420% of that normally present in an animal, and the animals were prepared for the generation of microclots in the renal glomerular capillaries by the administration of Thorotrast, EACA, or the combination of EACA and norepinephrine (Table 6 and 7). The administration of platelet factor 3 alone produces no activiation of intravascular coagulation worth mentioning, as EPSTEIN and QUICK already showed in 1953. EVENSEN and JEREMIC (1970) obtained similar results when they infused homologous "frozen-thawn" platelets to rabbits pretreated with Thorotrast; they were unable to induce any glomerular microclots. The authors did, however, observe an increased elimination rate of radio-labelled fibrinogen in rabbits pretreated with Thorotrast. These studies do not offer any conclusive proof of the significance of platelet factor 3 in the precipitation of intravascular coagulation, as it was not possible to produce any microclots with this experimental set-up, and as even the particulate com-

Table 6. Incidence of renal glomerular microclots in rabbits prepared by various agents. "Provoking" dose of endotoxin was substituted by different platelet factor 3 activities. (From MÜLLER-BERGHAUS, G. et al., 1967b)

Preparation (a)	Provocation (b)	Time between (a) and (b) hrs	Dose of provocation: Absolute amount	Dose of provocation: Relative amount of total platelet factor 3 activity	Duration of provoking infusion	Rabbits No.	Rabbits with glomerular thrombi No.
Thorotrast	Endotoxin	24	0.05 mg	—	—	6	4
Thorotrast	Inosithin	24	10 ml	85%	15 min	3	0
Thorotrast	Platelet factor 3	24	50 ml	50%	4 hrs	2	0
Thorotrast	Platelet factor 3	24	50 ml	100%	4 hrs	1	0
Thorotrast	Endotoxin	4	0.05 mg	—	—	11	11
Thorotrast	Thrombofax	4	30 ml	260%	2 hrs	4	0
Thorotrast	Inosithin	4	30 ml	260%	3 hrs	5	0
Endotoxin	Endotoxin	24	0.2 mg	—	—	12	11
Endotoxin	Thrombofax	24	30 ml	260%	2 hrs	4	0

ponents of platelet fragments alone could produce a very slight activation of intravascular coagulation, or the materials that make up the content of the platelets, as vasoactive amines, could impair the permeability with a consequent effect on the elimination rate of fibrinogen.

MÜLLER-BERGHAUS and LOHMANN (1974) attempted to gain an insight into the part played by platelet factor 3 in the initiation of intravascular coagulation by performing experiments on rabbits with a congenital deficiency of the sixth component of the complement system (C6). The platelets of animals with C6 deficiency cannot release platelet factor 3 after the addition of endotoxin to platelet-rich plasma (BROWN and LACHMANN, 1973). In the same way an injection of endotoxin does not result in the release of platelet factor 3 into the plasma in these animals, as it occurs in normal animals (BROWN and LACHMANN, 1973). In the decisive experiment, generalized intravascular coagulation with a fall in the platelet count and in the activity of both Factors V and VII was observed following the infusion of endotoxin into rabbits with C6 deficiency just as in normal animals (MÜLLER-BERGHAUS and LOHMANN, 1974). The same percentage of C6-deficient

Table 7. Effect of inosithin on occurrence of renal glomerular microclots in rabbit simultaneously infused with EACA and norepinephrine. Amount of inosithin infused represents 420% platelet factor 3 activity normally available in rabbit. In the control, inosithin was substituted by ellagic acid which activates Hageman factor. (Data from MCKAY, D. G. et al., 1969)

Ellagic acid	Inosithin	Epsilon-aminocaproic acid (EACA)	Norepinephrine	No. of rabbits	Incidence of glomerular microclots[a]
—	+	+	+	12	0/12
+	—	+	+	20	11/20

[a] Expressed as number of positive results over total number of rabbits studied.

Table 8. Incidence of renal glomerular microclots in normal and homozygous C6-deficient rabbits after i.v. infusion of endotoxin or saline. (From MÜLLER-BERGHAUS, G., and LOHMANN, E., 1974)

	Normal rabbits	Normal rabbits	C6-deficient rabbits
Treatment	Saline	Endotoxin	Endotoxin
Incidence of glomerular microclots[a]	0/10	8/10	9/10

[a] Expressed as number of positive results over total number of rabbits studied.

animals developed the generalized Shwartzman reaction with fibrin-rich microclots in the renal glomerular capillaries and formation of bilateral renal cortical necroses (Table 8). These studies do not exclude involvement of the platelets in generalized intravascular coagulation, but merely show that the first step in the activiation of intravascular coagulation is not initiated by platelet factor 3. If the coagulation process is already triggered the platelets can certainly assist in the further course of the coagulation process by acting as an accelerator, as the platelets of C6-deficient animals exhibit the same behavior as those of normal animals in relation to thrombin. The investigations of SLABBER et al. (1972) underline that platelets are of little importance in the initiation of intravascular coagulation. These authors were able to provoke a full-strength generalized Shwartzman reaction in rabbits even when the animals had been pretreated with platelet aggregation inhibitors, and by that treatment platelet counts did not fall after endotoxin administration in the same way as they did in normal animals. There is one important finding, however, that should not be overlooked in a discussion on the role of platelets with reference to the initiation of generalized intravascular coagulation. MARGARETTEN and McKAY (1969b) were able to prevent the generalized Shwartzman reaction by pretreating the animals with a platelet antiserum when the platelet count had fallen to extremely low values. The significance of the immune reaction in the production of thrombocytopenia should not be ignored in these investigations, as there may be cross-reactions with leukocytes or with the complement system.

Investigations with Liquoid support the assumption that platelets have little significance in the initiation of generalized intravascular coagulation. When thrombocytopenia was induced by pretreatment of the animals with busulphan, generalized intravascular coagulation with the generation of microclots was elicited despite platelet counts of below 9,000/μl (EVENSEN and JEREMIC, 1968).

b) Precipitation of Soluble Fibrin

LIPINSKI et al. (1968) as well as LIPINSKI and JELJASZEWICZ (1969) proposed the hypothesis that platelets play a part in the second phase of the generation of microclots, i.e. the precipitation and/or polymerization of soluble fibrin, in addition to accelerating the intravascular coagulation process. This is thought to come about by way of the release of basic proteins from the platelets; these proteins are known to be capable of precipitating soluble fibrin (LIPINSKI et al., 1968; KOPEC et al., 1968). It seems that particular significance in the precipitation of soluble fibrin is ascribed to platelet factor 4, which has a heparin-neutralizing effect (LIPINSKI et al., 1968). Platelet factor 4 is released from platelets during the release reaction (NIEWIAROWSKI et al., 1968) and can be detected in

Table 9. Effect of busulphan-induced thrombocytopenia or nitrogen mustard-induced granulocytopenia on precipitation of soluble fibrin by endotoxin. (Data from MÜLLER-BERGHAUS, G., and ECKHARDT, T., 1975; ECKHARDT, T., and MÜLLER-BERGHAUS, G., 1975)

	Thrombo-cytopenia	Control	Granulo-cytopenia	Control
No. of rabbits	10	9	10	13
Mean platelet counts (cells/μl)	7,992	305,000	—	—
Mean relative PMN counts (% of total WBC)	—	—	0–2	52.8
Incidence of glomerular microclots[a]	8/10	5/9	9/10	8/13

[a] Expressed as number of positive results over total number of rabbits studied.

the plasma in the course of generalized intravascular coagulation and of the generalized Shwartzman reaction (LIPINSKI et al., 1968; FUSTER et al., 1973). The significance of platelet factor 4 and other basic proteins released from platelets in the precipitation of circulating soluble fibrin was tested by ECKHARDT and MÜLLER-BERGHAUS (1975) in the generalized Shwartzman reaction following endotoxin (Table 9). It was found that circulating soluble fibrin was precipitated after endotoxin injection, even in animals with very low platelet counts (8,000/μl). Experiments showing that the endotoxin-induced precipitation of circulating soluble fibrin cannot be prevented by treating the animals with high doses of heparin have furnished a further indication that the heparin-neutralizing activity of the basic proteins is of little significance in this connection (MÜLLER-BERGHAUS and HOCKE, 1972, 1973).

The heparin-neutralizing activity released after platelet aggregation does not appear when animals are pretreated with acetylsalicylic acid (O'BRIEN et al., 1970). When rabbits received acetylsalicylic acid before the infusion of endotoxin it was not possible to prevent the generalized Shwartzman reaction (SLABBER et al., 1972). This observation also stresses that platelets and platelet factor 4 have little significance in the induction of the generalized Shwartzman reaction.

4. Leukocytes

The fall in neutrophilic leukocyte counts after the intravenous administration of endotoxin was first observed by SANARELLI (1924), and later by SHWARTZMAN and GERBER (1948) as well as STETSON (1951). Fig. 2 shows a typical leukocyte curve after the first and the second injection of endotoxin, as they were reported by THOMAS and GOOD (1952b). Particularly striking features of the curve are the rapid decline in leukocyte counts to values of less than 2,000/μl within 30 min after endotoxin injection, and the development of leukocytosis 24 hrs later. There is ample documentation of the observation that granulocytes are the principal target cells for endotoxin in the circulating blood, both in man and in various species of animal (for references see CLINE et al., 1968). Intravenous injection of small amounts of endotoxin regularly leads to a fall in the numbers of circulating granulocytes and is followed by rebound granulocytosis. The fall in leukocyte counts after the injection of endotoxin is independent of the coagulation system, as is seen from its occurrence even in animals pretreated with heparin to prevent the generalized Shwartzman reaction (GOOD and THOMAS, 1953).

THOMAS and GOOD (1952b) recognized the particular importance of granulocytes in the development of the generalized Shwartzman reaction following endotoxin. They showed that endotoxin does not provoke the generalized Shwartzman reaction when granulocytopenia has been induced in the animals by pretreatment with nitrogen mustard. The number of granulocytes before the second, provoking injection of endotoxin is the decisive factor. Treatment of the animals with nitrogen mustard can also prevent the induction of the generalized Shwartzman reaction by cortisone and endotoxin or Thorotrast and endotoxin (see Section D.I.1.) (THOMAS and GOOD, 1952a; GOOD and THOMAS, 1952; LERNER et al., 1968b). Pretreatment of the animals with nitrogen mustard does not prevent Liquoid from provoking the generalized Shwartzman reaction, however (THOMAS et al., 1955a). HORN and SPICER (1964, 1965) extended the concept of THOMAS et al. (1954, 1955b) when they detected sulfated acid mucopolysaccharides thought to have originated from the circulating leukocytes in the microclots together with a fibrinogen derivative.

The second theory on the role of the granulocytes in the generalized Shwartzman reaction was proposed by HORN and COLLINS (1968a, 1968b; for references see HORN, 1973). The authors postulated that granulocytes release a procoagulant substance if the cells are destroyed in the pulmonary capillaries by the action of endotoxin. According to HORN and COLLINS (1968a), the first injection of endotoxin induces leukocytosis, which raises the potential of granulocytes and thus the procoagulant activity that can be released from the granulocytes. The authors were able to support their hypothesis by an experiment showing that the infusion of peritoneal granulocytes into granulocytopenic animals restores their susceptibility to the development of the generalized Shwartzman reaction. HORN and COLLINS (1968a) obtained similar results when instead of granulocytes they administered the 400 ×g supernatant fraction of disrupted exudate granulocytes, which is rich in granulocyte granules, to the animals by *intra-aortal* infusion.

Other investigators' conclusions on the role of the granulocytes in the induction of the generalized Shwartzman reaction by endotoxin have been rejected by WENDT et al. (1967). According to their observations these authors claimed that the generalized Shwartzman reaction could be induced even in granulocytopenic animals if the injection of endotoxin was given four days after the administration of nitrogen mustard and not three days after. In this connection it should be mentioned that the authors assessed granulocytopenia before the first injection of endotoxin. Analysis of the findings of WENDT et al. (1967) obtained prior to the second injection of endotoxin reveals that granulocytopenia certainly did prevent the occurrence of the generalized Shwartzman reaction in these studies too. These results do not justify the authors' conclusions that the occurrence of the generalized Shwartzman reaction is not dependent on granulocyte counts, as at the time animal experiments were begun, i.e. 120 or 144 hrs after the administration of nitrogen mustard, the bone marrow has recovered the capacity for producing granulocytes (HERION et al., 1965).

The effect of nitrogen mustard in preventing the occurrence of the generalized Shwartzman reaction has been attributed to a possible influence of the drug on platelets. SMITH et al. (1968), however, were unable to produce the generalized Shwartzman reaction even in granulocytopenic animals whose platelet level was raised by transfusions of platelets, so that there can be no doubt about the findings of THOMAS and GOOD (1952a), especially as these findings have also been confirmed by more recent studies (FORMAN et al., 1969; GAYNOR, 1973; MÜLLER-BERGHAUS and ECKHARDT, 1975).

a) Activation of Intravascular Coagulation

Various authors have described a minimal procoagulant activity of leukocytes (LISIEWISZ, 1966a, 1966b; MCKAY et al., 1967a; RAPAPORT and HJORT, 1967; ERDOGAN, 1968; KOCIBA et al., 1972). When lysates of peritoneal leukocytes were infused to animals "prepared" for the generalized Shwartzman reaction by pregnancy, EACA, Thorotrast, cortisone or bacterial endotoxin, the leukocyte lysates did not provoke the reaction (MCKAY et al., 1967a). The detailed investigations of NIEMETZ (1969), NIEMETZ and FANI (1970, 1971, 1973), LERNER et al. (1971a, 1971b) as well as NIEMETZ (1972) revealed findings that proved the procoagulant activity of the leukocytes beyond all doubt. In particular, these authors were able to show that peritoneal leukocytes of rabbits develop thromboplastic activity *in vitro* when the cells are incubated with endotoxin in the presence of serum or plasma at 37°C. The increased activity after incubation with endotoxin can be more than ten times the initial activity. In view of the biological properties it is taken for granted that the procoagulant activity of the leukocytes corresponds to that of tissue thromboplastin. KOCIBA et al. (1972) were also able to release an activity similar to that of tissue thromboplastin when they incubated serum with canine peritoneal leukocytes or leukocytes taken from the peripheral blood of dog. Furthermore, the procoagulant activity of the leukocytesis increased many times, if platelet membranes are present in the reaction mixture at the same time (NIEMETZ and MARCUS, 1974).

If leukocytes with this procoagulant activity are intra-aortally infused together with endotoxin into rabbits, generalized intravascular coagulation occurs and the glomerular capillaries are lined with fibrin (NIEMETZ and FANI, 1971, 1973; KOCIBA and GRIESEMER, 1972). A striking feature of these studies is the observation that the infusion of leukocytes activated by endotoxin only leads to the generalized Shwartzman reaction if the infusion is given into the aorta, and not when the intravenous route is used, even though intravenous infusion of leukocytes does initiate generalized intravascular coagulation (KOCIBA and GRIESEMER, 1972).

The procoagulant activity of leukocytes, which is equivalent to that of tissue thromboplastin, has led, by analogy, to the conclusion that leukocytes are "thrombogenic". The studies of LERNER et al. (1974) have shown, however, that the formation of a thrombus in experimental venous thrombosis is not in any way dependent on the presence of leukocytes. This makes it clear that the formation of microclots in the generalized Shwartzman reaction has a different pathogenic mechanism than the development of thrombi on the vessel walls. The material in the renal glomerular capillaries should therefore not be referred to as microthrombi, but always as microclots.

b) Precipitation of Soluble Fibrin

In addition to their procoagulant activity leukocytes appear to have another role in the production of the generalized Shwartzman reaction. THOMAS et al. (1954, 1955b) suspected that the development of microclots in the renal glomerular capillaries comes about by way of a precipitation process. According to this theory, highly charged polymers are released from granulocytes, which may precipitate an altered fibrinogen caused by endotoxin (THOMAS et al., 1955b). In the current system of nomenclature, the fraction that THOMAS et al. (1954, 1955b) called heparin-precipitable protein can be equated with soluble fibrin (soluble fibrin monomer complexes). According to *in vitro* studies by KOPEC et al.

(1968, 1970) and HAWIGER et al. (1969), cellular basic proteins or lysosomal protein fractions of leukocytes are thought to precipitate soluble fibrin, which generates after thrombin has acted on the fibrinogen molecule. The soluble fibrin monomer complexes are also referred to by SHAINOFF and PAGE (1960, 1962) as cryoprofibrin or cryofibrinogen. In the generalized Shwartzman reaction and after the administration of endotoxin it was possible to detect these soluble fibrins in the circulating blood (SHAINOFF and PAGE. 1960; LIPINSKI et al., 1968; MÜLLER-BERGHAUS and HOCKE, 1973; MÜLLER-BERGHAUS and LOHMANN, 1974).

Certain cytoplasmic granules which are present in small numbers in neutrophilic granulocytes can increase substantially in number after endotoxin-induced leukocytosis (HORN and SPICER, 1964). It seems possible that these acid mucopolysaccharides are released from the granules after an injection of endotoxin, and precipitate soluble circulating fibrin. More recent investigations by ECKHARDT and MÜLLER-BERGHAUS (1974) and MÜLLER-BERGHAUS and ECKHARDT (1975) make it seem unlikely, however, that granulocytes are involved in the precipitation of soluble fibrin; for these authors showed that endotoxin produces precipitation of soluble fibrin, which was induced by infusion of the snake venom ancrod, even in animals with granulocytopenia (Table 9). Whether or not thrombin-induced soluble fibrin is also precipitated in the presence of leukocytes after injection of endotoxin has yet to be confirmed.

5. Vessel Wall

An intact vascular endothelium means a nonthrombogenic surface. Gaps between endothelial cells and endothelial defects are quickly filled up with blood platelets (MAJNO and PALADE, 1961; BAUMGARTNER et al., 1967). These adhere to the subendothelial structures (the basal membranes and other components of connective tissue). According to this, the endothelial surface is regarded as the first thrombogenic surface to come in contact with the circulating blood and thus initiate thrombosis. Apart from the effect of the subendothelial surface on the platelets (BOUNAMEAUX, 1961; HUGUES, 1962; WILNER et al., 1971), it is also possible for collagen and the subendothelial structures to activate surface-active plasma factors (NIEWIAROWSKI et al., 1965; WILNER et al., 1968). According to BAUMGARTNER'S studies (1973), the speed of the bloodstream also affects the reaction between subendothelial surface and platelets, or formation of fibrin. BAUMGARTNER'S experiments were concerned with the formation of thrombi adhering to the vascular wall, a pathologic phenomenon whose pathogenesis must be recognized to be completely separate from that of the formation of microclots.

The role of the endothelium in the initiation of generalized intravascular coagulation was examined by APITZ as long ago as 1934. He thought, on the basis of his observations, that damage to the vascular wall must be regarded as a primary cause of the changes observed after the injection of endotoxin into rabbits. In subsequent years, however, damage to the vascular wall was found to be demonstrable only in cases where there was a concomitant occurrence of microclots, so that cause and effect could not be distinguished. BRUNSON et al. (1955a) and PAPPAS et al. (1958) indicated that changes in the vascular wall can be detected by either light microscope or electron microscope examination before any fibrinoid material is deposited.

MCKAY et al. (1966) published a chronologic study on the occurrence of changes in the microcirculation after the administration of endotoxin to pregnant rats. The first changes visible under the electron microscope are aggregation and sequestration of the platelets in the pulmonary microcirculation; these phenomena are detected 15 min after the administration of endotoxin. One hour after the injection of endotoxin there are aggregates of polymorphonuclear leukocytes in the lungs, and in some parts there are destroyed leukocytes with released nuclear fragments and specific granules in the surrounding plasma. No fibrin strands are yet found at this point, at least according to the report by McKAY et al. (1966). Changes that might be connected with intravascular coagulation cannot be observed until two hours after the injection of endotoxin, when they are visible under the electron microscope. At this point fine fibrin strands are detected between platelets in lungs and liver. According to these studies by McKAY et al. (1966), the changes of the endothelial layer are secondary to platelet aggregation and the formation of fibrin in the microcirculation. The v. Kupffer's cells in the liver are obviously an exception, as they are swollen as little as one hour after the injection of endotoxin.

The theory that the generalized Shwartzman reaction might be triggered by primary changes to the vessel wall was not taken up again until 30 years after APITZ's studies (1934). Functional changes were observed in the endothelium of the aorta after the administration of endotoxin to rabbits. Even 15 to 30 min after the injection of endotoxin, these vascular segments had a higher procoagulant activity than the aortae of control animals (MÜLLER-BERGHAUS and LASCH, 1963). On the basis of these investigations the authors set up the hypothesis that activation of the coagulation system is initiated by damage to the vessel wall. This theory is supported by the findings of RUBINSTEIN et al. (1962), who found a cumulation of endotoxin in the vessel wall after injection of this bacterial toxin. The functional changes in the vessel wall described by MÜLLER-BERGHAUS and LASCH (1963) may reflect a release of procoagulant material from the endothelial cells and/or indicate that agglutination and aggregation of platelets and leukocytes have already taken place on the changed vessel wall.

The changes observed in the vessel wall 15 min after endotoxin injection (MÜLLER-BERGHAUS and LASCH, 1963) are matched by changes in the ultrastructure. HOFF et al. (1967) were the first to describe very early changes in the arterial walls after the injection of endotoxin. These authors found electron-dense particles in intra-endothelial vacuoles, in their opinion representing endotoxin. The morphologic studies of McGRATH and STEWART (1969) also revealed severe damage to the endothelial cells after injection of endotoxin, which occurred as early as one hour after the injection, i.e. at a point when functional changes in the vessel wall are also observed (MÜLLER-BERGHAUS and LASCH, 1963). The significance of the changes in the vessel wall in generalized intravascular coagulation is also supported by the studies of GAYNOR et al. (1970), who detected endothelial damage in the aorta with the electron microscope 30 to 60 min after the administration of endotoxin. At the same time, an increased number of circulating endothelial cells was found in the blood, correlating in the opinion of GAYNOR et al. (1970) with the vessel wall defect. Circulating endothelial cells are observed at the earliest 5 min after the injection of endotoxin. Damage to the vessel wall is apparent as little as 30 min after an injection of endotoxin, as HOFF et al. (1967) have described, and its occurrence cannot be prevented by the administration of heparin to the animals for anticoagulation (GAYNOR et al., 1970). This shows that the endothelial damage is a primary effect of endotoxin and develops independently of the coagulation system. More recent studies by GAYNOR (1973) are particularly interesting; they show that the damage to the vessel wall arises after the administration of endotoxin even in animals pretreated with nitrogen mustard. It seems obvious that the neutropenia induced by nitrogen mustard

Table 10. Incidence of renal glomerular microclots after infusion of thrombin into EACA-treated and normal rats. (Data from MARGARETTEN, W., et al., 1964)

Duration of infusion (min)	Total dose of thrombin (units)	EACA	Time sacrificed (hrs)	Incidence of glomerular microclots[a]
30	36– 40	−	0	6/6
30	36– 40	−	1	0/6
180	215–250	−	24	0/5
120	144–160	+	24	9/14

[a] Expressed as number of positive results over total number of rats studied.

does not prevent damage to the vessel wall, even though neutropenia does block the activation of intravascular coagulation after endotoxin injection (see Section F.II.4.). The importance of the thromboplastic activity of the vessel wall as the only activator of intravascular coagulation is also diminished by the findings of GARNER and EVENSEN (1974). They found that intravascular coagulation can be initiated by intraaortal infusion into Factor-VII deficient dogs even though the activation of coagulation was not as pronounced as in normal dogs. The studies in Factor-VII deficient animals are of great importance since Factor VII is the essential plasma factor for activation of thromboplastin-mediated activation of coagulation. All these studies considerably diminish the significance of vessel wall damage in the initiation of intravascular coagulation, unless we assume that leukocytes react with the vessel wall that has been damaged by endotoxin and that it is secondarily "activated" leukocytes that trigger the intravascular coagulation process.

On the basis of the studies of GAYNOR et al. (1970), it seems conceivable that circulating soluble fibrin precipitated after endotoxin injection (MÜLLER-BERGHAUS and HOCKE, 1972, 1973) finds a point for precipitation or polymerization in the vessel wall defect.

Injection of Liquoid is also followed by changes in the vessel wall which might be responsible for the activation of intravascular coagulation. Morphologic studies have not yielded any direct indication as to whether the damage to the vessel wall is caused by a direct effect of Liquoid or whether it is a secondary effect resulting from deposits of microclots that are rich in cells and fibrin (KRECKE, 1964; SKJØRTEN and EVENSEN, 1972). A 14-fold increase in the number of endothelial cells synthetizing DNA has been described after the injection of Liquoid (EVENSEN and SHEPRO, 1973), which gives further proof of massive endothelial damage but does not explain the causal connection with the occurrence of the damage to the vessel wall.

III. Fibrinolytic System

1. Activation of the Fibrinolytic System

MARGARETTEN et al. (1964) were the first to state the significance of fibrinolysis in the occurrence of microclots (Table 10). When nonpregnant rats were defibrinated by means of infusions of thrombin, it was possible to detect fibrin deposits in the renal glomerular capillaries immediately after thrombin infusion. When the animals were allowed to survive until one hour after thrombin infusion, the fibrin deposits had disappeared in nonpregnant animals, while fibrin clots were demonstrable in pregnant rats. When the nonpregnant rats were treated with the fibrinolysis inhibitor EACA in addition to the thrombin infusion, microclots were found in the glomerular capillaries 24 hrs after the infusion of thrombin, even in the nonpregnant animals. These studies allow the conclusion that the body can dissolve microclots in the renal glomerular capillaries but that this break-down mechanism for fibrin is at least partially inhibited during pregnancy (see Section F.VII.).

The elimination of fibrin from the kidney was demonstrated by BELLER et al. (1969) in the rabbit. These authors infused endotoxin over 14 hrs and then removed the left kidney; examination of this organ revealed microclots in the glomerular capillaries. If no further infusion of endotoxin was given, and if the animals were sacrificed 34 hrs later, no fibrin was demonstrable in the right kidney. As microclots develop simultaneously in both kidneys, these experiments prove that the body can spontaneously lyse microclots that have developed. The studies of GRAEFF et al. (1968) show that this is achieved by way of a local fibrinolytic activity. When these authors applied histochemical methods to the estimation of plasminogen tissue activator, they found that the tissue activator is no longer demonstrable in the outer medullary zone of the kidney when microclots have developed in the course of generalized intravascular coagulation. It is not known whether the reduction in the level of plasminogen activator should be attributed to inhibition or to consumption of the activator.

The demonstration of local fibrinolytic activity in the kidney leads to the assumption that fibrinolytic degradation products occur in the circulation and possibly contribute to the hemorrhagic diathesis as antithrombins or inhibitors of fibrin polymerization. NIEWIAROWSKI and KOWALSKI (1958) and TRIANTAPHYLLOPOULOS (1958) have shown in *in vitro* studies that fibrinogen derivatives that develop under the influence of plasmin have antithrombin properties. MÜLLER-BERGHAUS et al. (1963a, 1963b), however, did not find any disturbance of clot formation after two injections of endotoxin into rabbits that could be explained as interference caused by fibrinogen derivatives. The experiments indicate that secondary hyperfibrinolysis cannot decisively explain a hemorrhagic diathesis following the administration of endotoxin into rabbits, even when the euglobulin lysis time is minimally prolonged after the injection of endotoxin (LIPINSKI et al., 1968). Small amounts of fibrinolysis degradation products can be detected after the injection of endotoxin into rabbits by means of the more sensitive staphylococcal clumping test (FONG et al., 1974). After giving endotoxin by infusion, GRAEFF et al. (1968) observed a lowering of the plasminogen level, while the serum level of fibrinolysis split products rose only minimally (GRAEFF and BELLER, 1968).

Obviously, the changes in the fibrinolytic system after endotoxin administration are less pronounced in rabbits than in rats. PHILLIPS et al. (1968) observed a pronounced reduction of the plasminogen level after endotoxin injection as well as after thrombin infusion in pregnant and in nonpregnant rats. These results correspond with those of BELLER and THEISS (1973) who observed an increase in fibrinolysis split products after endotoxin administration to the rat.

2. Inhibition of the Fibrinolytic System

LEE (1962) simultaneously gave thrombin and EACA by infusion or endotoxin by injection and EACA by infusion to rabbits, and was able by these means to produce the generalized Shwartzman reaction. LEE interpreted his experiments and their results as an indication that EACA inhibits the phagocytic function of the reticulo-endothelial system and that the fibrin circulating after endotoxin injection or thrombin infusion is thus not adequately eliminated from the circulation (see Section D.I.1.f.). The significance of the fibrinolytic system in the development of the generalized Shwartzman reaction was first recognized by MARGARETTEN et al. (1964), when they showed that there was a causal connection between the inhibition of fibrinolysis by EACA and the preservation of microclots. These authors demonstrated that the generalized Shwartzman reaction can be evoked in the nonpregnant rat by infusion of thrombin and EACA. The generalized Shwartzman reaction is also produced by a single injection of endotoxin in the nonpregnant rat in which the fibrinolytic system is inhibited by the administration of EACA (PHILLIPS et al., 1968). The administration of the proteinase inhibitors aprotinin, soya bean trypsin inhibitor or ovomucoid protects experimentally induced microclots in rabbits from proteolysis, so that the animals develop the generalized Shwartzman reaction (BELLER et al., 1967).

MARGARETTEN et al. (1964) showed that the mechanism for degradation of fibrin in the kidney is impaired during pregnancy. This is in keeping with the observation made by EPSTEIN et al. (1968), that the tissue activator acitvity in the kidney is reduced during pregnancy. Therefore, there is some inhibition of the fibrinolytic system during pregnancy, which explains why pregnancy "prepares" the body for the induction of the generalized Shwartzman reaction by a single injection of endotoxin.

Inhibition of the fibrinolytic system is an essential mechanism in the generation of microclots. After the administration of endotoxin the lytic activity in the renal cortex is reduced in rabbits (LIPINSKI et al., 1968; BERGSTEIN and MICHAEL, 1973a).

Inhibition of the fibrinolytic activity in the renal tissue can be observed both after the first injection of endotoxin and after the second (BERGSTEIN and MICHAEL, 1973a). When the fibrin slide technique was used, no fibrinolytic activity was measured in the kidney even as little as one hour after endotoxin injection. Fibrinolytic activity was detected again in the kidney 24 hrs after a single injection of endotoxin. BERGSTEIN and MICHAEL (1973b) used the same technique, and were also able to observe an inhibition of the lytic activity in the renal cortex after the administration of Thorotrast, while injections of cortisone caused no inhibition. These studies were performed to examine the mechanism of action of Thorotrast and cortisone, as both substances "prepare" the body for the generalized Shwartzman reaction (see Section D.I.1.).

IV. Complement

1. Complement and Endotoxin

Increasing importance has been attached to the role of the complement system in generalized intravascular coagulation in recent years, as studies performed by different groups have shown that the complement system plays the part of a mediator in different reactions, not only after the administration of immune complexes or antisera, but also after the injection of endotoxin. The interactions of complement and endotoxin have been described in a review by MERGENHAGEN et al. (1969). PILLEMER et al. (1955) observed an inactivation of complement by lipopolysaccharides of gram-negative bacteria *in vitro*. GEWURZ et al. (1968) demonstrated that the inactivation of complement is really caused by consumption of individual components of complement. These authors observed consumption of all six terminal components of complement when guinea-pig serum was incubated with endotoxin, whereas only minimal consumption of components C1, C4, and C2 was recorded. In the same way, GILBERT and BRAUDE (1962) found a reduction of the complement level after the injection of endotoxin into the rabbit. The interactions between endotoxin and complement can themselves cause changes in the coagulation process, the reactivity of the vascular wall, the permeability and the platelet aggregation, as well as neutrophilic chemotaxis (for references see MERGENHAGEN et al., 1969; PFUELLER and LÜSCHER, 1972).

2. Complement and Generalized Intravascular Coagulation

The bearing of the complement system on intravascular coagulation came very much to the forefront of discussion when the experiments of ZIMMERMAN and MÜLLER-EBERHARD (1971) were published. These authors described a complement-dependent activation of *in vitro* coagulation initiated by bacterial endotoxin, and suggested that the activation of intravascular coagulation by endotoxin comes about by way of the alternate pathway of complement activation (GEWURZ et al., 1968).

Contradictory observations have been recorded under *in vivo* conditions. According to studies by POLÁK and TURK (1969), the local Shwartzman reaction occurs even when the level of total hemolytic activity of the complement is lowered by means of an antilymphocyte serum. The local Shwartzman reaction is suppressed, however, by an antiserum acting mainly against the third component of the complement system. According to the investigations of FONG and GOOD (1971), when rabbits are treated with cobra venom factor, both the local and the generalized Shwartzman reactions can be prevented. Cobra venom factor causes hypocomplementemia, which is conditioned mainly by the reduction in C3 activity (COCHRANE et al., 1970). BERGSTEIN and MICHAEL (1974) are not in agreement with FONG and GOOD (1971). They also induced hypocomplementemia by the administration of cobra venom factor, but were not able to prevent the occurrence of the generalized Shwartzman reaction after endotoxin by this means. They attribute the discrepancy between their results and those of FONG and GOOD (1971) to the use of different methods in the preparation of the cobra venom factor (BERGSTEIN and MICHAEL, 1974). It should be borne in mind during this discussion that apart from its effects on the complement system, cobra venom factor also affects the functions of the normal platelets (DODDS and PICKERING, 1972).

In an attempt to resolve the discrepancy between these two studies, MÜLLER-BERGHAUS and LOHMANN (1974) conducted investigations in rabbits with a congenital deficiency of the sixth component of the complement system (C6) (see Table 8). It was shown that the generalized Shwartzman reaction can be induced by infusion of endotoxin in these C6-deficient animals just as in normal animals, which proves that at least components C6 to C9 are not involved in the induction of the generalized Shwartzman reaction by endotoxin. Although generalized intravascular coagulation progresses in the same way in C6-deficient as in normal animals, the C6-deficient animals are particularly sensitive to endotoxin and die after much lower doses of endotoxin (JOHNSON and WARD, 1971).

The behavior of the platelets and leukocytes of C6-deficient animals after the administration of endotoxin is particularly interesting. Neither platelet counts nor leukocyte counts are any different from those seen in normal animals (MÜLLER-BERGHAUS and LOHMANN, 1974), from which it may be concluded that at least these parameters are unaffected by any interference with the reactions of blood cells and endotoxin. The fall in platelet counts during the infusion of endotoxin may not be conditioned by a direct effect of endotoxin on platelets but may reflect intravascular formation of thrombin, since BROWN and LACHMANN (1973) report that the immediate reaction of the platelets after endotoxin injection is disturbed in C6-deficient animals. According to these authors, the release of platelet factor 3 does not take place after intravenous administration of endotoxin (BROWN and LACHMANN, 1973); this confirms the findings of MÜLLER-BERGHAUS et al. (1967b), who observed that a primary release of platelet factor 3 does not lead to activation of intravascular coagulation with development of the generalized Shwartzman reaction.

V. Reticulo-Endothelial System

GOOD and THOMAS (1952) as well as SMITH et al. (1953) showed that if the phagocytic function of the reticulo-endothelial system (RES) had been inhibited by Thorotrast or trypan blue, a single injection of endotoxin is capable of inducing the generalized Shwartzman reaction. It was thought at first that the impaired function of the RES prevented elimination and inactivation of endotoxin (BEESON, 1947a; CREMER and WATSON, 1957; THOMAS, 1957; BENACERRAF and SEBESTYEN, 1957). BEESON (1947a, 1947b) observed in fact that after the administration of Thorotrast, animals that had built up a tolerance to endotoxin reacted to it again and developed the local Shwartzman reaction. Tolerance to endotoxin was achieved by BEESON (1947a, 1947b) by the administration of several doses of endotoxin.

Particular interest was aroused in the RES after the publication of reports by BRAUDE et al. (1955) and DOERING et al. (1965) indicating that the endotoxin given by injection was taken up by RES cells. When animals are pretreated with cortisone or X-ray irradiation, endotoxin is taken up by the RES in the normal way, but the decomposition and elimination of endotoxin by the RES is impaired (CREMER and WATSON, 1957). Thorotrast has a different mechanism of action. In contrast to cortisone, Thorotrast prevents endotoxin from being taken up into the cells of the RES. Thorotrast as well as cortisone are used to prepare the body for the generalized Shwartzman reaction (see Section D.I.1.).

The phagocytic function of the RES is limited only briefly after endotoxin injection (BENACERRAF and SEBESTYEN, 1957). As little as 24 hrs after the administration of endotoxin, the RES is able to eliminate carbon particles from the plasma at normal speed, or even better than before the injection. Thus the phagocytic function of the RES is restored to normal before the second injection of endotoxin. If the RES has any significance in the development of the generalized Shwartzman reaction, it lies in the concept that a RES with an impaired phagocytic function no longer effects an adequate elimination of activated coagulation factors (plasma Factors VII, IX, and X, as well as fibrinogen-fibrin intermediates) from the circulation. LASCH and RÓKA (1954), SPAET et al. (1961) and DEYKIN (1966) have shown that the RES is an important regulator in the phase of hypercoagulability, when activated coagulation products are released in the circulation (LASCH et al., 1957, 1958). LEE and MCCLUSKEY (1962) and PROSE et al. (1965) have shown in experiments with rabbits that the RES can eliminate fibrinogen derivatives from the bloodstream. On the basis of these findings, it is thought possible that animals could be "prepared" for the generalized Shwartzman reaction by thrombin administered by infusion (RODRÍGUEZ-ERDMANN, 1964a). Findings published by GOOD and THOMAS (1953) suggest that the inhibition of phagocytosis by coagulation products has no significance in the induction of the generalized Shwartzman reaction, however. These authors showed that heparinization before the first injection of endotoxin does not prevent the occurrence of the generalized Shwartzman reaction. If the coagulation process after the first injection had any effect on the phagocytic function of the RES, the prevention of intravascular coagulation following the first injection of endotoxin should prevent the appearance of the generalized Shwartzman reaction after the second injection of endotoxin. The studies of Pechet et al. (1969) also suggest that there is no connection between the activation of intravascular coagulation and the phagocytic function of the RES. Other investigations by Good and Thomas (1952) disclaim any significance of the RES, as substances such as glycogen and starch, which inhibit the RES, cannot be used instead of Thorotrast as a "preparatory" injection for the induction of the generalized Shwartzman reaction. The mechanism of action of substances that "prepare" animals for the induction of the generalized Shwartzman reaction by so-called inhibition of the RES must therefore be explained in some other way. Thus McGehee et al. (1966) and Levin and Beck (1966) showed that Thorotrast has a pronounced activating effect on the coagulation system as well as an inhibitory effect on the fibrinolytic system. Bergstein and Michael (1973b) reached a similar interpretation, as they observed a lowering of the fibrinolytic activity in the renal cortex after Thorotrast. Thus, the findings published to date cannot offer adequate documentation of any involvement of the RES (in the form of inhibited phagocytosis) in the induction of the generalized Shwartzman reaction. On the contrary, Fisher (1967) has come to the conclusion that more rapid uptake of endotoxin into the RES and slower disposal of endotoxin lodged in the RES contribute to the induction of the generalized Shwartzman reaction.

VI. Localizing Factors

1. Polymerization and Precipitation of Soluble Fibrin

If microclots are formed in the peripheral bloodstream in the course of intravascular coagulation, the distribution of the fibrin deposits is generally not homogeneous. The intensity of the formation of microclots can vary widely, both from one organ to another and within a single organ. As, in addition, there is no direct connection between an injury to the vessel wall and the occurrence of microclots, it seems unlikely in view of the concept on the pathogenesis of thrombus formation that microclots are formed by way of the development of thrombi adhering to the vessel walls. If endotoxin is given by intravenous injection, the formation of fibrin is certainly visible, but the fibrin strands are not fixed to the endothelium but floating freely in the plasma, as electron microscope studies reveal (McKay and Müller-Berghaus, 1967). It is not possible, then, to decide whether visible fibrin develops actually in the capillaries when intravascular coagulation processes are in progress, whether circulating soluble fibrin (soluble fibrin monomer complexes) polymerizes to visible fibrin in the capillaries, or whether fibrin strands are spread into the capillaries and deposited there as emboli. Studies by various experimenters make it seem likely that the activation of intravascular coagulation is generalized throughout the vascular system but that the formation of microclots is a disseminated process. It has been suggested that the disseminated formation of microclots is caused by "localizing factors".

Table 11. Incidence of renal glomerular microclots in rabbits treated with ancrod, endotoxin, and heparin in different combinations. Heparin cannot prevent microclot formation. (From MÜLLER-BERGHAUS, G., and HOCKE, M., 1972)

Treatment	No. of rabbits	Incidence of glomerular microclots[a]
Ancrod, —, —	10	0/10
Ancrod, endotoxin, —	10	8/10
—, endotoxin, —	10	0/10
Ancrod, endotoxin, heparin	10	7/10

[a] Expressed as number of positive results over total number of rabbits studied.

There are two stages in the development of microclots (MÜLLER-BERGHAUS and HOCKE, 1972, 1973):

1. The coagulation system has to be activated so that fibrin monomers are generated, which remain in the circulation due to the formation of soluble fibrin monomer complexes (soluble fibrin). These complexes can be eliminated from the circulation with no damage to the healthy body (MÜLLER-BERGHAUS and HOCKE, 1973);
2. When soluble fibrin cannot be adequately eliminated from the circulation it forms microclots at certain preferred points (MÜLLER-BERGHAUS and HOCKE, 1973; MÜLLER-BERGHAUS et al., 1973b; LIPINSKI et al., 1974b). This second stage may explain why the formation of microclots is a local process and varies from one organ to another.

The formation of soluble fibrin throughout the circulation, in conjunction with the absence of primary parietal fibrin thrombi, leads us to suspect that the activation of intravascular coagulation is generalized. Polymerization and/or precipitation of soluble fibrin can occur when the concentration of fibrin monomers exceeds a certain critical value (MÜLLER-BERGHAUS et al., 1972c, 1973b; MÜLLER-BERGHAUS and HOCKE, 1973; LIPINSKI et al., 1974a, 1974b). In heparinized rabbits, i.e. when the formation of thrombin is inhibited, the infusion of large amounts of soluble fibrin leads to the development of microclots in the renal glomerular capillaries and in other organs (MÜLLER-BERGHAUS et al., 1973b; LIPINSKI et al., 1974b).

Polymerization and/or precipitation of soluble fibrin can be brought out by endotoxin itself (MÜLLER-BERGHAUS and HOCKE, 1972, 1973). In anticoagulated animals, which are fibrinemic but in which further intravascular formation of thrombin is suppressed by the administration of heparin, endotoxin given by injection induces the formation of microclots (Table 11). Thus endotoxin exerts a second effect pertinent to the formation of microclots as well as its procoagulant effect. The polymerization and/or precipitation of soluble fibrin induced by endotoxin is not dependent on the presence of platelets or leukocytes, since even in thrombocytopenic or granulocytopenic rabbits endotoxin precipitates soluble fibrin (see Table 9) (ECKHARDT and MÜLLER-BERGHAUS, 1974, 1975; MÜLLER-BERGHAUS and ECKHARDT, 1975). The second stage in the formation of microclots does not always take place, which is in keeping with the frequent observation of an activation of intravascular coagulation, as opposed to the rare occurrence of microclots in the peripheral blood vessels.

The rest of this Section will be devoted to a discussion of the effects of catecholamines, glucocorticoids, and ACTH as they relate to the localization of micro-

Table 12. Incidence of renal glomerular microclots in rabbits after single injection of endotoxin and following infusion of norepinephrine or saline (control). (From MCKAY, D. G,. et al., 1969)

Infusions	Endotoxin mg.	Rabbits No.	Incidence of glomerular microclots[a]
Norepinephrine	0.4	8	5/8
Saline	0.4	8	0/8

* Expressed as number of positive results over total number of rabbits studied.

Table 13. Incidence of renal glomerular microclots in rabbit after infusions of ellagic acid, EACA and norepinephrine in different combinations. (Data from MCKAY, D. G. et al., 1969)

Group	Ellagic acid	Epsilon-amino-caproic acid	Norepi-nephrine	Rabbits No.	Incidence of glome-rular microclots[a]
I	+	+	+	15	8/15
II	−	+	+	12	0/12
III	+	+	−	5	0/5
IV	+	−	+	12	0/12

[a] Expressed as number of positive results over toal number of animals studied.

clots. Other effects of different hormones are also known (for references see SELYE, 1966).

2. Catecholamines

The level of catecholamines in the circulating blood rises steadily after the administration of endotoxin (HEIFFER et al., 1960; GILBERT, 1960). When rabbits are made resistant to epinephrine, the generalized Shwartzman reaction no longer occurs (HALL et al., 1964). The significance of catecholamines is further emphasized by the studies by PALMERIO et al. (1962) and LAMBERT et al. (1969), who prevented the occurrence of renal cortical necrosis by unilateral renal sympathectomy in the denervated kidney only. In a similar way, pretreatment of pregnant rats with an alpha-adrenergic blocking agent such as dibenamine or dibenzyline reduces the occurrence of the generalized Shwartzman reaction (see Table 4) (MÜLLER-BERGHAUS and MCKAY, 1967; MÜLLER-BERGHAUS et al., 1967a). If catecholamines are infused together with endotoxin, the generalized Shwartzman reaction occurs after only a single injection of endotoxin (Table 12) (ZELLER et al., 1967; MCKAY et al., 1969). In addition, the generalized Shwartzman reaction can be produced with ellagic acid or sodium stearate only when norepinephrine is infused as well as the procoagulant (ellagic acid) and the inhibitor of fibrinolysis (EACA) (Table 13) (MCKAY and MÜLLER-BERGHAUS, 1968; MCKAY et al., 1969; MÜLLER-BERGHAUS, 1969). In the gastrointestinal tract, stimulation of the alpha-adrenergic receptor sites appears to result in microclots in the capillaries with higher frequency, while stimulation of the beta-receptors localizes the microclots in the arterioles (MCKAY et al., 1971b). The stimulus for coagulation in these experiments was an infusion of thrombin. Additional infusion of histamine led to the localization of microclots in the capillaries and venules of the gastrointestinal tract.

Table 14. Incidence of renal glomerular microclots in the rabbit after administration of ancrod, aprotinin, and norepinephrine in different combinations. Norepinephrine infusion causes precipitation of ancrod-induced soluble fibrin. (From MÜLLER-BERGHAUS, G., and MANN, B., 1973)

Treatment	Rabbits No.	Incidence of glomerular microclots[a]
Ancrod, aprotinin, norepinephrine	22	15/22
Ancrod, aprotinin, —	18	5/18
Ancrod, — , norepinephrine	12	1/12
— , aprotinin, norepinephrine	10	0/10

[a] Expressed as number of positive results over total number of rabbits studied.

The effect of catecholamines is based on stimulation of the alpha-receptors of the adrenergic system, which leads to vasomotor changes in the peripheral blood vessels. These changes in flow in the microcirculation are obviously the immediate cause of the precipitation and/or polymerization of soluble fibrin, as circulating soluble fibrin could be converted to microclots by an infusion of catecholamines (Table 14) (MÜLLER-BERGHAUS and MANN, 1973). The precipitation of soluble fibrin is independent of the coagulation, as treatment of the animals with heparin does not prevent the development of microclots in this model (MÜLLER-BERGHAUS and MANN, 1973).

3. Corticoids

The response of the adrenal cortex to endotoxin seems to be very significant in the pathogenesis of the generalized Shwartzman reaction, for the administration of cortisone 3 to 4 days before the injection of endotoxin prepares the body for the reaction so that a single injection of endotoxin induces the generalized Shwartzman reaction (THOMAS and GOOD, 1951, 1952a; D'ANGELO et al., 1959; McKAY and MERRIAM, 1960). The effect of cortisone in preparing for the Shwartzman reaction is attributed to an impaired function of the RES according to the ideas of THOMAS and GOOD (1951, 1952b) and McKAY and MERRIAM (1960). It also seems possible that cortisone exerts its effect by way of inhibition of the fibrinolytic activity (RENAUD et al., 1966; BERGSTEIN and MICHAEL, 1973b). It is also known that corticosteroids potentiate the effect of catecholamines on blood vessels (ZWEIFACH et al., 1953; LEPRI and CRISTIANI, 1964; for references see LATOUR and McKAY, 1970). Changes in the renal microcirculation are of about the same intensity after cortisone treatment as 24 hrs after the first injection of endotoxin (McKAY and MERRIAM, 1960). These vasomotor changes are of decisive importance in the development of microclots in the renal glomerular capillaries, as the generalized Shwartzman reaction is completely prevented when the adrenal glands are surgically removed between the first and second injections of endotoxin (LATOUR and McKAY, 1970). If adrenalectomized rabbits receive substitution treatment with hydrocortisone, it becomes possible to induce the generalized Shwartzman reaction again. In the same way, LATOUR and McKAY (1970) were able to demonstrate that substitution treatment of adrenalectomized rabbits with norepinephrine also restored their susceptibility to induction of the generalized Shwartzman reaction. Further studies by this group led to the conclusion that the effect of the corticosteroids comes about by way of stimulation of the alpha-adrenergic receptor sites, which is essential to the localization of microclots in the kidney (MÜLLER-BERGHAUS and McKAY, 1967; MÜLLER-BERGHAUS et al., 1967a; McKAY and MÜLLER-BERGHAUS, 1968; McKAY et al., 1969; MÜLLER-BERGHAUS, 1969). Investigations conducted by LATOUR et al. (1971) showed that glucocorticoids (cortisone, triamcinolone) are suited to the preparation of rabbits for the generalized Shwartzman reaction, but mineralocorticoids such as desoxycorticosterone do not have the necessary properties for this purpose. The effect normally obtained with glucocorticoids can be prevented by pretreatment of the test animals with the alpha-receptor blocker dibenzyline, which leads to the conclusion that glucocorticoids exert their effect by stimulating the alpha-adrenergic receptor sites (LATOUR et al., 1971).

Preparation for the generalized Shwartzman reaction by means of glucocorticoids is only successful when a fairly high dose of the corticoid is given to the animals for four days. Quite a different effect of steroids with glucosteroid activity is obtained if a single dose of cortisone, triamcinolone or dexamethasone is given by injection two hours before the provoking injection of endotoxin, i.e. before the second injection of endotoxin in the rabbit, or before a single one in the pregnant rat. In this situation it is possible to block the appearance of the generalized Shwartzman reaction (D'ANGELO et al., 1959; BIANCO et al., 1960; LATOUR et al., 1972). Neither adrenocorticotropic hormones nor any mineralocorticoids have this effect of glucocorticoids. Various possible explanations have been offered by the authors, but the exact mechanism of effect is not known.

4. Adrenocorticotropic Hormone

When given in two intravenous injections, endotoxin occasionally induces hemorrhage in the adrenal glands. This phenomenon is known as the Waterhouse-Friderichsen syndrome (GRONCHI and CARNIELLI, 1934; KLEINMAIER et al., 1959). Adrenal hemorrhage can also be induced by the administration of Thorotrast followed by a single injection of endotoxin four hours later (LEVIN and CLUFF, 1965b). A particularly interesting point is that in this model Thorotrast can be replaced by ACTH, when a subsequent injection of endotoxin induces hemorrhage in the adrenal cortex. The administration of heparin during endotoxemia, like the induction of granulocytopenia with nitrogen mustard, can prevent the occurrence of hemorrhage in the adrenal cortex (LEVIN and CLUFF, 1965b). According to this group's investigations, the hemorrhage in the adrenal cortex is dependent to a particular degree on the phase of activity of the adrenal cortex. As the changes in the coagulation system after the administration of endotoxin are not so definitely pronounced in animals "prepared" for adrenocortical hemorrhage by ACTH as in the classic generalized Shwartzman reaction, LEVIN and BECK (1966) concluded that the mechanism behind the pathogenesis of the hemorrhage in the adrenal cortex is different from the mechanism involved in the pathogenesis of the generalized Shwartzman reaction, and they questioned the role of intravascular coagulation in the pathogenesis of adrenocortical hemorrhage (LEVIN and CLUFF, 1965b; LEVIN and BECK, 1966). MARGARETTEN et al. (1965) were able to demonstrate the involvement of intravascular coagulation in the development of adrenocortical hemorrhage in a unambiguous experiment, however (Table 15). These authors were able to induce microclots and hemorrhage in the adrenal cortex of rats by simultaneous infusion of ACTH and thrombin, while necrosis of the renal cortex occurred in only one case in this experiment. This seems to prove unequivocally that a raised level of metabolic activity in the adrenal cortex localizes microclots in the adrenal cortex in the presence of fibrinemia.

Table 15. Incidence of adrenal hemorrhage after infusion of thrombin and corticotropin (ACTH) into rats. (Data from MARGARETTEN, W. et al., 1965)

Group	Treatment	No. of rats	Adrenal hemorrhage
1	Thrombin	10	0
2	Corticotropin	6	0
3	Corticotropin + thrombin	6	6

VII. Pregnancy

Pregnant animals are particularly susceptible to the development of generalized intravascular coagulation and also of the generalized Shwartzman reaction. A single injection of endotoxin induces the generalized Shwartzman reaction in the pregnant rabbit and the pregnant rat (APITZ, 1935; TAKEDA and TSUCHIYA, 1953; McKAY et al., 1960; WONG, 1962; KALEY et al., 1962; McKAY and WONG, 1963; RODRÍGUEZ-ERDMANN, 1964b). Generalized intravascular coagulation with microclots in the renal glomerular capillaries can be induced in the pregnant hamster by administration of colchicine but not by administration of endotoxin (GALTON, 1963, 1964, 1966). A single injection of colchicine also induces the generalized Shwartzman reaction in the pregnant rat (MÜLLER-BERGHAUS and OBST, 1972). The generalized Shwartzman reaction can also be induced by feeding a diet rich in oxidized cod liver oil and a low vitamin E content (McKAY and WONG, 1962a).

The trigger mechanism of generalized intravascular coagulation in pregnant animals is not known, but it is probably similar to that in nonpregnant animals. The pregnant uterus, including the placenta and fetuses, seems to play no part in the induction of generalized intravascular coagulation either after endotoxin injection or after administration of colchicine, as in pregnant animals subjected to hysterectomy the generalized Shwartzman reaction can be induced in the same way as in pregnant animals not subjected to hysterectomy (Table 16) (MÜLLER-BERGHAUS and SCHMIDT-EHRY, 1972; MÜLLER-BERGHAUS and OBST, 1972). The difference between a pregnant and a nonpregnant animal in this respect obviously lies in the conditioning factors of the so-called additional mechansims. MARGARETTEN et al. (1964) induced microclots by the infusion of thrombin in both pregnant and nonpregnant rats. The microclots only persisted for any length of time in the pregnant rats, however, which led the authors to conclude that fibrinolytic activity in the kidney is reduced during pregnancy. These findings were confirmed by EPSTEIN et al. (1968). These authors found lower fibrinolytic activity levels in the renal cortex in pregnant than in nonpregnant animals of

Table 16. Incidence of renal glomerular microclots after i.v. injection of endotoxin into pregnant rats hysterectomized on the 20th or 6th day of gestation as well as into sham-operated animals. (From MÜLLER-BERGHAUS, G., and SCHMIDT-EHRY, B., 1972)

	Hysterectomy	Sham operation	Hysterectomy
Day of gestation	20	20	6
Incidence of glomerular microclots[a]	13/18	5/6	0/6

[a] Expressed as number of positive results over total number of rats studied.

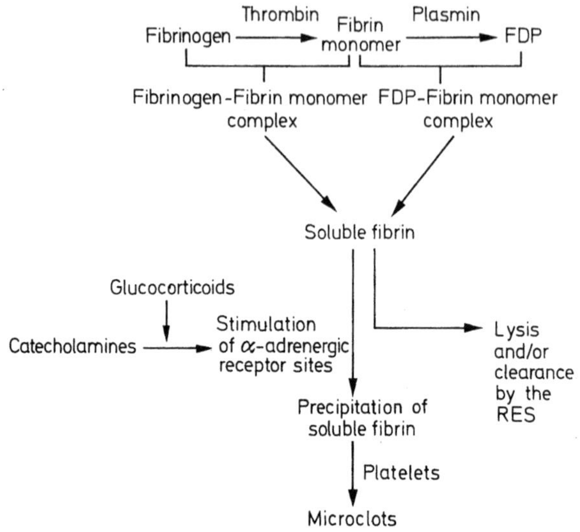

Fig. 35. Mechanisms for endotoxin-induced generation of renal glomerular microclots from soluble fibrin

various species. The RES seems to play no part in the preferential development of intravascular coagulation during pregnancy, however, as the phagocytic function of the RES tends to be better in pregnant than in normal animals (McKAY et al., 1964; WEXLER and KANTOR, 1966).

VIII. Theory of Pluricausality

The generalized Shwartzman reaction, defined as occlusion of the glomerular capillaries with fibrin-rich microclots persisting sufficiently long to lead to bilateral renal cortical necrosis, is a complex disorder of the microcirculation with changes in the coagulation system and gross impairment of fibrinolytic system and vasomotor apparatus. The development of microclots in the generalized Shwartzman reaction takes place in three reaction stages (MÜLLER-BERGHAUS and HOCKE, 1972; MÜLLER-BERGHAUS and LASCH, 1975):

1. The coagulation system has to be activated so that fibrin is formed and kept in solution by the development of soluble fibrin monomer complexes (soluble fibrin). These complexes can be eliminated from the circulation with no harm to a healthy body.

2. The soluble fibrin monomer complexes have to be precipitated in the renal glomerular capillaries to allow the generation of microclots. There, together with platelets which adhere to the fibrin strands, they thus form the typical microclots that can be detected by histologic or electron-microscopic examination.

3. The development of bilateral renal cortical necrosis requires that the microclots remain in the capillaries for some length of time and are not dissolved by fibrinolytic activity in the kidney. Reduced fibrinolytic activity in the kidney is therefore essential to the development of the generalized Shwartzman reaction.

These different pathophysiologic mechanisms involved in the development of the generalized Shwartzman reaction have been summed up in a theory of pluri-

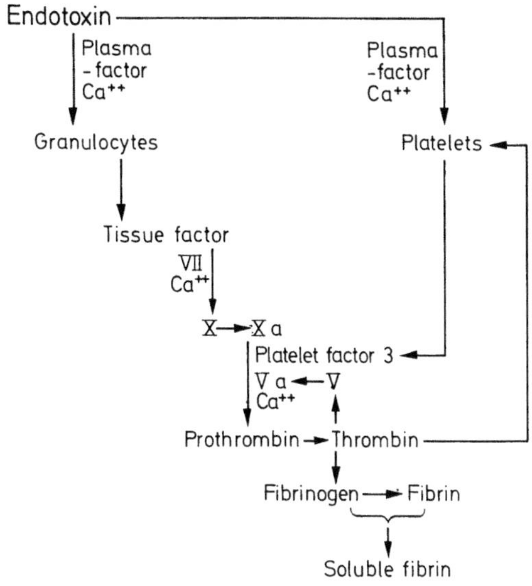

Fig. 36. Activation of generalized intravascular coagulation by endotoxin

causality (MÜLLER-BERGHAUS, 1969). Figure 35 illustrates the different events of pathogenetic reactions that lead to the generalized Shwartzman reaction after the administration of endotoxin. The changes following endotoxin are illustrated as an example since they are of great importance in clinical practice, and the pathophysiologic changes following the administration of endotoxin have been the subject of the most extensive investigations in animals.

1. Activation of Intravascular Coagulation

Generalized intravascular coagulation is central to the pathogenesis of the generalized Shwartzman reaction. In the presence of calcium and a plasma factor, endotoxin causes damage to the granulocytes and a release reaction (Fig. 36). The most important procoagulant released at this point is tissue thromboplastin, which activates the coagulation system by way of the extrinsic pathway. It is not possible to say whether the plasma factor is a complement factor. In a similar way endotoxin, together with calcium and a plasma factor, acts on platelets and initiates a release reaction. Platelet factor 3 is the component of platelet content that accelerates the coagulation, though it cannot be considered as the activator of coagulation. The real activator initiating generalized intravascular coagulation after endotoxin is the tissue thromboplastin released from the granulocytes. If thrombin is formed the system is further accelerated by means of a feedback mechanism. Thrombin itself acts on fibrinogen, and the fibrin monomers that develop form so-called soluble fibrin with the fibrinogen present in the plasma. The detection of soluble fibrin must be regarded as proof that intravascular coagulation has been activated.

2. Localization of Soluble Fibrin

A healthy body eliminates soluble fibrin from the circulation. Active fibrinolysis breaks down fibrin monomer into smaller fragments (fibrinolytic degradation

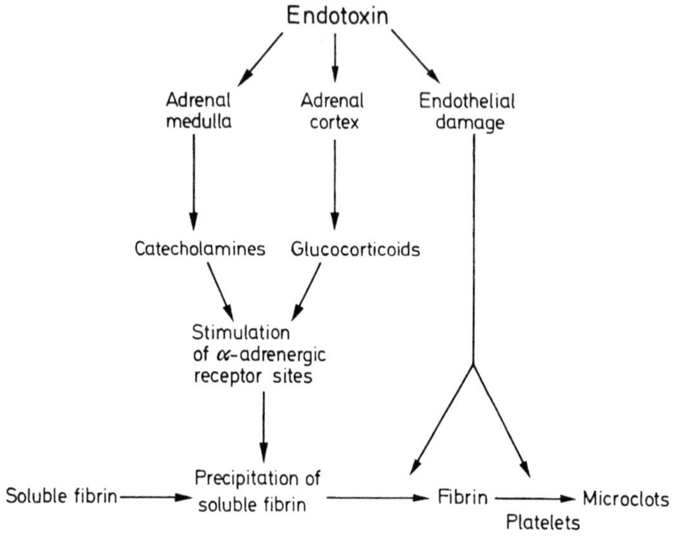

Fig. 37. Effects of endotoxin-induced adrenal stimulation and endothelial damage on precipitation of soluble fibrin

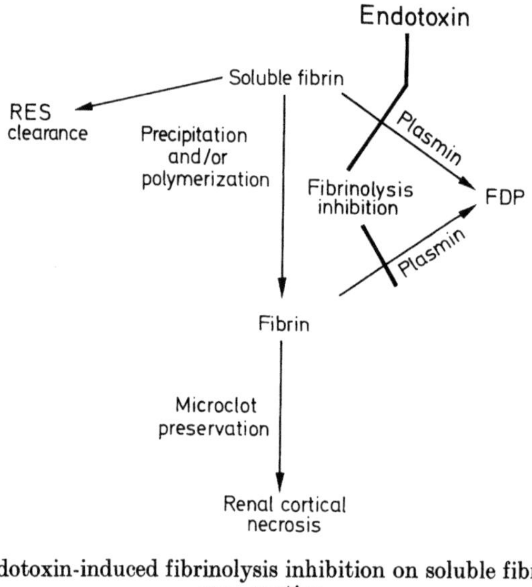

Fig. 38. Effect of endotoxin-induced fibrinolysis inhibition on soluble fibrin and on microclot preservation

products; FDP), which then form FDP-fibrin monomer complexes with further fibrin monomers. Before microclots generate in the renal glomerular capillaries, the soluble fibrin has to be precipitated or polymerized to long chains (Fig. 37). At this point fibrin can be detected by means of histologic and electron-microscopic examination. The precipitation of soluble fibrin in the renal glomerular capillaries is not dependent on either platelets or leukocytes, but it is caused by stimulation of the alpha-adrenergic receptor sites, which is brought about by interplay of catecholamines and glucocorticoids. No unequivocal statement is yet possible as to whether endothelial damage, which occurs independently of any activation of the coagulation system after the administration of endotoxin, is necessary to the generation of microclots.

3. Inhibition of the Fibrinolytic System

As the generation and lysis of soluble fibrin are subject to the laws of dynamics, any inhibition of fibrinolysis will limit the elimination of soluble fibrin from the circulation so that the level of soluble fibrin rises to a critical value in certain circumstances. If the critical concentration of soluble fibrin is exceeded, precipitation can follow as a result of this alone (MÜLLER-BERGHAUS et al., 1973b). Inhibition of fibrinolysis is also of decisive importance for the preservation of microclots in the glomerular capillaries, as ischemia and bilateral renal cortical necrosis develop only when the glomerular capillaries are occluded by microclots for some time (Fig. 38).

References

ALEXANDER, B., PECHET, L., KLIMAN, A.: Proteolysis, fibrinolysis, and coagulation. Significance in thrombolytic therapy. Circulation **26**, 596–611 (1962).

ALLARDYCE, D. B., GROVES, A. C.: Intravascular coagulation, hyperlipemia, and fatembolism: Their association during the generalized Shwartzman phenomenon in rabbits. Surgery **66**, 71–79 (1969).

APITZ, K.: Die Wirkung bakterieller Kulturfiltrate nach Umstimmung des gesamten Endothels beim Kaninchen. Virchows Arch. path. Anat. **293**, 1–33 (1934).

APITZ, K.: A study of the generalized Shwartzman phenomenon. J. Immunol. **29**, 255–266 (1935).

ARDLIE, N. G., HAN, P.: Enzymatic basis for platelet aggregation and release: The significance of the "platelet atmosphere" and the relationship between platelet function and blood coagulation. Brit. J. Haemat. **26**, 331–356 (1974).

BAUMGARTNER, H. R.: The role of blood flow in platelet adhesion, fibrin deposition, and formation of mural thrombi. Microvascular Res. **5**, 167–179 (1973).

BAUMGARTNER, H.-R., TRANZER, J.-P., STUDER, A.: An electron microscopic study of platelet thrombus formation in the rabbit with particular regard to 5-hydroxytryptamine release. Thrombos. Diathes. haemorrh. (Stuttg.) **18**, 592–604 (1967).

BEESON, P. B.: Tolerance to bacterial pyrogens. II. Role of the reticulo-endothelial system. J. exp. Med. **86**, 39–44 (1947a).

BEESON, P. B.: Effect of reticulo-endothelial blockade on immunity to the Shwartzman phenomenon. Proc. Soc. exp. Biol. (N. Y.) **64**, 146–149 (1947b).

BELL, W. R., MILLER, R. E., LEVIN, J.: Inhibition of the generalized Shwartzman reaction by hypofibrinogenemia. Blood **40**, 697–708 (1972).

BELLER, F. K., GRAEFF, H.: Deposition of glomerular fibrin in the rabbit after infusion with endotoxin. Nature (Lond.) **215**, 295–296 (1967).

BELLER, F. K., GRAEFF, H., GORSTEIN, F.: Disseminated intravascular coagulation during the continuous infusion of endotoxin in rabbits. Amer. J. Obstet. Gynec. **103**, 544–554 (1969).

BELLER, F. K., MITCHELL, P. S., GORSTEIN, F.: Fibrin deposition in the rabbit kidney produced by protease inhibitors. Thrombos. Diathes. haemorrh. (Suttg.) **17**, 427–439 (1967).

BELLER, F. K., THEISS, W.: Fibrin derivatives, plasma hemoglobin and glomerular fibrin deposition in experimental intravascular coagulation. Thrombos. Diathes. haemorrh. (Stuttg.) **29**, 363–374 (1973).

BENACERRAF, B., SEBESTYEN, M. M.: Effect of bacterial endotoxins on the reticuloendothelial system. Fed. Proc. **16**, 860–867 (1957).

BENNETT, J. M., YU, D., SUYEMOTO, J., PECHET, L.: The effects of infusing thrombin and its acetylated derivative. II. Observations on intravascular hemolysis with pathologic correlations. Thrombos. Diathes. haemorrh. (Stuttg.) **20**, 469–476 (1968).

BERGSTEIN, J. M., MICHAEL, A. F., JR: Renal cortical fibrinolytic activity in the rabbit following one or two doses of endotoxin. Thrombos. Diathes. haemorrh. (Stuttg.) **29**, 27–32 (1973a).

Bergstein, J. M., Michael, A. F., Jr.: The effect of Thorotrast and cortisone on renal cortical fibrinolytic activity in the rabbit. Amer. J. Path. **71**, 113–118 (1973b).

Bergstein, J. M., Michael, A. F., Jr.: Failure of cobra venom factor to prevent the generalized Shwartzman reaction and loss of renal cortical fibrinolytic activity. Amer. J. Path. **74**, 19–30 (1974).

Bianco, A. R., Mazzacca, G., D'Angelo, V.: Il desametazone e il fenomeno di Sanarelli-Shwartzman. Riv. Ist. sieroter. ital. **35**, 66–69 (1960).

Birndorf, N. I., Lopas, H.: Effects of red cell stroma-free hemoglobin solution on renal function in monkeys. J. appl. Physiol. **29**, 573–578 (1970).

Birndorf, N. I., Lopas, H., Robboy, S. J.: Disseminated intravascular coagulation and renal failure. Production in the monkey with autologous red blood cell stroma. Lab. Invest. **25**, 314–319 (1971).

Bleyl, U., Büsing, C. M., Graeff, H., Kuhn, W.: Perinatale Hämostase-Störung nach vorzeitiger Plazentarlösung. Virchows Arch. Abt. A **348**, 1–15 (1969a).

Bleyl, U., Büsing, C. M., Krempien, B.: Pulmonale hyaline Membranen und perinataler Kreislaufschock. Virchows Arch. Abt. A **348**, 187–204 (1969b).

Bleyl, U., Höpker, W. W.: Disseminierte intravasale Gerinnung und pulmonale hyaline Membranen bei connatalen cyanotischen Herzfehlern. Virchows Arch. Abt. A **350**, 225–239 (1970).

Bleyl, U., Kuhn, W., Graeff, H.: Retikuloendotheliale Clearance intravasaler Fibrinmonomere in der Milz. Thrombos. Diathes. haemorrh. (Stuttg.) **22**, 87–100 (1969d).

Bleyl, U., Sebening, H., Kuhn, W.: Morphologischer Nachweis von Fibrinmonomeren im histologischen Schnitt. Thrombos. Diathes. haemorrh. (Stuttg.) **22**, 68–86 (1969c).

Blombäck, M., Johansson, S.-A., Sjöberg, H.-E.: Coagulation factors and defibrination syndrome in anaphylaxis. Acta physiol. scand. **69**, 313–319 (1967).

Bohle, A., Krecke, H.-J., Miller, F., Sitte, H.: Über die Natur des sogenannten Fibrinoids bei der generalisierten Shwartzmanschen Reaktion. Elektronenmikroskopische Untersuchungen an Kaninchennieren. In: Immunopathologie, p. 339–350. I. Internat. Sympos. Basel/Seelisberg 1958. Basel: Schwabe, 1959.

Bohle, A., Sitte, H., Miller, F.: Elektronenmikroskopische Untersuchungen am Glomerulum des Kaninchens beim generalisierten Shwartzman-Phänomen. Verh. dtsch. path. Ges. **41**, 326–332 (1958).

Boivin, A., Mesrobeanu, I., Mesrobeanu, L.: Technique pour la préparation des polysaccharides microbiens spécifiques. C. R. Soc. Biol. (Paris) **113**, 490–492 (1933).

Bonameaux, Y.: L'accolement des plaquettes aux fibres sous-endotheliales. Thrombos. Diathes. haemorrh. (Stuttg.) **6**, 504–516 (1961).

Botti, R. E., Ratnoff, O. D.: Studies on the pathogenesis of thrombosis: An experimental "hypercoagulable" state induced by the intravenous injection of ellagic acid. J. Lab. clin. Med. **64**, 385–398 (1964).

Brain, M. C.: Microangiopathic haemolytic anaemia (MHA). Brit. J. Haemat. **23**, Suppl., 45–52 (1972).

Brain, M. C., Dacie, J. V., Hourihane, D. O'B.: Microangiopathic haemolytic anaemia: The possible role of vascular lesions in pathogenesis. Brit. J. Haemat. **8**, 358–374 (1962).

Brain, M. C., Esterly, J. R., Beck, E. A.: Intravascular haemolysis with experimentally produced vascular thrombi. Brit. J. Haemat. **13**, 868–891 (1967).

Brain, M. C., Hourihane, D. O'B.: Microangiopathic haemolytic anaemia: The occurrence of haemolysis in experimentally produced vascular disease. Brit. J. Haemat. **13**, 135–142 (1967).

Braude, A. I., Carey, F. J., Zalesky, M.: Studies with radioactive endotoxin. II. Correlation of physiologic effects with distribution of radioactivity in rabbits injected with lethal doses of E. coli endotoxin labelled with radioactive sodium chromate. J. clin. Invest. **34**, 858–866 (1955).

Brown, D. L., Lachmann, P. J.: The behaviour of complement and platelets in lethal endotoxin shock in rabbits. Internat. Arch. Allergy **45**, 193–205 (1973).

Brunson, J. G., Davis, R. L., Thomas, L.: Morphologic changes in rabbits following the intravenous administration of meningococcal toxin. III. The effects produced by endotoxin in association with certain high molecular weight acidic polymers. Amer. J. Path. **31**, 669–685 (1955c).

Brunson, J. G., Gamble, C. N., Thomas, L.: Morphologic changes in rabbits following the intravenous administration of meningococcal toxin. I. The effects produced in young and in mature animals by a single injection. Amer. J. Path. **31**, 489–499 (1955a).

Brunson, J. G., Thomas, L., Gamble, C. N.: Morphologic changes in rabbits following the intravenous administration of meningococcal toxin. II. Two appropriately spaced injections; the role of fibrinoid in the generalized Shwartzman reaction. Amer. J. Path. **31**, 655–667 (1955b).

BULL, B. S., BRAIN, M. C.: Experimental models of microangiopathic haemolytic anaemia. Proc. roy. Soc. Med. **61**, 1134–1137 (1968).

BULL, B. S., KUHN, I. N.: The production of schistocytes by fibrin strands (a scanning electron microscope study). Blood **35**, 104–111 (1970).

BUSCH, C., SALDEEN, T.: Amount of fibrin in different organs after intravenous, intraportal and intraaortal injection of thrombin in the rat. Thrombos. Diathes. haemorrh. (Stuttg.) **29**, 87–93 (1973).

CLINE, M. J., MELMON, K. L., DAVIS, W. C., WILLIAMS, H. E.: Mechanism of endotoxin interaction with human leucocytes. Brit. J. Haemat. **15**, 539–547 (1968).

COCHRANE, C. G., MÜLLER-EBERHARD, H. J., AIKIN, B. S.: Depletion of plasma complement *in vivo* by a protein of cobra venom: Its effect on various immunologic reactions. J. Immunol. **105**, 55–69 (1970).

COLLINS, R. D., ROBBINS, B. H., MAYES, C. E.: Studies on the pathogenesis of the generalized Shwartzman reaction. Production of glomerular thrombosis and renal cortical necrosis by intraaortic thrombin infusion in normal and leucopenic rabbits. J. Hopkins med. J. **122**, 375–379 (1968).

CONDIE, R. M., HONG, C. Y., GOOD, R. A.: Reversal of the lesions of the generalized Shwartzman phenomenon by treatment of rabbits with streptokinase. (Abstract) J. Lab. clin. Med. **50**, 803–804 (1957).

CONNOR, W. E., HOAK, J. C., WARNER, E. D.: The role of lipids in thrombosis. In: KOLLER, F., DUCKERT, F., STREULI, F. (eds.): Pathogenesis and treatment of thromboembolic diseases. p. 193–208. Stuttgart: Schattauer 1966.

CORRIGAN, J. J.: Effect of anticoagulating and non-anticoagulating concentrations of heparin on the generalized Shwartzman reaction. Thrombos. Diathes. haemorrh. (Stuttg.) **24**, 136–145 (1970).

CORRIGAN, J. J., JR., BELL, B. M.: Comparison between the polymyxins and gentamicin in preventing endotoxin-induced intravascular coagulation and leucopenia. Infect. Immun. **4**, 563–566 (1971).

CREMER, N., WATSON, D. W.: Influence of stress on distribution of endotoxin in RES determined by fluorescein antibody technic. Proc. Soc. exp. Biol. (N.Y.) **95**, 510–513 (1957).

CROWELL, J. W., READ, W. L.: In vivo coagulation—A probable cause of irreversible shock. Amer. J. Physiol. **183**, 565–569 (1955).

CROWELL, J. W., SMITH, E. E.: Effect of fibrinolytic activation on survival and cerebral damage following periods of circulatory arrest. Amer. J. Physiol. **186**, 283–285 (1956).

DAMUS, P. S., MARKLAND, F. S., JR., DAVIDSON, T. M., SHANLEY, J. D.: A purified procoagulant enzyme from the venom of the eastern diamond-back rattlesnake (Crotalus adamanteus): *In vivo* and *in vitro* studies. J. Lab. clin. Med. **79**, 906–923 (1972).

D'ANGELO, V., MAZZACCA, G., BIANCO, A. R.: Il cortisone e il fenomeno di Sanarelli-Shwartzman. Riv. Ist. sieroter. ital. **34**, 449–456 (1959).

DAVEY, M. G., LÜSCHER, E. F.: Release reactions of human platelets induced by thrombin and other agents. Biochim. biophys. Acta (Amst.) **165**, 490–506 (1968).

DAVIS, R. B., MEEKER, W. R., BAILEY, W. L.: Serotonin release by bacterial endotoxin. Proc. Soc. exp. Biol. (N. Y.) **108**, 774–776 (1961).

DAVIS, R. B., MEEKER, W. R., MCQUARRIE, D. G.: Immediate effects of intravenous endotoxin on serotonin concentrations and blood platelets. Circulat. Res. **8**, 234–239 (1960).

DENNIS, L. H., CONRAD, M. E.: Accelerated intravascular coagulation in a patient with Korean hemorrhagic fever. Arch. intern. Med. **121**, 449–452 (1968).

DENNIS, L. H., REISBERG, B. E., CROSBIE, J., CROZIER, D., CONRAD, D., CONRAD, M. E.: The original haemorrhagic fever: Yellow fever. Brit. J. Haemat. **17**, 455–462 (1969).

DES PREZ, R. M., HOROWITZ, H. I., HOOK, E. W.: Effects of bacterial endotoxin in rabbit platelets. I. Platelet aggregation and release of platelet factors *in vitro*. J. exp. Med. **114**, 857–873 (1961).

DES PREZ, R. M., MARNEY, S. R., JR.: Immunological reactions involving platelets. In: JOHNSON, S. A. (ed.): The circulating platelet, p. 415–471. New York-London: Academic Press 1971.

DEYKIN, D.: The role of the liver in serum-induced hypercoagulability. J. clin. Invest. **45**, 256–263 (1966).

DODDS, W. J., PICKERING, R. J.: Purified cobra venom factor: Effect on blood platelets. Proc. Soc. exp. Biol. (N. Y.) **140**, 429–434 (1972).

DOERING, P., CLEMENS, H., FRITZE, E.: Die Verteilung eines markierten Endotoxins im Organismus. Z. ges. exp. Med. **131**, 334–345 (1965).

ECKHARDT, T., MÜLLER-BERGHAUS, G.: Die Bedeutung der Granulocyten bei der intravasalen Präzipitation von löslichem Fibrin durch Endotoxin. Verh. dtsch. Ges. inn. Med. **80**, 1460–1463 (1974).

ECKHARDT, T., MÜLLER-BERGHAUS, G.: The role of blood platelets in the precipitation of soluble fibrin by endotoxin. Scand. J. Haemat. **14**, 181–189 (1975).
EGBERG, N., BLOMBÄCK, M., JOHNSSON, H., ABILDGAARD, U., BLOMBÄCK, B., DIENER, G., EKESTRÖM, S., GÖRANSSON, L., JOHANSSON, S.-A., MCDONAGH, J., MCDONAGH, R., NILSSON, S. E., NORDSTRÖM, S., OLSSON, P., WIMAN, B.: Clinical and experimental studies on reptilase. Thrombos. Diathes. haemorrh. (Stuttg.) Suppl. **47**, 379–387 (1971).
ENCKE, A., LASCH, H. G., PETERICH, I., SCHMIDT, H. D., SCHMIER, J.: Blood coagulation and fibrinolytic therapy in normotensive hemorrhagic shock of the dog. Z. Kreisl.-Forsch. **58**, 1298–1307 (1969).
ENCKE, A., PETERICH, I., SCHMIDT, H. D., SCHMIER, J.: Der Einfluß einer Fibrinolysetherapie auf die Überlebensquote im normotensiven hämorrhagischen Schock. Langenbecks Arch. klin. Chir. **316**, 677–680 (1966).
EPSTEIN, M. D., BELLER, F. K., DOUGLAS, G. W.: Kidney tissue activator of fibrinolysis in relation to pregnancy. Obstet. and Gynec. **32**, 494–504 (1968).
EPSTEIN, E., QUICK, A. J.: Effect of injecting platelet extract intravenously. Proc. Soc. exp. Biol. (N. Y.) **83**, 453–454 (1953).
ERDOGAN, G.: The thromboplastic activity of white blood cells. Blut **17**, 276–278 (1968).
EVENSEN, S. A., FOLLING ELGJO, R.: Antibody-induced platelet injury: Its potency as a trigger of intravascular clotting. Scand. J. Haemat. **9**, 61–72 (1972).
EVENSEN, S. A., FOLLING ELGJO, R., JORGENSEN, L., HUSBY, G.: Glomerular fibrin thrombi induced by antigen-antibody reactions: Protection by extreme thrombocytopenia. Microvasc. Res. **4**, 117–131 (1972).
EVENSEN, S. A., JEREMIC, M.: Intravascular coagulation with generalized Shwartzman reaction induced by Liquoid: Lack of protection by extreme thrombocytopenia. Thrombos. Diathes. haemorrh. (Stuttg.) **19**, 556–569 (1968).
EVENSEN, S. A., JEREMIC, M.: Platelets and the triggering mechanism of intravascular coagulation. Brit. J. Haemat. **19**, 33–46 (1970).
EVENSEN, S. A., JEREMIC, M., HJORT, P. F.: Intravascular coagulation with generalized Shwartzman reaction induced by a heparin-like anticoagulant (Liquoid). Thrombos. Diathes. haemorrh. (Stuttg.) **18**, 24–39 (1967).
EVENSEN, S. A., JEREMIC, M., HJORT, P. F.: Experimental thrombocytopenia induced by busulphan (Myleran) in rabbits: Extremely low platelet levels and intact plasma clotting system. Thrombos. Diathes. haemorrh. (Stuttg.) **19**, 570–577 (1968).
EVENSEN, S. A., SHEPRO, D.: Generalized Shwartzman reaction induced by Liquoid in the rat. Increased DNA-synthesis in aortic endothelium. Thrombos. Diathes. haemorrh. (Stuttg.) **30**, 347–351 (1973).
FINE, J., FRANK, E. D., RAVIN, H. A., RUTENBERG, S. H., SCHWEINBURG, F. B.: The bacterial factor in traumatic shock. New Engl. J. Med. **260**, 214–220 (1959a).
FINE, J., RUTENBURG, S., SCHWEINBURG, F. B.: The role of the reticulo-endothelial system in hemorrhagic shock. J. exp. Med. **110**, 547–569 (1959b).
FISHER, S.: Localization of radioiodinated endotoxin in organs of mice and rabbits: Effect of thorotrast, trypan blue, endotoxin and carbon administered intravenously. Nature (Lond.) **213**, 511–512 (1967).
FONG, J. S. C., GOOD, R. A.: Prevention of the localized and generalized Shwartzman reactions by an anticomplementary agent, cobra venom factor. J. exp. Med. **134**, 642–655 (1971).
FONG, J. S. C., ROTHER, K. O., GOOD, R. A.: The role of complement in localized Shwartzman reaction: Studies with congenitally C6-deficient rabbits. Clin. exp. Immunol. **16**, 77–88 (1974).
FORMAN, E. N., ABILDGAARD, C. F., BOLGER, J. F., JOHNSON, C. A., SCHULMAN, I.: Generalized Shwartzman reaction: Role of the granulocyte in intravascular coagulation and renal cortical necrosis. Brit. J. Haemat. **16**, 507–515 (1969).
FUSTER, V., KAZMIER, F. J., CASH, J. D., BOWIE, E. J. W., OWEN, C. A., JR.: Assay of platelet factor 4 in plasma. Mayo Clin. Proc. **48**, 103–106 (1973).
GAARDNER, A., JONSEN, J., LALAND, S., HELLEM, A., OWREN, P. A.: Adenosine diphosphate in red cells as a factor in the adhesiveness of human blood platelets. Nature (Lond.) **192**, 531–532 (1961).
GAGEL, C., LINDER, M., MÜLLER-BERGHAUS, G., LASCH, H. G.: Virus infection and blood coagulation. Thrombos. Diathes. haemorrh. (Stuttg.) **23**, 1–11 (1970).
GALTON, M.: Generalized Shwartzman reaction in the pregnant golden hamster. Science **139**, 923–924 (1963).
GALTON, M.: Studies of the generalized Shwartzman reaction in the pregnant golden hamster. Amer. J. Path. **44**, 613–627 (1964).
GALTON, M.: Thrombosis in the pregnant syrian hamster. Transact. N. Y. Acad. Sci. **28**, 423–438 (1966).
GANS, H., MATSUMOTO, K.: Are enteric endotoxins able to escape from the intestine? Proc. Soc. exp. Biol. (N. Y.) **147**, 736–739 (1974).

GARNER, R., EVENSEN, S. A.: Endotoxin-induced intravascular coagulation and shock in dogs: The role of Factor VII. Brit. J. Haemat. **27**, 655–668 (1974).

GAYNOR, E.: The role of granulocytes in endotoxin-induced vascular injury. Blood **41**, 797–808 (1973).

GAYNOR, E., BOUVIER, C., SPAET, T. H.: Vascular lesions: Possible pathogenetic basis of the generalized Shwartzman reaction. Science **170**, 986–988 (1970).

GERBER, I. E.: The Shwartzman phenomenon in the kidneys of rabbits. Observations on effects of intravenous administration of bacterial filtrates. Arch. Path. **21**, 776–796 (1936).

GEWURZ, H., SHIN, H. S., MERGENHAGEN, S. E.: Interactions of the complement system with endotoxic lipopolysaccharide: Consumption of each of the six terminal complement components. J. exp. Med. **128**, 1049–1057 (1968).

GILBERT, R. P.: Mechanisms of the hemodynamic effects of endotoxin. Physiol. Rev. **40**, 245–279 (1960).

GILBERT, V. E., BRAUDE, A. I.: Reduction of serum complement in rabbits after injection of endotoxin. J. exp. Med. **116**, 477–490 (1962).

GIROLAMI, A., AGOSTINO, D., CLIFFTON, E. E.: The effect of ellagic acid on coagulation *in vivo*. Blood **27**, 93–102 (1966b).

GIROLAMI, A., BRUNETTI, A., CELLA, G., PEDRAZZOLI, S., BERNARDI, R.: Disappearance of ellagic acid induced hypercoagulability in the dog after Trasylol administration. Thrombos. Diathes. haemorrh. (Stuttg.) **29**, 384–392 (1973).

GIROLAMI, A., CLIFFTON, E. E., AGOSTINO, D.: Hemorrhagic syndrome in dogs induced by intravenous thrombin. Thrombos. Diathes. haemorrh. (Stuttg.) **16**, 243–256 (1966a).

GIROLAMI, A., FIORETTI, D., CELLA, G., PEDRAZZOLI, G., BERNARDI, R.: The effect of fibrinolysis inhibitors on the ellagic acid activation of Hageman factor in the dog. Thrombos. Diathes. haemorrh. (Stuttg.) **26**, 557–564 (1971).

GLASER, E.: Die Bedeutung der intravaskulären Gerinnung für funktionelle und morphologische Organschädigungen unter besonderer Berücksichtigung von Lunge und Niere bei kontinuierlicher Endotoxin-Infusion. Tierexperimentelle Untersuchungen. Habil.-Schrift, S. 1–277. Gießen 1973.

GLASER, E., NEUHOF, H., HEY, D., OPPERMANN, C., LASCH, H. G.: Pathophysiologische Veränderungen im Endotoxinschock. Verh. dtsch. Ges. inn. Med. **77**, 157–161 (1971).

GODAL, H. C., ABILDGAARD, U.: Gelation of soluble fibrin in plasma by ethanol. Scand. J. Haemat. **3**, 342–350 (1966).

GOOD, R. A., THOMAS, L.: Studies on the generalized Shwartzman reaction. II. The production of bilateral cortical necrosis of the kidneys by a single injection of bacterial toxin in rabbits previously treated with Thorotrast or Trypan blue. J. exp. Med. **96**, 625–641 (1952).

GOOD, R. A., THOMAS, L.: Studies on the generalized Shwartzman reaction. IV. Prevention of the local and generalized Shwartzman reactions with heparin. J. exp. Med. **97**, 871–888 (1953).

GRAEFF, H., BELLER, F. K.: Hematological studies during endotoxin infusion in rabbits. Thrombos. Diathes. haemorrh. (Stuttg.) **20**, 420–429 (1968).

GRAEFF, H., BEZLER, H. M., IMMICH, H., KUHN, W.: Urokinase excretion during labor and in patients with disseminated intravascular coagulation sub partu. Int. J. Gynaec. Obstet. **9**, 141–151 (1971).

GRAEFF, H., HUGO, R. VON: Identification of fibrinogen derivatives in plasma samples. Thrombos. Diathes. haemorrh. (Stuttg.) **27**, 610–618 (1972).

GRAEFF, H., MITCHELL, P. S., BELLER, F. K.: Fibrinolytic enzyme system of the kidney related to renal function after infusion of endotoxin in rabbits. Lab. Invest. **19**, 169–173 (1968).

GRONCHI, V., CARNIELLI, P.: Ulteriori ricerche sulle iperplasie sperimentali della corteccia surrenale. Boll. Soc. ital. Biol. sper. **9**, 1035–1037 (1934).

HALL, D. L., BROOM, J. S., BRUNSON, J. G.: Effects of epinephrine tolerance on the Shwartzman phenomenon. Amer. J. Path. **44**, 431–439 (1964).

HANGER, F. M.: Effect of intravenous bacterial filtrates on skin tests and local infections. Proc. Soc. exp. Biol. (N. Y.) **25**, 775–777 (1927).

HARDAWAY, R. M.: Disseminated intravascular coagulation syndromes. Arch. Surg. **83**, 842–850 (1961).

HARDAWAY, R. M.: The role of intravascular clotting in the etiology of shock. Ann. Surg. **155**, 325–338 (1962).

HARDAWAY, R. M.: Syndromes of disseminated intravascular coagulation. With special reference to shock and hemorrhage. Springfield: Thomas 1966.

HARDAWAY, R. M., BRUNE, W. H., GEEVER, E. F., BURNS, J. W., MOCK, H. P.: Studies on the role of intravascular coagulation in irreversible hemorrhagic shock. Ann. Surg. **155**, 241–250 (1962).

Hardaway, R. M., Burns, J. W.: Mechanism of action of fibrinolysin in the prevention of irreversible hemorrhagic shock. Ann. Surg. **157**, 305–309 (1963).
Hardaway, R. M., McKay, D. G.: Disseminated intravascular coagulation: A cause of shock. Ann. Surg. **149**, 462–470 (1959).
Hardaway, R. M., McKay, D. G., Wahle, G. H., Tartock, D. E., Edelstein, R.: Pathologic study of intravascular coagulation following incompatible blood transfusion in dogs. 1. Intravenous injection of incompatible blood. Amer. J. Surg. **91**, 24–31 (1956).
Haslam, R. J., Rosson, G. M.: Aggregation of human blood platelets by vasopressin. Amer. J. Physiol. **223**, 958–967 (1972).
Hausman, R., Dreyfus, P. M.: Intracapillary precipitates produced in rabbits by means of sodium polyanetholsulfonate. Arch. Path. **56**, 597–606 (1953).
Haustein, K.-O., Markwardt, F.: Über den Einfluß von Hemmstoffen der Blutgerinnung und Fibrinolyse auf das Sanarelli-Shwartzman-Phänomen. Thrombos. Diathes. haemorrh. (Stuttg.) **13**, 60–64 (1965).
Hawiger, J., Collins, R. D., Horn, R. G.: Precipitation of soluble fibrin monomer complexes by lysosomal protein fraction of polymorphonuclear leukocytes. Proc. Soc. exp. Biol. (N. Y.) **131**, 349–353 (1969).
Hawiger, J., Niewiarowski, S., Gurewich, V., Thomas, D. P.: Measurement of fibrinogen and fibrin degradation products in serum by staphylococcal clumping test. J. Lab. clin. Med. **75**, 93–108 (1970).
Heene, D. L.: Gerinnungsanalytische Untersuchungen zum Verhalten des fibrinstabilisierenden Faktors bei Aktivierung des Gerinnungs- und Fibrinolyse-Systems. Ein Beitrag zur Diagnostik und Genese des erworbenen Mangels an fibrinstabilisierendem Faktor. Habil.-Schrift, p. 90–102. Gießen 1969.
Heene, D., Hoffmann-Fezer, G., Hoffmann, R., Weiss, E., Müller-Berghaus, G., Lasch, H. G.: Coagulation disorders in acute hog cholera. Beitr. path. Anat. **144**, 259–271 (1971).
Heiffer, M. H., Mundy, R. L., Mehlman, B.: Effect of lethal doses of bacterial endotoxin (E. coli) on sympathetic neurohormones in the rabbit. Amer. J. Physiol. **198**, 1307–1311 (1960).
Hellem, A. J.: The adhesiveness of human blood platelets in vitro. Scand. J. clin. Lab. Invest. **12**, Suppl. **51**, 1–117 (1960).
Herion, J. C., Walker, R. I., Herring, W. B., Palmer, J. G.: Effects of endotoxin and nitrogen mustard on leukocyte kinetics. Blood **25**, 522–540 (1965).
Herring, W. B., Herion, J. C., Walker, R. I., Palmer, J. G.: Distribution and clearance of circulating endotoxin. J. clin. Invest. **42**, 79–87 (1963).
Hilgard, P., Hohage, R., Schmitt, W., Köhle, W.: Microangiopathic haemolytic anaemia associated with hypercalcaemia in an experimental rat tumour. Brit. J. Haemat. **24**, 245–254 (1973).
Hirsch, R. L., McKay, D. G., Travers, R. I., Skraly, R. K.: Hyperlipidemia, fatty liver, and bromsulfophthalein retention in rabbits injected intravenously with bacterial endotoxins. J. Lipid. Res. **5**, 563–568 (1964).
Hjort, P. F., Rapaport, S. I.: The Shwartzman reaction: Pathogenetic mechanism and clinical manifestations. Ann. Rev. Med. **16**, 135–168 (1965).
Hocke, M., Maul, F.-D., Müller-Berghaus, G.: Hämolyse und Verbrauchskoagulopathie beim Kaninchen. Transfus. Immunhaem. **1**, 362–366 (1973).
Hoff, H. F., Gottlob, R., Blümel, G.: Ultrastructural changes in arteries induced by endotoxin. Naturwissenschaften **54**, 287–288 (1967).
Hoffmann, R., Hoffmann-Fezer, G., Kimeto, B., Weiss, E.: Mikrothromben als morphologischer Ausdruck einer Verbrauchskoagulopathie bei akuter Schweinepest. Zbl. Vet.-Med. B. **18**, 710–718 (1971).
Horn, R. G.: Evidence for participation of granulocytes in the pathogenesis of the generalized Shwartzman reaction: A review. J. infect. Dis. **128**, Suppl. 134–143 (1973).
Horn, R. G., Collins, R. D.: Studies on the pathogenesis of the generalized Shwartzman reaction. The role of granulocytes. Lab. Invest. **18**, 101–107 (1968a).
Horn, R. G., Collins, R. D.: Fragmentation of granulocytes in pulmonary capillaries during development of the generalized Shwartzman reaction. Lab. Invest. **19**, 451–459 (1968b).
Horn, R. G., Hawiger, J., Collins, R. D.: Electron microscopy of fibrin-like precipitate formed during the paracoagulation reaction between soluble fibrin monomer complexes and protamine sulphate. Brit. J. Haemat. **17**, 463–466 (1969).
Horn, R. G., Spicer, S. S.: Sulfated mucopolysaccharide and basic protein in certain granules of circulating heterophils of rabbits during endotoxin-induced leukocytosis. Amer. J. Path. **44**, 905–919 (1964).
Horn, R. G., Spicer, S. S.: Sulfated mucopolysaccharide in fibrinoid glomerular occlusions of the generalized Shwartzman reaction. Amer. J. Path. **46**, 197–213 (1965).

HOROWITZ, H. I., DES PREZ, R. M., HOOK, E. W.: Effects of bacterial endotoxin on rabbit platelets. II. Enhancement of platelet factor 3 activity *in vitro* and *in vivo*. J. exp. Med. **116**, 619–633 (1962).

HUGO, R. VON, GRAEFF, H., MÜLLER-BERGHAUS, G.: High molecular weight derivatives of fibrinogen and their relation to the total fibrinogen content following the infusion of endotoxin in pregnant rabbits. In: URBASCHEK, B., URBASCHEK, R., NETER, E. (eds.): Gram-negative bacterial infections and mode of endotoxin actions—Pathophysiological, immunological, and clinical aspects, p. 372–376. Wien-New York: Springer 1975.

HUGUES, J.: Accolement des plaquettes aux structures conjonctives périvasculaires. Thrombos. Diathes. haemorrh. (Stuttg.) 8, 241–255 (1962).

HUTH, K., BLUMENTHAL, J., MITTERMAYER, C., LASCH, H. G.: Experimentelle Verbrauchscoagulopathie nach Carragenin. Verh. dtsch. Ges. inn. Med. **72**, 287–291 (1966).

HUTH, K., KARLICZEK, G.: Die Endotoxin-induzierte Hyperlipämie des Kaninchens. In: BARTELHEIMER, H., HEISIG, N. (eds.): Aktuelle Gastroenterologie, p. 372–375. Verh. 24. Tag. dtsch. Ges. Verdauungs- und Stoffwechselkrankh., Hamburg 1967. Stuttgart: Thieme 1968.

HUTH, K., SCHOENBORN, W., KNORPP, K.: Experimentelle Verbrauchskoagulopathie nach intravenöser Zufuhr von Fett und Endotoxin. Thrombos. Diathes. haemorrh. (Stuttg.) **17**, 129–143 (1967).

IZAK, G., GALEWSKY, K.: Studies on experimentally induced hypercoagulable state in rabbits. Thrombos. Diathes. haemorrh. (Stuttg.) **16**, 228–242 (1966).

JACOBI, H., KARITZKY, D., MITTERMAYER, C., SESEKE, G., WITT, I., KÜNZER, W.: Intravasale Hämolyse und Blutgerinnung. Blut **22**, 244–254 (1971).

JANZARIK, H., KÖPPLER, E., LASCH, H. G.: Experimentelle Immunhämolyse und Blutgerinnung. Thrombos. Diathes. haemorrh. (Stuttg.) **26**, 22–28 (1971).

JOHNSON, K. J., WARD, P. A.: Protective function of C6 in rabbits treated with bacterial endotoxin. J. Immunol. **106**, 1125–1127 (1971).

JÜRGENS, R., STUDER, A.: Zur Wirkung des Thrombins. Helv. physiol. pharmacol. Acta **6**, 130–149 (1948).

KALEY, G., DEMOPOULOS, H., ZWEIFACH, B. W.: Occlusive vascular lesions induced by bacterial endotoxin in kidneys of pregnant rats. Proc. Soc. exp. Biol. (N. Y.) **109**, 456–459 (1962).

KEPPLER, D., LESCH, R., REUTTER, W., DECKER, K.: Experimental hepatitis induced by D-galactosamine. Exp. molec. Path. **9**, 279–290 (1968).

KLEBS, E.: Handb. Pathol. Anat. **2**, 114 (1876) (as quoted by SELYE, 1966).

KLEINMAIER, H., GOERGEN, K., LASCH, H. G., KRECKE, H.-J., BOHLE, A.: Untersuchungen zur Frage der Gerinnungsstörung beim Sanarelli-Shwartzman-Phänomen (sog. generalisierten Shwartzman-Phänomen) des Kaninchens. Z. ges. exp. Med. **132**, 275–294 (1959).

KLIMAN, A., MCKAY, D. G.: The prevention of the generalized Shwartzman reaction by fibrinolytic activity. Arch. Path. **66**, 715–719 (1958).

KOCIBA, G. J., GRIESEMER, R. A.: Disseminated intravascular coagulation induced with leukocyte procoagulant. Amer. J. Path. **69**, 407–420 (1972).

KOCIBA, G. J., LOEB, W. F., WALL, R. L.: Development of procoagulant (tissue thromboplastin) activity in cultured leukocytes. J. Lab. clin. Med. **79**, 778–787 (1972).

KOPEC, M., WEGRZYNOWICZ, Z., BUDZYNSKI, A. Z., LATALLO, Z. S., LIPINKI, B., KOWALSKI, E.: Interaction of fibrinogen degradation products (FDP) with platelets. Exp. Biol. Med. **3**, 73–79 (1968).

KOPEC, M., WEGRZYNOWICZ, Z., LATALLO, Z. S.: Effects of some basic proteins and acid mucopolysaccharides on fibrin deposition. In: KOLLER, F., BRINKHOUS, K. M., BIGGS, R., RODMAN, N. F., HINNOM, S. (eds.): Vascular factors and thrombosis. Thrombos. Diathes. haemorrh. (Stuttg.) Suppl. **40**, 253–258 (1970).

KOWALSKI, E., BUDZYNSKI, A. Z., KOPEC, M., LATALLO, Z. S., LIPINSKI, B., WEGRZYNOWICZ, Z.: Circulating fibrinogen degradation products (FDP) in dog blood after intravenous thrombin infusion. Thrombos. Diathes. haemorrh. (Stuttg.) **13**, 12–24 (1965).

KRECKE, H.-J.: Zum generalisierten Shwartzman-Phänomen (Sanarelli-Shwartzman-Phänomen) und seiner Bedeutung für die menschliche Pathologie. Stuttgart: Fischer 1964.

KUHN, W., GRAEFF, H.: Gerinnungsstörungen in der Geburtshilfe. Stuttgart: Thieme 1970.

KUSAMA, S.: Über Aufbau und Entstehung der toxischen Thrombose und deren Bedeutung. Beitr. path. Anat. **55**, 459–544 (1913).

KWAAN, H. C., BARLOW, G. H.: The mechanism of action of a coagulant fraction of Malayan pit viper venom, arvin, and of reptilase. Thrombos. Diathes. haemorrh. (Stuttg.) Suppl. **45**, 63–68 (1971).

LAMBERT, P. B., MING, S.-C., PALMERIO, C.: Vasomotor factors in the Shwartzman phenomenon. Amer. J. Path. **57**, 559–580 (1969).

Lambert, P. H., Salmon, J.: Réactions anaphylactiques du lapin et coagulation intravasculaire. C. R. Soc. Biol. (Paris) **160**, 1337–1340 (1966).
Landois, L.: Die Transfusion des Blutes. Leipzig: Vogel 1875.
Langdell, R. D., Hedgpeth, E. M.: A study of the role of hemolysis in the hemostatic defect of transfusion reactions. Thrombos. Diathes. haemorrh. (Stuttg.) **3**, 566–571 (1959).
Lasch, H. G.: Therapeutic aspects of disseminated intravascular coagulation. In: Mammen, E. F., Anderson, G. F., Barnhart, M. I. (eds.): Disseminated intravascular coagulation, p. 281–293. Stuttgart-New York: Schattauer 1969.
Lasch, H. G.: Pathophysiological and clinical aspects of diffuse intravascular coagulation. Excerpta Medica (Amsterdam) 1974, p. 275–281.
Lasch, H. G., Heene, D. L.: Diagnosis of intravascular coagulation and fibrinolysis. In: Brinkhous, K. M., Wright, I. S., Soulier, J. P., Roberts, H. R., Hinnom, S. (eds.): Platelets: Their role in hemostasis and thrombosis, p. 351–358. Stuttgart-New York: Schattauer 1967.
Lasch, H. G., Heene, D. L. (eds.): Microcirculation, hemostasis and shock. Stuttgart-New York: Schattauer 1970.
Lasch, H. G., Heene, D. L., Huth, K., Sandritter, W.: Pathophysiology, clinical manifestations and therapy of consumption-coagulopathy („Verbrauchskoagulopathie"). Amer. J. Cardiol. **20**, 381–391 (1967).
Lasch, H. G., Huth, K., Heene, D. L., Müller-Berghaus, G., Hörder, M.-H., Janzarik, H., Mittermayer, C., Sandritter, W.: Die Klinik der Verbrauchskoagulopathie. Dtsch. med. Wschr. **96**, 715–728 (1971).
Lasch, H. G., Krecke, H.-J., Rodriguez-Erdmann, F., Sessner, H. H., Schütterle, G.: Verbrauchskoagulopathien (Pathogenese und Therapie). Folia haemat. (N. F.) **6**, 325–330 (1961a).
Lasch, H. G., Mechelke, K., Nusser, E.: Über Änderungen der Gerinnungsfaktoren Prothrombin und VII bei hyper- und hypozirkulatorischen Kreislaufumstellungen der Katze. Dtsch. Arch. klin. Med. **204**, 1–21 (1957).
Lasch, H. G., Mechelke, K., Nusser, E., Daoud, F.: Der Einfluß der Fibrinolyse auf den Verlauf des hämorrhagischen Schocks. Klin. Wschr. **39**, 1137–1141 (1961b).
Lasch, H. G., Mechelke, K., Nusser, E., Sessner, H. H.: Über Beziehungen zwischen Blutgerinnung und Kreislauffunktion. Z. ges. exp. Med. **129**, 484–495 (1958).
Lasch, H. G., Rodríguez-Erdmann, F., Krecke, H.-J.: Quantitative und qualitative Veränderungen der Thrombocyten beim Sanarelli-Shwartzman-Phänomen. Verh. dtsch. Ges. inn. Med. **66**, 992–998 (1960).
Lasch, H. G., Rodríguez-Erdmann, F., Schimpf, K.: Antithrombin III und Anti-Blutthrombokinase bei experimenteller Verbrauchskoagulopathie (Am Beispiel des Sanarelli-Shwartzman-Phänomens). Klin. Wschr. **39**, 645–647 (1961c).
Lasch, H. G., Rodríguez-Erdmann, F., Westenhoefer, D.: Der Einfluß der Fibrinolyse auf den Verlauf des Sanarelli-Shwartzman-Phänomens, p. 469. Proc. 8th Congr. Europ. Soc. Haemat., Wien 1961. Basel-New York: Karger 1962.
Lasch, H. G., Róka, L.: Über den Bildungsmechanismus der Gerinnungsfaktoren Prothrombin und Faktor VII. Klin. Wschr. **32**, 460–464 (1954).
Lasch, H. G., Róka, L., Heene, D.: The defibrination syndrome. In: Brinkhous, K. M., Wright, I. S., Koller, F., Streuli, F., Duckert, F. (eds.): Diffuse intravascular clotting, p. 97–105. Stuttgart: Schattauer 1966.
Latour, J.-G., Bernard, F.: Prevention by aspirin of the classical generalized Shwartzman. (Abstract). Circulation **49/50**, Suppl. III (1974).
Latour, J.-G., McKay, D. G.: Requirement of the adrenal glands for provocation of the generalized Shwartzman reaction. Lab. Invest. **22**, 281–285 (1970).
Latour, J. G., McKay, D. G., Nasu, K.: Prevention of the generalized Shwartzman reaction by glucocorticoids. Amer. J. Obstet. Gynec. **113**, 863–867 (1972).
Latour, J.-G., Prejean, J. B., Margaretten, W.: Corticosteroids and the generalized Shwartzman reaction. Mechanisms of sensitization in the rabbit. Amer. J. Path. **65**, 189–202 (1971).
Leandoer, L., Niléhn, J.-E.: Effect of intravenous injection of stypven or thrombin on coagulation and fibrinolysis of blood and lymph in dogs. Acta chir. scand. **135**, 7–13 (1969).
Lee, L.: Reticuloendothelial clearance of circulating fibrin in the pathogenesis of the generalized Shwartzman rection. J. exp. Med. **115**, 1065–1082 (1962).
Lee, L.: Antigen-antibody reaction in the pathogenesis of bilateral renal cortical necrosis. J. exp. Med. **117**, 365–375 (1963).
Lee, L., McCluskey, R. T.: Immunohistochemical demonstration of the reticuloendothelial clearance of circulating fibrin aggregates. J. exp. Med. **116**, 611–617 (1962).
Lepri, G., Cristiani, R.: The ability of certain adrenocortical hormones to potentiate the vasoconstrictor action of nor-adrenaline on the conjunctival vessels in the rabbit and in man. Brit. J. Ophthal. **48**, 205–208 (1964).

LERNER, R., GOLDSTEIN, R., CUMMINGS, G.: The generation of coagulant activity by leukocytes. (Abstract). Fed. Proc. **30**, 479 (1971a).
LERNER, R. G., GOLDSTEIN, R., CUMMINGS, G.: Stimulation of human leukocyte thromboplastic activity by endotoxin. Proc. Soc. exp. Biol. (N. Y.) **138**, 145–148 (1971b).
LERNER, R. G., RAPAPORT, S. I., SIEMSEN, J. K., SPITZER, J. M.: Disappearance of fibrinogen-^{131}I after endotoxin: Effects of a first and second injection. Amer. J. Physiol. **214**, 532–537 (1968a).
LERNER, R. G., RAPAPORT, S. I., SPITZER, J. M.: Endotoxin-induced intravascular clotting: The need for granulocytes. Thrombos. Diathes. haemorrh. (Stuttg.) **20**, 430–443 (1968b).
LERNER, R. G., WIENER, J., GOLDSTEIN, R.: Experimental venous thrombosis in agranulocytic rabbits. Thrombos. Res. **4**, 165–175 (1974).
LEVIN, J., BANG, F. B.: The role of endotoxin in the extracellular coagulation of limulus blood. Bull. Johns Hopk. Hosp. **115**, 265–274 (1964).
LEVIN, J., BECK, E.: A re-appraisal of the role of blood coagulation and platelets in the generalized Shwartzman phenomenon. Thrombos. Diathes. haemorrh. (Stuttg.) **15**, 519–538 (1966).
LEVIN, J., CLUFF, L. E.: Platelets and the Shwartzman phenomenon. J. exp. Med. **121**, 235–246 (1965a).
LEVIN, J., CLUFF, L. E.: Endotoxemia and adrenal hemorrhage. A mechanism for the Waterhouse-Friderichsen syndrome. J. exp. Med. **121**, 247–260 (1965b).
LEVIN, J., TOMASULO, P. A., OSER, R. S.: Detection of endotoxin in human blood and demonstration of an inhibitor. J. Lab. clin. Invest. **75**, 903–911 (1970).
LIPINSKI, B., GUREWICH, V., NOWAK, A., WETMORE, R.: The effect of heparin and dipyridamole on the deposition of fibrin-like material in rabbits infused with soluble fibrin monomer or fibrinogen. Thrombos. Res. **5**, 343–358 (1974a).
LIPINSKI, B., JELJASZEWICZ, J.: A hypotesis for the pathogenesis of the generalized Shwartzman reaction. J. infect. Dis. **120**, 160–168 (1969).
LIPINSKI, B., NOWAK, A., GUREWICH, V.: The organ distribution of ^{125}I-fibrin in the generalized Shwartzman reaction and its relation to leucocytes. Brit. J. Haemat. **28**, 221–231 (1974b).
LIPINSKI, B., WOROWSKI, K., JELJASZEWICZ, J., NIEWIAROWSKI, S., REJNIAK, L.: Participation of soluble fibrin monomer complexes and platelet factor 4 in the generalized Shwartzman reaction. Thrombos. Diathes. haemorrh. (Stuttg.) **20**, 285–295 (1968).
LISIEWICZ, J.: Studies on the thromboplastic activity normal leukocytes. Acta physiol. pol. **17**, 287–297 (1966a).
LISIEWICZ, J.: Effect of extracts of normal leukocytes on thrombin generation in plasma. Acta physiol. pol. **17**, 627–636 (1966b).
LOPAS, H., BIRNDORF, N. I.: Haemolysis and intravascular coagulation due to incompatible red cell transfusion in isoimmunized monkeys. Brit. J. Haemat. **21**, 399–411 (1971).
LÜSCHER, E. F., PFUELLER, S. L., MASSINI, P.: Platelet aggregation by large molecules. Ser. Haematol. **6**, 382–391 (1973).
MACFARLANE, R. G.: An enzyme cascade in the blood clotting mechanism, and its function as a biochemical amplifier. Nature **202**, 498–499 (1964).
MAHN, I., MERKEL, H., SATTLER, E. L., MÜLLER-BERGHAUS, G.: Verhalten von ^{125}J-Fibrinogen und ^{131}J-Albumin bei der experimentellen Galaktosaminhepatitis. Verh. dtsch. Ges. inn. Med. **80**, 437–439 (1974).
MAJNO, G., PALADE, G. E.: Studies on inflammation. I. The effect of histamine and serotonin on vascular permeability: An electron microscopic study. J. biophys. biochem. Cytol. **11**, 571–605 (1961).
MARGARETTEN, W., ELTING, J., ROTHENBERG, J., MCKAY, D. G.: Experimental adrenal hemorrhage in the generalized Shwartzman reaction. Lab. Invest. **14**, 687–691 (1965).
MARGARETTEN, W., MCKAY, D. G.: The effect of leukocyte antiserum on the generalized Shwartzman reaction. Amer. J. Path. **57**, 299–306 (1969a).
MARGARETTEN, W., MCKAY, D. G.: The role of the platelet in the generalized Shwartzman reaction. J. exp. Med. **129**, 585–590 (1969b).
MARGARETTEN, W., MCKAY, D. G., PHILLIPS, L. L.: The effect of heparin on endotoxin shock in the rat. Amer. J. Path. **51**, 61–68 (1967).
MARGARETTEN, W., ZUNKER, H. O., MCKAY, D. G.: Production of the generalized Shwartzman reaction in pregnant rats by intravenous infusion of thrombin. Lab. Invest. **13**, 552–559 (1964).
MARSTEN, J. L., CHAN, K.-E., ANKENEY, J. L., BOTTI, R. E.: Antithrombotic effect of Malayan pit viper venom on experimental thrombosis of the inferior vena cava produced by a new method. Circulat. Res. **19**, 514–519 (1966).
MCGEHEE, W. G., HJORT, P. F., RAPAPORT, S. I.: Effects of thorium dioxide upon blood clotting and platelets. II. *In vivo* studies in rabbits. Thrombos. Diathes. haemorrh. (Stuttg.) **16**, 354–370 (1966).

McGrath, J. M., Stewart, G. J.: The effects of endotoxin on vascular endothelium. J. exp. Med. **129**, 833–848 (1969).
McKay, D. G.: A partial synthesis of the generalized Shwartzman reaction. Fed. Proc. **22**, 1373–1379 (1963).
McKay, D. G.: Disseminated intravascular coagulation. An intermediary mechanism of disease. New York: Hoeber, Harper and Row 1964.
McKay, D. G.: Progress in disseminated intravascular coagulation. Calif. Med. **111**, Part I 186–199; Part II 279–290 (1969).
McKay, D. G.: Vessel wall and thrombogenesis-endotoxin. Thrombos. Diathes. haemorrh. (Stuttg.) **29**, 11–26 (1973).
McKay, D. G., Gitlin, D., Craig, J. M.: Immunochemical demonstration of fibrin in the generalized Shwartzman reaction. Arch. Path. **67**, 270–273 (1959a).
McKay, D. G., Hardaway, R. M., Wahle, G. H., Jr., Edelstein, R., Tartock, D. E.: Alterations in blood coagulation mechanism after incompatible blood transfusion. Clinical and experimental observations. Amer. J. Surg. **89**, 583–592 (1955).
McKay, D. G., Kliman, A., Alexander, B.: Experimental production of afibrinogenemia and hemorrhagic phenomena by combined fibrinolysis and disseminated intravascular coagulation. New Engl. J. Med. **261**, 1150–1154 (1959b).
McKay, D. G., Latour, J.-G., Lopez, A. M.: Production of the generalized Shwartzman reaction by activated Hageman factor and α-adrenergic stimulation. Thrombos. Diathes. haemorrh. (Stuttg.) **26**, 71–76 (1971a).
McKay, D. G., Latour, J.-G., Parris, H. M. H.: Activation of Hageman factor by α-adrenergic stimulation. Thrombos. Diathes. haemorrh. (Stuttg.) **23**, 417–422 (1970).
McKay, D. G., Linder, M. M., Cruse, V. K.: Mechanisms of thrombosis of the microcirculation. Amer. J. Path. **63**, 231–241 (1971b).
McKay, D. G., Margaretten, W.: Disseminated intravascular coagulation in virus diseases. Arch. intern. Med. **120**, 129–152 (1967).
McKay, D. G., Margaretten, W., Csavossy, I.: An electron microscope study of the effects of bacterial endotoxin on the blood-vascular system. Lab. Invest. **15**, 1815–1829 (1966).
McKay, D. G., Margaretten, W., Phillips, L. L.: The role of leukocyte in the generalized Shwartzman reaction. Lab. Invest. **16**, 511–515 (1967a).
McKay, D. G., Margaretten, W., Rothenberg, J.: Blockade of the reticuloendothelial system induced by dietary lipids. Lab. Invest. **13**, 54–61 (1964).
McKay, D. G., Merriam, J. C.: Vascular changes induced by bacterial endotoxin during generalized Shwartzman reaction. Effect of cortisone. Arch. Path. **69**, 524–530 (1960).
McKay, D. G., Müller-Berghaus, G.: Therapeutic implications of disseminated intravascular coagulation. Amer. J. Cardiol. **20**, 392–410 (1967).
McKay, D. G., Müller-Berghaus, G.: Hageman factor (HF) and the generalized Shwartzman reaction (GSR). (Abstract). Fed. Proc. **27**, 436 (1968).
McKay, D. G., Müller-Berghaus, G., Cruse, V.: Activation of Hageman factor by ellagic acid and the generalized Shwartzman reaction. Amer. J. Path. **54**, 393–420 (1969).
McKay, D. G., Phillips, L. L., Kaplan, H., Henson, J. B.: Chronic intravascular coagulation in Aleutian disease of mink. Amer. J. Path. **50**, 899–916 (1967b).
McKay, D. G., Shapiro, S. S.: Alterations in the blood coagulation system induced by bacterial endotoxin. I. *In vivo* (generalized Shwartzman reaction). J exp. Med. **107**, 353–367 (1958).
McKay, D. G., Wong, T.-C.: Studies of the generalized Shwartzman reaction produced by diet. I. Pathology. J. exp. Med. **115**, 1117–1126 (1962a).
McKay, D. G., Wong, T.-C.: Studies of the generalized Shwartzman reaction produced by diet. III. Partial prevention by antibiotics. J. exp. Med. **115**, 1137–1140 (1962b).
McKay, D. G., Wong, T.-C.: The effect of bacterial endotoxin on the placenta of the rat. Amer. J. Path. **42**, 357–377 (1963).
McKay, D., Wong, T., Galton, M.: Effect of pregnancy on the disseminated thrombosis caused by bacterial endotoxin. (Abstract). Fed. Proc. **19**, 246 (1960).
Mergenhagen, S. E., Snyderman, R., Gewurz, H., Shin, H. S.: Significance of complement to the mechanism of action of endotoxin. Current Topics Microbiol. Immunol. **50**, 37–77 (1969).
Merskey, C., Johnson, A. J., Kleiner, G. J., Wohl, H.: The defibrination syndrome: Clinical features and laboratory diagnosis. Brit. J. Haemat. **13**, 528–549 (1967).
Mersky, C., Lalezari, P., Johnson, A. J.: A rapid, simple, sensitive method for measuring fibrinolytic split products in human serum. Proc. Soc. exp. Biol. (N. Y.) **131**, 871–875 (1969).
Minna, J. D., Robboy, S. J., Colman, R. W.: Disseminated intravascular coagulation in man. Springfield: Thomas 1974.
Mitchell, J. R. A., Sharp, A. A.: Platelet clumping "*in vitro*". Brit. J. Haemat. **10**, 78–93 (1964).

MITTERMAYER, C., VOGEL, W., BURCHARDI, H., BIRZLE, H., WIEMERS, K., SANDRITTER, W.: Pulmonale Mikrothrombosierung als Ursache der respiratorsichen Insuffizienz bei Verbrauchskoagulopathie (Schocklunge). Dtsch. med. Wschr. **95**, 1999–2002 (1970).

MORIAU, M., RODHAIN, J., NOEL, H., BEYS-COL, C. DE, MASURE, R.: Comparative effects of proteinase inhibitors, plasminogen antiactivators, heparin and acetylsalicylic acid on the experimental disseminated intravascular coagulation induced by thrombin. Thrombos. Diathes. haemorrh. (Stuttg.) **32**, 171–188 (1974).

MÜLLER-BERGHAUS, G.: Pathophysiology of disseminated intravascular coagulation. In: MAMMEN, E. F., ANDERSON, G. F., BARNHART, M. I. (eds.): Disseminated intravascular coagulation. Thrombos. Diathes. haemorrh. (Stuttg.) Suppl. **36**, 45–61 (1969).

MÜLLER-BERGHAUS, G.: Pathophysiologie der manifesten generalisierten intravaskulären Gerinnung. In: RÓKA, L. (ed.): Generalisierte intravaskuläre Gerinnung. Beeinflussung der Hämostase durch gefäßaktive Pharmaka. Thrombos. Diathes. haemorrh. (Stuttg.) Suppl. **50**, 5–32 (1971).

MÜLLER-BERGHAUS, G.: Trigger mechanism of endotoxin-induced intravascular coagulation. In: URBASCHEK, B., URBASCHEK, R., NETER, E. (eds.): Gram-negative bacterial infections and mode of endotoxin actions—Pathophysiological, immunological, and clinical aspects. p. 362–366. Wien-New York: Springer 1975.

MÜLLER-BERGHAUS, G., DAVIDSON, E., MCKAY, D. G.: Prevention of the generalized Shwartzman reaction in pregnant rats by alpha-adrenergic blockade. Effects on the coagulation mechanism. Obstet. and Gynec. **30**, 774–778 (1967a).

MÜLLER-BERGHAUS, G., ECKHARDT, T.: The role of granulocytes in the activation of intravascular coagulation and the precipitation of soluble fibrin by endotoxin. Blood **45**, 631–641 (1975).

MÜLLER-BERGHAUS, G., EHLERS, E., KÄUFER, P.: Das Verhalten der oberflächensensiblen Gerinnungsfaktoren XII und XI bei intravasaler Gerinnung. Verh. dtsch. Ges. inn. Med. **80**, 1458–1460 (1974).

MÜLLER-BERGHAUS, G., GOLDFINGER, D., MARGARETTEN, W., MCKAY, D. G.: Platelet factor 3 and the generalized Shwartzman reaction. Thrombos. Diathes. haemorrh. (Stuttg.) **18**, 726–735 (1967b).

MÜLLER-BERGHAUS, G., HEINRICH, D.: Fibrin monomer and platelet aggregation *in vitro* and *in vivo*. Brit. J. Haemat. **23**, 177–188 (1972).

MÜLLER-BERGHAUS, G., HOCKE, M.: Effect of endotoxin on the formation of microthrombi from circulating fibrin monomer complexes in the absence of thrombin generation. Thrombos. Res. **1**, 541–548 (1972).

MÜLLER-BERGHAUS, G., HOCKE, M.: Production of the generalized Shwartzman reaction in rabbits by ancrod ("Arvin") infusion and endotoxin injection. Brit. Haemat. **25**, 111–122 (1973).

MÜLLER-BERGHAUS, G., HOCKE, M., MANN, B., LASCH, H. G.: Entstehung von Mikrogerinnseln nach Infusion von Arvin. In: MARX, R., THIES, H. A. (eds.): Herzinfarkt und Blutgerinnung. Thrombos. Diathes. haemorrh. (Stuttg.) Suppl. **52**, 235–238 (1972c).

MÜLLER-BERGHAUS, G., HUTH, K., KRECKE, H.-J., LASCH, H.-G.: Blutlipide und intravasale Gerinnung in der Pathogenese des Sanarelli-Shwartzman-Phänomens. Schweiz. med. Wschr. **94**, 1519–1526 (1964).

MÜLLER-BERGHAUS, G., KRECKE, H.-J., LASCH, H.-G.: Thrombelastographic investigations on clot-formation in the generalized Shwartzman phenomenon. German Med. Res. **1**, 185–186 (1963a).

MÜLLER-BERGHAUS, G., KRECKE, H.-J., LASCH, H.-G.: Thrombelastographische Untersuchungen zum Gerinnselaufbau beim Sanarelli-Shwartzman-Phänomen. Klin. Wschr. **41**, 216–219 (1963b).

MÜLLER-BERGHAUS, G., LASCH, H.-G.: Untersuchungen über Beziehungen zwischen Gefäß- und Gerinnungsfaktoren beim Sanarelli-Shwartzman-Phänomen. Thrombos. Diathes. haemorrh. (Stuttg.) **9**, 335–346 (1963).

MÜLLER-BERGHAUS, G., LASCH, H. G.: Consumption of Hageman factor activity in the generalized Shwartzman reaction induced by Liquoid. Its prevention by inhibition of Hageman factor activation. Thrombos. Diathes. haemorrh. (Stuttg.) **23**, 386–404 (1970).

MÜLLER-BERGHAUS, G., LASCH, H. G.: Hageman factor activity in Liquoid-induced consumption coagulopathy. Failure to prevent the drop in Hageman factor activity by anticoagulation with a coumarin derivative. Thrombos. Diathes. haemorrh. (Stuttg.) **26**, 58–70 (1971).

MÜLLER-BERGHAUS, G., LASCH, H. G.: Consumption coagulopathy in the course of endotoxinemia. In: URBASCHEK, B., URBASCHEK, R., NETER, E. (eds.): Gram-negative bacterial infections and mode of endotoxin actions—Pathophysiological, immunological, and clinical aspects. p. 353–356. Wien-New York: Springer 1975.

Müller-Berghaus, G., Lohmann, E.: The role of complement in endotoxin-induced disseminated intravascular coagulation: Studies in congenitally C6-deficient rabbits. Brit. J. Haemat. **28**, 403–418 (1974).

Müller-Berghaus, G., Mann, B.: Precipitation of ancrod-induced soluble fibrin by aprotinin and norepinephrine. Thrombos. Res. **2**, 305–322 (1973).

Müller-Berghaus, G., Maul, F.-D., Hocke, M.: Die Bedeutung von intravasaler Hämolyse für die Auslösung einer Verbrauchskoagulopathie beim Kaninchen. (Abstract). In: Nowicki, L., Martin, H., Schubert, J. C. F. (eds.). Hämolyse — Hämolytische Erkrankungen. p. 250. München: Lehmann 1973a.

Müller-Berghaus, G., Maul, F.-D., Lasch, H. G.: Prevention of the Liquoid-induced consumption coagulopathy by the protease inhibitor aprotinin. Thrombos. Diathes. haemorrh. (Stuttg.) **27**, 396–406 (1972a).

Müller-Berghaus, G., Maul, F.-D., Lasch, H. G.: Effect of the protease inhibitor Trasylol on Liquoid-induced consumption coagulopathy. In: Brendel, W., Haberland, G. L. (eds.). New aspects of trasylol therapy **5**, 223–231 (1972b).

Müller-Berghaus, G., McKay, D. G.: Prevention of the generalized Shwartzman reaction in pregnant rats by α-adrenergic blocking agents. Lab. Invest. **17**, 276–280 (1967).

Müller-Berghaus, G., Mueller-Eckhardt, C.: Induction of consumption coagulopathy (disseminated intravascular coagulation) with special reference to Hageman factor activation by unrelated immune reactions. (Abstract). 13. Internat. Congr. Haemat. Munich 1970, Abstract Vol. p. 243.

Müller-Berghaus, G., Obst, R.: Induction of the generalized Shwartzman reaction in pregnant and nonpregnant rats by colchicine. Amer. J. Path. **69**, 131–138 (1972).

Müller-Berghaus, G., Reuter, C.: Disseminated intravascular coagulation in galactosamine-induced experimental hepatitis. Thrombos. Res. **1**, 473–486 (1972).

Müller-Berghaus, G., Róka, L., Lasch, H. G.: Induction of glomerular microclot formation by fibrin monomer infusion. Thrombos. Diathes. haemorrh. (Stuttg.) **29**, 375–383 (1973b).

Müller-Berghaus, G., Schmidt-Ehry, B.: The role of pregnancy in the induction of the generalized Shwartzman reaction. Amer. J. Obstet. Gynec. **114**, 847–849 (1972).

Müller-Berghaus, G., Schneberger, R.: Hageman factor activation in the generalized Shwartzman reaction induced by endotoxin. Brit. J. Haemat. **21**, 513–527 (1971).

Mueller-Eckhardt, C., Heene, D., Müller-Berghaus, G., Lasch, H. G.: Hämolytische Transfusionszwischenfälle mit „Verbrauchskoagulopathie" durch seltene Blutgruppenantikörper (Anti-Duffy (a)). Thrombos. Diathes. haemorrh. (Stuttg.) **22**, 336–343 (1969).

Mueller-Eckhardt, C., Müller-Berghaus, G.: Tierexperimentelle Untersuchungen zum Auslösungsmechanismus der Verbrauchskoagulopathie durch Immunreaktionen. Verh. dtsch. Ges. inn. Med. **77**, 1157–1159 (1971).

Nakai, H., Margaretten, W.: Effect of staphylococcal toxin on the rabbit kidney. Arch. Path. **76**, 38–43 (1963).

Nasu, K., Latour, J. G., McKay, D. G.: Modification of the generalized Shwartzman reaction by therapeutic agents. Amer. J. Obstet. Gynec. **109**, 991–996 (1971).

Nemerson, Y., Pitlick, F. A.: The tissue factor pathway of blood coagulation. In: Spaet, T. H. (ed.): Progress in hemostasis and thrombosis **1**, 1–38 (1972).

Nemerson, Y., Spaet, T. H.: The activation of factor X by extracts of rabbit brain. Blood **23**, 657–668 (1964).

Neuhof, H.: Changes in hemodynamics and gas metabolism after endotoxin injection. In: Urbaschek, B., Urbaschek, R., Neter, E. (eds.): Gram-negative bacterial infections and mode of endotoxin actions—Pathophysiological, immunological, and clinical aspects. p. 256–264. Wien-New York: Springer 1975.

Neuhof, H., Glaser, E., Hey, D., Lasch, H. G.: Pathophysiologic mechanisms in endotoxin shock and its therapeutic approaches. In: Shock: Biochemical, pharmacological, and clinical aspects. p. 159–170. Plenum Press 1970.

Neuhof, H., Hey, D., Glaser, E., Wolf, H., Lasch, H. G.: Hemodynamic reactions induced by streptokinase therapy in patients with acute myocardial infarction. Europ. J. Intensive Care Medicine **1**, 27–30 (1975).

Neuhof, H., Kaufmann, G.: Kreislaufveränderungen bei thrombozytenarmen Kaninchen nach Endotoxin- und Histaminverabreichung. Verh. dtsch. Ges. Kreisl-Forsch. **34**, 218–222 (1968).

Neuhof, H., Wolf, H., Rohtermundt, R., Glaser, E., Lasch, H. G.: Die Sauerstoffaufnahme des Organismus im hämorrhagischen Schock. Tierexperimentelle Untersuchungen. Z. Kardiol. **62**, 663–683 (1973).

Niemetz, J.: Thromboplastic activity of leukocytes from rabbits receiving endotoxin (Abstract). Fed. Proc. **28**, 442 (1969).

NIEMETZ, J.: Coagulant activity of leukocytes. Tissue factor activity. J. clin. Invest. **51**, 307–313 (1972).
NIEMETZ, J., FANI, K.: Procoagulant activity of leukocytes. Role in the generalized Shwartzman reaction (gSr). (Abstract). Blood **36**, 835 (1970).
NIEMETZ, J., FANI, K.: Role of leukocytes in blood coagulation and the generalized Shwartzman reaction. Nature (Lond.) New Biology **232**, 247–248 (1971).
NIEMETZ, J., FANI, K.: Thrombogenic activity of leukocytes. Blood **42**, 47–59 (1973).
NIEMETZ, J., MARCUS, A. J.: The stimulatory effect of platelets and platelet membranes on the procoagulant activity of leukocytes. J. clin. Invest. **54**, 1437–1443 (1974).
NIEWIAROWSKI, S., BAŃKOWSKI, E., ROGOWICKA, I.: Studies on the adsorption and activation of the Hageman factor (factor XII) by collagen and elastin. Thrombos. Diathes. haemorrh. (Stuttg.) **14**, 387–400 (1965).
NIEWIAROWSKI, S., GUREWICH, V.: Laboratory identification of intravascular coagulation. The serial dilution protamine sulfate test for the detection of fibrin monomer and fibrin degradation products. J. Lab. clin. Med. **77**, 665–676 (1971).
NIEWIAROWSKI, S., KOWALSKI, E.: Un nouvel anticoagulant dérivé du fibrinogène. Rev. Hémat. **13**, 320–328 (1958).
NIEWIAROWSKI, S., LIPIŃSKI, B., FARBISZEWSKI, R., POPLAWSKI, A.: The release of platelet factor 4 during platelet aggregation and the possible significance of this reaction in hemostasis. Experientia (Basel) **24**, 343–344 (1968).
NIEWIAROWSKI, S., STEWART, G. J., MARDER, V. J.: Formation of highly ordered polymers from fibrinogen and fibrin degradation products. Biochim. biophys. Acta (Amst.) **221**, 326–341 (1970).
NORDSTRØM, S.: Inhibition of blood coagulation by trasylol. *In vitro* and *in vivo* studies on dog blood. Coagulation **3**, 159–167 (1970).
NORDSTRØM, S., ZETTERQVIST, E.: Effects of epsilon aminocaproic acid (EACA) and Trasylol on thromboplastin-induced intravascular coagulation, studied in dogs with iodine-labelled fibrinogen. Acta physiol. scand. **76**, 93–105 (1969).
NOSSEL, H. L., RUBIN, H., DRILLINGS, M., HSIEH, R.: Inhibition of Hageman factor activation. J. clin. Invest. **47**, 1172–1180 (1968).
NOWOTNY, A.: Endotoxoid preparations. Nature (Lond.) **197**, 721–722 (1963).
NOWOTNY, A.: Molecular biology of gram-negative bacterial lipopolysaccharides. Ann. N. Y. Acad. Sci. **133**, 277–786 (1966).
NOWOTNY, A.: Relationship of structure and biological activity of bacterial endotoxin. Naturwissenschaften **58**, 397–409 (1971).
O'BRIEN, J. R.: A comparison of platelet aggregation produced by seven compounds and a comparison of their inhibitors. J. clin. Path. **17**, 275–281 (1964).
O'BRIEN, J. R., FINCH, W., CLARK, E.: Platelet-bound and soluble platelet factor 4: Effects of aggregating agents, of aggregation, and of aspirin. Proc. Soc. exp. Biol. (N. Y.) **134**, 1128–1131 (1970).
OBST, R., JANNAKOPULOS, E., URBASCHEK, B., HUTH, K., MÜLLER-BERGHAUS, G.: Blutgerinnung und Blutfette der trächtigen Ratte nach Endotoxininjection — Untersuchungen zum Sanarelli-Shwartzman-Phänomen. Thrombos. Diathes. haemorrh. (Stuttg.) **26**, 474–487 (1971).
PALMER, J. W., GERLOUGH, T. D.: A simple method for preparing antigenic substances from the typhoid bacillus. Science **92**, 155–156 (1940).
PALMERIO, C., MING, S. C., FRANK, E., FINE, J.: The role of the sympathetic nervous system in the generalized Shwartzman reaction. J. exp. Med. **115**, 609–612 (1962).
PAPPAS, G. D., ROSS, M. H., THOMAS, L.: Studies on the generalized Shwartzman reaction. VIII. The appearance, by electron microscopy, of intravascular fibrinoid in the glomerular capillaries during the reaction. J. exp. Med. **107**, 333–339 (1958).
PECHET, L., PECHET, G. S., MACDONALD, R. A.: Reticuloendothelial function and blood coagulation in rats. Thrombos. Diathes. haemorrh. (Stuttg.) **22**, 508–512 (1969).
PENICK, G. D., ROBERTS, H. R.: Intravascular clotting: Focal and systemic. Int. Rev. exp. Path. **3**, 269–328 (1964).
PENICK, G. D., ROBERTS, H. R., WEBSTER, W. P., BRINKOUS, K. M.: Hemorrhagic states secondary to intravascular clotting. An experimental study of their evolution and prevention. Arch. path. Anat. **66**, 708–714 (1958).
PFAU, P., LASCH, H. G., GÜNTHER, O.: Sanarelli-Shwartzman-Phänomen bei febrilen Fehlgeburten und schweren Schock- und Blutungszuständen in der Geburtshilfe. Gynaecologia (Basel) **150**, 17–33 (1960).
PFUELLER, S. L., LÜSCHER, E. F.: The effects of immune complexes on blood platelets and their relationship to complement activation. Immunochemistry **9**, 1151–1165 (1972).

PHILLIPS, L. L., MARGARETTEN, W., MCKAY, D. G.: Changes in the fibrinolytic enzyme system following intravascular coagulation induced by thrombin and endotoxin. Amer. J. Obstet. Gynec. **100**, 319–326 (1968).

PILLEMER, L., SCHOENBERG, M. D., BLUM, L., WURZ, L.: Properdin system and immunity. II. Interaction of the properdin system with polysaccharides. Science **122**, 545–549 (1955).

POLÁK, L., TURK, J. L.: Suppression of the haemorrhagic component of the Shwartzman reaction by anti-complement serum. Nature (Lond.) **223**, 738–739 (1969).

PROSE, P. H., LEE, L., BALK, S. D.: Electron microscopic study of the phagocytic fibrin-clearancing mechanism. Amer. J. Path. **47**, 403–417 (1965).

QUICK, A. J., GEORGATSOS, J. G., HUSSEY, C. V.: The clotting activity of human erythrocytes: Theoretical and clinical implications. Amer. J. med. Sci. **228**, 207–213 (1954).

QUICK, A. J., HUSSEY, C. V., HARRIS, J., PETERS, K.: Occult intravascular clotting by means of intravenous injection of thrombin. Amer. J. Physiol. **197**, 791–794 (1959).

RABINER, S. F., FRIEDMAN, L. H.: The role of intravascular haemolysis and the reticulo-endothelial system in the production of a hypercoagulable state. Brit. J. Haemat. **14**, 105–118 (1968).

RABINER, S. F., HELBERT, J. R., LOPAS, H., FRIEDMAN, L. H.: Evaluation of stroma-free hemoglobulin solution for use as a plasma expander. J. exp. Med. **126**, 1127–1142 (1967).

RAPAPORT, S. I., HJORT, P. F.: The blood clotting properties of rabbit peritoneal leukocytes *in vitro*. Thrombos. Diathes. haemorrh. (Stuttg.) **17**, 222–236 (1967).

RAPAPORT, S. I., HJORT, P. F., PATCH, M. J., JEREMIC, M.: Consumption of serum factors and prothrombin during intravascular clotting in rabbits. Scand. J. Haemat. **3**, 59–75 (1966).

RATNOFF, O. D., CONLEY, C. L.: Studies on afibrinogenemia. II. The defibrinating effect on dog blood of intravenous injection of thromboplastic material. Bull. Johns Hopk. Hosp. **88**, 414–424 (1951).

RAVIN, H. A., ROWLEY, D., JENKINS, C., FINE, J.: On the absorption of bacterial endotoxin from the gastro-intestinal tract of the normal and shocked animal. J. exp. Med. **112**, 783–792 (1960).

REGOECZI, E., GERGELY, J., MCFARLANE, A. S.: *In vivo* effects of Agkistrodon rhodostoma venom: Studies with fibrinogen-^{131}I. J. clin. Invest. **45**, 1202–1212 (1966).

REID, H. A., CHAN, K. E., THEAN, P. C.: Prolonged coagulation defect (defibrination syndrome) in Malayan viper bite. Lancet **1963I**, 621–626.

RELIHAN, M., LITWIN, M. S.: Effects of stroma-free hemoglobin solution on clearance rate and renal function. Surgery **71**, 395–399 (1972).

RENAUD, S., ALLARD, C., LATOUR, J. G.: The prevention by glucocorticoids of endotoxin-initiated thrombosis in rat, relation to fibrinolysis, coagulation, and lipemia. Amer. Heart. J. **72**, 797–805 (1966).

REUTER, C., MÜLLER-BERGHAUS, G.: Verbrauchscoagulopathie mit Auftreten von fibrinreichen Mikrogerinnseln bei experimenteller Hepatitis des Kaninchens. Verh. dtsch. Ges. inn. Med. **79**, 1340–1342 (1973).

REUTTER, W., LESCH, R., KEPPLER, D., DECKER, K.: Galaktosamin-Hepatitis. Naturwissenschaften **55**, 497 (1968).

RIFKIND, D., HILL, R. B., JR.: Neutralization of the Shwartzman reactions by polymyxin B. J. Immunol. **99**, 564–569 (1967).

RODRÍGUEZ-ERDMANN, F.: Blood clotting system in the pathogenesis of the Sanarelli-Shwartzman reaction of the rabbit. Experientia (Basel) **20**, 223 (1964a).

RODRÍGUEZ-ERDMANN, F.: Studies on the pathogenesis of the generalized Shwartzman reaction. I. Alterations in the coagulation system during the generalized Shwartzman reaction of the pregnant rabbit. Thrombos. Diathes. haemorrh. (Stuttg.) **12**, 452–461 (1964b).

RODRÍGUEZ-ERDMANN, F.: Studies on the pathogenesis of the generalized Shwartzman reaction. III. Trigger mechanism for the activation of the prothrombin molecule. Thrombos. Diathes. haemorrh. (Stuttg.) **12**, 471–483 (1964c).

RODRÍGUEZ-ERDMANN, F., KRECKE, H.-J., LASCH, H. G., BOHLE, A.: Über die morphologischen und gerinnungsanalytischen Veränderungen nach Liquoid. Ein Beitrag zur Pathogenese des Sanarelli-Shwartzman-Phänomens. Z. ges. exp. Med. **134**, 109–130 (1960).

ROTHER, K. O.: Experimentelle Nierenkrankheiten. Handb. exp. Pharmacologie **16/4**, 1–220 (1965).

ROTHER, K., ROTHER, U., VASSALLI, P., MCCLUSKEY, R. T.: Nephrotoxic serum nephritis in C'6-deficient rabbits. I. Study of the second phase of the disease. J. Immunol. **98**, 965–971 (1967).

ROTHER, K., TILL, G.: Experimentelle Glomerulonephritis durch Antikörper gegen Niere. In: ROTHER, K. (ed.): Komplement. Biochemie und Pathologie, p. 250–263. Darmstadt: Steinkopff 1974.

ROUX, E., YERSIN, A.: Contribution à l'étude de la diphtérie. Ann. Inst. Pasteur **2**, 629–661 (1888).

RUBINSTEIN, H. S., FINE, J., COONS, A. H.: Localization of endotoxin in the walls of the peripheral vascular system during lethal endotoxemia. Proc. Soc. exp. Biol. (N. Y.) **111**, 458–467 (1962).

SALMON, J., LAMBERT, P. H., HIERNAUX, M.: Coagulation intravasculaire et phénomènes anaphylactiques. N. Rev. franc. Hémat. **8**, 76–83 (1968).

SALMON, J., LAMBERT, P. H., LOUIS, J.: Pathogenesis of the intravascular coagulation syndrome induced by immunological reactions. In: DUCKERT, F., BRINKHOUS, K. M., HINNOM, S., KOLLER, F., SHERRY, S., STENGLE, J. M. (eds.): Immunological mechanisms in blood coagulation, thrombosis and hemostasis. Thrombos. Diathes. haemorrh. (Stuttg.) Suppl. **45**, 161–169 (1971).

SAMET, J., BOWMAN, H. S.: Fetomaternal ABO incompatibility: Intravascular hemolysis, fetal hemoglobinemia, and fibrinogenopenia in maternal circulation. Amer. J. Obstet. Gynec. **81**, 49–56 (1961).

SANARELLI, G.: Sur la pathogénie des états algides dans le choléra, les entérites et l'appendicite. Bull. Acad. nat. Med. (Paris) **90**, 204–210 (1923).

SANARELLI, G.: De la pathogénie du choléra (Neuvième mémoire). Le choléra expérimental. Ann. Inst. Pasteur **38**, 11–72 (1924).

SANDBERG, A. L., SIRAGANIAN, R. P., MERGENHAGEN, S. E.: Biological consequences of endotoxin interaction with complement. In: URBASCHEK, B., URBASCHEK, R., NETER, E. (eds.): Gram-negative bacterial infections and mode of endotoxin actions—Pathophysiological, immunological, and clinical aspects. p. 329–334. Wien-New York: Springer 1975.

SANDRITTER, W., LASCH, H. G.: Pathologic aspects of shock. Meth. Achievm. exp. Path. **3**, 86–121 (1967).

SCHIMPF, K., CIBELIUS, A.: Die physiologischen Inhibitoren der Blutgerinnung bei pathologisch gesteigerter Gerinnbarkeit *in vivo*. I. Verbrauchskoagulopathie beim Shwartzman-Sanarelli-Phänomen. Klin. Wschr. **42**, 431–435 (1964).

SCHIMPF, K., LENHARD, J., SCHAAF, G.: The influence of the polysaccharide Carrageenin on the clotting mechanism of the blood in the rabbit *in vitro* and *in vivo*. Thrombos. Diathes. haemorrh. (Stuttg.) **21**, 524–533 (1969).

SCHNEIDER, C. L.: The active principle of placental toxin: thromboplastin; its inactivator in blood: antithromboplastin. Amer. J. Physiol. **149**, 123–129 (1947).

SCHNEIDER, C. L.: "Fibrin embolism" (disseminated intravascular coagulation) with defibrination as one of the end results during placenta abruptio. Surg. Gynec. Obstet. **92**, 27–34 (1951).

SCHNEIDER, C. L.: Disseminated intravascular coagulation: Thrombosis versus fibrination, in clinical disease states. In: MAMMEN, E. F., ANDERSON, G. F., BARNHART, M. I. (eds.): Disseminated intravascular coagulation. Thrombos. Diathes. haemorrh. (Stuttg.) Suppl. **36**, 1–43 (1969).

SCHOENDORF, T. H., ROSENBERG, M., BELLER, F. K.: Endotoxin-induced disseminated intravascular coagulation in nonpregnant rats. A new experimental model. Amer. J. Path. **65**, 51–58 (1971).

SELYE, H.: Induced hypersensitivity to cold. Science **149**, 201–202 (1965).

SELYE, H.: Thrombohemorrhagic phenomena. Springfield: Thomas 1966.

SHAINOFF, J. R., PAGE, I. H.: Cofibrins and fibrin-intermediates as indicators of thrombin activity *in vivo*. Circulat. Res. **8**, 1013–1022 (1960).

SHAINOFF, J. R., PAGE, I. H.: Significance of cryoprofibrin in fibrinogen-fibrin conversion. J. exp. Med. **116**, 687–707 (1962).

SHAPIRO, S. S., MCKAY, D. G.: The prevention of the generalized Shwartzman reaction with sodium warfarin. J. exp. Med. **107**, 377–381 (1958).

SHEN, S. M-C., RAPAPORT, S. I., FEINSTEIN, D. I.: Intravascular clotting after endotoxin in rabbits with impaired intrinsic clotting produced by a factor VIII antibody. Blood **42**, 523–534 (1973).

SHIMAMOTO, T., YAMAZAKI, H., OHNO, K., UCHIDA, H., KONISHI, T., IWAHARA, S.: Effect of bacterial endotoxins on platelets and release of serotonin (5-hydroxytryptamine). I. Bacterial endotoxin on the number of circulating platelets. Proc. Japan. Acad. **34**, 444–449 (1958a).

SHIMAMOTO, T., YAMAZAKI, H., SAGAWA, N., IWAHARA, S., KONISHI, T., MAEZAWA, H.: Effect of bacterial endotoxins on platelets and release of serotonin (5-hydroxytryptamine). II. Appearance of platelet-agglutinating substance and serotonin (5-hydroxytryptamine) in the plasma of rabbit by administration of bacterial endotoxin. Proc. Jap. Acad. **34**, 450–455 (1958 b).

SHWARTZMAN, G.: A new phenomenon of local skin reactivity to B. typhosus culture filtrate. Proc. Soc. exp. Biol. (N. Y.) **25**, 560–561 (1927).

Shwartzman, G., Gerber, I. E.: Hemorrhagic manifestations of bacterial and virus infections: Experimental studies and pathological interpretations. Ann. N. Y. Acad. Sci. **49**, 627–640 (1948).

Skjørten, F., Evensen, S. A.: Disseminated intravascular coagulation induced by Liquoid in normal, thrombocytopenic and granulocytopenic rabbits. Light and electron microscope studies. Thrombos. Diathes. haemorrh. (Stuttg.) **27**, 377–388 (1972).

Slaastad, R. A., Eika, C.: Failure to trigger intravascular coagulation by water-induced haemolysis in rabbits. Scand. J. Haemat. **11**, 217–224 (1973).

Slaastad, R. A., Husby, G., Skjörten, F.: Soluble fibrin and fibrinogen-derived material in the kidneys during low-graded disseminated intravascular coagulation (DIC) in rabbits. Scand. J. Haemat. **13**, 152–159 (1974).

Slaastad, R. A., Jeremic, M.: The laboratory diagnosis of low-graded disseminated intravascular coagulation. A study in rabbits. Scand. J. Haemat. **11**, 50–58 (1973).

Slabber, C. F., Theiss, W., Beller, F. K.: The prevention of endotoxin-induced glomerular fibrin deposition by pyrimido-pyrimidine compounds. J. Med. **3**, 341–348 (1972).

Smith, S. P., Nuckolls, J. W., Horn, R. G., Collins, R. D.: Pathogenesis of the generalized Shwartzman reaction. Evaluation of platelets as a mediator of the suppressive effect of a nitrogen mustard. Arch. Path. **85**, 459–462 (1968).

Smith, R. T., Thomas, L., Good, R. A.: Generalized Shwartzman reaction. V. Intravenous injection of colloidal iron or carbon on response of rabbits to meningococcal toxin. Proc. Soc. exp. Biol. (N. Y.) **82**, 712–715 (1953).

Spaet, T. H., Horowitz, H. I., Zucker-Franklin, D., Cintron, J., Biezenski, J. J.: Reticuloendothelial clearance of blood thromboplastin by rats. Blood **17**, 196–205 (1961).

Steiner, P. E., Lushbaugh, C. C.: Maternal pulmonary embolism by amniotic fluid as a cause of obstetric shock and unexpected deaths in obstetrics. J. Amer. med. Assoc. **117**, 1245–1254 (1941) and **117**, 1340–1345 (1941).

Stetson, C. A., Jr.: Studies on the mechanism of the Shwartzman phenomenon. Certain factors involved in the production of the local hemorrhagic necrosis. J. exp. Med. **93**, 489–504 (1951).

Stewart, G. J., Niewiarowski, S.: Aggregation of fibrinogen and its degredation products by basic proteins. An electron microscope study. Thrombos. Diathes. haemorrh. (Stuttg.) **25**, 566–579 (1971).

Surgenor, D. M.: Erythrocytes and blood coagulation. Thrombos. Diathes. haemorrh. (Stuttg.) **32**, 247–259 (1974).

Tagnon, H. J.: The nature of the mechanism of the shock produced by the injection of trypsin and thrombin. J. clin. Invest. **24**, 1–10 (1945).

Takeda, Y., Tsuchiya, I.: Studies on the pathological changes caused by the injection of the Shwartzman filtrate and the endotoxin into pregnant rabbits. Jap. J. exp. Med. **23**, 9–16 (1953).

Theiss, W., Beller, F. K.: The effect of saline loading on endotoxin-induced disseminated intravascular coagulation. J. Lab. clin. Med. **81**, 431–442 (1973).

Thomas, L.: The role of the reticulo-endothelial system in the reaction to endotoxins. In: Halpern, B. N., Benacerraf, B., Delafresnaye, J. F. (eds.): Physiopathology of the reticulo-endothelial system, p. 226–244. Springfield: Thomas 1957.

Thomas, L., Brunson, J., Smith, R. T.: Studies on the generalized Shwartzman reaction. VI. Production of the reaction by the synergistic action of endotoxin with three synthetic acidic polymers (sodium polyanethol sulfonate, dextran sulfate, and sodium polyvinyl alcohol sulfonate). J. exp. Med. **102**, 249–261 (1955a).

Thomas, L., Good, R. A.: Bilateral cortical necrosis of kidneys in cortisone-treated rabbits following injection of bacterial toxins. Proc. Soc. exp. Biol. (N. Y.) **76**, 604–608 (1951).

Thomas, L., Good, R. A.: The effect of cortisone on the Shwartzman reaction. The production of lesions resembling the dermal and generalized Shwartzman reactions by a single injection of bacterial toxin in cortisone-treated rabbits. J. exp. Med. **95**, 409–428 (1952a).

Thomas, L., Good, R. A.: Studies on the generalized Shwartzman reaction. I. General observations concerning the phenomenon. J. exp. Med. **96**, 605–623 (1952b).

Thomas, L., Smith, R. T.: Effect of cortisone on response to endotoxin in mature rabbits. Proc. Soc. exp. Biol. (N. Y.) **86**, 810–813 (1954).

Thomas, L., Smith, R. T., Korff, R. von: Cold-precipitation by heparin of a protein in rabbits and human plasma. Proc. Soc. exp. Biol. (N. Y.) **86**, 813–818 (1954).

Thomas, L., Smith, R. T., Korff, R. von: Studies on the generalized Shwartzman reaction. VII. The role of fibrinogen in the deposition of fibrinoid after combined injections of endotoxin and synthetic acidic polymer. J. exp. Med. **102**, 263–278 (1955b).

Triantaphyllopoulos, D. C.: Anticoagulant effect of incubated fibrinogen. Canad. J. Biochem. **36**, 249–259 (1958).

TRIANTAPHYLLOPOULOS, E.: Hemoglobin, inhibitor of the contact phase of blood coagulation. Life Sci. **10**, 813–822 (1971).
URBASCHEK, B.: Addendum—The effects of endotoxins in the microcirculation. Microbial Toxins **5**, 261–275 (1971).
URBASCHEK, B., BRANEMARK, P.-I., NOWOTNY, A.: Lack of endotoxin effect on the microcirculation after pretreatment with detoxified endotoxin (endotoxoid). Experientia (Basel) **24**, 170–171 (1968).
URBASCHEK, B., NOWOTNY, A.: Endotoxin tolerance induced by detoxified endotoxin (endotoxoid). Proc. Soc. exp. Biol. (N. Y.) **127**, 650–652 (1968).
URBASCHEK, B., URBASCHEK, R., NETER, E. (eds.): Gram-negative bacterial infections and mode of endotoxin actions—Pathophysiological, immunological, and clinical aspects. Wien-New York: Springer 1975.
VASSALLI, P., MCCLUSKEY, R. T.: The pathogenic role of the coagulation process in rabbit Masugi nephritis. Amer. J. Path. **45**, 653–677 (1964).
VASSALLI, P., SIMON, G., ROUILLER, C.: Electron microscopic study of glomerular lesions resulting from intravascular fibrin formation. Amer. J. Path. **43**, 579–617 (1963).
VAZQUES, J. J.: Immunohistochemical analysis of "fibrinoid" in human and experimental conditions. (Abstract). Fed. Proc. **17**, 463 (1958).
VERMYLEN, J., GAETANO, G. DE, VERSTRAETE, M.: Round-the-table conference on normal and modified platelet aggregation. Acta med. scand. Suppl. **525** (1970).
VRIES, A. DE, DJALDETTI, M., COHEN, I., JOSHUA, H., BESSLER, H.: Coagulation disturbance induced by Echis colorata venom in vivo. In: KOLLER, F., DUCKERT, F., STREULI, F. (eds.): Pathogenesis and treatment of thromboembolic diseases. p. 565–569. Stuttgart: Schattauer 1966.
WALSH, P. N.: The effects of collagen and kaolin on the intrinsic coagulant activity of platelets. Evidence for an alternative pathway in intrinsic coagulation not requiring factor XII. Brit. J. Haemat. **22**, 393–405 (1972).
WALTHER, G.: Über die Gerinnungsaktivität hämolysierter menschlicher Erythrozyten. Blut **2**, 211–216 (1956).
WARDLE, E. N.: A study of intravascular coagulation in immune complex glomerulonephritis by use of ^{131}I-labelled fibrinogen and ^{125}I-labelled antigen. Clin. Sci. Molec. Med. **45**, 35–50 (1973).
WARDLE, E. N.: Studies during saline infusion of the effects of intravascular coagulation on rabbit kidney function. J. Lab. clin. Med. **84**, 525–535 (1974).
WEBER, E., MALESSA, S., LASCH, H. G.: Veränderungen der freien Thrombozytennukleotide beim Sanarelli-Shwartzman-Phänomen. Thrombos. Diathes. haemorrh. (Stuttg.) **9**, 304–316 (1963).
WEISS, H. J., ALLAN, S., DAVIDSON, E., KOCHWA, S.: A fibrinogenemia in man following the bite of a rattlesnake (Crotalus adamanteus). Amer. J. Med. **47**, 625–634 (1969).
WELCH, W. H., FLEXNER, S.: The histological changes in experimental diphtheria. Preliminary communication. Bull. Johns Hopk. Hosp. **2**, 107–110 (1891).
WELTI, E.: Über die Todesursachen nach Hautverbrennungen. Beitr. path. Anat. **4**, 520–555 (1889).
WENDT, F., KAPPLER, C., BURCKHARDT, K., BOHLE, A.: Production of generalized Shwartzman reaction in rabbits with nitrogen mustard-induced granulocytopenia. Proc. Soc. exp. Biol. (N. Y.) **125**, 486–488 (1967).
WESTPHAL, O., LÜDERITZ, O.: Chemische Erforschung von Lipopolysacchariden gramnegativer Bakterien. Angew. Chem. **66**, 407–417 (1954).
WESTPHAL, O., LÜDERITZ, O., BISTER, F.: Über Extraktion von Bakterien mit Phenol/Wasser. Z. Naturforsch. **7**, 148–155 (1952).
WEXLER, W. M., KANTOR, F. S.: Reticuloendothelial function in pregnancy. Yale J. Biol. Med. **38**, 315–322 (1966).
WHITACKER, A. N., BUNCE, I., NICOLL, P., DOWLING, S. V.: Interaction of angiotensin with disseminated intravascular coagulation. A possible mechanism in the genesis of acute renal failure. Amer. J. Path. **72**, 1–12 (1973).
WHITACKER, A. N., MCKAY, D. G.: Induction of hypotension in rhesus monkeys and rabbits by intravenous thrombin infusion. Lab. Invest. **20**, 79–86 (1969).
WILNER, G. D., NOSSEL, H. L., LEROY, E. C.: Activation of Hageman factor by collagen. J. clin. Invest. **47**, 2608–2615 (1968).
WILNER, G. D., NOSSEL, H. L., PROCUPEZ, T. L.: Aggregation of platelets by collagen: polar active sites of insoluble human collagen. Amer. J. Physiol. **220**, 1074–1079 (1971).
WONG, T.-C.: A study on the generalized Shwartzman reaction in pregnant rats induced by bacterial endotoxin. Amer. J. Obstet. Gynec. **84**, 786–797 (1962).
WOOLDRIGDE, L. C.: Ueber intravaskuläre Gerinnungen. Arch. Anat. Physiol. (Leipzig) 397–399 (1886).

ZANDER, J. (ed.): Septischer Abort und bakterieller Schock. Berlin-Heidelberg-New York: Springer 1968.

ZELLER, J., MARGARETTEN, W., MCKAY, D. G.: Effect of saline infusion and norepinephrine on response of the kidney to bacterial endotoxin. Proc. Soc. exp. Biol. (N. Y.) **126**, 446–449 (1967).

ZIMMERMAN, T. S., MÜLLER-EBERHARD, H. J.: Blood coagulation initiation by a complement-mediated pathway. J. exp. Med. **134**, 1601–1607 (1971).

ZIMMERMANN, H., HABERMANN, E., LASCH, H.-G.: Der Einfluß von Gift der Sandrasselotter (Echis carinata) auf die Hämostase. Thrombos. Diathes. haemorrh. (Stuttg.) **25**, 425–437 (1971).

ZUCKER, M. B., BORRELLI, J.: Platelet clumping produced by connective tissue suspensions and by collagen. Proc. Soc. exp. Biol. (N. Y.) **109**, 779–787 (1962).

ZWEIFACH, B. W., SHORR, E., BLACK, M. M.: The influence of the adrenal cortex on behavior of terminal vascular bed. Ann. N. Y. Acad. Sci. **56**, 626–633 (1953).

Author Index

Page numbers in *italics* refer to bibliography
Numbers shown in square brackets are the numbers in the bibliography

Subject Index

Handbuch der experimentellen Pharmakologie
Handbook of Experimental Pharmacology

Heffter — Heubner, New Series

Vol. 4:	**General Pharmacology**
Vol. 10:	**Die Pharmakologie anorganischer Anionen**
Vol. 11:	**Lobelin und Lobeliaalkaloide**
Vol. 12:	**Morphin und morphinähnlich wirkende Verbindungen**
Vol. 13:	**The Alkali Metal Ions in Biology.** Temp. out of print
Vol. 14:	
Part 1	**The Adrenocortical Hormones I**
Part 2	**The Adrenocortical Hormones II**
Part 3	**The Adrenocortical Hormones III**
Vol. 15:	**Cholinesterase and Anticholinesterase Agents**
Vol. 16:	**Erzeugung von Krankheitszuständen durch das Experiment Experimental Production of Diseases**
Part 1	**Blut/Blood.** In preparation
Part 2	**Atemwege**
Part 3	**Heart and Circulation**
Part 4	**Niere, Nierenbecken, Blase**
Part 5	**Liver.** In preparation
Part 6	**Schilddrüse.** In preparation
Part 7	**Zentralnervensystem**
Part 8	**Stütz- und Hartgewebe**
Part 9	**Infektionen I**
Part 10	**Infektionen II**
Part 11 A	**Infektionen III**
Part 11 B	**Infektionen IV**
Part 12	**Tumoren I**
Part 13	**Tumoren II**
Part 14	**Tumoren III.** In preparation
Part 15	**Kohlenhydratstoffwechsel, Fieber/Carbohydrate Metabolism, Fever**
Vol. 17:	
Part 1	**Ions alcalino-terreux I.** Systèmes isolés
Part 2	**Ions alcalino-terreux II.** Organismes entiers
Vol. 18:	
Part 1	**Histamine**
Part 2	**Anti-Histaminics.** In preparation

Vol. 19: **5-Hydroxytriptamine and Related Indolealkylamines**

Vol. 20:
- Part 1 **Pharmacology of Fluorides I**
- Part 2 **Pharmacology of Fluorides II**

Vol. 21: **Beryllium**

Vol. 22:
- Part 1 **Die Gestagene I**
- Part 2 **Die Gestagene II**

Vol. 23: **Neurohypophysial Hormones and Similar Polypeptides**

Vol. 24: **Diuretica**

Vol. 25: **Bradykinin, Kallidin, and Kallikrein**

Vol. 26: **Vergleichende Pharmakologie von Überträgersubstanzen in tiersystematischer Darstellung**

Vol. 27: **Anticoagulantien**

Vol. 28:
- Part 1 **Concepts in Biochemical Pharmacology I**
- Part 2 **Concepts in Biochemical Pharmacology II.** Out of print
- Part 3 **Concepts in Biochemical Pharmacology III**

Vol. 29: **Oral wirksame Antidiabetika**

Vol. 30: **Modern Inhalation Anesthetics**

Vol. 31: **Antianginal Drugs.** Out of print

Vol. 32:
- Part 1 **Insulin I**
- Part 2 **Insulin II**

Vol. 33: **Catecholamines**

Vol. 34: **Secretin, Cholecystokinin, Pancreozymin, and Gastrin**

Vol. 35:
- Part 1 **Androgene I**
- Part 2 **Androgens II and Antiandrogens/Androgene II und Antiandrogene**

Vol. 36: **Uranium-Plutonium-Transplutonic Elements**

Vol. 37: **Angiotensin**

Vol. 38:
- Part 1 **Antineoplastic and Immunosuppressive Agents I**
- Part 2 **Antineoplastic and Immunosuppressive Agents II**

Vol. 40: **Organic Nitrates**

Vol. 41: **Hypolipidemic Agents**

Vol. 42: **Neuromuscular Junction**

GPSR Compliance

The European Union's (EU) General Product Safety Regulation (GPSR) is a set of rules that requires consumer products to be safe and our obligations to ensure this.

If you have any concerns about our products, you can contact us on ProductSafety@springernature.com

In case Publisher is established outside the EU, the EU authorized representative is:

Springer Nature Customer Service Center GmbH
Europaplatz 3
69115 Heidelberg, Germany

Batch number: 10838062

Printed by Printforce, the Netherlands